Second Edition

CIRCULATORY PHYSIOLOGY:

Cardiac Output and its Regulation

ARTHUR C. GUYTON, M.D.
Professor and Chairman of the Department
of Physiology and Biophysics, University
of Mississippi Medical Center, Jackson, Mississippi

CARL E. JONES, Ph.D.
Assistant Professor of the Department of
Physiology and Biophysics, University of
Mississippi Medical Center, Jackson, Mississippi

THOMAS G. COLEMAN, Ph.D.
Associate Professor of the Department of
Physiology and Biophysics, University of
Mississippi Medical Center, Jackson, Mississippi

W. B. SAUNDERS COMPANY • Philadelphia • London • Toronto

W. B. Saunders Company: West Washington Square
                          Philadelphia, PA 19105

                          1 St. Anne's Road
                          Eastbourne, East Sussex BN21 3UN, England

                          1 Goldthorne Avenue
                          Toronto, Ontario M8Z 5T9, Canada

Circulatory Physiology: Cardiac Output and Its Regulation   ISBN 0-7216-4360-4

Print No: 9   8   7   6   5   4   3

PREFACE

The first edition of this monograph, which was published approximately ten years ago, had essentially a twofold purpose. The primary goal was to present an analysis of cardiac output regulation which had been developed largely in our department of physiology, and which has proved very useful in directing our thoughts regarding the principles of cardiac output regulation. A second goal was to offer an overall philosophy of the regulation of cardiac output, a philosophy which would explain principally the intimate relationship between the metabolic rate of the tissues of the body and cardiac output but which would also take into account the effects of cardiovascular reflexes, blood volume, blood viscosity, cardiac integrity, and other factors on cardiac output.

In the Second Edition of this monograph, the goals underlying the writing of the First Edition have been maintained. However, certain major changes have been made in the text itself. First, the results of a host of studies, both by ourselves and by others, which have been performed since the writing of the First Edition have been included, and an attempt has been made to show how these data fit into the scheme of cardiac output regulation. This portion of the revision was written mainly by Dr. Carl E. Jones. In this connection, we would like to emphasize that, although the physiological mechanisms involved in the regulation of cardiac output have been studied intensely during the past ten years, the basic concepts of cardiac output regulation have not been significantly altered. Rather, the new research has served more to substantiate the scheme of cardiac output regulation originally presented in this book.

The second major change appearing in this edition is the addition of three new chapters relating to topics which were not included in the first edition. The first two of these new chapters deal with the use of computers to simulate circulatory dynamics. Chapter 16 presents a computer analysis of ventricular function, showing particularly how one can determine the overall pumping ability of the left ventricle from such basic factors as anatomy of the heart, myocardial integrity, the physical laws governing fluid dynamics, degree of autonomic stimulation, input pressure to the ventricle, and output pressure. Chapter 17 shows how computers may be used to analyze function of the entire circulatory system. Presented in

iii

this chapter is a complex analysis which allows one to predict the effect of almost any circulatory change on cardiac output.

The third new chapter briefly reviews the problems which have been encountered in the search for a usable artificial heart and discusses the overall philosophy of cardiac output regulation when using an artificial heart. The major emphasis of this chapter is that the mechanisms regulating cardiac output from an artificial heart are essentially the same as those regulating cardiac output from the human heart.

It was stated in the Preface to the First Edition of this monograph that the attempt to formulate an overall picture of cardiac output regulation could have been considered by the reader to be premature. Indeed, ten years later and with a great quantity of additional data, such a statement is, perhaps, still appropriate. However, we believe that the research of the past decade has gone far toward validating the concepts presented in that text and in the present one. Therefore, we sincerely hope that the information, concepts, and philosophies offered in this monograph will be of value to the reader interested in cardiovascular physiology.

Since the revision of this book was the work of three authors, it is important to explain the division of labor. Most of the revision was accomplished by Dr. Carl E. Jones, including the literature search, updating most of the chapters, and rewriting major portions of many of the chapters. Chapter 16, which presents the computer analysis of ventricular function, was written by Dr. Thomas G. Coleman. And Chapter 17, which presents a computer analysis of the entire circulation, was written by Dr. Arthur C. Guyton.

The authors wish to express their deepest appreciation to the many persons who helped in the preparation of this book. Acknowledgment is given to the members of the Department of Physiology and Biophysics, whose experiments afforded much of the scientific basis of this monograph and whose thoughts and ideas were immensely useful. In this regard, special thanks is given to Drs. Jack W. Crowell, Elvin E. Smith, Aubrey E. Taylor, Harris J. Granger, Allen W. Cowley, Jr., and Luis G. Navar. We also extend wholehearted gratitude to Mrs. Billie Howard, Mrs. Linda Rice, and Mrs. Maryann Davila for their excellent secretarial help, to Miss Tomiko Mita and Mrs. Carolyn Hull for preparing the figures, and to the staff of the W. B. Saunders Company for their invaluable assistance in preparing the entire manuscript.

ARTHUR C. GUYTON
CARL E. JONES
THOMAS G. COLEMAN

CONTENTS

I

NORMAL VALUES AND METHODS FOR MEASURING CARDIAC OUTPUT

Chapter 1

NORMAL CARDIAC OUTPUT AND ITS VARIATIONS

Cardiac Output and the Mixing of Body Fluids

Each of the one hundred trillion cells of the body is a living automaton capable of existing, of continuing life functions, and in most instances even of regenerating as long as it remains in an appropriate and constant internal fluid environment. The heart supplies a motive power for mixing most of the body fluids, keeping a stream of fluid flowing continually through all parts of the body. Molecular diffusion allows fluid and dissolved substances to move back and forth between the flowing blood and the interstitial and intracellular fluids. Thus, a constant "internal environment" of the body is maintained.

To provide this mixing of the body fluids, the cardiac output normally moves all the blood completely around the circulation about once a minute. Then, to keep the blood mixed with the fluids in the interstitial spaces, diffusion occurs through the capillary membranes at a rate equal approximately to 45 times the total blood volume every minute (Pappenheimer, 1953). That is, 45 blood volumes of fluid diffuse both outward and inward through the capillary membranes per minute, which obviously allows almost instant interchange between the fluid of the blood and the fluid lying immediately outside the capillaries. Mixing is almost 100 per cent complete, even in the areas most remote from the capillaries, in less than 30 minutes (Elkinton, 1955).

Transport of Nutrients and Wastes

A corollary to the mixing function of cardiac output is the transport of nutrients and wastes from one part of the body to another. First, we might mention substances transmitted from organ to organ, such as acetoacetic acid from the liver to the cells elsewhere in the body, hormones from the endocrine glands to all regions of the body, fats from storage depots to the liver or directly to other functional cells of the body, and so forth. However, we usually consider the major function of cardiac output to be transport of nutrients from the input organs of the body, the gut and lungs, to the cells, and then transport of wastes from the cells to the output

3

organs of the body, the lungs and the kidneys. The principal nutrients that must be carried to the cells include oxygen, glucose, fatty acids, and amino acids, while the principal wastes are carbon dioxide and nitrogenous metabolic end products.

A sufficiently diminished cardiac output can kill the cells because of failure to transport adequate quantities of any single one of the nutrients or wastes, but transport of some of these is more important than transport of others. Normally there is a "safety factor" for the transport of each of them. For instance, even at normal cardiac output, oxygen can be transported to the cells at rates as great as three times the usual amount simply by removal of a larger proportion of the oxygen from the hemoglobin as it passes through the capillaries. In other words, the *utilization coefficient* for oxygen can rise to approximately three times normal even without an increase in cardiac output. Thus, the safety factor for delivery of oxygen to the tissues is approximately three fold.

If we calculate the safety factors for the other principal nutrients and wastes, they are approximately the following: glucose, thirty fold; fatty acid, twenty-eight fold; amino acids, thirty-six fold, carbon dioxide, twenty-five fold; and nitrogenous wastes, 480 fold. One sees immediately a major difference between the safety factor for transport of oxygen and the safety factors for the other substances, for oxygen is the one substance of them all that is most nearly "flow limited." If the cardiac output falls below one-third normal, the function of almost all of the tissues of the body will become seriously impaired because of oxygen lack, and yet transport of the other substances will not be significantly affected. For this reason, cardiac output must always be regulated at a level high enough to supply oxygen to the tissues, and, if this is achieved, then the transport of the other necessary substances will be insured.

RELATIONSHIP OF CARDIAC OUTPUT TO METABOLISM

Ever since the problem of cardiac output regulation began to be studied, research workers have recognized that output increases approximately in proportion to increase in body metabolism. The one physiological condition under which the body's metabolism increases the greatest is exercise; in extreme exercise in the well-trained athlete, this increase can be to as great as 15 to 20 times the basal level. Since the circulatory system has a safety factor for oxygen transport of only 3 to 1, more than a three fold increase in body metabolism would immediately cause a serious oxygen deficit in the functional tissues were it not for a simultaneous increase in cardiac output. However, the cardiac output does increase approximately in proportion to the degree of exercise, as shown by the solid curve of Figure 1–1. Assuming a normal cardiac output of slightly over 5 liters per minute, and noting that the cardiac output at the highest measured work output level is slightly over 30 liters per minute (Christensen, 1931), it is evident that the cardiac output can increase up to six times normal. Then, if we will recall that the utilization coefficient for oxygen can increase approximately three fold, we can calculate that delivery of oxygen to the tissues during the most severe exercise performed by the subject depicted

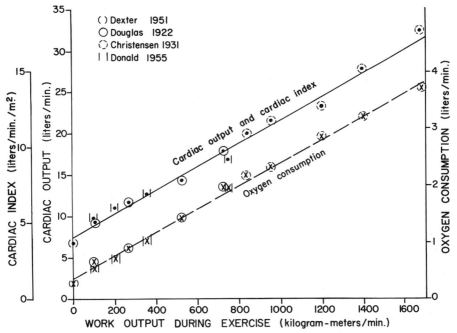

Figure 1–1. Relationship between cardiac output and work output (solid curve) and between oxygen consumption and work output (dashed curve) during exercise. [Data derived from studies by Douglas and Haldane (1922); Christensen and Mitteilung (1931); Dexter, Whittenberger, Haynes, Goodale, Gorlin, and Sawyer (1951); and Donald, Bishop, Cumming, and Wade (1955).]

in Figure 1–1 could have increased approximately eighteen fold. This fact is confirmed by the dashed curve of the figure, which shows the actual increase in oxygen usage. Furthermore, the body work output also increased approximately proportionately, as depicted by the abscissa.

DEPENDENCE OF CARDIAC OUTPUT REGULATION ON OXYGEN SUPPLY TO THE TISSUES

One can understand from the foregoing discussion that it would be highly desirable for the cardiac output to be regulated by the availability of oxygen to the tissues. This teleological reasoning leads us to suspect that oxygen availability to the tissues might well be one of the major factors controlling the overall total cardiac output. This subject will be discussed in detail later in this monograph, but to anticipate later discussions, particularly in Chapter 19, we can point out the following factors which indicate that cardiac output is regulated at least to a major extent by the availability of oxygen to the tissues. First, decreased oxygen concentration in the atmosphere (Grollman, 1930b; Cross, 1958; Gorlin, 1954), decreased ability of the blood to transport oxygen, such as results from anemia (Richardson, 1959), and decreased ability of the tissues to utilize oxygen in cyanide poisoning (Huckabee, 1960; Öberg, 1961) all cause the cardiac output to increase in proportion to the decrease in oxygen availability to the tissues up to the point at which the heart fails, thus illustrating that lack of oxygen *per se* will increase the cardiac output. Second, decrease in the arterial oxygen saturation (Yonce, 1959; Crawford, 1959; Ross, 1962) causes vascular dilatation, decreasing the peripheral resistance as much as four fold and causing a concomitant increase in cardiac output. Third, simple correlation studies have shown a very high correlation between oxygen consumption and cardiac output during increased body metabolism (Douglas, 1922; Christensen, 1931; Dexter, 1951; and Donald, 1955). For instance, Figure 1–1 illustrates that oxygen consumption and cardiac output both increase proportionately when the work output increases from zero up to maximum values during exercise.

After this brief introduction, we will leave for more complete discussion at later points in the book the mechanism by which cardiac output keeps in step with the metabolism of the body.

NORMAL VALUES FOR CARDIAC OUTPUT

CARDIAC OUTPUT IN MAN

Even though Harvey discovered the circulation of the blood over 300 years ago, accurate measurements of cardiac output in man have been made only during the last 30 years. Furthermore, only two methods have proved to be consistently accurate in measuring the output (Hamilton, 1944, 1945a, 1953). One of these has been the direct Fick procedure, the theory of which was propounded by Fick in the latter part of the eighteenth century (Fick, 1870) but was not applied to man until 1930 (Grollman, 1932). The second method has been the indicator-dilution method (Stewart, 1897), which is actually a special application of the Fick principle. Because of their importance, these two methods will be discussed in detail in Chapters 2 and 3. However, it is worth mentioning here that several other indirect methods utilizing the transfer of gases between the pulmonary alveoli and the pulmonary blood were utilized extensively between 1910 and 1940 for the measurement of cardiac output (Grollman, 1932). The most famous of these, the acetylene method, was used very actively from 1928 to 1940. Critical studies, however, in the last 25 years have proved that the acetylene method gives a cardiac output value in normal man approximately two-thirds that measured by either the Fick or the dilution method (Handbook of Circulation, 1959). Unfortunately, the percentage error of the gas methods may not remain the same under all conditions, so that their quantitative correctness, even when using a correction factor, is still doubtful. It is unfortunate that cardiac output measurements in man are much more difficult using either the Fick or the indicator-dilution method than when using some of the gas methods. For this reason, many of our concepts regarding the different factors that regulate cardiac output are still based on earlier measurements made by gas methods that were utilized in literally thousands of cardiac output measurements in man (Grollman, 1932) in contrast to much less common usage of the Fick and dilution methods in recent years.

The Cardiac Index Method for Expressing Cardiac Output in Man

Before giving normal values for cardiac output, it is necessary to point out that cardiac output is frequently expressed in terms of the *cardiac index*. In using this, a correction is made for the size of the individual based on the surface area of the body. The cardiac index mathematically is expressed by the following formula:

$$\text{Cardiac index (1./min./meters}^2) = \frac{\text{Cardiac output (1./min.)}}{\text{Surface area (meters}^2)}$$

The average normal man is usually considered to have a surface area of 1.73 square meters (Stead, 1950), and the surface area is calculated from the following formula developed by Dubois (1936) for use in metabolism studies:

$$\text{Body surface area} = \text{Weight}^{0.425} \times \text{Height}^{0.725} \times 0.007184$$
(square meters)   (kilograms)   (centimeters)

Figure 1–2 is a chart based on this formula from which the surface area can be determined within an accuracy of less than 2 per cent from a person's height and weight.

Inserting the average body surface area of 1.73 sq. meters into the above relationship between cardiac output and cardiac index, we find for the average normal man

$$\text{Cardiac output} = 1.73 \times \text{Cardiac index}$$

The validity of the cardiac index as a means for comparing cardiac outputs from individual to individual will be discussed later in the chapter.

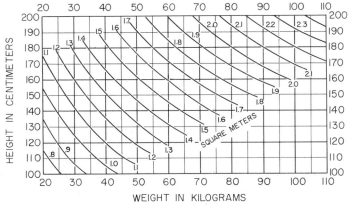

Figure 1–2. Chart for determining body surface area from height and weight (Dubois, 1936).

Cardiac Outputs Measured by the Fick and Indicator-Dilution Methods

Approximately 400 measurements of cardiac output made by the Fick and indicator-dilution methods in normal adult man have been collected in the Handbook of Circulation (1959). In these, the cardiac index averaged 3.52 liters per square meter per minute, which, for the average sized man, would be 6.08 liters per minute. These values have also been borne out almost exactly in still newer studies by Barratt-Boyes (1958), who have found a cardiac index of 3.5 in 26 subjects, and by Reeves (1961a), who found a cardiac index of 3.63 in 50 subjects. Furthermore, the average measurements by the Fick and dilution methods have been almost identical. In three different studies, the indicator-dilution and Fick methods have been compared in the same individuals. Hamilton and co-workers (1948) found in five individuals that the dilution method gave an 11 per cent greater cardiac output than the Fick method; Werko and coworkers (1949) found in six individuals that the dilution method gave a 6 per cent greater output; and Doyle and colleagues (1953) found in 53 individuals that the Fick method gave a 9 per cent greater output. If one considers the greater number of persons studied by Doyle, the two methods average out to give almost identical cardiac outputs.

Of historical importance is that the acetylene method in 151 different measurements (Handbook of Circulation, 1959) gave an average cardiac index of 2.24. If this is compared with the results using the Fick and indicator-dilution methods, the latter two give cardiac outputs averaging 55 per cent greater than those measured by the acetylene method.

Effect of Age on Cardiac Output

It is well known that body metabolism is affected greatly by age so that we would expect the cardiac output, which correlates very highly with body metabolism, also to be affected by age. Brandfonbrener and coworkers (1955) analyzed results from 77 different individuals in age groups from the teens through the eighties, with approximately equal representation in each of the decades. Figure 1–3 is constructed principally from Brandfonbrener's data with additional data for youths taken from Brotmacher (1957) and for newborn infants from Prec (1953, 1955).

Brandfonbrener's data show that the cardiac index decreases an average of 24.4 ml./sq. meter/min./year. Cournand (1945) found a similar figure of 26.2 ml./sq. meter/min./year in a less complete series of individuals. This decrease in cardiac output with age is to be expected because of the general decline in metabolic rate as one grows older (Boothby, 1929).

One might wonder why the cardiac index for the newborn baby as shown in Figure 1–3 is considerably less than that for older persons, particularly since we usually consider the metabolic rate per unit mass of tissue to be much greater in early childhood than at any other time of life. However, when one realizes the artificiality of the cardiac index as a means of expressing cardiac output, he can understand the low cardiac index for the newborn infant. The reason for this is that weight for weight, the newborn

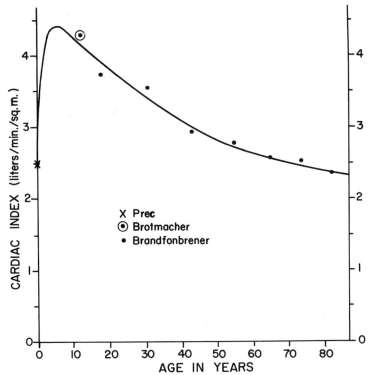

Figure 1–3. Cardiac index at different ages. Data mainly from Brandfonbrener, Landowne, and Shock (1955) but also from Brotmacher and Fleming (1957b) for youths and from Prec and Cassels (1953) for newborn infants.

infant has a far greater surface area than an adult. If the cardiac output is expressed on the basis of weight instead of surface area, we find the expected greater cardiac output per unit weight in the newborn infant (about two times as great) than in the adult. This phenomenon is also true in relation to metabolism; that is, the metabolic rate *per square meter* is less in a newborn infant than in the adult, but on a weight basis is much greater (Dubois, 1936).

Effect of Sex on Cardiac Ouput

Though one would expect the cardiac output of females to be less than that of males, there are not enough accurate data available to determine whether this is true. Furthermore, there would be real difficulty in deciding whether it is true because most females are considerably smaller than males, and comparison of cardiac outputs of persons of different weights and different sizes is still very artificial, as will be discussed later in the chapter in relation to the validity of the cardiac index.

However, if we assume that the cardiac index is proportional to the basal metabolic rate, we would expect the cardiac index of the female, except in early childhood, to be 7 to 10 per cent less than that of the male (Boothby, 1929).

The "Normal" Basal Cardiac Output

Earlier in the chapter it was pointed out that the average of many hundreds of cardiac output measurements in normal adult human beings, using the Fick and indicator-dilution methods, has been almost exactly 6 liters per minute. Whether or not these values are entirely basal is still a question, because a person would not be expected to be totally relaxed with a catheter in his heart or needles in a vein and an artery. Indeed measurements by a pulse-contour method for measuring cardiac output showed a considerable rise in output following insertion of a catheter into the heart, this presumably resulting from anxiety (Emmrich, 1958). Furthermore, by far the greater number of these measurements have been made on young adults rather than on a dispersed population of adults. Nevertheless, it is probably reasonable to assume that the cardiac output of the young, healthy adult of normal size either is 6 liters per minute or at least approaches this value.

On the other hand, the 6 liter value certainly is not valid for the average adult, whose average age, based on actuarial tables, is about 45 years. Probably the best data available on cardiac outputs at different ages are those of Brandfonbrener, Landowne, and Shock (1955), represented in Figure 1–3. These data show a cardiac index of almost exactly 3.0 liters/min./m.^{2} for the 45 year old human being and a cardiac output of 5.2 liters/min. (based on a surface area of 1.73 m.^{2}). If a single value for the normal adult cardiac output is required, this value of 5.2 liters/min. is probably as near to the true value as any presently available.

Normal Heart Rate, Stroke Volume, and Stroke Index

Brandfonbrener (1955), in the same study already quoted, found an average heart rate of 68 beats per minute, an average stroke volume output of 74 ml. per beat, and an average stroke index (stroke volume divided by surface area) of 43 ml. per beat. However, the stroke index decreased from an average of 50 ml. per beat at the age of 20 down to 37 at the age of 80. The heart rate, on the other hand, fell from an average of 75 at age 20 to an average of 61 at age 80. Thus, during the 60 year span from age 20 to 80, the stroke index decreased 26 per cent while the heart rate decreased 19 per cent. In other words, the cardiac output was reduced with age more by a decrease in stroke volume output than by a decrease in heart rate.

CARDIAC OUTPUT IN LOWER ANIMALS

Table 1–1 gives the cardiac output of nine lower animals, showing that the cardiac outputs correlate very well with body weight. The greatest cardiac output per kilogram of body weight is that of the rat with 0.26 l./kg./min. The least is 0.07 l./kg./min. found in the horse. The average cardiac output for all animals is 0.13 l./kg./min. with a mean deviation of ± 0.034. This value compares with an average cardiac output for the human being of 0.086 l./kg./min. In other words, the cardiac outputs measured for lower animals have ranged, on the average, almost 50 per cent

TABLE 1–1. CARDIAC OUTPUTS OF LOWER ANIMALS AND THEIR RELATIONSHIPS TO BODY SIZE

Animal	Average Weight (kg.)	Number Determinations	Cardiac Output (liters/min.)	C.O./Wt. (l./kg./min.)	C.O./Wt.$^{3/4}$	C.O./Wt.$^{2/3}$
Rat[1]	0.18	52	0.047	0.26	0.17	0.15
Ferret[1]	0.91	10	0.139	0.15	0.15	0.15
Chicken[2]	2.1	36	0.32	0.16	0.18	0.19
Rabbit[1]	2.6	53	0.28	0.11	0.14	0.15
Cat[1, 6, 8]	3.1	25	0.33	0.11	0.14	0.15
Dog[7]	19.3	149	2.3	0.12	0.24	0.31
Goat[1]	23.7	21	3.1	0.13	0.29	0.37
Sheep[3]				0.10		
Cattle[4]		22		0.11		
Cattle[5]		3	44.0			
Horse[1]	312	2	21.4	0.07	0.29	0.46
	Average			0.13	0.20	0.24
	Mean deviation			±0.034	±0.055	±0.104
	Per cent deviation from the mean			26%	27%	43%

1. Handbook of Circulation (1959)
2. Sturkie (1959)
3. Cross (1958)
4. Fisher (1959)

5. Doyle (1958)
6. Doi (1921)
7. Wiggers (1944)
8. Cross (1957)

more per kilogram of body weight than those for the human being. Table 1–1 also shows that if one uses the figure 0.13 liters per minute per kilogram in estimating cardiac output for animals of all sizes from the rat up to the horse, one will, on the average, be in error approximately 26 per cent. If one considers the tremendous range of size from the rat to the horse, nearly two thousand fold, it is easy to understand that an average error of 26 per cent in using this unified factor is indeed very slight.

It is interesting that the umbilical vein blood flow to fetal lambs is also 0.13 l./kg./min. (Cross, 1958) and that the total cardiac output of the fetal lamb is in the same range (Bancroft, 1934; Cross, 1958).

Experimental studies on lower animals have shown that precisely the same factors that affect cardiac output in human beings also affect cardiac output in lower animals. For instance, the cardiac output increases directly in proportion to the work output during exercise, the relationship being essentially linear as it is in the human being (Rushmer, 1959). Likewise, anemia (Richardson, 1959), anoxia (Gorlin, 1954), changes in body temperature (Brendel, 1958), and anxiety (Rushmer, 1954) all cause almost identically the same cardiac output responses in lower animals as in human beings. Therefore, it is reasonable to believe that cardiac output regulation in the lower animal is qualitatively identical to that in human beings, and the available data even suggest that quantitative regulation of cardiac output is not significantly different in the lower animal from that in the human being.

Cardiac Index in Lower Animals

Many investigators express the cardiac output in terms of the *cardiac index*, or cardiac output per square meter of surface area. To convert cardiac output into cardiac index, the surface area must first be calculated using some suitable formula, probably the best of which is that provided by Benedict's data as follows (Dubois, 1936):

$$\text{Surface area} = K \times \text{Weight}^{2/3}$$
(sq. meters)   (kilograms)

where K for most animals is about 0.1. For more precision the following values for K for common animals have been determined:

Mouse	0.090
Rat	0.091
Cat	0.100
Guinea pig	0.090
Rabbit	0.0975
Dog (over 4 kg.)	0.112
(under 4 kg.)	0.101
Sheep (sheared weight)	0.084
Swine	0.090
Cow and steer	0.090
Horse	0.100
Monkey	0.118
Man	0.11
Bird	0.10

Though cardiac outputs of most lower animals are reported on a per weight basis, the cardiac output of the dog is often reported in terms of cardiac index. Wiggers (1944a) tabulated the results from 14 separate studies, including a series of his own containing 149 determinations. His measurements, which seemed to be the most consistent of them all, gave an average cardiac index of $2.87 \pm$ S.D. 0.44 liter/sq.m./min.

VALIDITY OF THE CARDIAC INDEX

Obviously one would expect the cardiac output to be greater in a large than in a small person and likewise to be greater in a large than in a small animal. Therefore, a search has been made to find some valid relationship between the size of the animal and the cardiac output. The usual method for comparing cardiac outputs between human beings of different sizes, as has already been pointed out, is to use the cardiac index, which is the cardiac output per unit surface area of the body. Unfortunately the validity of the cardiac index for comparing cardiac outputs of persons or animals of different sizes is yet to be proved and is based entirely on spurious correlation rather than on actual correlation (Tanner, 1949b; Taylor, 1952). For instance, let us study Figure 1–4, which gives the cardiac outputs of over 100 normal adults having different surface areas (Brotmacher, 1956). Curve A in this figure represents the least squares regression line, when surface area of the body is considered to be the independent variable and cardiac output is considered to be the dependent variable. Curve B is the "sight" regression line, when neither cardiac output nor surface area is, considered to be dependent on the other, for actually there is no physiological reason to believe that one is dependent on the other. To be com-

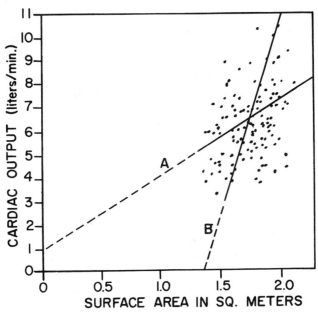

Figure 1-4. Relationship of cardiac output to surface area. [Data taken from figure published by Brotmacher and Deuchar (1956).] The two lines through the data represent regression curves determined in two different ways, neither of which prove the validity of the cardiac index as a measure of cardiac output.

pletely valid as a means of representing cardiac output in animals of different sizes, the regression Curve B of Figure 1-4 would have to fall precisely on all the points of the figure and would have to intersect the two axes at point 0,0. Obviously, neither of these two criteria is anywhere nearly fulfilled. Furthermore, the scatter of the points is so great that there is no statistical reason for believing that the correlation between cardiac output and surface area is better than the correlation between cardiac output and body weight.

In lower animals, the failure to confirm the validity of the cardiac index has been even more serious. Referring back to Table 1-1 we note that there is reasonable correlation between body weight and cardiac output. If we assume that all animals have essentially symmetrical shapes, then the surface areas of the different animals will be proportional to weight$^{2/3}$. In the last column of Table 1-1 the relationship between the cardiac output and weight$^{2/3}$, or, in other words, the relationship between cardiac output and the surface area, is shown for each of the animals. After averaging these values and determining the mean deviation, we find that use of this relationship would lead to an average error of 43 per cent. This compares with an average error of 26 per cent when using cardiac output per unit weight.

The original reason for using the cardiac index as a means for expressing cardiac output for human beings of different sizes was that the basal metabolic rate in human beings is expressed in terms of surface area, and this is done because a better correlation has been found in human beings between basal metabolic rate and surface area than between basal metabolic rate and weight (Berkson, 1936). However, a far better correlation between the metabolic rate and weight$^{3/4}$ has been found by Kleiber (1947) in lower animals ranging in size from the mouse to the ox. Likewise, studies on many different respiratory functions, such as minute respiratory volume, velocity of air flow in the respiratory passages, tidal volumes, and so forth (Guyton, 1947a, 1947b), showed in animals ranging in size from the mouse to man that essentially all these respiratory values also vary almost directly in proportion to weight$^{3/4}$. If we assume that the A-V oxygen differences are the same for all animals, it would be necessary, likewise, to assume that the cardiac outputs vary from animal to animal in proportion to weight$^{3/4}$.

Therefore, we can probably come to the following conclusions: On the basis of present data, use of the cardiac index in expressing cardiac outputs in either lower animals or human beings has not proved to be more valid than expression of cardiac output on the basis of weight. However, we have very poor statistics for correlating cardiac output with any function of body size. On the other hand, the statistics available for correlating body size and metabolic rate have been collected in great detail (Kleiber, 1947), and the correlation is very good between basal metabolic rate and weight$^{3/4}$. Because cardiac output follows metabolic rate, it would probably be best to assume, at least for the present, that cardiac output is similarly related to body size. If we can make this assumption, the most valid relationship between body size and cardiac output would be the following:

$$\text{Cardiac output} \propto \text{Weight}^{3/4}$$

On the basis of the data in Table 1–1, the use of this formula would provide almost as accurate a prediction of cardiac output as would a prediction on the basis of body weight (27 per cent versus 26 per cent mean error). Unfortunately, though, thousands of cardiac measurements, all made by completely accurate methods, would be required to determine the best factor to use in correlating cardiac output with body size.

One might easily argue that within any one species of animals the cardiac output could be proportional to surface area while in the entire animal kingdom it is proportional to weight$^{3/4}$. However, the statistical validity for correlations even within any single animal species is infinitely poorer than for the entire animal kingdom because the sizes within one species vary far too little for statistical accuracy. Therefore, for the present, there is no real justification for believing that the cardiac index is a valid means for relating cardiac output to body size. Yet, since this method for expressing cardiac outputs is very prevalently used, especially in human beings, it will also be used at many points in the present monograph.

VARIATIONS IN CARDIAC OUTPUT

The principal purpose of this monograph is to discuss the regulation of cardiac output. For this reason almost the entire book will be concerned with variations in cardiac output. The discussion in the next few paragraphs will give a brief preview of some of the variations and their ranges in different physiological and pathological conditions.

PHYSIOLOGICAL VARIATIONS

Exercise

Exercise can cause the cardiac output in human beings to increase as much as six fold in well trained athletes (Christensen, 1931)—or at least this is true if we can accept earlier studies using the acetylene method for measuring cardiac output. The cardiac output has probably never been measured in the human being by either the direct Fick or the dilution method while the subject was exercising at his greatest possible work load, but measurements at approximately two-thirds maximal work loads and at about two-thirds maximal rates of oxygen consumption have given about four fold increases in cardiac output (Chapman, 1954; Bevegard, 1960; Reeves, 1961b), thus supporting the six fold increase measured by the acetylene method at maximum work load.

Anoxia

Mild and moderate degrees of anoxia increase the cardiac output as much as two fold (Cross, 1958; Gorlin, 1954), while further degrees of anoxia cause the cardiac output to fall (Oberg, 1961). The increased cardiac output results from decreased resistance throughout the peripheral circulatory system even though the anoxia causes a decrease in the strength of cardiac contraction (Öberg, 1961). The total peripheral resistance decreases in severe anoxia to as little as one-fifth normal. However, beyond a certain stage of anoxia, the heart becomes so weak that despite the decreased peripheral resistance, the cardiac output then declines. Thus, the effect of anoxia on cardiac output is biphasic: (1) an increase in output in the lesser degrees of anoxia resulting from effects on the peripheral circulation and (2) a decrease in cardiac output in the later phases, resulting from weakening of the heart.

In the case of anoxia of the peripheral tissues but without anoxia of the heart itself, one would expect a considerable increase in cardiac output in all stages of anoxia. Exercise is a condition that causes relative anoxia of the skeletal muscles without causing cardiac anoxia. Therefore, it is possible that much of the increase in cardiac output during exercise is caused by relative anoxia of the muscles.

Anesthesia

It is difficult to state the effect of anesthesia on cardiac output because both increases and decreases, as well as no change, have been reported when cardiac output is measured before and after the onset of anesthesia. In a series of cardiac output measurements in dogs collected by Wiggers (1944a)—the outputs having been measured in both unanesthetized dogs and dogs anesthetized with morphine, ether, barbital, urethane, chloralo-sone, or pentobarbital—the ranges observed in the unanesthetized dogs almost exactly overlapped the ranges in the anesthetized dogs.

Most research workers have generally found that deep barbiturate anesthesia reduces cardiac output (Remington, 1949; Quilligan, 1957), but with light anesthesia, Esten (1954, 1955), using the dye-dilution method for measuring cardiac output, showed that thiopental anesthesia in human beings does not significantly change the output. Korner (1954) showed no effect of barbiturate anesthesia in rabbits, and Holman (1938) showed no effect of pentobarbital anesthesia in dogs. In our laboratory, long experi-ence with sodium pentobarbital anesthesia has brought us to the following conclusions: Light anesthesia with this agent apparently does not affect the cardiac output while very deep anesthesia can reduce the output as much as 25 to 40 per cent. However, it is unfortunate that the dosage difference between light and very deep anesthesia when using sodium pentobarbital is very slight so that one must use the agent with care, or otherwise the results will be lower than one would expect in the unanesthetized prepara-tion.

Using halothane anesthesia, Payne (1959) showed no significant differ-ence between the cardiac output before and after induction of surgical anesthesia. Robbins (1938) and Quilligan (1957), using cyclopropane, reported a slight increase in cardiac output in dogs under moderate sur-gical anesthesia, though under very deep anesthesia the animals often had a decreased cardiac output. Finally, Charlier (1948b) found that chloroform anesthesia decreases the cardiac output as much as 20 to 30 per cent, and Remington (1949), Greisheimer (1954b, 1956), and Vidt (1959) all found that ether markedly elevates the cardiac output, some-times as much as 50 to 70 per cent.

To summarize, no one has proved, except perhaps in the cases of chloroform which lowers and ether which raises cardiac output, that light to moderate anesthesia has any significant effect on cardiac output. Yet it cannot be questioned that deep anesthesia of any type that approaches the lethal level can reduce the cardiac output severely.

Posture

When the human being rises from the lying to the sitting position, the cardiac output decreases 5 to 20 per cent (Donald, 1953; Lawrence, 1927; Scott, 1936; Gladstone, 1935a; Bevegard, 1960).

In several different studies to determine the effect of rising from the recumbent or sitting position to the standing position, the Fick, the indicator-dilution, and the less accurate respiratory methods have all shown the cardiac output to decrease 20 to 30 per cent on standing, provided the subject is passively or very quietly changed to the standing position (Law-rence, 1927; Scott, 1936; Gladstone, 1935a; Stead, 1945). On the other hand, if the subject rises to the standing position while simultaneously preparing for walking or other action, the tensing of his muscles can cause a rise in cardiac output instead of a fall. For instance, in Figure 1–1 the cardiac output at the zero work output level was 7.4 liters per minute, which would represent the mean cardiac output for a human being in the standing position ready and expecting to do work. In contrast to this value, however, when the human being is tilted from the recumbent almost to the standing position on a tilt table to which he is strapped, and provided he himself does not perform any muscular activity whatsoever, the cardiac output will decrease an average of approximately 23 per cent and sometimes much more than this (Stead, 1945).

Body Temperature and Climatic Factors

The effect of body temperature on cardiac output has not been studied adequately in the human being, but in anesthetized dogs very exact measurements are available (Brendel, 1958). Figure 1–5 illustrates the average relationship of cardiac output to body temperature found in five dogs. This curve is plotted on a semilogarithmic scale and extends over a range of 18 degrees centigrade or approximately 33 degrees Fahrenheit. Note that the cardiac output bears a direct semilogarithmic relationship to body temperature. Figure 1–5 also shows that the increase in cardiac output is 2.45 fold for each 10° C. rise in body temperature. When one remembers that the Q_{10} for body metabolism is 2.3 to 2.65 (Dubois, 1936), it becomes immediately evident that the data represented in Figure 1–5 are further proof of the intimate relationship between cardiac output and metabolism.

In the human being, no true correlation between body temperature and cardiac output has been established. However, isolated studies of the cardiac output under various climatic conditions have shown general changes in cardiac output in the human being similar to those in lower animals (Asmussen, 1940; Grollman, 1930c; Scott, 1940; Barcroft, 1923)

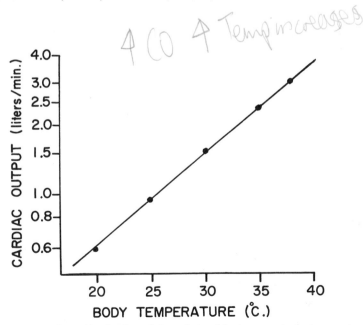

Figure 1–5. Semilogarithmic plot of the relationship between body temperature and cardiac output. [Data obtained from Brendel, Albers, and Usinger (1958), representing studies in five dogs with an average weight of 24.6 kilograms.]

except that when a person shivers, his cardiac output often rises despite a fall in body temperature (Barcroft, 1923). Also, especially important have been Burch's studies (1957) on the cardiac output in both normal persons and patients with cardiac failure under very hot and humid conditions, showing that cardiac output can often increase as much as two to four fold under these conditions, presumably mainly because of large increases in skin blood flow.

Anxiety

Emotional factors are a major cause of changes in cardiac output. The one emotional condition in which cardiac output has been studied to a major extent is anxiety. For instance, Stead and his coworkers (1945) showed that persons showing overt signs of anxiety while having their cardiac outputs measured by the Fick procedure with inlying cardiac catheters had an average cardiac output 67 per cent greater than normal. This same effect was also shown in anxiety resulting from other causes when the ballistocardiographic method was utilized for measuring cardiac output, though in some instances the anxiety caused circulatory collapse with a concomitant fall in cardiac output (Hickam, 1948b).

From these data one can readily see that measurement of cardiac output in man or animals under conditions that create anxiety could cause serious error in the estimation of basal cardiac output. Indeed it is very likely that the basal cardiac output measured in the human being both by the Fick procedure (which requires catheterization of the heart) and by indicator-dilution methods (which require arterial puncture) is in error because of the anxiety factor. Thus, although we believe both of these methods to be entirely accurate in measuring the actual output, it is questionable whether the true basal level of cardiac output is as high as 6 liters per minute even in young adults, as one would believe from the average of measurements made to date.

Other Physiological Factors That Affect Cardiac Output

In earlier days, when the acetylene method for measuring cardiac output was in vogue, the cardiac output was measured in almost all types of physiological conditions. Though far fewer measurements have been made by the more accurate Fick and indicator-dilution methods, if we can believe the relative changes as measured by the acetylene method, one finds (1) that ingestion of a heavy meal can increase the cardiac output approximately 25 per cent (Grollman, 1929; Gladstone, 1935c); (2) that the cardiac output decreases to approximately 25 per cent below his daytime basal value when a person sleeps (Grollman, 1930d); (3) that the cardiac output rises during premenstrual days, falls slightly during the menstrual period, rises slightly again during the postmenstrual days, and falls slightly at the time of ovulation (Grollman, 1932); and (4) that the cardiac output can increase as much as 50 to 100 per cent when a person takes a bath in water of moderate temperature (Grollman, 1932). These data are probably directionally correct even though the acetylene method for measuring cardiac output is not accurate enough for us to be sure of the precise percentage changes that have been quoted for these various conditions.

PATHOLOGICAL VARIATIONS IN CARDIAC OUTPUT

The detailed effects of different pathological conditions on cardiac output will be discussed in later chapters of this monograph. Many tabulations of cardiac output in disease are available, both in the older literature, utilizing mainly respiratory methods for measuring cardiac output (Grollman, 1932; Starr, 1933, 1934, 1935; Lequime, 1940), and in the modern literature, utilizing the more accurate indicator-dilution and Fick methods (Stead, 1947b; Kattus, 1955; Handbook of Circulation, 1959). Figure 1–6 shows the average effects of certain pathological conditions, and the following few paragraphs present a brief synopsis of some of the more important of these effects. The data in Figure 1–6 were derived from averages of values collected in the Handbook of Circulation (1959) and do not represent the extreme ranges of values that can on occasion be observed in the different clinical conditions.

Beriberi is shown in Figure 1–6 to be the worst offender in increasing the cardiac output (see Chapter 27). This results from a decrease in peripheral resistance, for it is also known that beriberi directly affects the heart to make it a weaker pump rather than a stronger pump (Sodeman, 1961). This effect is analogous to the increase in cardiac output which occurs in anoxia, as described earlier, even though the heart is weakened (Öberg, 1961).

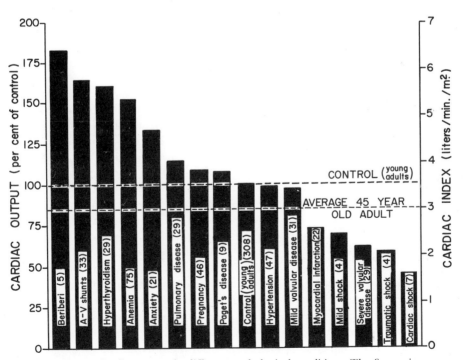

Figure 1–6. Cardiac output in different pathological conditions. The figures in parentheses represent numbers of patients from which the average values were obtained. [Constructed from data in the Handbook of Circulation (1959).]

A-V shunts also frequently cause increases in cardiac output as great as two or more times normal (see Chapter 23). Here again, the primary effect is a reduced peripheral resistance.

Hyperthyroidism, on the average, increases the cardiac output about 60 per cent but can more than double it (Stead, 1950). The basic factor involved in hyperthyroidism is an increase in metabolism with a concomitant increase in cardiac output presumably caused by the link between metabolism and cardiac output, which was discussed earlier in the chapter (see also Chapter 19).

Anemia in 75 patients caused an average increase in cardiac output of slightly more than 50 per cent. However, anemia has been known to increase the cardiac output as much as two to three fold (see Chapter 22). This effect of anemia probably results from at least two peripheral factors: first, decreased viscosity of the blood, which reduces the total peripheral resistance, and, second, decreased delivery of oxygen to the tissues, which causes vasodilatation and in turn increases venous return to the heart with consequently increased cardiac output.

Anxiety increased the cardiac output, on the average, about 35 per cent in 21 persons (see Figure 1–6), this presumably resulting from sympathetic stimulation with resultant contraction of the veins and translocation of blood into the heart to cause an increased cardiac output.

Pulmonary disease can increase the cardiac output up to two fold, but, on the average in 29 patients (Figure 1–6), increased the output about 15 per cent. This again could be a result of decreased oxygen delivery to the tissues, though the precise factors involved have not been completely elucidated.

Pregnancy increases the cardiac output about 8 per cent, correlating very well with the increased metabolism in this condition.

Paget's disease increases the cardiac output slightly because of increased blood flow through the bones.

The cardiac output is completely normal in *hypertension* (Holman, 1938), a fact that has concerned students of hypertension for a long time because it would be easy to explain some of the mechanisms of hypertension if the cardiac output were increased rather than normal.

Factors that reduce the cardiac output are mainly those having to do with decreased blood volume (see Chapter 20) or damage to the heart itself (see Chapters 26 and 27). Mild damage to the heart such as *mild valvular disease* or *mild myocardial infarction* can often be adequately compensated by increased pumping force of other parts of the heart so that the cardiac output will be completely normal. Yet, in *moderate acute myocardial infarction,* the cardiac output is usually reduced as much as 30 per cent and in *severe acute myocardial infarction* as much as 50 to 60 per cent. In *chronic, severe valvular disease* the cardiac output often remains reduced as much as 35 to 40 per cent over a period of many months, illustrating that a human being can live with a cardiac output of less than two-thirds normal almost indefinitely. However, severe shock usually ensues when the cardiac output remains less than one-half normal for any significant period of time.

Chapter 2

MEASUREMENT OF CARDIAC OUTPUT BY THE DIRECT FICK METHOD

THE FICK PRINCIPLE

Adolph Fick spent his lifetime in scholarly study of work and heat production in muscles (Rose, 1956). Yet, out of his thoughts came a diversion in 1870 into the field of cardiac output measurement, this leading to a brief report of an idea by which the cardiac output could be calculated (Fick, 1870). Thus, the "Fick principle" was enunciated, but Fick himself never used this principle to measure the cardiac output in an actual animal. Instead, it was first used by Grehant and Quinquant in 1886 to measure the cardiac output in six dogs. Subsequently, one of the most famous early uses of the Fick principle occurred in 1898 when Zuntz and Hagemann (1898) measured the cardiac output of two horses both at rest and while exercising, thus demonstrating for the first time that the cardiac output increases automatically during exercise. However, it was not until catheterization of the right heart in the human being was popularized in the early 1940's that the Fick principle began to be widely used for measurement of the output in the human being (Cournand, 1945a, 1945b; Richards, 1945; Stead, 1945; McMichael, 1944, 1945; Charlier, 1946). Since that time, literally tens of thousands of measurements of cardiac output have been carried out by the procedure in the human being.

The Fick principle has become so important in the field of cardiac output measurement and is now so often used as a standard reference for measurement of cardiac output that the original description of this principle deserves reproduction in this monograph:

Hr. Fick hält einen Vortrag über die Messung des Blutquantums, das in jeder Systole durch die Herzventrikel ausgeworfen wird, eine Grösse, deren Kenntniss ohne Zweifel von grösster Wichtigkeit ist. Gleichwohl sind darüber die abweichendsten Ansichten aufgestellt. Während Th. Young die in Rede stehende Grösse auf etwa 45^{ccm} anschlägt cursiren in den neueren Lehrbüchern der Physiologie meist sehr viel höhere Angaben, weche, gestützt auf die Schätzungen von Volkmann und Vierordt, sich bis auf 180^{ccm} belaufen. Bei dieser Sachlage ist es seltsam, dass man noch nicht auf folgenden naheliegenden Veg gekommen ist, auf dem diese wichtige Grösse wenigstens an Thieren direkter Bestimmung zugänglich ist. Man bestimme, wie viel Sauerstoff ein Thier während einer gewissen Zeit aus der Luft aufnimmt und wie viel Kohlensäure es abgibt. Man nehme ferner dem Thiere während der Versuchszeit eine Probe arteriellen und eine Probe venösen Blutes. In beiden ist der Sauerstoffgehalt und der Kohlensäuregehalt zu ermitteln. Die Differenz des Sauerstoffgehaltes ergibt, wie viel Sauerstoff jedes Cubiccentimeter Blut beim Durchgang durch die Lungen aufnimmt, und da man weiss, wie viel Sauerstoff im Ganzen während einer bestimmten Zeit aufgenommen wurde, so kaun man berechnen, wie viel Cubiccentimeter Blut während diester Zeit die Lungen passierten, oder wenn man durch die Anzahl der Herzschläge in dieser Zeit dividirt, wie viel Cubiccentimeter Blut mit jeder Systole des Herzens ausgeworfen wurden. Die entsprechende Rechnung mit den Kohlensäuremengen gibt eine Bestimmung desselben Werthes, welche die erstere controllirt.

Da zur Ausführung dieser Methode 2 Gaspumpen gehören, so ist der Vortragende leider nicht in der Lage, experimentelle Bestimmungen mitzutheilen. Er will daher nur noch nach dem Schema der angegebenen Methode eine Berechnung der Blutstromstärke des Menschen geben, gegründet auf mehr oder weniger willkürliche Data. Nach den von Scheffer in Ludwig's Laboratorium ausgeführten Versuchen enthält 1^{ccm} arterielles Hundeblut 0,146^{ccm} Sauerstoff (gemessen bei 0° Temperatur und 1^{m} Quecksilber Druck), 1^{ccm} venöses Hundeblut enthält 0,0905^{ccm} Sauerstoff. Jedes Cubiccentimeter Blut nimmt also beim Durchgang durch die Lungen 0.0555^{ccm} Sauerstoff auf. Nehme man an, das wäre beim Menschen gerade so. Nehme man ferner an, ein Mensch absorbirte in 24^{h} 833^{gr} Sauerstoff aus der Luft. Sie nehmen bei 0° und 1^{m} Druck 433200^{ccm} Raum ein. Demnach würden in den Lungen des Menschen jede Secunde 5^{ccm} Sauerstoff absorbirt. Um diese Absorption zu bewerkstelligen müssten aber der obigen Annahme gemäss $\frac{5}{0.0555^{ccm}}$ Blut die Lungen durchströmen, d. h. 90^{ccm} Angenommen endlich, dass 7 Systolen in 6 Secunden erfolgten, würden mit jeder Systole des Ventrikels 77^{ccm} Blut ausgeworfen.

The basic Fick principle can be further explained by Figure 2–1. This figure shows a flowing stream into which an indicator substance is being injected at a rate $\frac{\Delta S}{\Delta t}$. The concentration of this substance in the flowing stream before the point of injection is $C_1 S$ and the concentration after mixing with the injected substance is $C_2 S$. By simple mathematical procedures we can see that the rate of entry of the substance into the flowing fluid $\left(\frac{\Delta S}{\Delta t}\right)$ will equal the change in concentration $(C_2 S - C_1 S)$ times the rate of flow (F). That is,

$$\frac{\Delta S}{\Delta t} = F\ (C_2 S - C_1 S) \tag{2-1}$$

On rearranging, equation 2–1 becomes

$$F = \frac{\dfrac{\Delta S}{\Delta t}}{C_2 S - C_1 S} \tag{2-2}$$

This is the familiar mathematical expression of the Fick principle, and it states very simply that the flow in a given period of time is equal to the

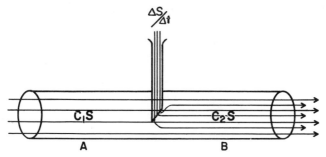

Figure 2–1. Demonstration of the basic Fick principle.

amount of substance entering the stream of flow in the same period of time divided by the difference between the concentrations of the substance before and after the point of entry.

One of the most important points that must be understood about the Fick principle is that it can be applied to any flowing stream of fluid when a substance either enters or leaves the stream, provided the rate of entry or exit of the substance and its concentrations on the two sides of entry or exit can all be measured. We shall see later that the Fick principle has been employed for measuring cardiac output in several different ways, utilizing both entry of an indicator substance into the flowing blood or removal of a substance from the blood stream.

Thorough Mixing as a Basic Requirement for Measuring Cardiac Output by the Fick Principle

A basic requirement of the Fick principle as described in Figure 2–1 is that the indicator substance must be thoroughly mixed with the flowing fluid at each point of sampling. Otherwise the sample's concentration might not be representative of that throughout the entire cross section of the stream; this obviously could cause a very significant error in the calculation of cardiac output. There are only two places in the circulation where all the parallel vascular pathways become confluent and where the blood becomes adequately mixed for use in the determination of cardiac output. The first of these is in the right heart, and the second is in the left heart. Therefore, all procedures utilizing the Fick principle for determination of cardiac output have depended upon measurement of blood concentrations of substances in one or both sides of the heart or in the arteries beyond these two mixing chambers.

THE DIRECT FICK METHOD FOR MEASURING CARDIAC OUTPUT UTILIZING OXYGEN AS THE INDICATOR SUBSTANCE

From the earliest use of the Fick principle for measuring cardiac output, it was realized that oxygen entering the blood through the lungs is an almost ideal indicator for employing the Fick principle to measure cardiac output, because both the rate of oxygen uptake through the lungs and the blood's concentrations of oxygen on each side of the lungs can be measured with ease. Thus the formula for measuring cardiac output becomes

$$\text{Cardiac output (liters/min.)} = \frac{O_2 \text{ consumption (ml./min.)}}{\text{Arterial } O_2 - \text{Venous } O_2 \text{ (ml./liter)}} \qquad (2\text{-}3)$$

This formula means very simply that the cardiac output is equal to the oxygen consumed through the lungs each minute divided by the anterio-venous oxygen difference.

DETERMINATION OF THE ARTERIOVENOUS OXYGEN DIFFERENCE

One can easily obtain a sample of mixed blood leaving the lungs by simply removing blood from any one of the systemic arteries. The reason this gives an appropriate, representative sample is the following: Blood coming from all the parallel channels of the lungs mixes in the left heart and then is distributed into all the systemic arteries with neither loss nor gain of oxygen from the blood after it is originally mixed in the left heart. Consequently, the concentration of oxygen in the blood of any artery is exactly the same as that of any other artery, so that obtaining a sample of mixed blood distal to the lungs with equally distributed oxygen concentration is a very simple matter.

On the other hand, the most difficult of all the problems in utilizing the Fick method for determining cardiac output has been to obtain an adequate sample of mixed venous blood prior to its entry into the lungs. The only segment of the circulation from which this can be done is the right ventricle or pulmonary arterial system. Unfortunately, one can never be sure that the blood in the right atrium is adequately mixed, because the inflows from the superior and inferior venae cavae, as well as from the coronary sinus, are likely to streamline in the right atrium rather than becoming mixed. In sampling the atrial blood, therefore, one is likely to be in serious error because of sampling from a single streamline. In studying this problem, Shore (1945) and Warren (1946) separately found that right atrial oxygen concentrations are often markedly different from those of mixed venous blood removed from the ventricle. On the other hand, Cournand (1945b) found that if the investigator removes blood through a catheter whose tip is placed precisely at the mid-point of the right atrium near the tricuspid valve, little error is likely to occur. Yet, to be completely safe in obtaining mixed venous blood, the sample must be taken either from the right ventricle or the pulmonary artery, and some investigators have even questioned whether too much stream-lining might not occur in the right ventricle for complete accuracy (Warren, 1948a).

The usual method for removing blood from the right ventricle or pulmonary artery is through a catheter. Forssmann (1929) first proved the innocuousness of catheterizing the right heart, and Klein (1930) first showed that an adequate sample of mixed venous blood for determining cardiac output can be removed from the right heart through a catheter. However, this procedure was not popularized until Cournand (1941) began making extensive cardiac output measurements by the catheter method. Catheters have been left in place in the right hearts of human beings for over two days (Cournand, 1945b) and in dogs for as long as 21 days (Frieden, 1952). [Historically, it should also be noted that in the early 1930's mixed venous blood for measuring cardiac output was also obtained in a few persons by direct needle puncture of the right ventricle through the anterior chest wall (Grollman, 1932).]

The technique for introducing the catheter into the right ventricle of the human being is basically the following: The catheter itself is radiopaque and has a slight curvature near its end. It is inserted under aseptic conditions into an antecubital vein and then upward to the innominate vein, the superior vena cava, right atrium, and right ventricle. The catheter is guided under fluoroscopic control past any obstructive point along the venous system by rotating it so that the curved tip is directed in the proper direction. By use of this procedure, and by pulling back and pushing forward again whenever an obstruction is met, passage of the catheter into the right atrium is ordinarily uneventful. Here, under fluoroscopic guidance again, the tip of the catheter is rotated toward the tricuspid valve, and further passage leads the catheter directly into the right ventricle. For detailed description of some of the precautions, materials, and precise precedures, the reader is referred to Cournand's (1945) and Warren's (1948) complete descriptions of their procedures for cardiac catheterization and determination of the cardiac output in the human being.

In the animal, catheterization is usually performed in the same manner as for the human being except that the catheter is more often inserted down the external jugular vein into the right atrium and thence into the right ventricle rather than through a limb vein.

Ordinarily a slow drip of fluid into the catheter will prevent clotting for many hours, and samples of mixed venous blood can be removed whenever desired. When fluoroscopic guidance is not available to tell whether the catheter is in the right ventricle, one can usually determine this by opening the exterior end of the catheter to the air and raising its level upward and downward. As long as the cardiac tip of the catheter is in the right atrium, the level of the blood in the external part of the catheter will be approximately at the level of the heart, whereas once the catheter is in the right ventricle, the level of blood will be 8 to 15 cm. above the level of the heart.

Only two significant untoward effects have resulted from leaving catheters in the heart for many hours at a time; these are (1) thrombosis of the peripheral veins through which the catheter had been inserted and (2) occasional arrhythmias of the heart resulting from pressure of the catheter tip against the intracardiac surface. In very rare instances ventricular fibrillation has occurred, though not more than once during many thousands of cardiac catheterizations in human beings.

Analysis of the Blood Oxygen Concentration

The oxygen content of the blood samples is most often determined by the manometric Van Slyke apparatus, the use of which has been described in detail by Peters and Van Slyke (1932). However, other methods available for analyzing the blood oxygen are the Roughton-Scholander micromethod (1943), the Haldane blood gas analyzer method (Courtice, 1947), and various photometric methods (Drabkin, 1950). The details of a special automatic photometric method that we have developed in our laboratory will also be presented later in this chapter in a description of a continuous cardiac output recorder we have used for the past several years.

MEASUREMENT OF OXYGEN CONSUMPTION

Measurement of oxygen consumption for the determination of cardiac output is usually made by one of two methods called the "open circuit" and the "closed circuit" methods. In the open circuit method, the subject's expired air is collected over a given period of time in a Douglas bag or a Tissot spirometer. Then a Haldane gas analyzer is used to measure the concentration of oxygen in both the expired and the normal inspired air. To calculate the total oxygen consumed during the given interval of time, the concentration difference between the inspired and expired airs is multiplied by the total quantity of air collected in the bag or spirometer.

A modified open circuit method which we have developed for measuring oxygen consumption continuously, utilizing the Pauling oxygen meter, will also be described in the following section of this chapter in connection with the description of a continuous cardiac output recorder.

The usual application of the closed circuit method for measuring oxygen consumption is to use the standard metabolism apparatus. Ordinarily the metabolism apparatus is filled with oxygen, and the rate of oxygen usage is determined by the rate at which the rebreathing chamber of the metabolism apparatus empties.

A CONTINUOUS CARDIAC OUTPUT RECORDER

During the past dozen years, we have developed and used extensively in our laboratory a continuous cardiac output recorder that utilizes the Fick principle (Guyton, 1959f, 1962b; Crowell and Guyton, 1962; Granger and Guyton, 1969; Prather, 1969; Dobbs, 1971). Figure 2–2 illustrates the apparatus. A person or an animal breathes into the breathing tube and the expired gases are conducted into an appropriate oxygen analyzer to measure rate of oxygen utilization. Simultaneously, blood is conducted through catheters into respective venous and arterial cuvettes, and an appropriate photoelectric circuit measures the arteriovenous oxygen difference. Finally, the information from both of these sources is fed into an analog computer that continuously computes the cardiac output. These three basic components of the continuous cardiac output recorder are as follows:

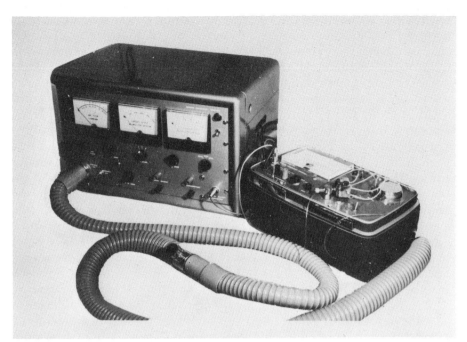

Figure 2–2. A photograph of the continuous cardiac output recorder. For complete description, see text.

The Arteriovenous Oxygen Difference Recorder

Figure 2–3 illustrates the basic principles of the arteriovenous oxygen difference recorder. Venous and arterial bloods, taken from appropriate catheters in the human being or animal, are pumped through the two respective cuvettes. Two separate light sources transmit light beams through the two respective cuvettes, and the beams in turn impinge on a single photomultiplier tube. The two light sources are neon glow bulbs excited by an electronic circuit that causes light emission during only

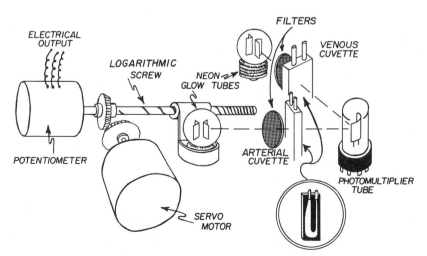

Figure 2–3. The basic components of the arteriovenous oxygen difference recorder. See text for explanation.

one-half of each cycle of the 60 cycle alternating power source. Furthermore, the two lights are excited 180 degrees out of phase with each other. That is, during each complete cycle, one of the lights will be on during the first half of the cycle and the other on during the second half, this process repeating itself indefinitely. If the light beams passing through the two cuvettes and impinging on the photomultiplier tube are of equal brightness, this fact is detected by the photomultiplier tube and nothing happens. However, if one is brighter than the other, the servomotor of the analyzer moves the arterial light source along a tract. If the light passing through the arterial cuvette is weaker than that through the venous cuvette, the servomotor runs in the direction to bring the arterial light source closer to the cuvette. Conversely, if the light passing through the arterial cuvette is brighter than that through the venous cuvette, the light source moves away from the cuvette, and movement continues until the two lights transmitted through the two respective cuvettes become of exactly equal brightness. The screw that moves the arterial light source forward or backward is a "corrected" semilogarithmic screw and has been corrected at each point along its extent so that the A-V oxygen difference can be read directly from the number of turns that the screw must make to move the light source. The screw is also connected directly to a potentiometer and this in turn is connected to an appropriate electronic circuit and meter so that the A-V oxygen difference can be read linearly on the recording meter; or it can be recorded on any appropriate D.C. recorder.

The light that is transmitted through the two cuvettes is a filtered dark red light. In this color range the optical density of venous blood is approximately two times that of arterial blood, which is the characteristic that allows a photoelectric system such as this to be accurate in measuring A-V oxygen difference.

The advantages of using two separate cuvettes for arterial and venous bloods and having these balanced against each other are the following: First, changes in hematocrit do not affect the output reading. Second, changes in the amount of reduced hemoglobin in the arterial blood have no effect on the output of the recorder. Third, incidental optical density changes caused by such factors as abnormal color of the plasma and so forth also have essentially no effect on the output. The reason why these different factors do not affect the reading of the instrument is that all of them change exactly the same in both the venous and the arterial blood. Therefore, their effects on the reading of the instrument are completely nullified, and the instrument detects only *differences* between the two cuvettes. Since the only difference between venous and arterial bloods that causes a significant optical density difference is the difference between reduced and oxygenated hemoglobin, the instrument reads the A-V oxygen difference itself rather than some other function of oxygen saturation in the blood.

The Oxygen Consumption Analyzer

Figure 2–4 illustrates diagrammatically the basic principles of the oxygen consumption analyzer. This instrument consists of two essential

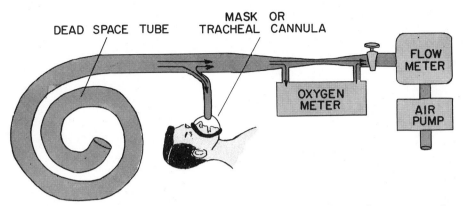

Figure 2–4. The basic components of the oxygen consumption analyzer. See text for explanation.

parts: first, an airflow device that pulls air through a breathing tube at a fixed rate and, second, an oxygen analyzer that measures the decrease in oxygen in the air passing through the instrument. When a person or an animal breathes into the breathing tube, the air that he inhales is fresh air that is flowing through the breathing tube. When he exhales, his expired air also enters this flowing stream of air, and it, mixed with the flowing air, enters the instrument. The presence of the expired air reduces the concentration of oxygen in the air entering the instrument. A small sample of this air is pulled continuously through the oxygen analyzer, which detects the reduction in oxygen concentration below the control oxygen concentration of the air. For instance, if 10 liters of air is flowing through the tube per minute and the oxygen analyzer detects a 2.5 volume per cent decrease in oxygen concentration in the air below that of normal room air, the rate of oxygen consumption is 250 ml./minute. Corrections are made for respiratory exchange ratio, water vapor in the air, and air temperature. The rate of oxygen consumption is calibrated directly onto the meter face.

Factors that can cause the greatest error in this system for measuring oxygen consumption are water vapor and changes in the respiratory ratio. Within usual ranges of water vapor changes, an error as great as ± 4 per cent might occur. This error can be avoided by use of an air drying system, but in practice the results do not seem to be improved significantly by this procedure. In relation to the respiratory ratio, one calculates that a change in the usual range between 0.7 and 1.0 will cause a maximum error of approximately ± 3.5 per cent, which is small enough to be ignored. For extra short transient periods, such as when a person greatly overbreathes, the respiratory ratio can change beyond the usual normal range, in which case errors as great as ± 10 per cent can theoretically occur. However, such errors cannot last long because the respiratory ratio soon comes into equilibrium with the respiratory quotient, which almost never goes beyond the normal limits of 0.7 to 1.0.

The oxygen analyzer utilizes a new type of paramagnetic unit capable of measuring *difference* between oxygen in the same air and oxygen in normal air. This unit is illustrated in Figure 2–5, which shows a very thin

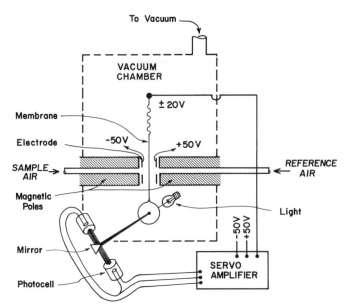

Figure 2–5. A diagram of the paramagnetic unit used in the oxygen consumption analyzer. See text for explanation.

aluminum membrane suspended in a powerful magnetic gap. The membrane is encased in a closed chamber, and its movement is detected by a beam of light impinging on photocells. A slight vacuum is applied to the closed chamber, and air is pulled through holes in the two respective magnetic poles onto the two sides of the suspended membrane, with sample air impinging on one side of the membrane and room air on the opposite side. Since oxygen exhibits paramagnetic properties, it tends to crowd into the strong magnetic field. Therefore, if more oxygen is on one side of the membrane than on the other, the crowding of oxygen on that side will push the membrane to the opposite side. By use of an electronic servo feedback mechanism excited by the photocells, the membrane is moved back to its original position by electrostatic force. The electrical voltage required to cause this electrostatic return of the membrane to its neutral position is a direct measure of the force on the membrane caused by the difference in oxygen concentration between the two sides. Therefore, the voltage on the membrane is also a direct measure of the difference between the Po_2 of the sample air and that of the room air. The paramagnetic analyzer itself has a capability of detecting oxygen concentration differences as small as 0.02 volume per cent, and its output is linear within approximately ± 2 per cent.

The Computer

Computation of cardiac output from the outputs of the A-V oxygen difference recorder and oxygen consumption recorder is performed by usual analog techniques. A voltage derived from the oxygen consumption analyzer is fed into the computer, and resistance coupled to the drive screw of the A-V oxygen difference analyzer is also fed into the computer. Utilizing these two values, the computer can compute oxygen consumption divided by A-V oxygen difference with an accuracy of less than 1 per cent. Considering possible errors in the other two instruments, however, the overall cardiac output measurement error is believed to be within ± 7 per cent.

The principal advantages of using a continuous cardiac output recorder are two fold. First, when errors do occur in the measurement technique, these are usually compensated within a few seconds to a few minutes (for instance, return of very high respiratory ratios toward normal), and one can also detect that errors have occurred because of the shape of the curve. Second, cardiac output changes markedly from minute to minute; therefore, when measurements are made by single measurement techniques, the measured cardiac output may be as great as 25 per cent above or below the average cardiac output value. By having a continuous record, one can prevent this type of error.

Figure 2–6 shows a typical recording of cardiac output, oxygen consumption, and A-V oxygen difference during an experiment in which 300 ml. of whole blood was infused into a dog. Additional records appear throughout the book.

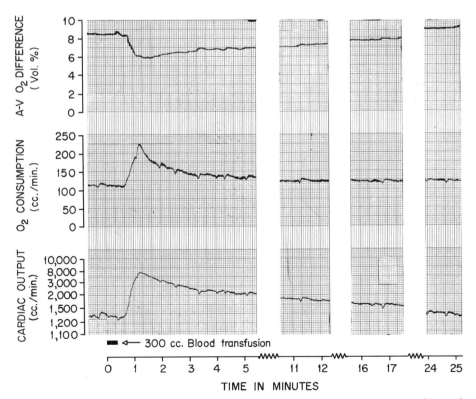

Figure 2–6. A representative recording of cardiac output, oxygen consumption, and A-V oxygen difference using the continuous recorder.

ERRORS OFTEN ENCOUNTERED WHEN MEASURING CARDIAC OUTPUT BY THE OXYGEN-FICK METHOD

Measurement of cardiac output by the oxygen-Fick method can sometimes be in error by more than 100 per cent. This, however, is not caused by any basic error in the principle itself but instead by misapplication of the principle. The types of errors involved can be classified into three categories: (1) errors in sampling and analysis, (2) errors caused by a changing cardiac output, and (3) errors caused by changing respiratory conditions (Visscher, 1953; Nahas, 1953).

Errors in Sampling and Analysis

Earlier in the chapter it was pointed out that it is essential to obtain adequately mixed venous blood before attempting to calculate the cardiac output by the oxygen-Fick procedure.

Another problem related to sampling has to do with the precise time of sampling, because the right ventricular blood oxygen content increases and decreases constantly, even within the space of a few seconds (Warren, 1946, Griffin, 1951; Wood, 1955). Therefore, a sample of blood taken at one second may not be representative of an average sample of blood over a period of time. To avoid this difficulty, blood is usually removed from the right ventricle slowly, over a period of 5 to 10 seconds or longer, so that the sample represents an average sample rather than an instantaneous sample.

A similar error occurs sometimes in sampling blood from the arteries, though not usually. Ordinarily, blood that has passed through normally respired lungs is approximately 97 per cent saturated with oxygen, and even moderate changes in alveolar Po_2 usually will not significantly alter this degree of saturation. However, when the average Po_2 in the alveoli falls very low, in the range of 40 to 50 mm. Hg, a very slight change in pulmonary Po_2 will cause a marked change in saturation of the systemic arterial blood. Under these conditions, the degree of arterial blood saturation can change as much as several volumes per cent during each respiratory cycle, and the slower the respiratory cycle, the greater will this change be. Therefore, an arterial blood sample taken at one second during the respiratory cycle under anoxic conditions may not be representative of the average hemoglobin saturation over a period of time; this might account partially for the poor results that have been reported in measuring cardiac output by the Fick method during anoxia (Nahas, 1953; Fishman, 1952). Here again, it is important to remove the arterial sample at a steady rate over a period of many seconds in order to obtain a representative average sample of systemic arterial blood rather than an instantaneous sample.

The errors in the methods for measuring oxygen contents of the venous and arterial bloods are mainly obvious, but these should be listed to remind one of possible pitfalls: When photometric methods are used, the oxygen dissolved in the fluid of the blood is not measured. At normal alveolar P_{O_2}'s this will cause an error of less than 4 per cent because the amount dissolved in the blood is only 0.3 volume per cent in the arterial blood and only 0.12 volume per cent in the venous blood; this is a very small A-V difference for the dissolved oxygen and is usually insignificant. On the other hand, if the subject breathes pure oxygen, the dissolved arterial oxygen then becomes about 2.0 volumes per cent, and the A-V difference becomes approximately 1.9 volumes per cent. This represents as much as 40 per cent of the normal A-V difference of oxygen that fails to be measured by the method, thus giving a very serious error in the measurement of cardiac output by photometric methods under these conditions.

Another obvious error in measuring blood oxygen content, which unfortunately is often forgotten, is that the Van Slyke method for measuring oxygen causes release not only of oxygen from the blood but also of most anesthetic gases that might be present in the blood (Prime, 1952). Therefore, when the subject is anesthetized by gaseous anesthesia, errors in the measured oxygen content of the blood by the Van Slyke procedure may cause as much as a 20 to 50 per cent error in the computed cardiac output. Under these conditions a chemical method for measurement of oxygen should be employed rather than a gaseous method.

Errors in sampling and measurement of oxygen consumption can also occur, though these usually are not nearly so serious as those relating to measurement of blood oxygen content. A minor error can occur when collecting expired air in a Douglas bag or Tissot spirometer if the collection is begun in expiration and ends in inspiration, or vice versa. However, this error will be minimized if the expired air is collected over a prolonged period of time. And, in using the open circuit method, the assumption that the inspired air has a constant oxygen concentration can lead to errors as much as 20 to 30 per cent, for certainly this is not true in a poorly ventilated room. The best precaution against this is to have the subject breathe air brought immediately from the outside. Even then, changes in barometric pressure can cause errors unless appropriate allowances or control determinations are made.

Errors Caused by a Changing Cardiac Output

If the cardiac output is changing while the cardiac output is being measured by the Fick method, the measurement will usually be in error, sometimes by as much as 100 per cent or more. For instance, let us assume that the oxygen consumption remains constant while the A-V oxygen difference slowly changes at a steady rate. One might suspect that the average cardiac output could be measured quite adequately by simply averaging venous and arterial blood oxygen contents during the period of the change. However, the cardiac output does not change directly with a change in A-V oxygen difference but instead inversely. Because of this fact, an average A-V oxygen difference is not adequate to calculate the cardiac output during the interval of time. Instead the cardiac output must be calculated from the following formula:

$$F = \frac{O_2 \; \log_e \frac{(\Delta O)_2}{(\Delta O)_1}}{(\Delta O)_2 - (\Delta O)_1} \tag{2-4}$$

in which F is the average cardiac output for the interval of time, O_2 is the oxygen consumed during the interval of time, $(\Delta O)_2$ is the A-V oxygen difference at the end of the interval, and $(\Delta O)_1$ is the A-V oxygen difference at the beginning of the interval.

Under most circumstances, this error will be negligible. For instance, let us assume that the oxygen consumption remains constant at 200 ml./min. and that the A-V oxygen difference at the beginning of an interval of time is 40 ml./liter of blood but then rises at a steady rate up to 80 ml./liter at the end of the interval. The average A-V oxygen difference during this period of time is 60 ml./liter, which would give an average cardiac output calculation of 3.33 liters per minute. However, using the above formula the actual average cardiac output is 3.465 liters per minute. In other words, by simply taking an average A-V oxygen difference the error would be 4 per cent.

Since the cardiac output rarely changes more than double during intervals of measurements, this type of error is rarely significant, but now let us assume that a great change occurs in cardiac output, with the A-V oxygen difference changing at a steady rate from 10 ml./liter up to 100 ml./liter. The average cardiac output calculated from the average A-V oxygen difference would be 3.6 liters per minute, though the true average cardiac output calculated by the above formula is 5.1 liters per minute. Thus, the error in this case would be 30 per cent. Some of the conditions in which this type can occur are (a) during a Valsalva maneuver, (b) during rapid transfusion or hemorrhage, or (c) at the onset or cessation of stimulation of one of the circulatory reflexes.

Another type of error that can result from a changing cardiac output occurs when the cardiac output rises very high, then falls very low, then rises high again, and repeats this cycle again and again while the rate of oxygen consumption remains constant. The A-V oxygen difference will approach zero during high cardiac output and will approach some high value during low cardiac output. However, because of the nonlinear relationship between cardiac output and A-V oxygen difference, one cannot calculate the average cardiac output by using the A-V oxygen difference, and the precise formula for calculating the average cardiac output would depend upon the pattern of the flow curve. If this pattern is rectilinear, with the cardiac output suddenly increasing to a certain level, holding this level for a period of time, then falling suddenly and holding the lower level for the same period of time, thus repeating the cycle again and again, the cardiac output would be calculated from the following formula:

$$F = \frac{O_2 \left[\frac{1}{(\Delta O)_2} + \frac{1}{(\Delta O)_1} \right]}{2} \tag{2-5}$$

in which $(\Delta O)_2$ is the A-V oxygen difference at minimum cardiac output, and $(\Delta O)_1$ is the A-V oxygen difference at maximum cardiac output. Let us assume, for instance, that the oxygen consumption remains constant at 200 cc./minute, while the A-V oxygen difference varies between a lower limit of 10 ml./liter and an upper limit of 100 ml./liter, with equal cycles of low and high levels. The true average cardiac output as calculated by the above formula would be 11 liters per minute. However, the average A-V oxygen difference, $(10 + 100)/2$, is 55 cc./liter. If we should use this value in the usual formula for calculating cardiac output, the result would be 3.63 liters per minute or 7.37 liters less than the true average cardiac output. Thus, the true cardiac output would be about 200 per cent greater than the measured value.

This type of error can result from the rise and fall in cardiac output that occurs with very deep respiration, particularly when the respiration is very slow.

One of the principal advantages of the continous cardiac output recorder described earlier in this chapter has been that it minimizes and almost completely eliminates the errors that result from a changing cardiac output. The reason for this is that the cardiac output is calculated each second from the instantaneous A-V oxygen difference, and then one can average the recorded cardiac outputs rather than first averaging the A-V oxygen differences and then calculating the cardiac output, which leads to the errors just discussed.

Errors Caused by Changing Respiratory Conditions

CHANGES IN MEAN PULMONARY VOLUME. Probably the most serious of all errors in the oxygen-Fick method for determining cardiac output result from a changing mean pulmonary volume. To explain this, let us return to the basic Fick formula, which states that the cardiac output is calculated from two values: first, the amount of oxygen entering the blood each minute and, second, the A-V oxygen difference. However, the methods for measuring oxygen consumption *do not necessarily measure the amount of oxygen entering the blood each minute* but instead measure the amount of oxygen *entering the lungs each minute,* and the lungs themselves are a large reservoir between the pulmonary airway and the alveolar membrane. Very often the amount of oxygen entering the lungs becomes, for temporary periods of time, far greater or far less than the amount of oxygen entering the blood.

Let us assume, for instance, that the oxygen consumption is being measured by a standard basal metabolism apparatus and that a change in position of the patient or some other physical change causes him to increase his mean pulmonary volume. This increase is measured by the metabolism apparatus as an increase in oxygen consumption although this is not true. As an example, if a person is consuming 250 ml. of oxygen per minute but over a period of one minute he progressively increases his mean pulmonary volume by 500 ml., which is well within reason, then the measured oxygen consumption would be 750 ml. per minute, while only

250 ml. of this would actually be entering the blood. As a result, the calculated cardiac output would be 200 per cent above the true cardiac output.

Significant error from this cause can still result even when the cardiac output is averaged over periods of time as long as 5 minutes, for a subject can easily change his mean pulmonary volume as much as 1 liter during this period of time. Assuming an actual consumption of 250 ml. per minute, a 1 liter increase in mean pulmonary volume over a 5 minute period of time would give 80 per cent too high a measurement for cardiac output.

The error is even more dramatic when the mean pulmonary volume decreases during a 5 minute interval by as much as 1 liter while 250 ml. of oxygen is actually entering the blood each minute. In this case a total of 1250 ml. will be consumed in 5 minutes while the mean pulmonary volume is being reduced by 1000 ml. Therefore, the metabolism apparatus measures an oxygen consumption of 250 ml. for the 5 minutes, or one-fifth normal, giving a cardiac output only one-fifth of the true value. In this instance, the true cardiac output is 400 per cent greater than the measured cardiac output. Thus, in use of the standard metabolism apparatus for measurement of cardiac output, very slight changes in the mechanics of respiration can alter the calculated cardiac output drastically.

RELATIVE ERRORS WHEN BREATHING AIR VERSUS BREATHING OXYGEN. The error in measurement of cardiac output caused by a mean pulmonary volume change is about five times less when an open circuit method is used and the respiratory gas is air rather than pure oxygen. The reason for this is that when air is used, four-fifths of the gas that becomes stored or is removed from the lung when the mean pulmonary volume changes is nitrogen. For instance, if the mean pulmonary volume increases by 1 liter while the subject is breathing air, the error in the oxygen measurement will be 200 ml. rather than 1000 ml., which would be the case when using the oxygen metabolism apparatus.

CHANGES IN RATE OF PULMONARY VENTILATION. Another type of respiratory change that can cause the measured value to be different from the true value of cardiac output is a change in rate of pulmonary ventilation. Mathematically, this error is about the same in using the open circuit method as in using the metabolism apparatus method, and it can be explained as follows: If the rate of alveolar ventilation is increased to double the normal, assuming that the rate of oxygen entry into the blood remains constant, the alveolar oxygen P_{O_2} will rise from approximately 104 mm. Hg up to 126 mm. Hg. This represents an increase of about 90 ml. of oxygen stored in the lungs and, therefore, causes the measured value of oxygen consumption to be 90 ml. greater than the amount that actually enters the blood. This can cause an error as great as 15 to 20 per cent when the oxygen consumption is measured over an interval of several minutes or an error as much as several hundred per cent when the oxygen consumption is measured over a period of only a few seconds.

In using the continuous cardiac output recorder, the pulmonary types of errors appear on the record as tremendous spikes in the recording, completely out of accord with the remainder of the record; therefore, they usually can be ignored because the recorded cardiac output returns to its true value just as soon as the new respiratory state has been reached.

Another value of the continuous cardiac output recorder is that when pulmonary ventilation or mean pulmonary volume is increasing and decreasing, the errors in the recorded cardiac output are nullified by compensatory errors in the recording when the respiration changes back in the opposite direction.

Necessity for Steady State Conditions in Using the Fick Principle

From the foregoing discussion of the possible errors and the magnitudes of these errors, one can readily see why physiologists have always emphasized the necessity for steady state conditions when using the oxygen-Fick method for determining cardiac output. It is generally stated that one should allow two minutes after a change in circulatory or respiratory conditions before making a determination of cardiac output by this procedure. However, when using the continuous cardiac output recorder, which utilizes an open circuit method for measuring oxygen consumption, it is rare that the cardiac output is in error for more than 30 to 45 seconds after a change in steady state conditions has occurred. On the other hand, if one uses the oxygen filled metabolator to measure oxygen consumption, and if changes are occurring slowly, often too slowly to be observed, the measurements can remain as much as 100 per cent in error for as long as 4 minutes at a time. Therefore, the most important of all precautions is to be sure that steady state conditions, especially with regard to mean pulmonary volume, prevail when making a measurement of cardiac output by the oxygen-Fick method.

Accuracy of the Oxygen-Fick Method

One will never know the true accuracy of the oxygen-Fick method. If absolutely steady state conditions could be achieved, then the Fick principle should be infallible for measurement of cardiac output, but one can readily see from the above cautionary paragraphs that plenty of opportunities are available for error. Our best reason for believing that the Fick method, as usually applied with normal precautions, is a truly accurate method for measuring cardiac output is that Fick measurements of cardiac output compare very favorably with measurements of cardiac output by other methods that are believed to be equally accurate. For instance, Seely and coworkers (1950a, 1950b) and Huggins and coworkers (1950) have compared Fick measurements with direct rotameter measurements of cardiac output, with the rotameters inserted respectively in the pulmonary artery and in the venous input circuit to the heart. In both instances, the measurements compared within the limits of accuracy of the rotameters themselves. Furthermore, a very large number of comparisons have been made between the oxygen-Fick method and the indicator-dilution method, which will be described in the following chapter (Moore, 1929; Hamilton, 1948; Etsten, 1954, Eliasch, 1955; Cross, 1957; Doyle, 1953). These comparisons have been made both in man and in animals. Some of these different comparative studies have shown the indicator-dilution method to give a slightly higher measurement than the Fick method, and others have shown the opposite effect, but the average results show almost identical values for both methods. Furthermore, repetitive determinations of cardiac output in the same animal or human being under constant conditions gives almost exactly the same result (Wood, 1955; Selzer, 1958; Thomasson, 1957; Howell, 1959). Therefore, it is believed that the oxygen-Fick method for measuring cardiac output is accurate within a few per cent when appropriate precautions for establishment of steady state conditions are observed.

OTHER DIRECT FICK METHODS FOR MEASURING CARDIAC OUTPUT

The term "direct" Fick method for measuring cardiac output, as opposed to "indirect" Fick method, means that all factors necessary for calculating cardiac output are directly measured, whereas, in applying an indirect Fick method, some of the factors are inferred from other factors rather than being measured directly. For instance, in the oxygen-Fick method, oxygen consumption and A-V oxygen difference are directly measured, whereas in the indirect oxygen-Fick method, oxygen consumption is measured, but the A-V oxygen difference is inferred from measurements of the respiratory gases rather than from direct measurements of the A-V oxygen difference in the blood itself.

However, there are other types of direct Fick methods besides the oxygen-Fick method (Cournand, 1945; Grossman, 1953; Sapirstein, 1954a, 1954b; Love, 1958). Two of these deserve particular comment: (1) the use of carbon dioxide instead of oxygen as the indicator, and (2) the use of para-aminohippuric acid as an indicator. Each of these has some advantages and disadvantages in relation to the oxygen-Fick method.

The Carbon Dioxide Direct Fick Procedure

It is not necessary to explain the details of the carbon dioxide direct Fick procedure because they parallel almost exactly those of the oxygen-Fick procedure. Arteriovenous carbon dioxide difference and the amount of carbon dioxide exhaled during a given period of time are measured, either gasometrically or chemically, and, using the general Fick formula, the cardiac output can be calculated.

The advantages of the carbon dioxide method over the oxygen method are mainly the ease of measurement of carbon dioxide both in blood and in expired air. However, the carbon dioxide method has all of the same potential errors of the oxygen method plus another very serious error that is manifest only very slightly by the oxygen method. This is the following: a very slight change in alveolar P_{CO_2} will alter tremendously the rate of carbon dioxide transfer from the blood to the alveoli (Hamilton, 1953). For instance, if pulmonary ventilation is reduced by only 10 per cent, the amount of carbon dioxide released from the lungs during the next minute or so will be reduced by about 200 ml. because of storage of this amount of carbon dioxide in the body fluids resulting from the rise in alveolar Pco_2. When one considers that pulmonary ventilation can change as much as several fold under different conditions, one immediately realizes the capriciousness of the carbon dioxide method for measurement of cardiac output. This does not invalidate the basic principle of the carbon dioxide procedure, for if absolute steady state conditions are achieved, one would expect as accurate measurements of cardiac output by this procedure as by the oxygen-Fick procedure. The only problem is that the steady state conditions need to be far steadier for the carbon dioxide method than for the oxygen method (Cournand, 1945a).

The Para-aminohippuric Acid Fick Method

Several different investigators have used para-aminohippuric acid as an indicator substance for measuring the cardiac output. Grossman and coworkers (1953) used this in almost identically the same manner that oxygen is used, as follows: A catheter is inserted into the pulmonary artery, another into the right ventricle, and a needle into an artery. Para-aminohippuric acid is injected at a steady rate into the pulmonary artery until reasonably steady state conditions ensue. Arterial blood is removed from any systemic artery in the same manner as with the oxygen-Fick method, and mixed venous blood is removed from the right ventricle. Since almost one-fifth of the PAH is removed from the blood by the kidneys each time the blood goes around the circulatory circuit, it is very easy to maintain a large A-V oxygen difference. Therefore, knowing the rate of injection of PAH and measuring its A-V oxygen difference, one can calculate the cardiac output from the general Fick formula.

An even more interesting use of PAH for measuring cardiac output was developed by Sapirstein (1954a, 1954b), this method not requiring catheterization of the heart. Instead the PAH is injected continuously into a peripheral vein, and systemic arterial PAH measurements are made until the arterial PAH concentration becomes essentially constant. Then, suddenly, the infusion of PAH into the vein is stopped, while the arterial sampling is continued. Just as quickly as blood can pass from the veins to the arteries, the PAH concentration in the arterial blood falls suddenly to a much lower level. Sapirstein has produced evidence that this new level is equal to the mixed venous PAH concentration. Therefore, by using the arterial PAH measurements taken before and after stopping the infusion, the A-V oxygen difference can be calculated without the necessity for removing mixed venous blood from the heart. Comparative studies using this method and the indicator-dilution method showed very good agreement. Therefore, this method deserves serious consideration when it is not feasible or desirable to catheterize the subject.

Chapter 3

INDICATOR-DILUTION METHODS FOR DETERMINING CARDIAC OUTPUT

In the simplest of the indicator-dilution methods for determining cardiac output, an indicator substance is injected rapidly into the venous blood, and then its concentration in the blood is measured continuously as it passes into the arterial system. The greater the cardiac output, the more rapidly the "dilution" curve of the substance appears and disappears in the arterial blood. This is the origin of the term "indicator-dilution" method. Any type of substance that can be injected into the circulation without altering circulatory dynamics, that does not disappear from the blood as it passes to the point of sampling, and that can be analyzed in the blood can be used as the indicator.

Two different types of indicator-dilution methods have been used with success by many different investigators: (1) the *single injection method* in which the indicator substance is injected in a single rapid injection, and (2) the *continuous infusion method* in which a continuous infusion of an indicator substance is suddenly begun and continued for a third of a minute or more. Later in the chapter we shall see that by rather simple mathematical procedures one can use the same analytical procedures for both these methods, so that in reality they are merely variations of the same procedure.

Other names besides "indicator-dilution" have been used for these methods, including the "Stewart" method, the "Stewart-Hamilton" method, the "Hamilton" method, and the "dye-dilution" method. These names have originated principally from the names of persons most prominent in the development of the method or from the fact that the indicator substance most frequently used is a dye.

HISTORY OF THE INDICATOR-DILUTION METHOD

Stewart (1897) was the first to use an indicator-dilution method for measuring cardiac output; he used the continuous infusion procedure. In his early experiments, he used as indicators different dyes or glucose, but because of technical difficulties, he later chose hypertonic saline solution as his preferred indicator. He determined its concentration in the arterial blood by measuring the change in electrical conductivity of the blood. Basically Stewart's procedure was the following: He began a sudden infusion by hypertonic saline solution directly into the input side of the heart or directly into the left ventricle and recorded the time of appearance of the solution in a peripheral artery by use of electrodes on the artery that measured changes in electrical conductivity. Also, using this same device he was able to tell when the saline concentration in the peripheral artery reached a "plateau." During the interval of this plateau, he collected blood from the artery and later analyzed its concentration of hypertonic saline in a specially constructed conductivity cell. By applying the Fick principle he was then able to calculate the cardiac output as follows: The venous blood prior to injection of the saline had zero concentration of the injected indicator, whereas the arterial blood had a definite, measurable concentration, which remained constant during the "plateau." Knowing the rate of injection of the indicator, he used the Fick formula presented in the previous chapter to calculate the cardiac output; that is, rate of infusion divided by the A-V difference of the indicator equals cardiac output. The mathematics of this will become evident later in the chapter.

Though Stewart (1921a) stated in a second paper written in 1921 that he had used the single injection technique for measuring cardiac output in his studies during the 1890's, he did not describe this method in his publication of 1897. Instead, the first recorded use of the single injection method was by Henriques (1913). Henriques derived the formula that is used today in the single injection dilution method and also recognized and discussed the importance of recirculation of indicator as a possible error in the method.

After several forays by other investigators (Bock and Buchholtz, 1920; and Gross and Mittermaier, 1926) into the use of both the single injection and continuous infusion methods, Hamilton and his colleagues (1928a, 1928b, 1932, 1944, 1945a, 1947a, 1948, 1953; Kinsman, 1929; Moore, 1929; Howard, 1953; Dow, 1946, 1955, 1956) in 1928 began a long series of studies to prove the validity of the single injection indicator-dilution method for accurate measurement of cardiac output. In his many studies, Hamilton has investigated essentially all suggested possibilities of error in the method, and very early in his work he made a particularly important contribution to the procedure by devising a technique to correct for recirculation of the indicator (Kinsman, 1929), thereby greatly improving the accuracy of the method.

Though the single injection technique now is used almost universally in cardiovascular laboratories, Stewart's original continuous infusion technique has received little emphasis, having reappeared only a few times— for instance, Wiggers (1944a), Holt (1944a), Rashkind (1949), and Shepherd (1955)—over the period of the past 30 years. Yet, even so, the continuous infusion method can be employed as satisfactorily as the single injection method if adequate technical and analytical procedures are used. One of the problems has been to devise a simple method to correct for recirculation of indicator. Later in the chapter, such a method will be presented.

THE SINGLE INJECTION INDICATOR DILUTION METHOD

The Procedure

Perhaps a hundred different variations of the single injection indicator-dilution method have been employed for determining cardiac output, the variations including different choices of indicator substances, different injection sites, different sampling sites, and different procedures for measuring the indicator concentration in the arterial blood. Therefore, it will be impossible to give a single procedure for all of them, though they usually differ from each other only in minute details and not in principle. Two necessities must always be met if the measurement of cardiac output is to be successful: First, the indicator substance must go through a portion of the central circulation where all of the blood flow of the body becomes mixed. It was pointed out in the previous chapter in relation to the Fick procedure that all the blood flow becomes mixed only in the right heart or in the left heart. If the procedure is applied anywhere else in the circulation except across one or both of these mixing areas, the flow that is measured will be something else besides cardiac output. Second, most of the indicator substance must pass the site of sampling before recirculation of the indicator begins. Otherwise an accurate calculation of cardiac output cannot be made. This will be discussed in greater detail below.

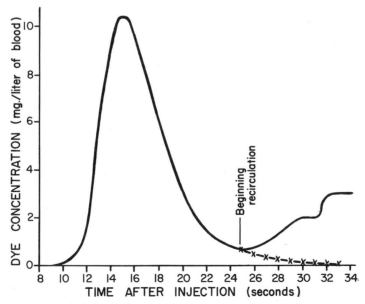

Figure 3–1. Typical single injection indicator-dilution curve, illustrating recirculation of indicator after the 25 second mark and correction of the curve by the semilog replot method.

The following is a typical procedure for measuring cardiac output by the single injection method (see also Warren, 1958): A small polyethylene tube is inserted through a needle into the subject's radial artery, and the other end of the tube is connected to a cuvette densitometer capable of measuring the concentration of dye in blood. Also, a catheter is inserted through an antecubital vein into the right atrium, right ventricle, or pulmonary artery. Then 6 mg. of tricarbocyanine green dye is injected through the cardiac catheter as rapidly as possible, and constant rate withdrawal of arterial blood through the cuvette densitometer is begun immediately. The solid curve of Figure 3–1 illustrates a typical time course of the concentration changes in the arterial blood as recorded by the densitometer, showing in this instance that the dye first made its appearance in the arterial blood approximately 9 seconds after injection, reached a maximum concentration at 15 seconds, and then fell almost back to the baseline at 25 seconds. However, at this point the dye concentration began to rise again, indicating that some of it was by then passing a second time through the circulation. From the curve recorded in Figure 3–1, the cardiac output can be calculated, but to be accurate in this calculation it is first necessary to correct the curve for the recirculated dye, as will be explained below.

Correction for Recirculation of Indicator by the Semilog Plot Method

One of the principal contributions of Kinsman, Hamilton, and their colleagues, made over 40 years ago, is a procedure to correct the recorded curve for recirculation of the indicator (Kinsman, 1929). In Figure 3–1, the dye concentration returns near enough to the baseline so that one could reasonably extend the downslope of the curve by sight and come out with a reasonably accurate total curve. Very often, however, recirculation of the indicator begins before the arterial concentration of the indicator has fallen back to anywhere near the baseline. Under these conditions, it is extremely difficult to extend the curve in an appropriate manner simply by sight.

The method proposed by Kinsman, Hamilton, and their coworkers for correcting the curve depends upon plotting the curve on semilog graph paper, as shown in Figure 3–2. Note that the downslope of this curve to the point of beginning recirculation is essentially a straight line. To correct for recirculation, it can be assumed that the true curve will continue along a linear downslope on the semilog coordinates. Therefore, the dashed line of the figure is extrapolated linearly to the base of the graph, and then, using the extrapolated line, one can replot on Figure 3–1, as indicated by the x's, what would have happened to the remainder of the concentration curve had recirculation not occurred.

To validate this method of correcting for the recirculated indicator, Hamilton and his coworkers (1932; Kinsman, 1929) constructed several different types of models that simulated the various anatomical units of the central circulation, namely, the cardiac chambers and the vascular beds of the lungs. Then flow measurements were made through the models by the

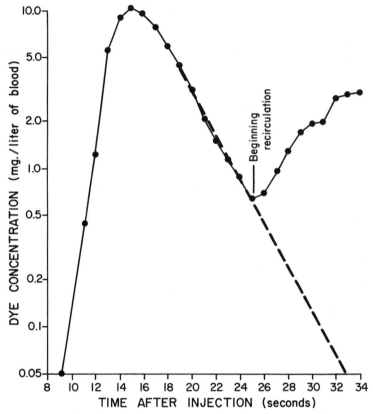

Figure 3–2. Semilog plot of the same curve shown in Figure 3–1, illustrating that recirculation begins at 25 seconds and showing by the dashed curve an extrapolation of the downslope almost to the zero (0.05) indicator concentration level.

indicator-dilution method. When recirculation was prevented and the flow kept constant, the downslopes of the curves invariably followed a semilog pattern. Later these same procedures were applied in heart-lung preparations in which recirculation of blood was prevented, and here again the downslopes were of the semilog nature. Thus, both in models and in the central circulation of animals in which recirculation was prevented, the semilog nature of the downslope of the curve was proved. Therefore, since that time, the semilog method for correcting the curve has been considered to be almost completely accurate.

Alternate Semilog Method to Correct for Recirculation of Indicator

In modern use of the single injection technique for determining cardiac output, the arterial concentration of indicator is often, if not usually, recorded by a continuous recording apparatus, which will be discussed in more detail later in the chapter. The resulting curve is a smooth, continuous curve instead of a plot of individual points. To correct for recirculation of indicator by the semilog replot method, appropriate measurements

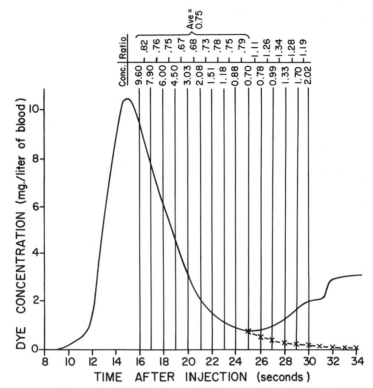

Figure 3–3. Alternate method for correcting the curve shown in Figure 3–1 for recirculation of indicator.

must be made on the original recording and the curve replotted on semilog graph paper. However, one can bypass this extra step in the procedure in the following way:

Figure 3–3 illustrates the same curve as that recorded in Figure 3–1 but shows time lines drawn at each second from 16 through 30 seconds. Immediately above each time line is written the *concentration* of the dye at that particular instant, and immediately above these concentrations are written the *ratios* of each two successive concentrations. If the downslope of the curve is describing a semilog plot, the ratios will remain constant, but if the downslope is not describing a semilog function, the ratios will be changing. We note that from the 16 second mark to the 25 second mark the ratios were reasonably constant and average 0.75. However, beyond the 25 second mark these ratios suddenly become erratic. Therefore, even without plotting this curve on semilog graph paper one can readily see that recirculation begins at the 25 second mark. Now, to correct the curve beyond the 25 second mark, we simply take the last value of the correct curve which occurred at 25 seconds, 0.7 mg./l. in this instance, and continue the same ratio of decrease in concentration during the succeeding seconds. Thus, at 26 seconds, the value would be 0.75 times 0.7, or 0.52 mg./l.; at 27 seconds the value would be 0.75 times 0.52, or 0.39; and so forth. The corrected curve is shown by the x's and the dashed line in

Figure 3–3. Note that the correction in this case is so nearly identical to that in Figure 3–1 that one would not be able to distinguish between the two.

This alternate method for correcting the curve is particularly advantageous when one is reasonably sure that recirculation occurs only at the tail end of the curve, for under these conditions one need mark off only two or three intervals along the downslope in order to obtain the extrapolated curve. For instance, instead of using once every second, one could have done a completely adequate job in the example of Figure 3–3 by using intervals of once every three seconds. After a little practice, only a few minutes' manipulation of the slide rule are needed to correct a curve.

Calculation of the Cardiac Output

Once the corrected indicator-dilution curve is available, one can calculate the cardiac output from the following formula:

$$\text{Cardiac output} = \frac{I}{\int_0^\infty C\ dt} \tag{3-1}$$

where I is the quantity of indicator injected, C is the concentration of indicator in the arterial blood, and t is time. This formula can be rewritten:

$$\text{Cardiac output (in liters per minute)} = \frac{60I}{\overline{C}T} \tag{3-2}$$

where T is the total duration of the curve in seconds, $\overline{C}$ is the average concentration of the indicator in mg./liter during time T, and I is the injected quantity of indicator in milligrams. This formula is based on the following two basic considerations: (1) By dividing the average concentration of the indicator into the total amount of indicator injected, one obtains the total volume of blood passing into the arterial tree during the duration of the curve. (2) Then, to determine the cardiac output per minute, this volume is multiplied by 60 and divided by the number of seconds' duration of the curve.

Formulas 3–1 and 3–2 are essentially the same as the basic formula originally used by Henriques (1913) and subsequently by Stewart (1921a), Hamilton (1928a), and many others in the calculation of cardiac output by the single injection indicator-dilution method.

Now, let us use Formula 3–1 to calculate the cardiac output from the curve depicted in Figure 3–1. First, we can obtain the total area beneath the corrected curve by planimetry, this giving a value of 65.8 mg. seconds/liter. Second, the total amount of dye injected was 6 mg. Putting these values into the formula we obtain the following calculation of cardiac output:

$$\text{Cardiac output} = \frac{6\ \text{mg.}}{65.8\ \text{mg. sec./liter}} = 0.09\ \text{liter/sec.} = 5.47\ \text{liters/min.} \tag{3-3}$$

(The reason for expressing the integrated area beneath the curve in mg. seconds/liter is that the abscissa units are seconds and the ordinate units are mg./liter; seconds times mg./liter gives mg. seconds/liter.)

THE TRIANGLE METHOD FOR CALCULATION OF THE CARDIAC OUTPUT. In a series of studies, Nicholson and Wood (1951) and Warner and Wood (1952b) developed an empirical method by which the cardiac output can be calculated far more rapidly than by using the semilog plot method. This simplified procedure is based on reducing the uncorrected dye-dilution curve to one large triangle, as shown in Figure 3–4, then calculating the area of this, and finally using an empirical correction factor to determine the total area. One of the apices of the triangle is drawn to lie at the origin of the curve at point x. A second apex is drawn at the peak of the curve at point y, and the third apex is z, which is determined by extending a line from point y down the "best line of sight" along the downslope and extrapolating to the zero level. One can calculate the area of the triangle by the formula: area equals one-half the height of the triangle times the length of its base. In a large series of measurements made by both the usual semilog plot and this triangular method, Warner and Wood found the true area to average 24.4 per cent greater than the area of the triangle. Therefore, the following empirical formula has been developed for determining the total area under the curve by this method:

$$\int_0^\infty C\ dt = 0.622\ C_p T_b \qquad (3\text{–}4)$$

where C_p is the concentration at the peak of the curve and T_b is the time

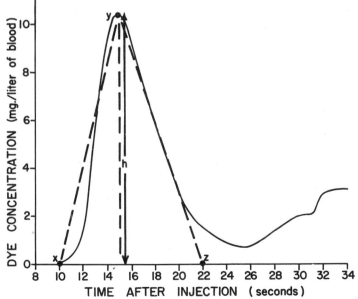

Figure 3–4. The triangle method for computing cardiac output from the indicator-dilution curve.

represented by the $\overline{xz}$ of the triangle. Formula 3–4 and Formula 3–1 can then be combined as follows for calculation of cardiac output:

$$\text{Cardiac output} = \frac{60I}{0.622 \ C_p T_b} \qquad (3\text{–}5)$$

where cardiac output is in liters per minute, I is in mg. of dye injected, C_p is in mg./liter, and T_b is in seconds.

If Formula 3–5 is used to calculate cardiac output from the curve represented in Figure 3–1 and Figure 3–3, the calculated value is 4.8 liters per minute, a value 13 per cent below that calculated by the semilog method. This moderate discrepancy between the results of the two methods of calculation illustrates the difficulty in applying empirical methods for analyzing these curves even though the empirical methods do save a great amount of time. In a large series of studies, Warner and Wood (1952b) calculated that the variance of the results will on the average be increased approximately 3 per cent when the triangular method of analysis is used in place of the semilog plot method, and because the normal variance when using the semilog method is about 11 per cent, the additional 3 per cent is not truly significant.

CALCULATION OF CARDIAC OUTPUT FROM ATYPICAL CURVES. Atypical curves that have no well defined semilogarithmic downslope frequently occur in subjects having cardiac disease or anomalies of the central circulation. In these cases, the curves are often prolonged so greatly that recirculation of the indicator causes too much distortion of the downslope for one to extrapolate the curve to the zero baseline. For this reason, several different statistical efforts have been made to develop empirical formulae for calculating the cardiac output entirely from the upslope portion of the dilution curve. One of these methods is another triangle method devised by Wood and his colleagues (Ramirez, 1956; Hetzel, 1958), which may be explained as follows (refer once again to Figure 3–4): A perpendicular is dropped from point y to the baseline, and the area of the left-hand triangle is determined. In many different records which could be analyzed by usual methods. Ramirez found the area of this "forward" triangle to be 0.37 times the area inscribed by the complete curve when the indicator is injected into the heart. Therefore, the following formula was developed for cardiac output:

$$\text{Cardiac output} = \frac{60I}{\dfrac{C_p}{2} \cdot T_f} \cdot 0.37 \qquad (3\text{–}6)$$

where T_f is the time represented by the base of the forward triangle.

Benchimol (1963) evaluated the use of formula 3–6 for calculation of cardiac output in 152 indicator-dilution curves from 48 patients. He found that the average difference between cardiac outputs estimated by Formula 3–6 and by the conventional technique (Formulas 3–1 and 3–2) was 14 per cent. He also found that if a proportionality constant of 0.34 instead of 0.37 was used, the average difference between cardiac outputs calculated by the "forward triangle" method and the conventional method was reduced to 10 per cent.

Dow (1955), also by analyzing a large series of curves, derived another empirical formula for calculating the area of an atypical curve:

$$\text{Cardiac output} = \frac{601}{C_p \times T_{pc}/(3.0 - 0.9\ T_{pc}/T_a)} \qquad (3\text{--}7)$$

where cardiac output is in liters per minute, I is mg. of indicator injected, C_p is the peak concentration of indicator in mg./liter, T_{pc} is the time in seconds from injection to peak concentration, and T_a is the time in seconds from injection to appearance of indicator at the sampling site.

Oriol (1967) compared cardiac output values obtained by the conventional technique with those obtained by use of Dow's formula for area calculation in 130 "normal" dye-dilution curves. He found that cardiac output estimated by Dow's formula was within 10 per cent of the value obtained by the conventional technique in 90 per cent of the curves and was within 15 per cent in all curves.

Both of these formulas have proved to be adequate when tested against other methods for calculating or measuring cardiac output, and Thorburn (1961) and Williams (1966) have proposed new formulas that may prove to be even better. The absolute errors of these formulas will probably never be known, because many multitudes of curve shapes can and do occur, thus seriously altering the empirical relationships with each type of curve. Dow undoubtedly correctly points out that empirical formulas such as these will probably be more accurate in determining cardiac output than the usual semilog plot method when recirculation of indicator occurs before the indicator concentration falls below 50 per cent of its peak concentration. Even theoretically, the upper portion of the curve's downslope is not semilogarithmic in character; therefore, any attempt to use this portion of the curve for extrapolation to the baseline can cause very serious error.

USE OF COMPUTERS FOR CALCULATION OF CARDIAC OUTPUT. It should be obvious that the calculation of cardiac output from indicator-dilution curves by any of the methods described above is tedious and time consuming, especially when a large number of curves is to be analyzed. For this reason, and because of the increasing availability of electronic computers, many researchers and clinicians have resorted to the use of computers for these calculations (Skinner and Gehmlich, 1959; Moody, 1961; Hara and Bellville, 1963; Wessel, 1964; Benchimol, 1965a; Sinclair, 1965; Hamer, 1966; Kunz and Smith, 1967; Starmer and Clark, 1970; Coleman and Criddle, 1970a). The primary difficulty in automating the calculation of cardiac output has been the necessity of correcting for indicator recirculation, and the computer techniques employed to date have utilized various means for rapidly removing the distortion due to recirculation and for integrating the corrected curve. Essentially four types of computer systems have been used for this purpose. The first three to be described employ electronic analog circuitry, and the last makes use of the digital computer.

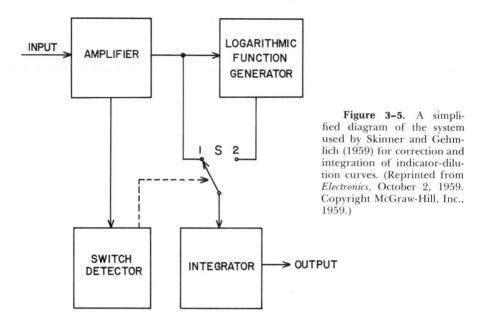

Figure 3–5. A simplified diagram of the system used by Skinner and Gehmlich (1959) for correction and integration of indicator-dilution curves. (Reprinted from *Electronics*, October 2, 1959. Copyright McGraw-Hill, Inc., 1959.)

System 1. This type of system is exemplified by that of Skinner and Gehmlich (1959), who were the first to demonstrate the feasibility of using the analog computer for the calculation of cardiac output from dilution curves. A simplified diagram of the system used by Skinner and Gehmlich for correction and integration of dilution curves is illustrated in Figure 3–5 and is essentially described as follows: The output voltage of the detector used to measure the arterial concentration of indicator serves as the input to the computer. A typical input signal is illustrated by the solid line in Figure 3–6. This signal is fed into an amplifier and to an integrator through switch S which is normally in position 1. At some time after the curve peaks, it begins to decay exponentially. The beginning of exponential decay is shown at t_0 in Figure 3–6. This point is detected by the switch detector circuit, which, after a preset delay, causes the switch to move to position 2. This occurs at time t_1 in Figure 3–6. Between times t_0 and t_1 a logarithmic function generator senses the waveform of the

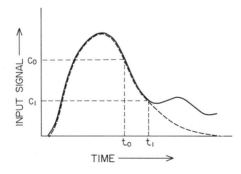

Figure 3–6. A typical input signal (solid curve) to computer systems used for analysis of indicator-dilution curves, and the same signal (dashed curve) as it appears after correction by the computer system.

actual input signal, and when the switch moves to position 2, the function generator generates an exponentially decaying curve having the same exponent as the actual signal during the time interval t_0 to t_1 and with an initial value of C_1. Thus, the signal fed into the integrator is the corrected dilution curve, indicated by the dashed line in Figure 3–6, and the output of the integrator is the area under this curve. This area is used for the calculation of cardiac output by the formula:

$$\text{Cardiac output} = 60I\ \alpha/A \qquad (3-8)$$

where I is the quantity of the indicator injected, α is the calibration factor (volts/unit quantity of indicator/liter), and A is the integrator output (volts $\times$ seconds).

An essential part of the analog system of Skinner and Gehmlich is the function generator circuit, which obtains the exponent of the actual indicator curve and generates an ideal curve having this same exponent. In order to obtain this exponent, the circuit performs a basic mathematical procedure which is described as follows: Between times t_0 and t_1 (refer to Figure 3–6), the actual curve is described by the equation:

$$C = C_0 e^{-kt} \qquad (3-9)$$

where C is the value of the signal at any time t between t_0 and t_1, C_0 is the value of the signal at time t_0, e is the base of natural logarithms, and k is the decay constant or exponent. Taking the natural logarithm of both sides of this equation, we find:

$$/nC = /nC_0 - kt \qquad (3-10)$$

Now by taking the derivative of both sides of Equation 3–10, we see that

$$\frac{d/nC}{dt} = -k \qquad (3-11)$$

These equations illustrate that the necessary exponent k can be obtained by first taking the logarithm of the exponential curve and then differentiating the result. This operation is performed by a logarithmic function generator and an associated differentiator circuit.

Analog systems very similar to the one described above have been used by Hara and Bellville (1963) and Benchimol (1965a). The major difference between the system used by Skinner and Gehmlich and those used in these more recent studies is that in the first system the point at which the generation of the ideal curve begins is selected as a function of time after the actual curve starts to decay exponentially; in the latter systems this point is selected as a function of the peak value of the actual curve. In the computer circuit of Hara and Bellville, generation of the ideal curve begins when the actual curve has decayed to 40 per cent of its peak value, and in the analog circuit used by Benchimol, generation begins when the actual curve has fallen to 60 per cent of its peak value.

Hara and Bellville (1963) compared cardiac output values calculated by the computer with cardiac output values obtained by the conventional hand method. In over 20 comparisons, the results of computer calculations did not vary from the results of conventional calculations by more than 4 per cent. In most cases the difference between the results of the two methods was much less than this. Since Hara and Bellville recorded the output of the densitometer on magnetic tape before feeding it into the computer, they were able to obtain repeated calculations of cardiac output from the same dye-dilution curve. Repeated calculations of cardiac output from any one recorded dye-dilution curve usually did not vary by more than 1 per cent, which indicates the precision of this computer system.

System 2. A somewhat different analog system for automatic computation of the area under indicator-dilution curves is that devised by Wessel (1964). This system also assumes an exponential downslope of the curve but allows the total area to be computed as the sum of the two areas A_1 and A_2. A_1 is the area under the actual curve from the time of its appearance to the time t_0 (refer again to Figure 3–6). A_2 is the area under the ideal, nondistorted dilution curve from time t_0 until the curve decays to zero, and is computed by the formula:

$$A_2 = \frac{C_0}{(C_0 - C_1)} \int_{t_0}^{t_1} Cdt \tag{3-12}$$

where C_0 and C_1 are values on the exponential downslope of the dilution curve.

Formula 3–12 for the computation of area A_2 can be derived as follows: Since the exponential downslope of the curve is described by Equation 3–9, it is obvious that area A_2 from time t_0 to infinity is given by the equation:

$$A_2 = \int_{t_0}^{\infty} Cdt = \frac{C_0}{k} \tag{3-13}$$

and the area under the curve between the times t_0 and t_1 is given by the equation:

$$\int_{t_0}^{t_1} Cdt = \frac{(C_0 - C_1)}{k} \tag{3-14}$$

Therefore, multiplying equation (3–14) by the quantity $(C_0/C_0 - C_1)$ yields equation 3–12.

The analog system used by Wessel obtains A_1 by integrating the actual signal from the time of its appearance until time t_0. To obtain A_2, the peak value of the actual curve is detected and held for comparison with the downslope. C_0 and C_1 are selected as fixed percentages of the peak value; C_0 is selected as 60 per cent of the peak value and C_1 as 30 per cent of the peak value. With these values for C_0 and C_1, the ratio $C_0/(C_0 - C_1)$ becomes simply 2. Thus, when the actual signal decays to value C_0 the integrator gain is doubled. Integration continues until the actual signal is reduced to value C_1, at which time the integration is stopped.

The output of the integrator then represents the area under the ideal curve and can be used for calculation of cardiac output. Wessel compared cardiac outputs obtained from this system with cardiac outputs calculated by the conventional hand method, and a mean difference between the results of the two methods of only 1.9 ± 2.5 per cent indicates its reliability.

System 3. Another analog system which has been used on at least three occasions (Sinclair, 1965; Hamer, 1966, Kunz and Smith, 1967) consists basically of an integrator and a continuous predictor in parallel. The input to these circuits is the output of the detector monitoring the arterial concentration of indicator, and their outputs are fed into a summing amplifier which provides the computer's output.

The manner in which this system operates is as follows: It can be shown by mathematical procedures that the area under an exponentially decaying curve from any time t to infinity may be "predicted" by the equation;

$$\text{Predicted area} = \frac{C^2}{-dC/dt} \qquad (3-15)$$

where C is the value of the signal at the time t. The predictor circuit continuously differentiates the input signal and solves Equation 3-15. The output of the predictor is essentially, therefore, the predicted area under the exponential downslope from the time t to infinity. This signal is then summed with the output of the integrator. The output of the summing amplifier is, therefore:

$$\text{Total area} = I + \frac{C^2}{-dC/dt} \qquad (3-16)$$

where I is the integrator output up to the time t. Equation 3-16 is solved continuously during the entire dilution curve. However, the output of the predictor is functionally useful only during the exponentially decaying part of the curve, since only during this time is equation 3-15 true. It follows that the output of the summer is meaningful only during the exponential portion of the curve.

A typical input and output signal from this type of system is illustrated in Figure 3-7. Curve C in this figure represents a typical indicator-dilution

Figure 3-7. Typical input and output signals of the computer system used by Sinclair (1965), Hammer (1966), and Kunz (1967) for analysis of indicator-dilution curves. Curve C is the input signal, and curve I is the output of the integrating circuit. Curve P represents the computer output and is the sum of the outputs of an integrator circuit and a predictor circuit. [Modified from Kunz (1967).]

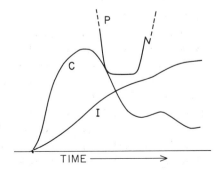

curve. Curve I represents the output of the integrator, and curve P represents the output of the integrator summed with the output of the predictor circuit. Curve P is, therefore, the continuous solution of Equation 3–16. Note that during the initial rise in the dilution curve, curve P is off scale. However, during the exponential decay of the dilution curve, curve P reaches a constant value. This constant value obtained by curve P represents the asymptote approached by curve I and is a measure of the area under curve C extrapolated to zero concentration if no recirculation occurs. Note also in Figure 3–7 that when recirculation occurs, curve P once again reads off scale. Thus, it is evident that this analog system not only provides an immediate value for the area under the indicator-dilution curve, but it also evaluates the validity of the exponential downslope, since only during this time will its output reach a plateau, and signals the onset of recirculation. Results using this system have compared excellently with the results obtained by the conventional hand method in dogs (Sinclair, 1965; Hamer, 1966; Kunz and Smith, 1967) and in humans (Sinclair, 1965).

System 4. Digital computers have only recently been used for the analysis of indictor-dilution curves (Coleman and Criddle, 1970a; Starmer and Clark, 1970). In order to use the digital computer for this purpose, the graphical records of indicator concentration must first be converted to digital data by use of an analog-to-digital converter. A general purpose digital computer then performs the necessary computations. In order to convert the graphical information to digital numbers, Coleman and Criddle (1970a) constructed an inexpensive curve tracer which is connected to the analog-to-digital conversion channels of a digital computer. As the recorded dilution curve is traced with this device, it provides an output which consists of voltages proportional to the vertical and horizontal displacement of the actual dilution curve. These voltages are then converted to digital numbers by the analog-to-digital converter. The area under the indicator-dilution curve and the cardiac output are then calculated by essentially a computerized version of the conventional hand method described earlier in this chapter. The slope of the curve during its exponential decay is obtained, and the curve is extrapolated to zero and integrated. Cardiac output is then calculated using this extrapolated area.

It is evident from the above discussion that computers may be employed to circumvent what has been one of the primary deterrents to the use of indicator-dilution techniques for the estimation of cardiac output; i.e., the necessary long delay between injection of the indicator and the availability of the result. However, it should be pointed out that the use of computers does not eliminate the primary sources of error inherent in the indicator-dilution technique. These will be discussed fully later in this chapter.

Effect of Injection Site and Sampling Site on the Indicator-Dilution Curve

Ordinarily any site in the arterial system is satisfactory for sampling blood when recording the indicator-dilution curve (Hertzel, 1954). Usually blood for this purpose is removed either from the radial or femoral artery or, in experimental animals, often from the carotid artery. Occasionally blood is even sampled from the pulmonary artery when the indicator is injected into a peripheral vein (Fritts, 1957; Carnell, 1961).

The injection site, on the other hand, plays a much more important role than the sampling site in determining the shape of the curve, principally because blood flow on the venous side of the heart is slower and more variable than on the arterial side. The usual sites of injection are a peripheral vein, the right atrium, the right ventricle, the pulmonary artery, or the left ventricle. Obviously injection into the right heart or pulmonary artery requires venous catheterization of the heart, and injection into the left ventricle requires retrograde catheterization of the left ventricle through an artery.

To give an idea of the shapes of the indicator-dilution curves when different injection sites are used, Figure 3–8 shows four curves recorded after dye injection into respectively (a) the root of the aorta, (b) a pulmonary vein, (c) the pulmonary artery, and (d) the right atrium (from Pearce, 1953). Note that each added segment of the central circulation through which the dye had to pass increased the duration of the curve proportionately. In general, passage of the indicator through the arteries does not disperse the curve greatly (Peterson, 1954), whereas passage through each side of the heart and through the lungs causes fairly great dispersion. Passage through the peripheral veins is also likely to cause considerable dispersion of the curve, partly because of the slow velocities of blood flow in peripheral veins and partly because of variable flow in some veins.

There is only one significant consideration that must be kept in mind

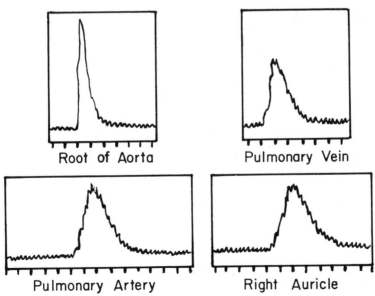

Figure 3–8. Four separate indicator-dilution curves, illustrating effect of the injection site on the form of the curve.

in choice of sampling and injection sites: the greater the distance between these sites, the longer will be the duration of the indicator-dilution curve, and, therefore, the greater will be the likelihood of difficulty with indicator recirculation. Other than for this consideration, the injection and sampling sites seem to make little difference in the final calculation of cardiac output. This was shown particularly in a series of studies by Hetzel and Wood (1954) comparing cardiac outputs measured by right heart injection versus peripheral vein injection and was confirmed by Gunnells and Gorten (1961), Bousvaros (1962), and Samet (1965). On the other hand, Lawson (1954b) found in a series of five dogs a slightly lower cardiac output when the injection site was peripheral than when it was intracardiac. However, the differences were so slight that one questions their significance.

Different Indicator Substances Employed

From the time of Stewart's earliest studies (1897), it has been realized that the nature of the indicator makes very little difference in the results obtained from indicator-dilution measurements of cardiac output. The only two criteria which must be applied are that the indicator remain in the blood between the points of injection and sampling and that it be capable of dispersing uniformly in the blood. Different indicators that have been employed include a long list of dyes [vital red (Stewart, 1921a); brilliant blue (Davis, 1958): Evans blue (Hamilton, 1948); Fox green (Fox, 1957; Merriman, 1958); indigo carmine (Lacy, 1955); bromsulfalein (Wassen, 1956; Mellette, 1958); rose bengal (Vidt, 1955); and Coomassie blue (Phinney, 1963; Zitnik, 1965)], hypertonic saline (Stewart, 1897), decholin (Conn, 1957), radioactively tagged plasma albumin, radioactively tagged red cells (Dow, 1946; Lawson, 1952), radioactive krypton gas in solution, dissolved hydrogen (Klocke, 1968), ethyl ether (Bachofen, 1971a), glucose solution, heat or cold (measured in terms of thermal dilution—Fegler, 1954; Evonuk, 1961; Hosie, 1962; Khalil, 1966; Branthwaite and Bradley, 1968), and normal plasma (measured in terms of hematocrit dilution).

A substance employed frequently in the past has been the dye T-1824, also called Evans blue, which is the dye that has been employed most extensively for the measurement of blood volume. The principal characteristics which make it very satisfactory for this purpose are: (a) it is nontoxic, (b) it combines readily with the plasma proteins and, therefore, leaks out of the circulation only very slowly (Baker, 1961), and (c) it can be analyzed readily in the plasma and with care even in whole blood. However, there are two unfortunate problems with Evans blue. First, use of more than 50 mg. of the dye in a single person will cause bluish discoloration of his skin, which will last for many weeks. This limits the total number of cardiac output determinations using this indicator usually to eight or less, the exact number depending on methods of sampling and analysis. Second, the wave length of maximum light absorption by Evans blue is 620 millimicrons, a wave length at which hemoglobin also absorbs a large amount of light. Therefore, hemoglobin often interferes with or even causes serious error in the determination of the dye in the blood.

Another dye, tricarbocyanine green, also known as "cardiogreen" or as "Fox green" (Fox, 1957), has been introduced to obviate some of the difficulties inherent with Evans blue and at present is probably the most frequently used dye for indicator-dilution. This dye, like Evans blue, is nontoxic and combines with the proteins. However, its point of maximum light absorption is approximately 800 millimicrons in comparison with 620 millimicrons for Evans blue. At 800 millimicrons the light absorption by oxyhemoglobin and reduced hemoglobin is the same, and, furthermore, the light absorption of both types of hemoglobin is far less at 800 millimicrons than at 620 millimicrons. For these reasons Fox green can (a) be analyzed in whole blood at far smaller concentrations than can Evans blue and (b) can be analyzed without significant error even when hemolysis has occurred or when the ratio of oxy- to reduced hemoglobin is altered in the blood. Therefore, much more accurate and greater numbers of cardiac output determinations can be made with this dye than with Evans blue.

Some indicator substances, such as hypertonic saline, glucose, thiocyanate ion, and other small molecular weight substances, leak partially out of the circulation as they pass through capillary beds. Measurements both by White (1947) and by Hamilton and Remington (1947a) have demonstrated that approximately 10 per cent of such indicators is lost from the circulation during their first passage through the lungs, thereby giving a cardiac output estimate 11 per cent too high. Lawson (1954a), on the other hand, did not find measurable loss of diffusible substances during first passage through the lungs. Nevertheless, the error from this cause is undoubtedly variable and unknown, which makes it desirable not to use diffusible indicator substances for indicator-dilution methods of cardiac output determination except when the points of injection and sampling are such that the indicator does not pass through either the pulmonary or systemic capillary beds.

Use of radioactive krypton gas as an indicator (Cornell, 1961; Rochester, 1961) deserves special comment because of its particular properties. This gas passes so rapidly through the respiratory membrane that about 95 per cent of it is lost from the blood in one passage through the pulmonary circulation. Therefore, it cannot be used in measuring cardiac output when the injection site is before the pulmonary circulation and the sampling site is after the pulmonary circulation. However, it can be used for measuring cardiac output when the point of injection is a peripheral vein and the point of sampling is the pulmonary artery, or it can be used when the point of injection is the left heart and the point of sampling is a peripheral artery. In using this indicator, the radioactive krypton gas is first dissolved in a solution, which is then injected into the blood. After sampling, the concentration is measured by usual radioactive techniques. Advantages of the krypton gas method are two fold. First, there is essentially no problem with recirculation of the indicator because almost all the indicator is lost on the first passage through the lungs. Second, determination of cardiac output can be repeated as many times as desired, because the indicator substance is rapidly removed from the circulation.

Although radioactive krypton has been the most frequently used inert gas for the estimation of cardiac output by indicator dilution, Chidsey (1958) suggested that recirculation could be avoided by using any dissolved inert gas with a low solubility in blood, since it would be quantitatively excreted by the lungs. In this respect, Klocke (1968) has recently demonstrated the feasibility of using dissolved hydrogen as an indicator. Hydrogen dissolved in saline is either injected into the inferior or superior vena cava and its concentration measured in the pulmonary artery, or it is injected into the left atrium and its concentration measured in a systemic artery. The concentration of hydrogen in arterial blood is determined with a platinum electrode catheter inserted into the artery. Since hydrogen is only 25 per cent as soluble in blood as is krypton gas, it is excreted by the lungs more rapidly than krypton. Indeed, the work of Klocke demonstrates that 97 per cent of the hydrogen injected is removed from the blood in one passage through the pulmonary circulation.

A particularly interesting indicator substance that has been employed on at least four occasions for measurement of cardiac output is whole plasma or dextran solution (Guyton, 1951; Heller, 1951; Lochner, 1957; Goodwin, 1957). This dilutes the red blood cells and is responsible for a dilution curve, in reverse, as the diluted red blood cells pass into the arterial tree. The curve can be recorded either by the increase in conductivity of the blood as measured by a conductivity cell or by the increase in light transmission as measured by an optical densitometer. Ten to 15 ml. of plasma thus injected is usually sufficient to give an adequate measurement of cardiac output.

In the past twenty years a great variety of thermodilution methods have also been used for measuring cardiac output (Fegler, 1954, 1957; Klussman, 1959; Evonuk, 1961; Hosie, 1962; Mohammed, 1963; Wessel, 1971; Branthwaite and Bradley, 1968). For instance, a few milliliters of either warm or cold solution can be injected into a vein and the change in blood temperature at the sampling site can be measured by use of a thermal registering device such as a thermistor, a thermocouple, or a platinum wire resistance. The sampling site can be in the pulmonary artery or in a systemic artery. Obviously, a large amount of heat will be transferred between the blood and the surrounding tissues; this is particularly true when the blood passes through the lungs before it reaches a systemic arterial sampling site. However, heat that is exchanged with the surrounding tissues is re-exchanged during the downslope portion of the dilution curve, and the total amount of heat transferred from injection site to sampling site is approximately equal to the amount of heat originally injected. Therefore, experience has shown that the thermodilution method is a reasonably accurate method for measuring cardiac output (probably within ± 15 per cent), but a few investigators feel that a small amount of heat is unrecoverable, which would give slightly elevated cardiac output measurements.

Types of Sampling Devices

Obviously, to record the indicator-dilution curve, only rapid sampling devices can be employed. If one is certain that recirculation will not occur, he can simply withdraw a sample of blood at a steady rate throughout the period of passage of the indicator. In this way, he obtains a single sample of blood which already has an average concentration of indicator in it. This is the procedure originally used by Henriques (1913) in his first measurement of cardiac output by this method.

When it was realized that recirculation of the indicator is a serious problem, it then became important to record the entire indicator-dilution curve second by second so that correction for the recirculation could be made. With this purpose in mind, Hamilton and his colleagues (1928b; see also Rothe, 1954) devised a rapid sampling device which functioned as follows: A series of small test tubes were strapped to the side of a kymograph drum. During the measurement of the indicator-dilution curve, this drum was set to run at a speed such that a new sampling tube would automatically pass approximately once every one to two seconds under a stream of blood flowing from the sampling artery. Then, after analysis of the dye in each of the tubes, the concentrations were plotted on graph paper.

More recently, the tendency has been to use continuous recording methods with the blood from the artery flowing continuously through a sampling device that automatically records the indicator concentration (for a comparison of several systems, see Marshall, 1961). When dyes are used as the indicator, this automatic recording device is an optical densitometer utilizing light passing through a blood cuvette and impinging on a photo cell (Nicholson, 1951; Guyton, 1951b; Friedlich, 1950; Shadle, 1953; Greisheimer, 1954a, 1954b, 1955a, 1955b; Falholt, 1956, 1958; Theilen, 1955a; Wiederhielm, 1956; Van Thiel, 1958; Richardson, 1959; Hansen, 1962; Scheel, 1969; Cohn, 1969). When hypertonic saline or whole plasma is used, the sampling device is then a conductivity cell (Goodwin, 1957). When a radioactive substance is used (MacIntyre, 1952; Pritchard, 1952; Conn, 1955; Cross, 1957), the sampling device is usually a well-scintillation counter.

Some of the continuous sampling devices allow the blood to return to the subject, while others simply utilize a constant rate withdrawal syringe. It is especially important in using continuous sampling devices that the rate of blood flow through the sampling device remain constant. Otherwise, a distortion in the time scale of the curve will occur, which will grossly affect the calculated cardiac output; this will be discussed in more detail later in the chapter.

A method which has recently been refined for the assessment of dye-dilution curves employs the relatively new concept of fiberoptics (Hugenholtz, 1965, 1969; Wagner, 1968; Singh, 1970). This concept is based on the principle that light entering optically clad glass fibers will be transmitted along their length with only a small loss of energy. In using this technique, a catheter containing two fiberoptic bundles is inserted into an artery. Following the injection of dye into the right side of the heart, light of appropriate wave length is directed through one of these bundles. It has been shown that the intensity of the light reflected by the arterial blood is proportional to the concentration of the dye within the blood. This reflected light is picked up by the second fiberoptic bundle and transmitted to the external end of the catheter, where its intensity is determined with a photomultiplier. Although the use of the fiberoptic method has not been widespread, it does offer a means for direct measurement of blood dye concentration without the necessity of blood withdrawal.

Several other types of intravascular types of sampling devices have also been used. For dilution with electrolytes, such as saline, electrical conduction between two electrodes placed in the blood can be used as a sampling technique (Stewart, 1897; White, 1947). In the thermodilution method, a very minute resistance thermometer wound around a catheter tip has been used by Khalil (1963a, 1963b; 1966), as will be described in more detail later in the chapter. Also, a very useful system has been devised by Korner (1965), in which minute thermistors are placed on the very tips of catheters with diameters less than 1 mm. These thermistors can be calibrated before being placed in an artery, but they can be left in the artery for at least several weeks without significant change in calibration, thus allowing chronic measurements of cardiac output by the thermodilution method. Furthermore, the Korner catheter-tip sensor is so small that the method is readily applicable to animals as small as the rabbit.

INDIRECT METHODS OF SAMPLING. Two indirect methods of sampling have been widely tested in the last few years. One of these is optical recording of dye-dilution curves by light transmission through the ear lobe (Beard, 1950, 1951; Milnor, 1953; Gilmore, 1954; Sekelj, 1958a, 1958b; McGregor, 1961; Phinney, 1963; Reed and Wood, 1967; Barr and Bradley, 1968; Sekelj, 1970). The other has been registration of indicator-dilution curves from radioactive isotopes passing into the arterial circulation. A standard ear oximeter can be employed for registering dye-dilution curves from the ear lobe provided other factors such as oxygenation of the blood, rate of blood flow through the ear, and so forth remain constant. Wood and his associates, especially, have had success in recording dye-dilution curves by this method, and McGregor et al. (1961), in a comparative study of ear oximetric and cuvette oximetric techniques found that the two give almost exactly the same cardiac output measurements. Furthermore, Phinney (1963) reported that cardiac output values obtained by ear densitometry compared excellently with simultaneous values obtained by the direct Fick method. Radioactive indicator-dilution curves have been recorded by placing the head, arm, or a finger in a special radioactive counter, or they have been recorded by use of scintillation detectors collimated to pick up radioactivity from one or both chambers of the heart or from the great vessels of the thorax (Prinzmetal, 1948; Huff, 1955; Crane, 1956; Ziff, 1957; Mack, 1957; Pritchard, 1958; MacIntyre, 1958; Van Der Feer, 1958; Bozer, 1958; Seldon, 1959; Sevelius, 1959; Weinberg, 1959; Akesson, 1959; Gorten, 1959; Murphy, 1963; Gorten, 1965; Hernandez, 1967; Kloster, 1969).

The greatest problem in use of an indirect method for sampling is not in the primary registration of the indicator-dilution curve itself but instead is in calibrating the instrument. To do this, an additional step in the procedure is required. First, only an indicator that will remain in the circulatory system for a prolonged period of time can be used. After registration of the indicator-dilution curve, one waits an additional period of time until the indicator has become completely mixed with the blood. During this period of time the operator attempts to maintain exactly the same geometry of the ear vasculature in the case of the oximeter method and of the radioactive counting system in the case of the radioactive methods. Once the mixing has been accomplished, a sample of blood is removed from a vessel, and its concentration of indicator is determined by some standard in vitro method. At the same time that the sample is taken, the reading of the optical or radioactive device is also recorded. If the device is linear in its recording characteristics, a single sample of blood such as this can be used to calibrate the instrument.

A further problem in the radioactive methods is background count, which must be accounted for in the calibration procedures.

A particularly interesting development has been an automatic computing cardiac output instrument utilizing an ear device that is capable of measuring the dye-dilution curve and can be calibrated without removing a sample of blood (Sekelj, 1958a, 1958b). After the dilution curve is run, the instrument is calibrated by essentially the same procedures used for calibrating the ear oximeter for the determination of the per cent oxygen saturation of the arterial blood, namely, by comparison of optical densities of the ear under different conditions and at different wave lengths. The readings from these different measurements enter an analog computer along with the recorded dye-dilution curve, and the cardiac output is then automatically computed. Though the absolute accuracy of the method is not yet established, and though it is doubtful that it is as accurate as conventional methods utilizing direct sampling of arterial blood, nevertheless the procedure should be very valuable in measuring cardiac output during operative procedures or when it is not advisable to disturb the arterial circulation.

Recently, the reliability of the ear as a recording site for dye-dilution curves has been greatly increased by the development of the dichromatic earpiece densitometer (Sinclair, 1961; Sutterer and Wood, 1962; Reed and Wood, 1967; Barr and Bradley, 1968). This device provides compensation for changes in blood content of the ear pinna and changes in hematocrit of the blood flowing through the ear. The dichromatic densitometer contains two photocells: One is sensitive to changes in dye concentration and the other is insensitive to changes in dye concentration. However, both photocells are approximately equally sensitive to changes in optical density of the ear caused by changes in blood content or hematocrit. Compensation for changes in the transilluminance of the ear which are unrelated to changes in dye concentration is, therefore, obtained by using the two photocells in reverse polarity to each other. Such compensation results in a stable baseline, even though the blood content of the ear or the hematocrit is altered substantially. Furthermore, since this instrument automatically compensates for differences in ear transilluminance not due to changes in dye concentration, a previously calibrated ear piece can be used for the estimation of cardiac output without the necessity of blood withdrawal (Reed and Wood, 1967).

MATHEMATICAL BASIS OF THE SINGLE INJECTION LINE

The Semilog Decay of the Downslope

In an effort to make the mathematical analysis of cardiac output even more accurate than can be afforded by the semilog plot method, biophysicists and mathematicians have attempted during the past 25 years to delineate mathematically the factors that determine the shape of the indicator-dilution curve. However, before attempting to give a mathematical derivation of the shape of the curve, it is first important to understand the original thinking behind the semilog plot method for correcting the curve for recirculated indicator.

The logic of Kinsman, Hamilton, and their coworkers (Kinsman, 1929) in originally proposing the semilog plot method for correcting the downslope of the indicator-dilution curve was essentially the following: When fluid is flowing through a mixing chamber and a foreign substance then suddenly becomes distributed in the mixing chamber, one finds that a certain percentage of the indicator will be washed out of the mixing chamber the first second, the same percentage of that remaining in the chamber will be washed out the second second, the same percentage of that remaining will be washed out the third second, and so forth. In other words,

$$\frac{dC}{dt} = -KC \qquad (3\text{--}17)$$

where C is the instantaneous concentration at the point of outflow from the chamber, t is time, and K is a constant depending upon the rate of fluid flow, the size of the chamber, and the mixing characteristics within the chamber. On solving the differential equation we find

$$C = C_0 e^{-Kt} \qquad (3\text{--}18)$$

where C_0 is the initial concentration. Figure 3–9 illustrates by the solid curve this exponential decay of concentration during the period of washout.

Kinsman, Hamilton, and their associates recognized from the beginning that the washout curve would not explain any of the features of the upslope of the dye-dilution curve or of the peak, but they reasoned that, after a period of time, sufficient mixing of the indicator would occur in the heart and pulmonary circulation to allow the washout curve to apply to the more distal portions of the downslope of the indicator-dilution curve. Their experimental evidence, and that of many others since their time, amply justifies their original view that most of the downslope of an indicator-dilution curve is essentially described by the typical washout decay curve. To illustrate this point, a typical indicator-dilution curve is shown in Figure 3–9; its downslope parallels the decay of the washout curve.

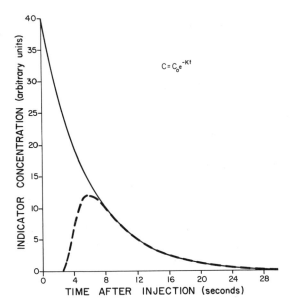

Figure 3–9. Comparison of a typical indicator-dilution curve (dashed curve) with the typical exponential washout curve, the formula for which is given in the figure.

Derivation of the Indicator-Dilution Curve from the Normal Curve of Random Distribution

Sheppard (1952, 1962) has pointed out that the shapes of most indicator-dilution curves can be calculated on the basis of random distribution of indicator substance in the flowing blood. Though analyses based generally on this principle have taken several different forms (Sheppard, 1952, 1962; Newman, 1951; Stow, 1954; Korner, 1961; Zierler, 1962), the following is a simple analysis which will give almost precisely the shape of the indicator-dilution curve as it is usually measured in cardiac output determinations.

This analysis begins with the following four basic assumptions: (1) The indicator is injected as a single slug requiring essentially zero time to be injected into the flowing stream. (2) The average velocity of movement of the indicator along with the flowing stream is equal to the average velocity of fluid flow. (3) The indicator is continually dispersing from the time of original injection, some of the dye moving ahead of the average velocity of flow and some lagging behind. It is assumed that this dispersion occurs in random fashion, with the same quantities of dye moving ahead and moving behind, and that the curve of distribution of the random movement is the usual normal distribution curve. This is the effect that one would observe for turbulent flow of blood in the circulation. (4) The degree of dispersion is proportional to the average distance that the blood and indicator have moved.

Starting with these basic assumptions, we can now construct the distribution of an indicator along the axis of a vessel at different time intervals following injection into the vessel when the blood is flowing at an average velocity of 1 cm. per second. Figure 3–10 illustrates that, at the point of injection, the concentration is infinite and the horizontal disper-

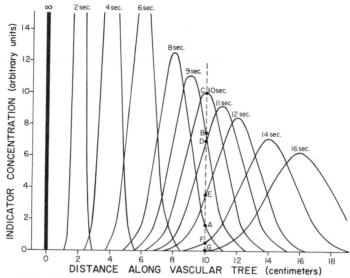

Figure 3–10. Progressive dispersion of an indicator as it is washed along a vessel beginning with infinite concentration at zero time and with the peak concentration decreasing inversely with the distance traveled, while at the same time the horizontal dispersion increases proportionately with the distance traveled.

sion of the indicator is zero. However, after a period of 2 seconds, the concentration has fallen to some finite value, and the indicator has begun to disperse in both directions from the point of peak concentration. At 4 seconds, the dispersion is twice that at 2 seconds, but the peak concentration is only one-half as great. At 6 seconds, the dispersion is three times as great as that at 2 seconds, and the peak concentration one-third as great. At 10 seconds, the dispersion is five times that at 2 seconds, but the peak concentration is one-fifth as great.

Now let us assume that we are sampling blood 10 cm. down the vessel and that we take samples at 8 seconds, 9 seconds, 10 seconds, 11 seconds, 12 seconds, 14 seconds, and 16 seconds. At 8 seconds, only the beginning of the dispersed dye has reached the 10 cm. point, and its concentration will be that illustrated by point A in the figure. At 9 seconds a much larger proportion of the dye will have reached the 10 cm. mark and its concentration will be represented by point B. At 10 seconds the peak of the curve will have reached the 10 cm. mark, and its concentration is illustrated in the figure by point C. Similarly for 11, 12, 14, and 16 seconds, points D, E, F, and G represent the respective concentrations which would be recorded. Now let us plot these points on a time scale as shown in Figure 3–11. On drawing the indicator-dilution curve through these points, we observe the characteristic curve which has been recorded thousands of times under normal experimental conditions. The formula for this curve can be derived as follows:

Let:

t = time following injection
M = mass of indicator injected
C = instantaneous concentration at the sampling site
k = constant for the rate of dispersion of the indicator

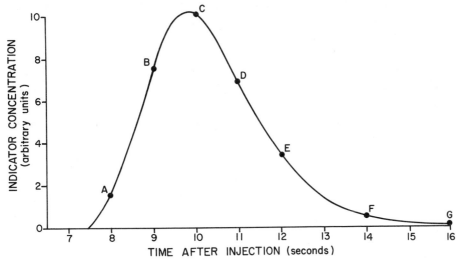

Figure 3–11. The derived indicator-dilution curve determined from Figure 3–10 when sampling at a distance 10 cm. away from the injection site.

D = distance along the vascular tree from injection to sampling site
V = velocity of blood flow
T = distance from the peak of the concentration curve to the sampling site in terms of standard deviations of the indicator dispersion
K = proportionality constant

The normal distribution curve is described by the following formula:

$$C = \frac{1}{\sqrt{2\pi}}\, e^{-T^2/2} \tag{3-19}$$

As the distribution curve moves along the vascular tree and approaches the sampling site, the distance of the peak of the distribution curve from the sample site will be D − Vt, and the degree of dispersion of the distribution curve will be kt. Therefore,

$$T = \frac{D - Vt}{kt} \tag{3-20}$$

Furthermore, the peak concentration of the distribution curve is decreasing with time, or, in other words, peak concentration is equal to M/kt. Putting this together with the above value of T and with the normal distribution curve we can derive a formula for the complete dye concentration curve as follows:

$$C = \frac{KM}{\sqrt{2\pi}\ kt}\, e^{-\left(\frac{D-Vt}{kt}\right)^2 / 2} \tag{3-21}$$

The curve of Figure 3–11 was derived from this formula by using arbitrary units. To use actual units instead of arbitrary units one needs to define the cross-sectional area of the flowing system.

To see whether the curve derived graphically in Figures 3–10 and 3–11 and algebraically by Formulas 3–19 through 3–21 is approximately equivalent to that usually recorded under experimental conditions, we can test its downslope by the semilog plot method. Figure 3–12 illustrates such a test, showing that the downslope of the curve in Figure 3–11 does fall along a typical exponential decay curve.

One can readily see from Figure 3–12 why a semilog plot can be used very accurately to correct for recirculation of an indicator. However, it should be pointed out that the semilog downslope does not fit the derived curve very satisfactorily until the concentration has fallen below approximately one-half the peak concentration. Therefore, on the basis of this mathematical derivation, it is probably unreasonable ever to use the semilog plot method for extrapolating the downslope of an indicator-dilution curve if recirculation of the indicator begins before the halfway mark on the recorded downslope. This is the same conclusion that was reached by Dow (1955) from empirical considerations.

Another analysis of the indicator-dilution curve, which was very similar to the present one, was offered by Stow and Hetzel (1954). These authors started with the assumption that the indicator-dilution curve is

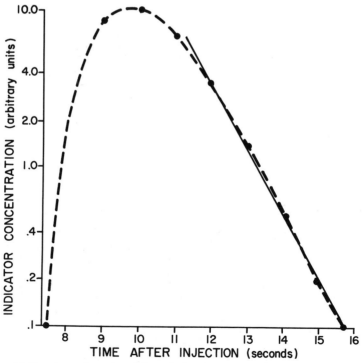

Figure 3–12.   A semilog plot of the calculated indicator-dilution curve in Figure 3–11, illustrating that the downslope of the calculated curve is essentially semilogarithmic in nature.

depicted by a log-normal distribution curve. The formula derived above is not precisely that of a log-normal distribution curve, but when the value D is large in relation to the value k, such would usually be almost the case.

Nevertheless, Stow found that use of his curve to correct for recirculation of indicator gave an average calculation of cardiac output only 3.5 per cent different from that found by use of the semilog plot method. This amount of difference is within the limits of experimental error, though it is possible that it was caused by an error in the basic assumption that the true curve obeys a log-normal function or an error in the basic assumption that the downslope of the curve is a semilog function. However, because of too many variables, further refinements in mathematical derivations of indicator-dilution curves probably will not make our use of such curves for measuring cardiac output significantly more accurate than it already is. A monograph by Sheppard (1962) on tracer methods and their mathematical basis gives the many different theoretically possible variations in shapes of indicator-dilution curves, though he too points out the practical limitations in accuracy that can be achieved despite our modern development of mathematical theory.

THE CONSTANT INFUSION METHOD FOR MEASURING CARDIAC OUTPUT

Stewart's original procedure (1897) for measuring cardiac output was a constant infusion indicator-dilution method. This was actually derived from the Fick method for measuring output; later the single injection procedure was in turn derived from the constant infusion method. Because of greater technical simplicity, the single injection method has become very widely used, whereas the constant infusion method has been used only on rare occasions (Wiggers, 1944a; Holt, 1944a; Rashkind, 1949; Shepherd, 1955; Pavek, 1964; Klocke, 1968) since its initial introduction by Stewart.

The Procedure

The procedure in the constant infusion method differs from that in the single injection method in the following way: Instead of injecting all the indicator substance suddenly, as in the single injection method, a constant infusion of the indicator is suddenly begun and then continued until an appropriate record is obtained for measuring the cardiac output. Figure 3–13 illustrates a record replotted from Shepherd (1955) of arterial dye concentration following sudden onset of T-1824 dye infusion into the right ventricle at zero time at a rate of 0.76 mg. per second. Simultaneously with the onset of the infusion, arterial blood was allowed to flow at a constant rate through a cuvette densitometer. This figure shows the dye first making its appearance in the arterial blood at approximately 11 seconds and its concentration rising steadily thereafter over a period of 20 seconds to approach an asymptote. The record is divided into two-

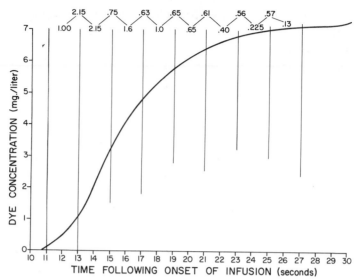

Figure 3–13. A typical continuous infusion concentration curve recorded from a peripheral artery [replotted from Shepherd, Bowers, and Wood (1955)]. The figures above show that the upper portion of the curve is essentially semilogarithmic in nature; this is discussed in the text.

second intervals, and the *increase* in concentration is noted for each one of the intervals. Then the *ratio of the successive increases* is shown above. Note that, except for the first two intervals, the ratios of the successive increases remained essentially constant. These results illustrate that the upper portion of the curve is a semilogarithmic function similar to the distal portions of the single injection indicator-dilution curve. This is an important fact because, as we shall see later, it can be used to correct the curve for recirculation of the indicator.

Calculation of Cardiac Output from the Continuous Infusion Dye Concentration Curve

The real advantage of the continuous infusion method over the single injection method is the simplicity of calculation of cardiac output. The following formula gives the calculation by this method.

$$\text{Cardiac output} = \frac{I_r}{C_p} \tag{3-22}$$

where C_p is concentration of the dye on the asymptotic plateau and I_r is the rate of infusion of the indicator. If the concentration is given in milligrams of indicator per liter and the rate of infusion in terms of milligrams per minute, then the cardiac output will be in liters per minute. This formula is actually a derivation of the Fick equation (Formula 2–2 in the previous chapter). C_p is analogous to the arterial concentration of the substance in the Fick formula, and I_r is the same as the numerator of the Fick equation. The only factor missing from Formula 3–22 that is present in the Fick equation is a factor for the venous concentration of the indicator. The reason this factor is missing is that the venous concentration of the indicator in the indicator infusion method is zero, or at least this is true before recirculation of the indicator occurs, and, when recirculation does occur, appropriate procedures can be used, as will be discussed below, to correct for this recirculation so that the venous concentration still need not be considered.

Using Formula 3–22, we can now calculate the cardiac output measured by the curve shown in Figure 3–13. The level of the plateau was 7.0 mg./liter and the rate of infusion was 45.6 mg./min. Therefore, the cardiac output was 45.6/7 or 6.5 liters per minute.

Correction for Recirculation of Indicator

If the indicator substance begins to recirculate too soon while the curve is being recorded, no significant plateau will develop in the arterial concentration of indicator, so that one will be unable to determine the level of the plateau merely by inspection of the curve. Therefore, a correction procedure is required to derive the true curve.

Figure 3–14 illustrates a curve that has been replotted from Howard, Hamilton, and Dow (1953), illustrating recirculation of dye long before an adequate plateau has developed. The problem here is to correct for recirculation and to determine the asymptotic level that the plateau would have reached. To do this we proceed in the following manner. First, one can be quite certain that no plateau is developing as long as the *slope* of the curve is progressively increasing. Therefore, we need not worry about the early portion of the curve. However, once the upward slope of the curve begins to decrease, which occurs at approximately 8 seconds in Figure 3–14, we must then test the curve to determine whether or not it is approaching an asymptote. Since the approach to the asymptote is a semilogarithmic function, as pointed out in the previous discussion of the

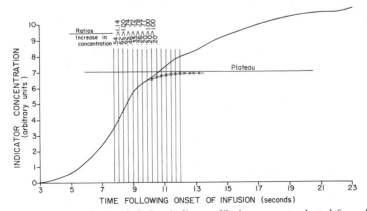

Figure 3–14. A continuous infusion indicator-dilution curve replotted from Howard, Hamilton, and Dow (1953), showing recirculation of indicator before a plateau can be obtained. The numbers and the dashed curve illustrate a method for determining the level of the plateau; this is discussed in the text.

typical curve, we can use a method very similar to the alternate semilog method given earlier in the chapter to correct the single injection curve.

Second, once the upward slope of the curve begins to decrease, the curve is marked off in equidistant time intervals. The precise choice of these intervals is immaterial as long as there is a sufficient number of them. In Figure 3–14, the marked intervals are one-third of a second, beginning approximately 8 seconds following the onset of infusion. The increase in concentration during each one of these time intervals is then recorded above, and above these intervals the *ratios* of each two successive increases are recorded. Note that the ratio between the first two intervals is 1.14 and that between the second two intervals is 0.74. Then the following four ratios are approximately equal and average 0.75. However, at approximately 10 seconds the ratio suddenly increases back to 1.0. Thus, we see that for the period between 8.4 and 9.9 seconds the curve describes a semilogarithmic course. If we assume that it should continue along the semilogarithmic course, we can begin at 10 seconds, immediately before recirculation begins, and calculate the subsequent course of the true curve. Note that during the interval between 9.6 and 9.9 seconds the concentration increased 0.20 units. Using the ratio found during the semilogarithmic portion of the curve, 0.75, we can calculate that the true curve should have increased 0.75×0.2, or 0.15 units, during the next interval; it should have increased 0.75×0.15, or 0.11 units, during the next interval, and so forth. In this way, the cross marks on Figure 3–14 were calculated, and one can readily see that the curve approaches a well defined plateau.

To simplify this procedure still further, one can use the following formula for determining the level of the plateau:

$$C_p = C_m + \Delta C_s + r\Delta C_s + r^2\Delta C_s + \ldots + r^\infty\Delta C_s \qquad (3\text{–}23)$$

In using this formula a large part of the semilogarithmic portion of the curve is first divided into two equal time zones. Then the concentration of the indicator at the plateau, C_p, is calculated from the concentration of the indicator at the mid-point between the two equal time zones, C_m, the increase in concentration of the indicator during the second time zone, ΔC_s, and the ratio of the concentration increase, r, during the second time zone to the concentration increase during the first time zone, $\frac{\Delta C_s}{\Delta C_f}$. This formula can be simplified as follows:

$$C_p = C_m + \frac{\Delta C_s}{1 - \dfrac{\Delta C_s}{\Delta C_f}} \qquad (3\text{–}24)$$

Applying Formula 3–24 to Figure 3–14, we can divide the semilog portion of the curve into the following two time zones: 8.7 to 9.3 seconds, and 9.3 to 9.9 seconds. Then C_m, measured at 9.3 seconds, is 5.92; ΔC_s is 0.46; and ΔC_f is 0.79. Placing these values in Formula 3–24, we obtain a plateau concentration (C_p) of 7.01. This also is the level of the plateau which the extrapolated curve is approaching in Figure 3–14.

Most continuous infusion curves will not be nearly so difficult to correct for recirculation as the one illustrated in Figure 3–14. Indeed this particular curve was first published (Howard, 1953) to emphasize the difficulty in using the continuous infusion method for calculating cardiac output. This curve was chosen to illustrate that even a curve as distorted as this one can still be corrected for recirculation of indicator by a simple procedure.

MATHEMATICAL BASIS OF THE CONSTANT INJECTION PROCEDURE

The Continuous Infusion Curve as the Integral of the Single Injection Curve

Figure 3–15 illustrates the single injection curve which was derived in Figure 3–11 from basic theoretical considerations and which has essentially the same shape as the single injection curve recorded experimentally under many different conditions. The other curve of Figure 3–15 is the integral of the area subtended by the single injection curve. This integral was obtained by the usual graphic method for integrating the area under a curve, whereby each successive point on the integral curve rises a constant proportion of the instantaneous concentration on the single injection curve.

Note that the integral in Figure 3–15 is essentially identical with the continuous infusion curve illustrated in Figure 3–13 and also with the corrected continuous infusion curve in Figure 3–14. However, it is not

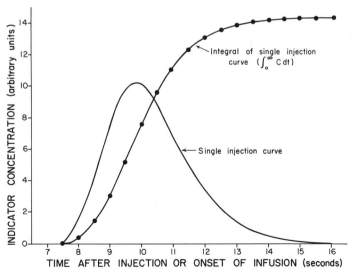

Figure 3–15. A single injection-dilution curve and the integral of the area subtended by the curve, illustrating that the continuous infusion curve has precisely the same characteristics as the integral of the single injection curve.

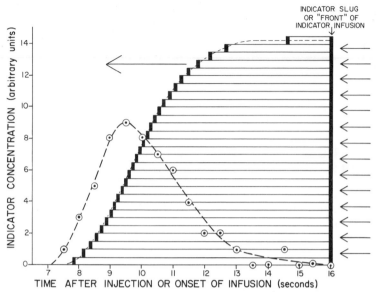

Figure 3–16. Diagram to show theoretically why the continuous infusion curve is the integral of the single injection curve; explanation in the text.

sufficient simply to point out the similarity between the integral and the continuous infusion curve. Therefore, let us use Figure 3–16 to illustrate logically why the continuous infusion curve is the integral of the single injection curve.

Far to the right in the figure is a solid bar, which represents one of two different conditions: sudden injection of a slug of indicator or sudden onset of infusion of an indicator. In the case of sudden injection of a slug of indicator, different particles of the indicator will move toward the left at different velocities because of the random dispersion of the indicator; this effect was discussed earlier in the derivation of the single injection curve. The small, dark bar segments moving across the graph represent these particles of indicator moving in the left-hand direction. In the case of the continuous infusion of indicator, many minute columns of indicator move to the left, and the small dark bars now represent the "fronts" of the moving columns of indicator. Note that if one plots a curve through the fronts of these columns, he obtains the typical continuous infusion curve, as illustrated in Figure 3–15. To determine the concentration curve of the single injection method, we simply count the number of dark slugs in each time interval. Thus, between the limits of 7 and 8 seconds on the abscissal scale we count one slug passing the point of sampling. Between the limits of $7\frac{1}{2}$ and $8\frac{1}{2}$ seconds we count three slugs passing the point of sampling. Between the limits of 8 and 9 seconds we count five slugs. This process is continued until all the slugs have passed the sampling site, which will have occurred by approximately 16 seconds. The encircled dots in Figure 3–16 illustrate a plot of the number of slugs passing the sampling site during each 1 second interval, and the dashed curve drawn through these dots is the total curve. If we compare these two derived curves with

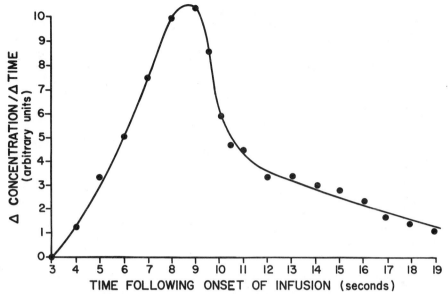

Figure 3–17.   Differential of the contunuous infusion curve of Figure 3–14, showing an example of conversion of a continuous infusion curve into a single injection curve.

those illustrated in Figure 3–15, we see that they are identical with the differential and integral curves, respectively, of the previous figure.

Therefore, by integrating the single injection curve, one can obtain the continuous infusion curve that would have been recorded had the infusion method been used instead of the injection method. Likewise, by differentiating the continuous infusion curve, one can obtain the single injection curve that would have been recorded had the single injection method been used instead of the continuous infusion method.

CONVERSION OF A REPRESENTATIVE CONTINUOUS INFUSION CURVE INTO A SINGLE INJECTION CURVE.   Let us return to the curve in Figure 3–14. By using a typical graphical differentiating procedure, the corresponding single injection curve derived from Figure 3–14 is that shown in Figure 3–17. Now let us replot Figure 3–17 on semilog coordinates, and we find the curve shown in Figure 3–18, which has a semilog downslope during its early portion; this curve can be extrapolated to zero by the usual method.

The reason for choosing the very "poor" curve of Figure 3–14 is to illustrate that precisely the same principles and problems exist in using the continuous infusion method as in using the single injection method for calculation of cardiac output. If we observe Figure 3–18 carefully, we will see that recirculation occurred, at least to some extent, before the curve had fallen to a concentration less than one-half of its peak. In the discussion earlier in the chapter of the single injection method for determining cardiac output, it was pointed out that curves which leave the semilog function prior to falling in a concentration one-half the peak value cannot be used with accuracy in determining the cardiac output. Thus, the poor curve of Figure 3–14, which was very difficult to use in

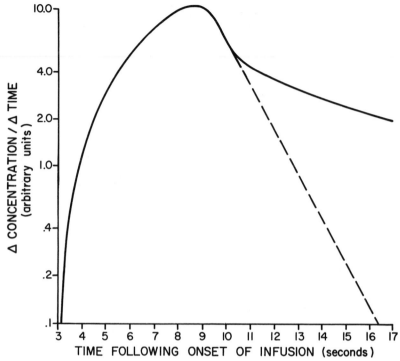

Figure 3–18. Semilog plot of the curve in Figure 3–17, illustrating that the semilog method for correcting the curve can be applied to the differential of the continuous infusion curve.

calculating the cardiac output from the continuous infusion method, actually represented extremely early recirculation and not an error in the continuous infusion method itself; this is evident from the fact that the differential of the curve in Figure 3–14, as illustrated in Figures 3–17 and 3–18, shows that a single injection curve recorded in the same experiment at the same time would likewise have given a curve that would have been very difficult, if not impossible, to analyze accurately.

THE KHALIL CATHETER-TIP CONTINUOUS INFUSION THERMODILUTION METHOD

Figure 3–19 illustrates a special application of the continuous infusion method for measuring cardiac output. This method, developed by Khalil (1966), utilizes heat as the indicator substance and employs nothing more than a single specially made catheter. This catheter is provided with a resistance thermometer which consists of copper wire wrapped around the last inch or so of the catheter. This catheter is passed preferably upward through the inferior vena cava and its tip is positioned in the pulmonary artery and its branches. Around the shank of the catheter, where it passes upward through the vena cava, is wrapped a heater winding. In using this method, electrical current is applied to the heater winding at a constant

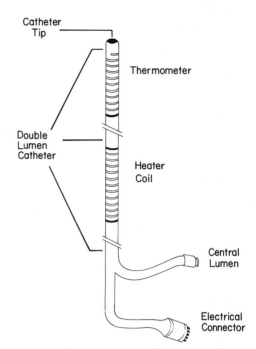

Figure 3–19. A simplified diagram of the Khalil thermodilution catheter, showing the thermometer winding at the catheter tip, and the heater winding on the catheter shank. The electrical connections are directed through the outer lumen of the double lumen catheter. The center lumen remains unobstructed and may be used for pressure measurements or blood sampling. [Modified from Khalil (1966).]

rate, which constitutes a sudden onset of continuous heat infusion. A second or so later, the temperature measured by the tip of the catheter begins to increase, and this temperature reaches a plateau after approximately another 8 to 10 seconds, as illustrated in Figure 3–20. Once the plateau is reached the electrical current is turned off, whereupon isothermal conditions are usually reestablished within about 30 seconds. After this time another measurement can be made.

The Khalil catheter can be left in an animal for several days, and it has also been used successfully in human beings. The problems with the catheter thus far have been mainly difficulty of manufacture.

In a double blind study using this method and the continuous cardiac output Fick method described in Chapter 2, the mean deviation between measurements made by the two methods was approximately 6 per cent. This is about as satisfactory a result as has been achieved in comparison

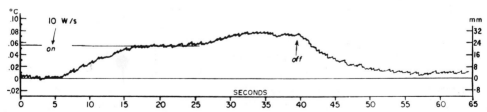

Figure 3–20. A record of temperature in the pulmonary artery of a dog following the application of heat at the heater winding of the Khalil thermodilution catheter. Heat was applied at a rate of 10 watts. The plateau in temperature 10 seconds after the onset of heating is evident. The second rise in temperature is due to recirculation of the heated blood. [From Khalil (1966).]

of any two methods. Thus, it is obvious that this catheter tip method deserves special consideration, since its simplicity and accuracy made it a likely candidate for widespread use in the future.

COMPARISON OF THE SINGLE INJECTION AND CONSTANT INFUSION INDICATOR-DILUTION METHOD

Hamilton and coworkers maintained up until 1953 (Howard, 1953) that the constant infusion method could not be used accurately for measuring cardiac output, because, they stated, no satisfactory method had been devised to correct for recirculation of the indicator. However, from the foregoing discussion, one can see that mathematically sound methods are available for correcting for recirculation of the indicator. Indeed, should one wish, he could actually differentiate the continuous infusion curve and then use the semilog plot method to correct the continuous infusion curve for recirculation of indicator. This would be a rather laborious procedure in comparison with the simplified method using Formula 3–24.

Since 1953 the integral-differential relationship between continuous infusion and single injection curves has been pointed out (Lewis, 1953a, 1953b; Cleempoel, 1957), and it has become evident that whatever error is inherent in one of the methods is also inherent in the other (Meier and Zierler, 1954). Also, each mathematical procedure for correcting one of these types of curves has its counterpart for correcting the other one. Therefore, we must conclude that, from the point of view of accuracy, the single injection and the continuous infusion methods for measuring cardiac output have almost identical possibilities. If anything, the continuous infusion method might be slightly ahead of the single injection method, because it is impossible to inject a slug of indicator into the circulation in zero time. Yet the very slight error that is entailed by taking as much as one-half or even as much as 2 seconds in injecting the slug of indicator is not a matter of real significance.

From a technical point of view, however, the single injection method has been greatly preferred over the continuous infusion method. Its widespread use has made its vagaries and its difficulties far better understood than those of the continuous infusion method. Furthermore, to record adequate concentrations of indicator in the arterial blood, approximately twice as much indicator must be infused into the subject when using the continuous infusion method as when using the single injection method. And a caution that must be observed in using the continuous infusion method is to infuse the indicator at an absolutely constant rate (Wiggers, 1944a); this is comparable to the analogous precaution in the single injection method, that the indicator slug must be injected *in toto* within a very short period of time and must become mixed very rapidly with the flowing blood.

POSSIBLE ERRORS IN USING INDICATOR-DILUTION METHODS

If all technical aspects of either of the indicator-dilution methods are carried out properly, there are only two factors that can ordinarily cause errors in the measurement of cardiac output. These are (a) recirculation of the indicator and (b) changes in rate of blood flow while the indicator-dilution curve is being recorded. The first of these two possible errors has already been discussed in detail for both the single injection and the continuous infusion methods. Therefore, the present discussion will concern errors relating to changing blood flow during the course of measurement.

Two types of errors can result from changing rates of blood flow: (a) changing rate of flow through the sample catheter into the sampling device and (b) changing rate of cardiac output.

When the rate of flow from the artery into the sampling device changes, regardless of whether a continuous or discontinuous method of sampling is used, the precise time relationships of the curves will not be recorded. Therefore, if recirculation of indicator occurs, it will be impossible to extrapolate either the single injection or the continuous infusion curve to determine the true curve. If recirculation does not occur, failure to keep the rate of flow constant will not cause an error at all when using the continuous infusion method, because the concentration will eventually reach exactly the same plateau level irrespective of variations in the time scale of the recording. However, in the case of the single injection method, variations in the time scale caused by varying sample flow will cause an error in the total area subtended by the curve, and an error that cannot be corrected in any way.

Even when the rate of flow from the artery into the sampling device is precisely constant, it is still possible to have an error of this type under the following conditions: On rare occasions the percentage of the total cardiac output going to the sampling artery changes from moment to moment. If the percentage flow to the sampling artery changes while the indicator-dilution curve is being recorded, this would also cause a changing time scale, with the same errors in measurement of cardiac output as discussed above. For instance, Lange (1960) showed that blood flow to the brachial artery is often quite variable and that this can cause considerable error. In contrast, the flow to the femoral artery is reasonably uniform.

The second principal way in which flow changes can cause errors in the measurement of cardiac output is for the entire cardiac output to change while the measurement is being made. This is analogous to the same type of error that occurs under similar conditions when using the Fick method, which was discussed in the previous chapter. Let us suppose, for instance, that a single injection dye-dilution curve is being recorded at the same time that a cardiac output is changing, and let us suppose that the cardiac output during the passage of the first half of the injected dye is 2 liters per minute and during the passage of the second half of the dye is 20 liters per minute. The average cardiac output during the same time would be 11 liters per minute, but let us calculate what the single injection method would have measured the cardiac output to be. Let us assume that a total of 4 mg. of dye is injected and that the first 2 mg. of this dye passes into the arteries during the first 10 seconds of the test. During the first 10 seconds we record an arterial dye concentration of 6 mg. per liter so that we can calculate the average cardiac output during this 10 seconds as $(60 \times 2) / (6 \times 10)$, or 2 liters per minute. However, during the second 10 seconds of the test we record an average arterial concentration of dye of 0.6 mg. per liter, and we can calculate that the average cardiac output for this second half is $(60 \times 2) / (0.6 \times 10)$, or 20 liters per minute. Now let us average the dye concentration over the total 20 second period of time, which gives an average concentration of 3.3 mg./liter. Using the usual formula for calculating cardiac output, Formula 3–2, we find that the cardiac output is 3.6 liters per minute in comparison with the true average cardiac output of 11 liters per minute during the course of recording the dye curve.

Obviously, such serious errors as this will not ordinarily occur, because the cardiac output almost never changes ten fold in a matter of a few seconds' time. On the other hand, cardiac outputs do change as much as two to three fold in this period of time, and this change can easily cause errors of 20 to 30 per cent. Therefore, this could be one of the most common of all the errors that occur in use of indicator methods for recording cardiac output.

Another type of error, which is actually a technical error rather than a basic theoretical error, in the use of indicator-dilution methods for measuring cardiac output is illustrated in Figure 3–21. This shows an effect, pointed out by Howard, Hamilton, and Dow (1953), that frequently

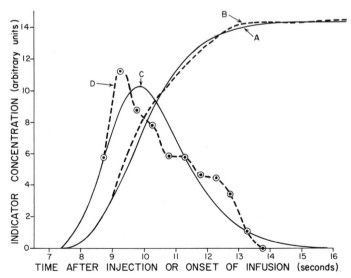

Figure 3–21. A typical continuous infusion curve (A) and its differential (C) (which is also a typical single injection curve), compared with atypical curves (B and D) caused by rhythmical alterations in blood flow during the period of recording the curves, illustrating that such rhythmical changes in blood flow sometimes make it impossible to distinguish recirculation of the indicator from other distortions in the curves.

occurs when the cardiac output changes rhythmically as a result of deep respiration or any other condition. Figure 3–21 illustrates the same continuous infusion and single injection curves (A and C, respectively) as those shown in Figure 3–15. The dashed curve B is a slightly different continuous infusion curve, depicting a less smooth curve resulting from changing cardiac output during the course of recording the curve. The difficulty with this curve is that one would not be able to extrapolate it to an accurate plateau level. For instance, after the first hump in the curve one might well consider that the curve is already approaching a plateau and therefore extrapolate from this point to a plateau that would be much too low.

Curve D in Figure 3–21 illustrates the differential of Curve B and, therefore, represents the character of the single injection dye-dilution curve that one would record if these same variations in cardiac output were occurring while the curve was being recorded. Note that it would be impossible in this case also to determine when recirculation of indicator occurs. Actually one might suspect from this curve that recirculation had begun when the downslope had fallen to only 40 per cent of the peak concentration, whereas actually no recirculation has occurred at all.

In either curve B or D, if one is completely certain that recirculation of indicator has not occurred at all, the calculation of cardiac output would be completely accurate by either method, but the difficulty lies in the fact that from these curves one cannot tell when or where recirculation begins, or in some instances the curve might lead to a false assumption of the point at which recirculation does begin, thus leading to errors that can be as great at 50 per cent or more. The object of Figure 3–21 is that one should not attempt to extrapolate curves that do not have reasonably typical shapes.

Errors Resulting from Parallel Flow Channels of Different Flow Velocities

In calculating the theoretical indicator-dilution curve in Figures 3–10 and 3–11 and in integrating this to determine the continuous infusion curve in Figure 3–15, we made the assumption that progressive and continuous mixing of the indicator occurs all along the course from the point of injection to the point of sampling. In general, this is a reasonable assumption, but if anywhere between the points of injection and sampling, part of the blood takes an entirely separate course from the other part of the blood, as occurs in the pulmonary circulation, and a portion of the blood travels and disperses at a completely different rate from that which travels through the other parallel circuit, then the indicator concentration curve recorded from the peripheral artery can have a downslope which will not describe a semilog function. This is particularly true if the velocity of flow through one of the channels is many times that through another channel. Unfortunately, on recombination of these separate channels of blood flow, it is possible for them to recombine in such a way to give a downslope that has a semilog function in a portion of the slope. If this should occur in the upper portion of the curve and recirculation of indicator should obscure the lower downslope, one might falsely extrapolate the curve to the zero level. This point is made simply for the following reason: Even when the downslope of the curve appears to be semilogarithmic in its upper portion, this sometimes results from fortuitous circumstances rather than because of a true exponential washout. Under these conditions the extrapolation would be in error; how much in error would never be known.

COMPARISON OF CARDIAC OUTPUTS MEASURED BY THE INDICATOR-DILUTION AND FICK PROCEDURES

Through the years, the Fick method for measuring cardiac output has become the standard for testing the validity of other methods, this having occurred despite the serious technical errors that can appear in Fick measurements, as discussed in the previous chapter. Nevertheless, in numerous comparisons of the Fick method with the two indicator-dilution methods, the results have been almost identical (Hamilton, 1948; Werkö, 1949; Doyle, 1953; Wilson, 1953; Eliasch, 1955; MacCanon, 1955; Phinney, 1963; Klocke, 1968), one sometimes measuring slightly higher than the other and at other times the opposite being the case, but averaging the same.

Because of this excellent agreement between the two methods, both methods, when used correctly, are now accepted as about equally valid. Yet because the single injection-dilution method can be used more easily than the Fick method under most conditions, it is now used much more widely in most surveys of cardiac outputs, for instance, in the newborn (Prec, 1953, 1955), in normal adults (Brandfonbrener, 1955; Lagerlöf, 1950), in patients with cardiac disease (Kattus, 1955), and in many other studies that will be cited throughout this book.

Chapter 4

THE INDIRECT FICK AND THE FOREIGN GAS METHODS FOR ESTIMATING CARDIAC OUTPUT

The technical difficulties of the direct Fick method described in Chapter 2 and of the different indicator-dilution procedures described in Chapter 3 have led a great host of investigators to seek simpler methods for determining cardiac output. Each of the methods to be described in this and the following chapter is based on a different mathematical relationship between cardiac output and some secondary factor that can be measured easily. Once the secondary factor has been measured, it can then be converted with varying degrees of accuracy to cardiac output. In the *indirect* Fick methods, one simply measures the quantities and concentrations of carbon dioxide or oxygen in the respiratory gases collected under special conditions and then calculates the cardiac output from the measurements. In the case of the pulse pressure method, one records the aortic pressure pulse contour and, utilizing known data for pressure-volume relationships of the arterial vascular tree, calculates the cardiac output. Similarly, the foreign gas and roentgenographic methods require very simple measurements, and easily applied mathematical relationships between these measurements and cardiac output then allow one to compute the cardiac output.

In general, these indirect methods have proven to be less accurate in measuring cardiac output than have the direct Fick and indicator-dilution methods. On the other hand, some of them are exceedingly simple to apply, and others allow quantitation of cardiac output from heart beat to heart beat or from breath to breath, which is not true of either the direct Fick or the indicator-dilution method. Because a large amount of literature on cardiac output has been amassed in the past describing the use of some of these indirect methods, an understanding of the methods is important in judging the reliability of much of what is known about cardiac output.

81

THE INDIRECT FICK METHODS

Before discussing the different indirect Fick methods for measuring cardiac output, it is necessary that we first recall the principle of the direct Fick method, which was discussed in detail in Chapter 2. The usual Fick procedure is to measure simultaneously (1) the rate of oxygen uptake by the lungs and (2) the difference between the concentrations of oxygen in the arterial blood and in the venous blood. From these values, the cardiac output can be calculated by using the following formula:

$$\text{Cardiac output (l./min.)} = \frac{O_2 \text{ uptake (ml./min.)}}{\text{Arteriovenous } O_2 \text{ difference (ml./l.)}} \quad (4\text{--}1)$$

In making the measurement of arteriovenous oxygen difference, it is necessary to sample mixed venous blood from the right heart, which requires cardiac catheterization, and to sample arterial blood from a systemic artery, which requires arterial puncture. An investigator prefers not to use either of these procedures on a human being if he can easily obtain the information any other way. For this reason, many different investigators, beginning with Loewy (1903), progressively developed procedures by which the Fick formula could be utilized to calculate cardiac output from measurements of carbon dioxide or, in some instances, oxygen concentrations in alveolar air derived from the lungs under special conditions (Plesch, 1909; Christiansen, 1914; Henderson, 1917; Douglas, 1922; Meakins, 1922; Field, 1924; Burwell, 1924a, 1924b; Collier, 1956; Defares, 1958, 1961; Ashton and McHardy, 1963; Jernerus, 1963; Kim, 1966; Cerretelli, 1966a; Jones, 1967). All of these various procedures are of two basic types. In the first type, the subject is required to rebreath from a rubber bag, during which time gas samples are taken either from the expired air or from the bag. Such methods are appropriately termed "rebreathing methods." In the second and more recent type of procedure, gas analyses are performed on a single expiration, and this method is termed "the single breath method."

REBREATHING METHODS

The basic principles of the rebreathing methods that utilize carbon dioxide as the indicator are the following:

Step 1.   The amount of carbon dioxide expired from the lungs in a given period of time is measured by collecting the expired air in a Douglas bag or Tissot spirometer, then analyzing the carbon dioxide concentration in the expired air, and multiplying this by the volume of air collected per minute. The value obtained, in milliliters per minute, is then used as the numerator in the Fick equation.

Step 2.   The carbon dioxide concentration in systemic arterial blood is determined next. To do this, the experimenter makes use of the fact that systemic arterial blood is almost exactly in equilibrium with normal alveolar air. Therefore, a sample of normal alveolar air is collected, and

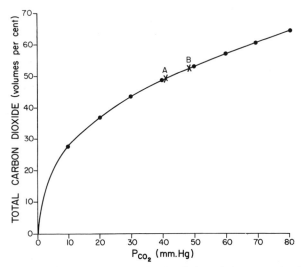

Figure 4–1. A standard carbon dioxide–blood dissociation curve. Point A represents the determination of carbon dioxide concentration in arterial blood and point B in venous blood as explained in the text.

its partial pressure of carbon dioxide is measured by any convenient method. Then, referring to a dissociation curve for carbon dioxide with whole oxygenated blood, as illustrated in Figure 4–1 (Christiansen, 1914; Root, 1958), one can determine the volumes per cent of carbon dioxide in the arterial blood. For instance, assume that the partial pressure of carbon dioxide measures 41 mm. Hg; from point A in the figure one finds that this is equivalent to 49 volumes per cent. In using the carbon dioxide-blood dissociation curve, however, one must realize that the curve is different for each person's blood because of differences in hemoglobin concentration and blood pH. Gray, Bing, and Vandam (1947), however, have pointed out that a carbon dioxide dissociation curve can be simply constructed for each person's blood provided two factors are known, the hemoglobin concentration of the blood and a single carbon dioxide concentration in the blood at a single known P_{CO_2}.

The usual method for obtaining a sample of normal alveolar air is the following (Haldane, 1905): First, the subject takes a normal inspiration; at the end of inspiration he suddenly expires forcefully, and a sample of the last portion of the expired air is taken. This sample is called "inspiratory alveolar air." Second, at the end of a normal expiration the subject again expires very forcefully, and the last portion of this expired air is also collected; this sample is called "expiratory alveolar air." Third, the concentrations of carbon dioxide in these two samples of alveolar air are measured, and the average is considered to be the carbon dioxide concentration in normal alveolar air.

Step 3. The determination of carbon dioxide concentration in mixed venous blood is considerably more difficult. It is based on a principle first established by Loewy and von Schroetter (1903) and further developed by Plesch (1909) that if one breathes his own expired air long enough, the carbon dioxide partial pressure in the alveolar air will become equal to the carbon dioxide partial pressure of the mixed venous blood. In practice, however, rebreathing cannot continue too long, for otherwise recirculation of blood during the course of rebreathing will change the venous carbon dioxide concentration before equilibrium can be established. For this reason, several different procedures have been devised since 1903 by different investigators for obtaining alveolar air equilibrated with mixed venous blood and yet without prolonged rebreathing. The earlier procedures required serial sampling of the expired air, followed by chemical analysis of this air and plotting of the results. These procedures naturally were time consuming. The advent of rapid CO_2 analyzers have greatly simplified the technique. A method which is currently in wide use is exemplified by that introduced by Collier (1956), which is as follows: The subject is allowed to rebreath from a rubber bag which initially contains 0.5 to 1.0 liter of 7 to 8 per cent carbon dioxide in oxygen. During rebreathing, a portion of the air flowing to and from the bag is directed through an infrared carbon dioxide analyzer. This analyzer provides an output which is proportional to the instantaneous partial pressure of carbon dioxide in this air. With each successive breath, the gas in the bag mixes with the alveolar air to produce a carbon dioxide tension more closely approximating that of the oxygenated mixed venous blood. Eventually the partial pressure of carbon dioxide in the bag becomes equal to the partial pressure of carbon dioxide in alveolar air. At this point, the carbon dioxide pressure within the alveoli is in equilibrium with that of oxygenated mixed venous blood, and the P_{CO_2} detected by the carbon dioxide analyzer represents the oxygenated mixed venous P_{CO_2}.

Figure 4–2 illustrates a typical determination of mixed venous P_{CO_2} by this method. Note that before the rebreathing procedure was begun, the expired air had a P_{CO_2} of approximately 41 mm. Hg, and the inspired

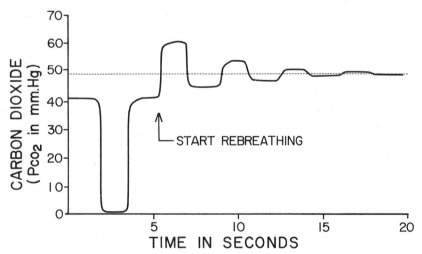

Figure 4–2. Carbon dioxide partial pressure of inspired air and expired air during the course of the rebreathing procedure of Collier (1956). The dashed line represents the value at which inspired air P_{CO_2} is equal to expired air P_{CO_2}. This value represents the oxygenated mixed venous P_{CO_2}.

air had a Pco_2 of about zero. Immediately after the initiation of the rebreathing procedure, the air inspired from the bag had a Pco_2 of 61 mm. Hg, and the first gas expired had a Pco_2 of 45 mm. Hg. With each additional breath, the Pco_2 of the air inspired from the bag was reduced, and that of the gas expired into the bag was increased, until after approximately 13 seconds of rebreathing the two had become equal. In this case, the "plateau" Pco_2 was 48.5 mm. Hg, which is assumed to be the Pco_2 of the oxygenated mixed venous blood. Referring again to the carbon dioxide dissociation curve for oxygenated whole blood shown in Figure 4–1, we find at point B that a Pco_2 of 48.5 mm. Hg is equivalent to 52.3 volumes per cent of carbon dioxide in the mixed venous blood.

Step 4. Now, to calculate the cardiac output, let us assume that the amount of carbon dioxide exhaled in one minute as determined in step 1 was 225 cc., that the arterial carbon dioxide concentration was 49.0 volumes per cent as determined in step 2, and that the venous concentration was 52.3 volumes per cent as determined in step 3. We can calculate the cardiac output, using the Fick formula, as follows:

$$\text{Cardiac output} = \frac{225}{52.3 - 49.0} = 68 \text{ deciliters/min.} = 6.8 \text{ liters/min.}$$

When using the rebreathing method of Collier, it is often found that a distinct plateau cannot be obtained before recirculation of blood causes the mixed venous Pco_2 to rise abruptly. Such a failure to obtain a distinct plateau is generally due to an initial carbon dioxide partial pressure in the bag which is too high. However, if the initial carbon dioxide pressure in the rebreathing bag is no more than 10 to 20 mm. Hg above the partial pressure of carbon dioxide in mixed venous blood, a distinct plateau can nearly always be obtained (Collier, 1956; Ashton and McHardy, 1963; Farhi and Haab, 1967). For this reason, most users of this method often prepare several rebreathing bags of various carbon dioxide partial pressures, and employ a trial and error procedure until the proper gas mixture is found.

Another rebreathing method which has been used frequently in recent years was introduced by Defares (1958, 1961). This method utilizes the principle first recognized by Dubois (1952) that if a person rebreathes from a bag, the CO_2 tension within the bag increases exponentially with the number of expirations and gradually approaches a limiting value, this limiting value being the Pco_2 of the mixed venous blood. In order to determine mixed venous Pco_2 by this method, the subject is allowed to rebreath deeply and rapidly from a rubber bag for approximately five breaths. The exponential rise of Pco_2 within the bag is then ascertained, and the mixed venous Pco_2 is interpolated.

Possibilities of Error in Using the Rebreathing Methods

Though the indirect Fick method is sound in principle, unfortunately the necessary measurements cannot be made with enough precision to achieve a high degree of accuracy. The most likely errors are the following:

1. The difference between arterial Pco_2 and venous Pco_2 is only a few millimeters of mercury. Therefore, a very light error in the physical or chemical determinations of carbon dioxide in the alveolar air can cause a marked error in the calculated cardiac output.

2. One cannot be sure that an average between "inspiratory alveolar air" and "expiratory alveolar air" is the true average Pco_2 of the arterial blood, because this average might well be weighted in favor of one or the other of these two alveolar airs, depending upon the character of the respiratory cycle and local conditions in the lungs. Furthermore, abnormal perfusion-ventilation ratios in different parts of the lungs can readily cause a serious error in this measurement.

3. The method for measuring the mixed venous blood Pco_2 is subject to many possible errors, the most important of which is that the mixed venous Pco_2 can rise during the rebreathing procedure. The principle cause of this is recirculation of the blood before the procedure can be completed. As has been discussed above, when using the method of Collier or one of its modifications, recirculation of blood can prevent the occurrence of a normal plateau. Fahri (1967) has claimed that this absence of a plateau prevents the record from being misread, but Ashton (1963) has pointed out that if the carbon dioxide tension in the lung-bag system is too high for equilibrium to have been possible by the time recirculation occurs, a later equilibrium may still be obtained with mixed venous blood containing a portion of recirculated blood. In this case the plateau will give an overestimate of mixed venous carbon dioxide partial pressure. Fortunately, this problem of recirculation is not as severe as it might at first appear, because as the blood passes through the systemic circulation, its Pco_2 becomes equilibrated with the Pco_2 of the tissues. In this way, the tissues prevent most of the excess carbon dioxide in the arterial blood from returning to the venous blood. Nevertheless, the error still exists and could cause a falsely low cardiac output calculation.

4. Another possibility of error during the rebreathing process is that the deep respirations, such as are required in the method of Defares, can alter the cardiac output.

5. A final source of error that occasionally is important is that the indirect Fick method measures only the pulmonary capillary flow, and any flow through a pulmonary shunt is not measured. Indeed, Bing, Vandam, and Gray (1947) have estimated the blood flow through pulmonary shunts by subtracting the indirect Fick measurement of cardiac output from the direct Fick measurement, which difference theoretically equals the shunt flow.

Variations in Rebreathing Methods

A considerably different variation in the rebreathing method was that first used by Burwell (1924a, 1924b), in which oxygen instead of carbon dioxide was used as the indicator. Burwell's method was to determine the arterial concentration of oxygen in a sample of arterial blood and to determine the mixed venous oxygen concentration by a respiratory procedure. To make this second determination, the subject was required to rebreath from a rubber bag containing 0.7 to 2 per cent oxygen and 6 to 7 per cent carbon dioxide. The subject breathed deeply in and out of this bag two times, this process requiring not over 10 to 15 seconds. At the end of these two breaths, the concentration of oxygen in the bag would obviously be a little closer to equilibrium with that in the mixed venous blood than was true at the beginning of the rebreathing. A sample of the last portion of air exhaled was, therefore, taken for analysis. After the subject had reestablished normal breathing some 15 to 30 seconds later, two more deep breaths were taken from the bag, and another sample of air was taken. This process was repeated several times, usually 4 to 6 times, and the concentrations of oxygen in the samples of air were recorded. After several repetitions of the rebreathing, the oxygen concentration in the alveolar air samples was usually stable and the Po_2 of this air was then considered to be essentially equivalent to the Po_2 of the mixed venous blood. To be as accurate as possible in determining the mixed venous concentration of oxygen, a sample of the last expired air following the equilibration procedure was then taken and placed in a tonometer with a small amount of blood obtained from the subject. The oxygen of the blood was equilibrated with that of the expired air, and the blood oxygen concentration was then determined by usual chemical methods. Subtracting this value for the venous oxygen concentration from the value for arterial concentration, the A-V oxygen difference was readily obtained, and the usual Fick formula could be used for calculating the cardiac output.

More recently, Cerretelli (1966a) and Farhi (1966) have demonstrated that if a person is allowed to rebreath a gas mixture of 7 to 8 per cent carbon dioxide in nitrogen from a 1 liter rubber bag, a well defined Po_2 plateau can be obtained which is similar to the Pco_2 plateau obtained in the rebreathing method of Collier described above. This Po_2 plateau is assumed to represent the value of mixed venous Po_2. Cerretelli, in the original description of the method, employed a respiratory gas mass spectrometer for the determination of oxygen tensions in the rebreathing apparatus. The requirement for such a device would naturally limit the use of this method, and Farhi later demonstrated that a rapidly responding oxygen electrode could be used with satisfaction in this procedure.

Results

Cardiac output values obtained in the earlier studies employing various rebreathing techniques with carbon dioxide as the indictor were, in general, consistently below or equal to those obtained by the direct Fick method (Hayasaka, 1927; Lawrence, 1927; Grollman, 1932; Kroetz, 1930; Ewig, 1931). Furthermore, these earlier techniques were often unreliable. This is shown in a comparative study of the indirect Fick method employing a rebreathing technique and the direct Fick method used in the same subjects (Gray, Bing, and Vandam, 1947). In this study the two procedures gave nearly equal values in many persons, though a discrepancy of as much as 40 to 50 per cent was not uncommon. In these instances of major discrepancy, the indirect Fick method usually gave the higher values.

Unfortunately, the modern advances in technology have improved neither the accuracy nor the reliability of the rebreathing methods. Modern rebreathing techniques continue to provide cardiac output values which are consistently lower than those obtained by the direct Fick method (Jernerus, 1963; Muiesan, 1965, 1968; Ferguson, 1968; Clausen, 1970), and in a more recent comparative study similar to that of Gray (1947), Clausen, (1970) frequently found discrepancies of as much as 30 to 50 per cent between the values obtained by a rebreathing method and those obtained by the direct Fick method; in all of these instances, the rebreathing technique provided the lowest cardiac output value. Thus, from the above discussion it would appear that although the rebreathing methods using carbon dioxide as the indicator are sound in principle and although advanced technology has reduced the labor involved in their performance, the technique is still somewhat less reliable and less accurate than the direct Fick or dye-dilution methods.

Since rebreathing methods with oxygen as the indicator have not been used extensively in the past, it is difficult to evaluate their accuracy. Burwell's oxygen method (1924b) usually gave values about 20 per cent below those commonly obtained with the direct Fick method. However, the more recent studies (Cerretelli, 1966a; Cruz, 1969) have provided values for cardiac output which agree well with what is usually considered normal cardiac output. Thus, although this technique has not been fully tested, it appears that it may eventually prove to be a valuable tool for the measurement of cardiac output.

THE SINGLE BREATH METHOD

The single breath method is not in reality a completely new technique for determining cardiac output. Rather, it is but an additional step in the evolution of the indirect Fick method. Portions of the basic concept of the method can be seen in studies by Douglas and Haldane (1922), and later by Fenn and Dejours (1954) and Knowles, Newman, and Fenn (1960). However, it was not until the studies of Kim, Rahn, and Farhi (1966) that the theory and application of the technique were fully described. The major differences between the single breath method and the rebreathing methods described earlier are the following: (1) The single breath method does not require rebreathing procedures for the determination of mixed venous P_{CO_2}. Rather, mixed venous P_{CO_2} is determined by analysis of a single prolonged expiration. (2) The method does not determine oxygenated mixed venous P_{CO_2} as in the rebreathing methods, but it provides an estimation of the true mixed venous P_{CO_2}. (3) The single breath method provides an indirect approach to the estimation of arterial P_{CO_2} and, therefore, does not require the direct sampling of "normal alveolar air."

The basic theory of the single breath method is as follows: If the normal rate of expiration is retarded, or if the breath is held, the alveolar and arterial concentrations of carbon dioxide begin to rise. During this time the mixed venous carbon dioxide concentration as well as the arterial oxygen concentration remains essentially unchanged. The rise in alveolar carbon dioxide concentration, and consequently in arterial carbon dioxide concentration (arterial P_{CO_2} is equal to alveolar P_{CO_2}), is assumed to reflect changes in the carbon dioxide output of the blood perfusing the lung. Therefore, the continuing rise in the alveolar carbon dioxide concentration is a measure of a reduction in the respiratory exchange ratio, R, which is the ratio of carbon dioxide output to oxygen uptake by the lung. Under normal steady state conditions, R has a value of approximately 0.80. However, as alveolar and arterial carbon dioxide concentrations rise, the arterial concentration approaches and will eventually become equal to the mixed venous carbon dioxide concentration. At this point, the exchange of carbon dioxide between the pulmonary blood and the alveoli ceases, and R becomes zero. Since when R is zero, the concentration of carbon dioxide in arterial blood is equal to that in venous blood, and since the oxygen content of arterial blood is higher than that of venous blood, the P_{CO_2} of arterial blood must be greater than the P_{CO_2} of venous blood by virtue of the Haldane effect. When it is recalled that mixed venous P_{CO_2} is normally greater than arterial P_{CO_2}, it becomes evident that at some time during the prolonged expiration, or during the apnea, the P_{CO_2} of arterial blood must equal that of venous blood. Such equality of venous and arterial carbon dioxide partial pressures must occur when R is equal to 0.32, since for every unit volume of oxygen taken up by the hemoglobin of the venous blood, 0.32 volumes of carbon dioxide is displaced without a change in

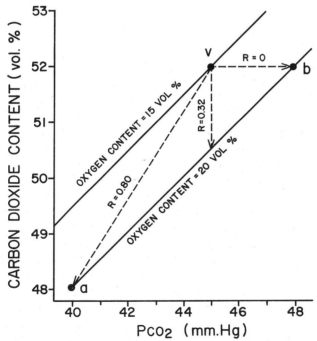

Figure 4–3. Portions of carbon dioxide dissociation curves for normal venous blood and normal arterial blood. Normal venous values for carbon dioxide and oxygen are represented by point a. Point b represents the carbon dioxide and oxygen values of arterial blood when carbon dioxide concentration in arterial blood is equal to that in venous blood. The dashed lines represent the respiratory exchange ratios for various values of arterial carbon dioxide concentration. Note that when R has a value of 0.32, venous P_{CO_2} is equal to arterial P_{CO_2}. [Modified from Kim (1966).]

Pco_2. Thus, if the respiratory exchange ratio is measured continually throughout a prolonged expiration, the alveolar (arterial) Pco_2 which exists at the time R is reduced to 0.32 represents the true mixed venous Pco_2.

The basic concepts described above are illustrated diagrammatically in Figure 4–3, which shows a portion of a carbon dioxide dissociation curve for venous blood and a portion of the curve for arterial blood. Normal venous blood is represented by point v with a carbon dioxide concentration of 52 volumes per cent and an oxygen concentration of 15 volumes per cent. Normal arterial blood is represented by point a with a carbon dioxide concentration of 48 volumes per cent and an oxygen concentration of 20 volumes per cent. The normal respiratory exchange ratio is 0.80, as shown on the dashed line connecting points v and a. During the prolonged expiration, or during breath holding, the arterial point moves along the normal arterial carbon dioxide dissociation curve and approaches point b, at which time arterial and venous carbon dioxide concentrations are equal, and R is zero. As shown in this graph, when R is equal to 0.32, arterial, and alveolar, Pco_2 is equal to venous Pco_2.

In the performance of the method according to the original description by Kim (1966), the following steps are taken:

Step 1. The subject is allowed to breathe into a Tissot spirometer, and oxygen uptake and carbon dioxide output are determined in the conventional manner. From the carbon dioxide output and the oxygen uptake, the normal respiratory exchange ratio is computed.

Step 2. The subject then inspires a tidal volume larger than normal and expires through a high resistance airway which prolongs the expiration for a period of approximately 10 seconds or longer. After approximately 2 to 3 seconds of expiration, samples of air are taken from the airway at 1 second intervals, and the partial pressures of oxygen and carbon dioxide in these gas samples are determined.

Step 3. The Pco_2 of each gas sample is plotted against its Po_2 and the points are connected by a smooth curve as shown in Figure 4–4A. The slope of this curve at any point is equal to the instantaneous respiratory exchange ratio at that point after corrections for the changes in lung volumes are considered. Therefore, tangents to the curve at various points are corrected for changes in lung volume, and the results are plotted against the respective alveolar Pco_2 as shown in Figure 4–4B. Note the relationship between R and Pco_2 is approximately linear within the range of Pco_2 shown here. This is expected, since the carbon dioxide dissociation curve is approximately linear between carbon dioxide partial pressures of 35 to 60 mm. Hg.

Now, referring to Figure 4–4B we see that at a respiratory exchange ratio of 0.32, the corresponding arterial Pco_2 is 46.7 mm. Hg, and for the reasons discussed above, this is also assumed to be the true mixed venous Pco_2. If we assume that the normal respiratory exchange ratio determined in step 1 is 0.80, referring to Figure 4–4B we find that the corresponding arterial Pco_2 is 40.0 mm. Hg. This is considered to be the normal arterial Pco_2. These values for venous and arterial Pco_2 may be converted to concentrations by referring to venous and arterial carbon dioxide dissociation curves. For example, by referring again to Figure 4–3 we see that a

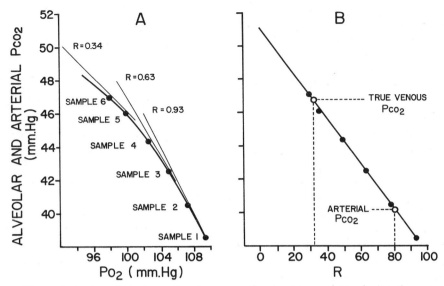

Figure 4-4. Graph A shows the changes in alveolar P_{CO_2} and P_{O_2} during the course of a prolonged expiration. From the slopes of this curve at various points, the respiratory exchange ratios at those points may be calculated. The respiratory exchange ratio which exists at specific points along this curve is illustrated on the tangents to these points. Graph B shows the $R-P_{CO_2}$ relationship obtained from the curve illustrated in graph A. True venous P_{CO_2} and arterial P_{CO_2} are obtained from this curve as explained in the text. [Modified from Kim (1966).]

venous P_{CO_2} of 46.7 mm. Hg represents a carbon dioxide concentration of 52.8 volumes per cent, and an arterial P_{CO_2} of 40.0 mm. Hg represents a carbon dioxide concentration of 48.0 volumes per cent.

Step 4. Cardiac output may now be calculated. Assuming a carbon dioxide output, as determined in step 1, of 225 cc. per minute, cardiac output is calculated as follows;

$$\text{Cardiac output} = \frac{225}{52.8 - 48.0} = 4.7 \text{ liters per minute}$$

The method of Kim has been greatly simplified since its original description (Cerretelli, 1966b; Bickel, 1970; Hlastala, 1971). Cerretelli and Bickel measure alveolar P_{O_2} and P_{CO_2} continuously with a mass spectrometer during the course of the prolonged expiration. Values of P_{CO_2} and P_{O_2} are fed into an X–Y recorder which provides the moment by moment relationship between these two partial pressures. From this relationship, the $R-P_{CO_2}$ curve and the true venous P_{CO_2} may be obtained as described above. Furthermore, the use of a rapidly responding spirometer permits the determination of respiratory flow rate during the prolonged expiration. With this flow rate and with the simultaneously determined values of carbon dioxide and oxygen concentrations, the oxygen uptake and the carbon dioxide output can be computed for each breath. To obtain the normal arterial P_{CO_2}, the normal respiratory exchange ratio is computed from carbon dioxide output and oxygen uptake during a normal breath. Thus, once the normal respiratory exchange ratio is known, all the information necessary for the calculation of cardiac output can be obtained during the course of one prolonged breath. Bickel (1970) and Hlastala (1917) have carried the automation of the procedure one step further, since they fed the information obtained during each expiration into a digital computer for the actual calculation of cardiac output. In this way, cardiac output was measured almost breath by breath.

Possibilities of Error in Using the Single Breath Method

The single breath method is based on several assumptions which have not yet been completely justified and may, therefore, cause considerable error in the results. The major assumptions are the following:

1. A crucial assumption is that the changes in alveolar gas composition during prolonged expiration reflect changes in the gas exchange between the pulmonary blood and the alveoli. It should be noted that such changes could be due to sequential emptying of alveoli with various ventilation-perfusion ratios. However, recent work on normal subjects (Sikand, 1966) has shown that although the various components of the lung, indeed, have a wide range of ventilation-perfusion ratios, they seem to contribute to the expired air in a constant proportion. Thus, the basic assumption seems to be valid, but Kim (1966) has pointed out that in cases in which the uniformity of alveolar gas composition is in doubt, changes in the composition of expired gas during the prolonged expiration may reflect only sequential emptying of alveoli. Under such conditions, application of the single breath method is dangerous.

2. As in rebreathing methods, recirculation of blood during the course of the prolonged expiration could cause an error. Although this is unlikely during the 10 second period required for the expiration, the possibility still exists.

3. It is assumed that the carbon dioxide dissociation curve is linear between partial pressure of 35 and 60 mm. Hg. Although this is not strictly correct, the slope is so nearly linear within this range that the error involved in assuming perfect linearity is small. However, assuming linearity of the carbon dioxide dissociation curve when the mixed venous P_{CO_2} is considerably reduced, such as at high altitude, could cause a significant error.

4. An additional assumption which could possibly produce an error in the calculation of cardiac output is that the respiratory exchange ratio measured in the alveolar gas is equal to or very nearly equal to that in the blood. This would only be true if the quantity of carbon dioxide which is actually stored in the alveolar wall during the expiration is small. Kim (1966) stated that the quantity of carbon dioxide which is liberated by the blood and is actually stored in the alveolar wall is only approximately 1 per cent of the total carbon dioxide liberated. If this is true, the error caused by this factor is negligible.

5. A final source of error stems from the assumption that at a respiratory exchange ratio of 0.32, the displacement of carbon dioxide from hemoglobin by oxygen does not alter the P_{CO_2}. Varying values for this respiratory exchange ratio are given by different investigators. However,

it is obvious that another value could easily be substituted, if proven correct, without altering the basic principle of the method.

Results

Although the single breath method is relatively new and has not been employed extensively to date, the values for cardiac output obtained with the method by some investigators appear to agree satisfactorily with established values of cardiac output. In the combined results of Cerretelli (1966b), Kim (1966), and Hlastala (1971), resting cardiac output values varied from approximately 4 to 6 liters per minute. In addition, Hlastala repeatedly determined cardiac output on three subjects and found that two cardiac output values from the same subject never varied by more than 13 per cent. On the other hand, Gilbert and Auchincloss (1970) compared cardiac outputs obtained by the single breath method with those obtained by a standard indicator-dilution technique and found that the regression coefficient between the results of the two methods was only 0.85, and that the standard error of the estimate was 2.9 liters per minute. Thus, it is obvious that although some investigators believe that the single breath method is both accurate and reliable, this definitely has not been established, and the method must undergo more extensive examination before its validity can be universally accepted.

THE ACETYLENE AND OTHER FOREIGN GAS METHODS FOR DETERMINING CARDIAC OUTPUT

Basic Principles of the Foreign Gas Methods

Many gases are so highly diffusible through the pulmonary membrane that the gas pressure in the pulmonary capillary blood comes to equilibrium with that in the alveoli during the very brief interval that the blood remains in the lungs. If we assume that none of the cardiac output is shunted through channels other than the pulmonary capillaries, the gas pressure in the systemic arterial blood will equal that in the pulmonary alveoli. Furthermore, the concentration of the gas in the systemic arterial blood can be calculated by using the following formula:

$$C_{sa} = P_{al} \times k \tag{4-2}$$

where C_{sa} is the concentration in the systemic arterial blood in ml./liter, P_{al} is the partial pressure of the gas in the alveoli in mm. Hg, and k is the solubility coefficient for the gas in ml./liter/mm. Hg. The solubility coefficient for the gas can be determined by in vitro measurements. Therefore, if one simply knows the gas pressure in the alveoli, he can calculate the gas concentration in the systemic arterial blood.

To determine the blood flow through the pulmonary capillaries, the subject is required to breathe a foreign gas, and special procedures are instituted to obtain, first, the average concentration of the gas in the alveoli over a period of time and, second, the average rate of gas absorption during the same period of time. Then cardiac output can be calculated by using the following formula:

$$\text{Cardiac output (l./min.)} = \frac{Q_g}{k \cdot P_{al}} \qquad (4\text{--}3)$$

where Q_g is the rate of gas absorption in ml./minute.

The problem with all foreign gas methods have been two fold. First, it has been difficult to devise techniques whereby precise measurements of alveolar gas concentrations and rates of gas absorption can be made completely accurately. Second, Formula 4–3 holds only in case there is no gas already dissolved in the venous blood entering the pulmonary capillaries. Therefore, the entire measurement must be made before blood can recirculate through the systemic circulation and back into the pulmonary capillaries again. Since recirculation ordinarily begins within 8 to 12 seconds, it has been almost impossible to devise procedures that can sample alveolar gases accurately within such a short period of time.

Foreign Gases That Have Been Employed

The first foreign gas to be employed for measurement of cardiac output was nitrous oxide, which has also been used in recent years (Markoff, 1911; Krogh, 1912; Lindhard, 1925; Cander and Forster, 1959; Wasserman and Comroe, 1961; Becklake, 1962; Ayotte, 1970). This was followed later by the use of ethylene (Marshall, 1928), ethyl iodide (Henderson, 1925; Starr, 1927, 1928; Donal, 1934), and acetylene (Grollman, 1929; Cander and Forster, 1959; Klausen, 1965), all of which have special properties that made them progressively more adaptable to the foreign gas method. In addition, Bornstein (1910) used essentially the same principle as that described above but measured the excretion of nitrogen through the lungs when the subject breathed pure oxygen rather than measuring the uptake of a foreign gas. By making various assumptions by which he could calculate the mixed venous P_{N_2}, he was able to devise a method that gave some indication of changes in cardiac output but did not give satisfactory absolute measurements.

Though acetylene is the foreign gas that has been most extensively used for measuring cardiac output (this gas will be discussed at greater length below), ethyl iodide also deserves particular mention because it has properties different from those of most other foreign gases that have been employed (Henderson, 1925; Starr, 1928). The principal advantage of ethyl iodide is that most of it is destroyed as it circulates through the systemic circulation. Therefore, even when the subject breathes ethyl iodide for a prolonged period of time, its concentration in the mixed venous blood remains relatively low so that the problem with recirculation is not nearly so acute as it is with some of the other foreign gases that have been employed. Unfortunately, though, ethyl iodide is highly soluble in fats, and this causes its solubility coefficient to change greatly with changes in blood lipids, thus often introducing serious error. Also the concentration of ethyl iodide in mixed venous blood is highly variable from subject to subject and from time to time, and chemical methods for its measurement are very difficult; these considerations led to the abandonment of the ethyl iodide method in the late 1930's. Yet this gas is mentioned because it is still possible that some investigator will find a foreign gas that will be totally removed from the systemic blood before it can return to the heart. If such a gas can be discovered, it should be very simple to devise a completely satisfactory foreign gas method for measuring cardiac output.

THE ACETYLENE METHOD

In a search for the ideal foreign gas for determining cardiac output, Grollman (1929) found acetylene to fit more nearly the criteria for the perfect gas than any of many others which he tried. First, acetylene is not excessively lipid-soluble so that its solubility coefficient does not change with changing lipid concentration in the blood. Second, it is highly diffusible through the pulmonary membrane. Third, it is soluble enough in blood that reasonable quantities of it are removed from the alveoli in only a few seconds' time (which allows accuracy in measurement), and yet it is not so soluble that it is difficult to establish satisfactory equilibrium in the alveoli in the few seconds that are available for the test. Fourth, by a simple modification of the Haldane gas analysis apparatus, the concentration of acetylene in alveolar gas samples can be measured very easily.

One of the difficulties in using a foreign gas method for measuring cardiac output is to measure the precise time that the foreign gas remains in contact with the pulmonary membrane. For instance, if samples of expired alveolar air are taken only 5 seconds apart and one of the expirations is prolonged 2 seconds longer than the other expiration, it is almost impossible to determine whether the gas actually remains in contact with the pulmonary membrane for 5 seconds, 4 seconds, 3 seconds, or for some other period of time. Therefore, very early in the use of foreign gases for measuring cardiac output a procedure was developed which does not require the measurement of the time that the gas remains in contact with the pulmonary membrane (Krogh, 1912; Lindhard, 1925). In this procedure one measures the rate of oxygen absorption at the same time that the rate of foreign gas absorption is measured. Then from the *ratio* of these two rates of absorption one can calculate the arteriovenous oxygen difference and can use the Fick formula (Chapter 2) to calculate cardiac output. In the acetylene method, this is accomplished by the following procedure (Grollman, 1932);

1. The subject rebreathes a mixture of air and acetylene from a bag for a few seconds to equilibrate his alveolar air with the air in the bag. Then, at the end of a deep expiration, a small sample of the last expired air is taken.

2. The subject continues to breathe from the bag for another few seconds, and a second sample is removed in a similar manner.

3. The concentration of oxygen in the first sample and that in the

second sample are measured using the Haldane apparatus; likewise, the concentrations of acetylene in both samples are measured.

4. From the above measurements one calculates arteriovenous oxygen difference by the following formula:

$$\text{A-V O}_2 \text{ difference} = \frac{(O_{2_I} - O_{2_{II}})\,(C_2H_{2_I} + C_2H_{2_{II}})\,(B - 48.1)\,(0.00974)}{2(C_2H_{2_I} - C_2H_{2_{II}})} \qquad (4\text{-}4)$$

where O_{2_I} is the percentage of oxygen in the first sample, $O_{2_{II}}$ is the percentage of oxygen in the second sample, $C_2H_{2_I}$ is the percentage of acetylene in the first sample, $C_2H_{2_{II}}$ is the percentage of acetylene in the second sample, B is the barometric pressure in mm. Hg, 48.1 is the vapor pressure of water in the lungs, and 0.00974 is a factor including the solubility coefficient for acetylene in blood at body temperature. The derivation of this formula is given in detail by Grollman (1932) as well as a review of all the work that led to development of the acetylene method for measuring cardiac output.

It is important to note that one need not time the interval between the first and second samples because the arteriovenous oxygen difference is calculated from the *ratios* of oxygen and acetylene in the samples and not from the actual absorption of acetylene per unit time. Combining Formula 4–4 with the usual Fick equation, we obtain the following formula for cardiac output:

$$\text{Cardiac output} = \frac{2(O_2 \text{ consumption})\,(C_2H_{2_I} - C_2H_{2_{II}})}{(O_{2_I} - O_{2_{II}})\,(C_2H_{2_I} + C_2H_{2_{II}})\,(B - 48.1)\,(0.00974)} \qquad (4\text{-}5)$$

where O_2 consumption is the rate of oxygen uptake by the lungs in ml./minute as measured by any of the usual procedures for measuring oxygen utilization.

In practice, the acetylene method has taken several different forms. In his original procedure, Grollman made it a point to complete the entire rebreathing process in less than 23 seconds, assuming that only an insignificant amount of blood recirculation occurs during this period of time. The first 10 to 15 seconds were consumed in mixing the alveolar air with the gases in the bag, and the last few seconds of the procedure were consumed in taking the samples. Other forms of the procedure have been to take three or more samples and to calculate the arteriovenous oxygen difference from each two successive samples. Indeed, Adams (1941) took as many as six samples and calculated the arteriovenous oxygen difference during the five intervals between the six samples. Unless he found a stable arteriovenous oxygen difference in two or more of the intervals, he considered the measurement to be unreliable, but, if he did find a stable value, he used this value in calculating the cardiac output.

In still another procedure devised by Nielson (Espersen, 1941a), the subject breathed a very high concentration of acetylene for a few seconds at the beginning of the breathing process to bring the alveolar acetylene to equilibrium very rapidly with that in the bag. This shortened the time required for the test and presumably made equilibrium of the gases more nearly complete before the samples were taken. Finally, Gladstone (1935b) attempted other modifications to allow completion of the entire rebreathing process in less than 10 seconds, but his results, in light of present-day measurements of cardiac output, show that he was unsuccessful.

Results and Errors in Using the Acetylene Method

In spite of the many different modifications of the acetylene method that have been offered, the errors that apply to all foreign gas methods, as discussed above, have never been completely remedied (Keys, 1941). Thus, no one has yet devised a method by which acetylene can be brought to equilibrium in the alveolar air and two successive samples of accurately obtained alveolar air removed in the 10 seconds before blood recirculation begins. For this reason the accuracy of almost all foreign gas methods has been compromised by extending the length of the procedure to a period long enough to obtain adequate alveolar air samples, in the hope that the quantity of recirculation of blood is not significant. Unfortunately, direct measurements of the quantity of recirculation show that as much as 52 per cent of the blood has completely recirculated within 23 seconds (Starr, 1930), which is the period that Grollman allowed for completion of his procedure. Because of this fact, undoubtedly a large and indeterminate amount of acetylene is already present in the mixed venous blood prior to obtaining the two samples of alveolar air required for the measurement. The presence of acetylene in the mixed venous blood greatly reduces the rate of acetylene absorption so that the calculated cardiac output is, therefore, considerably less than the true value, thus explaining why many different investigators have found the acetylene method to give considerably lower values for the output than either the direct Fick procedure or the indicator-dilution procedure. For instance, Berseus (1950) found the acetylene method to give values 45 per cent lower than the Fick method when the two methods were applied simultaneously, and Chapman (1950) also found the values to be 31 per cent too low in similar studies. In a collection of several hundred acetylene, Fick, and indicator-dilution studies summarized in the Handbook of Circulation (1959), the average cardiac output for the average human adult as measured by the acetylene method was 35 per cent below that measured by the other two methods. In a study in dogs, Maltby (1936) found the acetylene method to give values averaging 32 per cent below those determined simultaneously by the direct Fick method. Finally, in a recent comparative study, Klausen (1965) found that a carbon dioxide rebreathing method and the acetylene method for determining cardiac output provided almost exactly the same values in resting subjects. It should be recalled that the carbon dioxide rebreathing methods usually provide cardiac output values lower than those obtained with either the direct Fick or the indicator-dilution technique.

Yet the acetylene method, as well as the ethyl iodide and other foreign gas methods, should not be discarded lightly, for two reasons: First, a very large segment of our knowledge of the field of cardiac output has been amassed through studies using foreign gas methods (Grollman,

1932; Starr, 1933, 1934, 1935; Maltby, 1934; Gladstone, 1935a, 1935b; Scott, 1940; Bersius, 1943; and many others). Second, it is possible, if not probable, that the error remains reasonably constant from subject to subject and that by applying an appropriate correction factor one can still use the foreign gas method to measure *changes* in cardiac output. Certainly the ease of applying these methods is a tremendous advantage over the Fick and indicator-dilution procedures. It should also be noted that in at least one comparative study of the dye-dilution method and the acetylene method (Asmussen, 1952), the acetylene results averaged only 5 per cent below the dye-dilution results in 23 comparisons made under resting conditions, and during exercise the results averaged almost exactly the same in a total of 58 comparisons. In this particular study Asmussen was especially careful to complete his measurements in the shortest possible time, and this could have accounted for the difference between his results and those of others.

One final point should be considered regarding the acetylene method. Though many different investigators have emphasized the error that can be introduced by recirculation of the blood before completion of rebreathing, it is likely that only part of the error can be accounted for by this factor alone, for the following reasons: Acetylene is a highly diffusible substance so that most of the gas probably diffuses out of the blood as it passes through the systemic circulation, leaving rather little acetylene to return to the pulmonary capillaries during the period of measurement, even though the total quantity of blood returning might be very significant. If we cannot be sure that all the error is caused by recirculation of blood containing acetylene, we must look for other possibilities of error. A likely error is that the alveolar air does not become satisfactorily equilibrated with the acetylene in the rebreathing bag during the period of the determination. This could be true especially if the gases in certain portions of the lung are slow to equilibrate, as is well known to occur in many pulmonary diseases and even to a less extent in the normal lung. Some modern investigator, having more recent knowledge of pulmonary function not available to Grollman when he devised his acetylene method and knowing the physiological properties of additional types of gases, could very possibly devise a completely satisfactory foreign gas method for accurate measurement of cardiac output. The problem is not insurmountable, even though many investigators who extoll the virtues of the Fick and indicator-dilution methods would have one believe that these two methods are the final answer.

Chapter 5

INDIRECT ESTIMATION OF CARDIAC OUTPUT BY PHYSICAL METHODS: THE PULSE CONTOUR AND ROENTGENOGRAPHIC METHODS

ESTIMATION OF CARDIAC OUTPUT FROM THE ARTERIAL PRESSURE PULSE CONTOUR

None of the methods considered thus far for measuring or estimating the cardiac output has been capable of measuring the output from beat to beat. Instead, most give only a mean cardiac output value over a period of 20 seconds to a few minutes. In a search for a method that would give the stroke volume output of the heart with each beat, many different investigators have recognized that the arterial pressure pulse contour is physically related to the stroke volume output and that, if appropriate physical relationships could be found, one would have a very valuable method for recording cardiac output from heart beat to heart beat. Attempts by different investigators to establish these physical relationships have met with varying degrees of success, but, unfortunately, the different investigators have yet to agree that any one of them has developed a completely accurate procedure. The discussion that is to follow mainly describes Warner's method (1953) for estimating cardiac output from the pressure pulse contour, but the basic principles apply almost equally as well to several of the other methods, especially to the Hamilton and Remington procedure (1947) from which it was partially derived.

BASIC PRINCIPLES OF ALL THE PRESSURE PULSE CONTOUR METHODS

Estimation of Diastolic Blood Flow from the Decline in Diastolic Pressure

All of the different methods for estimating stroke volume output from the pressure pulse contour have some basic features in common. For

99

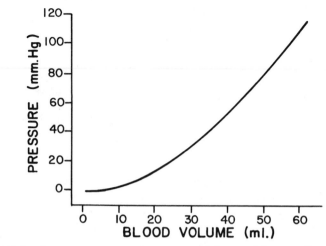

Figure 5-1. Average pressure volume curve of the arterial system for the 12 kg. dog. [From data in Guyton, Armstrong, and Chipley (1956b).]

instance, almost all of them record the pressure pulse contour from the root of the aorta rather than from some other part of the arterial system, and they all make use of a principle first suggested by Hürthle in 1896 that during diastole the rate of blood drainage out of the arterial tree to the veins is proportional to the arterial pressure decline. This principle can be explained by referring to the pressure-volume curve of the arterial system illustrated in Figure 5-1. This curve was derived from live, normal dogs in our laboratory (Guyton, 1956b) by rapidly measuring the blood volume decrease in the entire arterial tree as the arterial pressure fell following the onset of cardiac fibrillation. Note that in the normal arterial pressure range the pressure-volume curve is almost linear, a fact also demonstrated on isolated arteries (Green, 1950). The curve of Figure 5-1 shows that reduction in the arterial pressure from 118 mm. Hg down to 60 mm. Hg is equivalent to the removal of approximately 18 ml. of blood from the arterial tree.

Now, to explain Hürthle's concept, let us observe Figure 5-2, which shows a normal arterial pressure pulse contour. During diastole, between points L and M on the pressure pulse contour, the aortic valve is closed, and the only blood leaving the arterial tree is that which drains through the peripheral vessels into the veins. Therefore, if we know the pressure-volume curve of the arterial tree of this particular animal, we can calculate the volume of blood which drains from the arteries to the veins during the interval of time between points L and M, using the following formula:

$$D_d = C \cdot \Delta P \tag{5-1}$$

in which D_d is the diastolic drainage, C is the capacitance of the arterial tree which is the change in volume of the arterial tree for each unit change in pressure, and ΔP is the pressure drop from point L to point M in the figure. If we assume that the pressure between points L and M falls twice

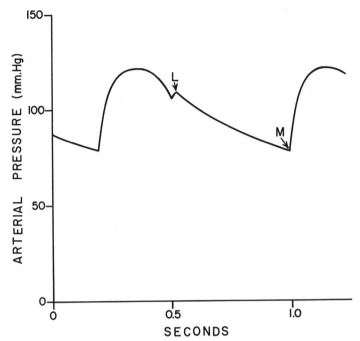

Figure 5–2. A normal arterial pressure pulse contour, showing the interval of diastolic drainage between points L and M.

as much during one heart cycle as during the next heart cycle, and if we assume that the pressure-volume curve is entirely linear, then the diastolic drainage would be twice as great during the first cycle as during the second cycle. Therefore, the rate of decline of the pressure during diastole is at least a rough measure of the cardiac output from heart beat to heart beat.

To estimate even more accurately the amount of blood drainage through the peripheral vessels during diastole, almost all investigators have made use of a finding first reported by Whittaker and Winton (1933) that in the normal animal the blood flow from the arteries to the veins is proportional to the arterial pressure in millimeters of mercury minus 20 mm., or in mathematical terms:

$$\frac{dV}{dt} \propto P - 20 \qquad (5\text{--}2)$$

where dV/dt is rate of blood flow and P is pressure in millimeters of mercury. Though this formula is not precise, nevertheless it is accurate enough for estimating drainage through the systemic tree. Combining Formulas 5–1 and 5–2, we can see that the diastolic drainage is proportional to the mean diastolic pressure ($\overline{P}_d$) minus 20 times the duration of diastole (T_d), or in mathematical terms:

$$D_d \propto (\overline{P}_d - 20) \, T_d \qquad (5\text{--}3)$$

Estimation of Systolic Drainage

In a manner similar to the calculation of diastolic drainage we can see that the systolic drainage (S_d) is proportional to the mean systolic pressure ($\overline{P}_s$) minus 20 times the duration of systole (T_s); that is:

$$S_d \propto (\overline{P}_s - 20)\, T_s \tag{5-4}$$

From Formulas 5–3 and 5–4 we can establish the ratio of systolic drainage to diastolic drainage as follows:

$$\frac{S_d}{D_d} = \frac{(\overline{P}_s - 20)\, T_s}{(\overline{P}_d - 20)\, T_d} \tag{5-5}$$

Rearranging this formula, we find systolic drainage:

$$S_d = \frac{(\overline{P}_s - 20)\, T_s}{(\overline{P}_d - 20)\, T_d} \cdot D_d \tag{5-6}$$

However, the determination of systolic drainage is not quite as simple as one would expect from the above description, for the following reason. At the very end of systole the pressure at the capillaries is not the same as the pressure in the aortic end of the aorta. Instead, a certain period of

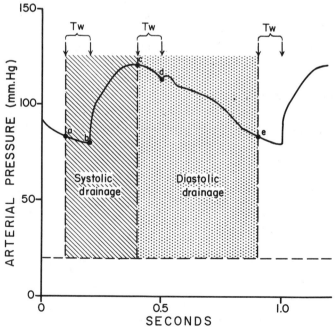

Figure 5–3. A central arterial pressure pulse divided into segments and areas for calculating cardiac output by Warner's method, which is explained in the text.

time is required for transmission of the pulse wave to the periphery. In the following few sections a method will be described, which is essentially the one developed by Warner (1952a, 1953), that allows us to correct for this time lag.

First, let us observe Figure 5-3, which shows another central pulse contour illustrating the end of systole at point d. In this figure the transmission time of the pulse wave to the periphery is indicated by the symbol T_w. At the end of systole, the pressure in the small peripheral vessels will be the pressure at point c in Figure 5-3 because of the lag time in the transmission of the pressure wave to the periphery. Likewise, point e represents the pressure in the small vessels at the end of diastole. The blood flow through the small vessels is proportional to the pressure in these small vessels and is not proportional to the pressure in the proximal aorta. Therefore, the true pressure contour during diastole is represented by the segment of the pressure pulse contour between points c and e in Figure 5-3, and the true pressure pulse contour in the peripheral vessels during systole is that represented between points a and c in the figure. One can readily see that the denominator in Formula 5-5 is proportional to the dotted area (D_a) *under the curve* of Figure 5-3 and that the numerator is proportional to the cross-hatched area (S_a) *under the curve.* Therefore, we can simplify Formula 5-6 as follows:

$$S_d = \frac{S_a}{D_a} D_d \qquad (5\text{–}7)$$

The transmission time, T_w, can be estimated by applying an appropriate correction factor after measuring one of the following: (a) the interval of time between the appearance of the pressure wave in the carotid artery and in the femoral artery, (b) the interval of time between the apex beat of the heart and the appearance of the wave in the femoral artery, or (c) the interval of time between the pressure pulse recorded in the central aorta and in some peripheral artery. In the normal human being under normal conditions, the value for T_w averages 105 msec., which is usually an adequate value to use in the calculation; however, for more exact determination of this factor under different conditions the reader is referred to Warner (1953).

Calculations of Stroke Volume Output and Cardiac Output

From Formula 5-1 we have the diastolic drainage during each cardiac cycle, and from Formula 5-7 we have the systolic drainage during each cardiac cycle. The total drainage during the cardiac cycle, which is also equal to the stroke volume output (SV), is the combination of these two. In other words:

$$SV = (C \cdot \Delta P) + \frac{S_a}{D_d} D_d$$

or

$$SV = (C \cdot \Delta P) + \frac{S_a}{D_a}(C \cdot \Delta P) \qquad (5\text{--}8)$$

or

$$SV = (C \cdot \Delta P)\left(1 + \frac{S_a}{D_a}\right)$$

In using this formula, we must evaluate ΔP, which is the change in pressure in the arterial tree during diastole. Unfortunately, the pressures are not exactly the same everywhere in the arterial tree at the end of systole or at the end of diastole. Therefore, we must estimate these pressures from the pressure pulse contour, as follows: It was discussed above that the pressure wave more distally in the arterial tree lags behind the pressure wave in the proximal aorta. Therefore, to estimate the average systolic and diastolic pressures throughout the arterial tree at the ends of systole and diastole, we must utilize portions of the pressure pulse contour immediately prior to the ends of systole and diastole. Referring again to Figure 5–3 we can assume that the pressure in the proximal aorta at the end of systole is equal to the pressure at point d, whereas the pressure in the peripheral portions of the arterial bed is equal to the pressure at point c, which was explained above. In various parts of the arterial tree, the pressures will be respectively represented by a continuous series of points along the segment cd of the pressure pulse contour. Therefore, we can estimate the average pressure in the arterial tree at the end of systole ($\overline{P}_{cd}$) as being equal to the average pressure of segment $\overline{cd}$. Likewise, we can estimate the average pressure in the arterial tree at the end of diastole ($\overline{P}_{ab}$) to be the average of the pressures along the segment $\overline{ab}$. Now, to determine ΔP as used in Formulas 5–1 and 5–8, we use the following formula:

$$\Delta P = \overline{P}_{cd} - \overline{P}_{ab} \qquad (5\text{--}9)$$

Combining Formulas 5–8 and 5–9, we have a composite expression for stroke volume:

$$SV = C\,(\overline{P}_{cd} - \overline{P}_{ab})\left(1 + \frac{S_a}{D_a}\right) \qquad (5\text{--}10)$$

To calculate the cardiac output (CO), we simply need to multiply the stroke volume output times the frequency of heart beats per minute (F):

$$CO = CF\,(\overline{P}_{cd} - \overline{P}_{ab})\left(1 + \frac{S_a}{D_a}\right) \qquad (5\text{--}11)$$

Estimation of the Capacitance (C) of the Arterial Tree

Although up to this point most of the different procedures for estimating cardiac output from the pressure pulse contour are basically the same, we still have one term in Formula 5–11, the capacitance of the arterial tree (C), which cannot be determined directly from the pressure pulse contour. Furthermore, different investigators have used at least three entirely different methods for estimating the value of the capacitance, as follows:

I. Broemser and Ranke (1930, 1933), Aub (1932), Bazett and his coworkers (1935, 1936, 1941), Wezler and Böger (1939), Deppe and Wetterer (1939), and Evans (1958) all used methods for measuring cardiac output, each of which estimated the capacitance of the arterial tree either from the following relationship described by Bramwell and Hill in 1922 or from a similar relationship derived by Frank in 1899:

$$C = k \frac{V}{v^2} \qquad\qquad (5\text{--}12)$$

in which C is the capacitance $\left(\frac{\Delta V}{\Delta P}\right)$ of the total arterial system, V is the initial volume of the tube, v is the velocity of transmission of the pulse wave, and k is a constant. To use this formula, the different investigators measured the velocity of transmission of the pulse wave to the periphery in several different ways: by measuring the interval of time between the apex beat of the heart and the appearance of the pressure wave in a peripheral artery, by measuring the interval of time between the appearance of the pulse wave in a central artery such as the carotid artery and in a more peripheral artery such as the femoral artery, or by measuring the time lag in the transmission of the pressure wave as measured directly from arteries at different distances from the heart.

II. The second procedure for calculating the value of C was that used by Hamilton and Remington in which they simply measured the capacitances of different segments of the arterial tree or tension-length relationships of arterial rings in *dead* dogs and extrapolated this information to calculate the capacitances of different arterial segments in *live* dogs (Hamilton, 1947b; Remington, 1945a, 1945b, 1947, 1948, 1949, 1952). These authors considered this procedure to be justified because they found that the capacitance of a small segment of vessel does not change significantly when the vasomotor tone changes; the factor that does change is the basic diastolic volume of the vessel rather than the capacitance. On the basis of these theoretical considerations, Hamilton and Remington worked out various tables, based on the surface area of the dog and on the diastolic pressure, for the capacitances of different arterial segments. Then, utilizing a complicated but logically derived procedure, they estimated the diastolic drainage of blood from a combination of capacitances of the respective portions of the arterial tree and pressures measured at specific points on the pressure pulse contour.

III. The simplest and probably the most accurate method for determining the value of the capacitance was a more direct procedure used by Warner and his coworkers (1952a, 1953). These investigators considered that the physical factors which determine the capacitance of the arterial tree are probably far too variable ever to allow prediction of the arterial capacitance without actually measuring it. Therefore, they simply made a measurement of the capacitance of the arterial tree in each person in whom they used the pressure pulse contour method for measuring cardiac output. To do this they proceeded essentially as follows: They made a measurement of cardiac output by some accepted method, such as the Fick or indicator-dilution method, and made a simultaneous recording of the central aortic pressure pulse contour. Then they put the measured value of cardiac output into Formula 5–11, measured all the other values in the formula from the pressure pulse contour besides that of C, and then calculated the value of C. They found that the value of C remained essentially constant in any one individual, so that once C had been determined, it was possible to measure the cardiac output from beat to beat by utilizing this value of C in Formula 5–11.

RESULTS OF USING PRESSURE PULSE CONTOUR METHODS FOR MEASURING CARDIAC OUTPUT

Early results using pressure pulse contour methods for measuring cardiac output were very poor. The first pressure pulse method used to any significant extent for estimating cardiac output was one suggested by Erlanger and Hooker (1904) and later used by Dawson and Gorham (1908) and Rosen and White (1926) in which it was assumed that cardiac output is directly proportional to the pulse pressure times the pulse rate. Unfortunately, these authors did not compare their measurements with measurements made by some reliable method. Subsequent studies by many other workers have shown that estimation of the cardiac output from the pulse pressure is generally unreliable. More recently, Starr (1954a, b, c) proposed a modification of the Erlanger and Hooker method, taking into consideration age as well as pressure measurements. However, Starr's own estimations using this method did not accord well with Fick measurements of output, and Reubi and Schmid (1956) and Brotmacher (1957a) came to the conclusion that the method is much too inaccurate for general use.

Most of the different methods which have utilized pulse wave velocity to determine the capacitance of the arterial tree have also failed to give reliable results when tested critically under widely varying conditions. For instance, Bazett's results (1935) agreed reasonably well with results obtained by use of the acetylene method for measuring cardiac output, but unfortunately the acetylene method has been proved since that time to give values that are far too low. Likewise, the Wezler-Boger method gives cardiac output values that are only about 60 per cent of those measured by the Fick procedure (Schmid, 1951, 1953; Reubi, 1956). In general, the other pulse wave velocity procedures have either been similarly unreliable or have not yet been critically and extensively examined.

On the other hand, the results with the Hamilton and Remington method and with Warner's method have been quite satisfactory in the hands of certain individuals, though unfortunately not universally so. Five different studies comparing the Hamilton and Remington procedure with direct Fick, dye injection, or rotameter measurements of cardiac output revealed an average difference between the values of less than 13 per cent

(Hamilton, 1947b; Remington, 1949; Huggins, 1948, 1949; Longino, 1951). However, the ranges of the differences were from -50 up to $+59$ per cent, which is a very considerable range. A sixth group of investigators (Duomarco, 1948) used a differential flowmeter in open-chest animals to measure cardiac output continuously and at the same time measured the output by the Hamilton and Remington procedure. These workers found the average difference between cardiac output measured by the Hamilton and Remington procedure and by the differential flowmeter to be ±142 per cent, which is a tremendous error. Furthermore, they found the range to vary from -14 per cent up to $+374$ per cent. Still more damning to the procedure was the fact that in certain types of physiological procedures the cardiac output as measured by the differential flowmeter went up, while it went down as measured by the Hamilton and Remington procedure. More recently, Brotmacher (1957a) found that the Hamilton and Remington procedure as applied to man does not give results that are accurate enough to be trusted as a measure of cardiac output.

The method employed by Warner (1953), in which the capacitance of the arterial tree is directly measured in each experimental subject, seems to have had considerable success, at least in human beings. However, it has not been subjected to the same scrutiny as has the Hamilton and Remington method. In Warner's own studies, comparison of his method with the Fick method under a wide range of physiological conditions showed the two measurements to differ from each other by a standard deviation of only ±9 per cent. This is by far the best report on the use of any pressure pulse contour method that has been recorded in the human being. If other investigators substantiate this degree of accuracy, and especially if they substantiate this degree of accuracy in far more widely varying conditions than those studied by Warner, the method will then deserve extensive use in clinical investigative studies, because it allows one to estimate the cardiac output from beat to beat rather than simply estimating mean cardiac output over a period of time. The study of many physiological mechanisms of the circulation could be tremendously benefited by a beat-to-beat cardiac output measurement should this become available in a form that is completely accurate.

ROENTGENOGRAPHIC METHODS FOR DETERMINING CARDIAC OUTPUT

The first successful physical method for measuring cardiac output was the roentgenographic method, which was introduced by Bardeen in 1918. Since that time the procedure has been used in at least four different ways: (1) by exposing serial x-ray plates to determine the difference between systolic and diastolic size of the heart, (2) by recording roentgenokymograms for the same purpose, (3) by recording the changing x-ray density of the heart during the cardiac cycle, which is called the electrokymographic procedure, and (4) by cinefluorographic methods.

Roentgen methods for determining cardiac output are unfortunately limited by the degree of exposure to which the animal or human being can reasonably be subjected and by the expense of the apparatus.

CARDIAC OUTPUT MEASURED BY SERIAL X-RAY PICTURES

Bardeen's original method for measuring cardiac output (1918) was to record two x-ray pictures, one immediately before contraction of the ventricles and one immediately after emptying of the ventricles. Bardeen attempted to take the first x-ray during the isometric contraction period of the heart and the second during the isometric relaxation period. To do this, he used a device that detected the carotid pulse to trigger the two x-ray exposures. Both exposures were on the same x-ray plate and thus permitted immediate comparison of the sizes of the heart before and after ventricular emptying. Yet, because of the double exposure, it was at times difficult to make precise measurements of the systolic and diastolic silhouettes on the same plate.

Bardeen studied x-ray shadowgraphs of the heart in dead persons in whom he was able to control the volumes of fluid in the heart. On the basis of these direct measurements of fluid volumes and of the corresponding measurements of the silhouettes from the x-ray films, he developed a formula for estimating the total heart volume as follows:

$$\text{Heart volume} = 0.53A^{3/2} \qquad (A = \text{silhouette area}) \qquad (5\text{--}13)$$

He used this formula to calculate the heart volume at the end of diastole and then again at the end of systole, and considered the difference between the two to represent the volume of blood removed from the heart during cardiac contraction. (He assumed blood volume in the atria to be essentially the same at the beginning of ventricular contraction as at the end of contraction.) Since the output from one ventricle would be equal to one-half this total volume difference, he used the following formula for calculating stroke volume:

$$\text{Stroke volume} = 0.265 \left(A_{\text{diastolic}}^{3/2} - A_{\text{systolic}}^{3/2} \right) \qquad (5\text{--}14)$$

Measurement of cardiac output in a series of 24 determinations using this procedure gave stroke volume outputs ranging from approximately 40 to 100 ml./beat, which is the range we know to be normal from our modern measurements of cardiac output and stroke volume.

Eyster and Meek (1920), colleagues of Bardeen, improved Bardeen's method by constructing a rapid cassette changer so that two separate x-ray plates could be exposed of the end-diastolic and end-systolic cardiac silhouettes during the same cardiac cycle. However, there was still difficulty in timing the x-ray pictures precisely so that they could be recorded immediately after ventricular contraction. Therefore, Hodges, working at the same university, developed in 1928 a photoelectric procedure whereby movement of the string of an electrocardiograph would trigger the exposure of the x-ray pictures. In this way, it then became possible to record the cardiac shadowgraphs at the appropriate and precise times in the cardiac cycle.

Eyster and Meek (1920) and Hodges (1928) used Bardeen's formula for calculating cardiac output and obtained almost the same results as those first reported by Bardeen. Their values were approximately in the range of those measured by the Fick and dye-dilution procedures. In addition, Meek (1923) showed that the method was useful in measuring cardiac output during different physiological states. For instance, measurements made during exercise showed that the stroke volume output increased only a small amount while the heart rate increased greatly, indicating that by far the major portion of the cardiac output increase in exercise results from a change in heart rate rather than from a change in stroke volume. Other methods which we now know to be accurate have demonstrated this point to be completely correct.

In the years since the original work of Bardeen and associates, the serial exposure of x-ray plates has become one of the most widely used roentgenographic methods for measuring the changes in cardiac volume and, therefore, cardiac output (Soloff, 1956, 1966; Dodge, 1960, 1966; Jones, 1964; Miller and Swan, 1964; Sanmarco, 1966a). However, continued efforts have been made to improve further the reliability and accuracy of the method, and recent developments in instrumentation have outdated the relatively crude apparatus used by Bardeen. Consequently, several changes have been made in the method, although the basic principle has remained unaltered. The major changes are as follows:

More recently developed instrumentation now permits the simultaneous exposure of two x-ray plates in different planes, and most users of the serial exposure technique prefer to take pictures of the heart in two planes for the determination of cardiac volumes. One picture is usually taken of the frontal plane of the heart; a second, of the anterior-posterior plane. Since these two exposures are made at the same time, they permit the visualization of the heart as a three dimensional figure. It would seem probable that biplane exposures of the heart would permit a more accurate assessment of cardiac volumes. However, some persons still prefer to use single plane exposures, and comparative studies of single plane and biplane techniques indicate that both provide values for cardiac volumes and cardiac output which are of comparable accuracy (Sandler, 1965; Dodge, 1966; Sanmarco, 1966a). In techniques employing x-ray exposure in only one plane, the anterior-posterior plane is usually chosen.

Another improvement in the technique which has been brought about primarily by a refinement in instrumentation is that the rate of film exposure has been greatly increased. Modern biplane or single plane serial film changers permit exposures to be taken at rates of approximately 4 to 12 frames per second. Such rapid exposure rates are usually continued over a period of several seconds so that changes in cardiac volume may be visualized throughout the course of several cardiac cycles. This obviously allows more precise evaluation of the changes in cardiac volume during the cardiac cycle.

A third major change is that it is now common practice to inject a radiopaque contrast medium into the heart prior to the exposure of x-ray films. Probably the most commonly used contrast media are sodium and methyl glucamine diatrizoate. Use of these materials allows direct visualization of the interior dimensions of the cardiac chamber, and one would expect that in this way a more accurate estimation of changes in cardiac volume could be obtained than by the visualization of the external dimensions of the heart. However, some recent studies indicate that changes in cardiac volume based on changes in external dimensions are as accurate as those based on changes in internal dimensions (Davila, 1966a; Sanmarco, 1966a). Nevertheless, it is reasonable to expect that methods based on internal dimensions of the cardiac chamber are more accurate, since in these methods such factors as changes in ventricular wall thickness do not have to be considered.

Unfortunately, the various contrast media used for the roentgenographic determination of cardiac output are not without cardiovascular side effects which may cause errors in the estimation of true cardiac output (Kawai, 1964; Vandenberg, 1964; Brown, 1965; Friesinger, 1965; Rahimtoola, 1967; Zelis, 1970; Bove, 1971a). The changes reported following injection of contrast media are highly varied, but in general they include either a decrease or an increase in cardiac work, an increase in heart rate, and in some cases an increase in stroke volume output. Dodge (1966), however, states that the changes which occur after injection of contrast material are evident only after several seconds or minutes following the injection and, therefore, do not affect the heart volume during the actual filming procedure.

Calculations of Heart Volumes and Cardiac Output from Internal Cardiac Chamber Dimensions

In recent years a number of methods have been used to calculate chamber volumes from biplane x-ray films (Chapman, 1958; Dodge, 1960, 1966; Arvidsson, 1961; Hallerman, 1963; Sanmarco and Stuart, 1966b). Most of these methods assume that the left ventricle can be represented by a three dimensional geometrical figure and that the dimensions of this reference figure may be obtained from the biplane x-ray exposures. One of the most accurate methods is that of Dodge (1960), which assumes the left ventricle to be an ellipsoid. The volume of the left ventricle during systole and during diastole is, therefore, calculated by the equation:

$$\text{Volume} = \frac{4}{3} \times \pi \times \frac{L}{2} \times \frac{D_{AP}}{2} \times \frac{D_F}{2} = \frac{\pi}{6} \times L \times D_{AP} \times D_F \qquad (5\text{--}15)$$

where L is the longest measured axis, D_{AP} is the transverse diameter in the anterior-posterior plane, and D_F is the transverse diameter in the frontal plane. In the method of Dodge, the two transverse diameters are

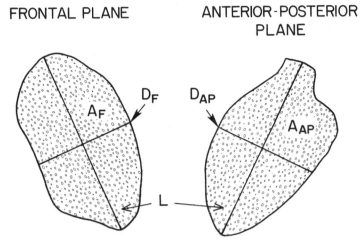

Figure 5–4. Outlines of an opacified left ventricle in the frontal and anterior-posterior planes. The dimensions used in the method of Dodge (1960) for calculation of ventricular volume are indicated. [Modified from Sanmarco and Stuart (1966).]

not measured directly but are calculated from the planimetered area of the ventricle in each plane by the equation:

$$D = \frac{4A}{\pi L} \qquad (5\text{–}16)$$

where A is the projected area of the ventricle in that plane. These dimensions are illustrated in Figure 5–4. In the studies of Dodge, it was shown that volumes calculated by this method in postmortem hearts regularly exceeded the known volumes of these hearts. This discrepancy may be explained in part by the fact that an ellipsoid figure does not accurately represent the actual shape of the left ventricle and in part by the fact that the volume occupied by papillary muscles and cardiac trabeculae are not considered in the calculated volume. However, Dodge recognized that there was a constant relationship between the true volume of the ventricle and the calculated volume. This relationship is as follows:

$$\text{True volume} = 0.928 \text{ Calculated volume} - 3.8 \text{ ml.} \qquad (5\text{–}17)$$

This equation is used to correct all volumes calculated by equations 5–15 and 5–16.

Sanmarco and Stuart (1966b) compared the accuracy of six different methods for calculating chamber volume in excised dog hearts and found that the method of Dodge was by far the most accurate. Using this method, the difference between the calculated volume and the true volume was less than 15 per cent at true volumes between 20 and 30 ml. At true volumes above 30 ml., the difference was only 8 per cent.

To calculate cardiac volume from a single plane exposure, a method similar to that of Dodge (1960) may be used. However, it must be assumed that the transverse diameter of the left ventricle in the plane perpendicular to the exposed plane is equal to the transverse diameter in the exposed plane. In other words, it must be assumed that D_{AP} is equal to D_F (Sandler, 1965; Dodge, 1966). With this assumption, Equation 5–15 becomes:

$$\text{Volume} = \frac{\pi}{6} \times L \times D^2 \qquad (5\text{–}18)$$

where D is the transverse diameter in the exposed plane as calculated from the x-ray.

Results

Although the roentgenographic determination of cardiac volumes and cardiac output has been questioned, primarily on the basis of the geometric considerations employed in calculating ventricular volume and because of the uncertainty of the influence of contrast media on ventricular performance, serial exposure of x-ray plates remains a widely used technique for this purpose. Stroke volume and cardiac output determined by this method are well within the range established by the direct Fick and dye-dilution techniques. Dodge (1962) found that stroke volumes determined by the serial exposure of x-ray plates compared excellently with those determined by an indicator-dilution method. In this study, the mean stroke volume determined by the roentgenographic method was only 2.3 ml. greater than the mean volume determined by the indicator-dilution method. The results of the two methods had a correlation coefficient of 0.98 and a standard error of only 4.2 ml. Similarly, Miller and Swan (1964) showed that the correlation coefficient between the results of the same two methods was 0.92 with a standard error of only 6.9 ml. Furthermore, good correlations between cardiac output determined by serial exposure of x-ray plates and that determined by the direct Fick method have been observed (Gribbe, 1960). Thus it appears that despite reasonable objections, the serial exposure of x-ray plates does provide a suitable means for determining cardiac output, and the widespread use of the method is justified.

MEASUREMENT OF CARDIAC OUTPUT BY ROENTGENKYMOGRAPHY

Roentgenkymography is a method by which movement of an organ can be recorded on a single x-ray plate. The basis of this procedure is the following: A lead plate is placed between the subject and the x-ray film. However, this lead plate has very long 1 mm. slots cut in it, approximately one per centimeter, to allow lines of x-rays to impinge on the plate. During exposure of the subject to x-rays, the film is moved perpendicular to the slots so that it will traverse a distance of approximately 0.9 cm. in about 2 seconds. During these 2 seconds the heart will normally go through at least two complete cardiac cycles while the exposure is being made. The moving borders of the heart will cause the shadows in the lines of x-rays

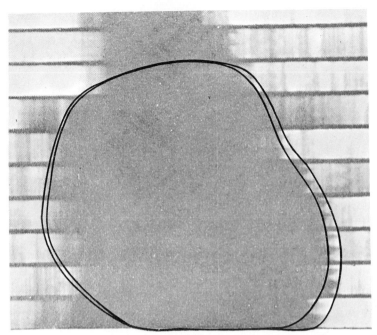

Figure 5–5. An x-ray kymograph of the heart, showing outlines drawn on the heart shadow to designate diastolic and systolic heart size.

to elongate and shorten during the cardiac cycle, and these will be recorded on the film as shown in Figure 5–5. By drawing lines around the heart shadow at the bases of these movements and again around the apices of these movements, one can outline the shadowgraphs for the systolic and diastolic cardiac silhouettes (Johnson, 1937; Keys, 1939; Mayerson, 1943).

On the basis of comparisons between roentgenkymographic determinations of cardiac output and determination by the acetylene method, Keys (1939) developed the following formula, slightly different from Bardeen's formula, for stroke volume output:

$$\text{Stroke volume} = 0.64 \left(A_{\text{diastolic}}^{1.45} - A_{\text{systolic}}^{1.45} \right) \qquad (5\text{--}19)$$

Keys found the average difference between acetylene and roentgenkymographic determinations of cardiac output to be only ±5 per cent, which illustrates that the roentgenkymographic method for measuring cardiac output can give very constant results, whether they are correct or not.

ELECTROKYMOGRAPHIC MEASUREMENTS OF CARDIAC OUTPUT

The electrokymograph is composed of three parts: an x-ray source, a small fluorescent screen, and a very sensitive photomultiplier pickup

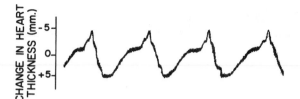

Figure 5–6. An electrokymogram, showing the changes in cardiac thickness during the heart cycle.

placed adjacent to the fluorescent screen. In determining cardiac output, Ring (1949, 1950a, 1950b, 1952) and his associates used a collimated beam of x-rays approximately 3 cm. in diameter, and the beam was passed posteroanteriorly directly through the middle of the ventricles. The thickness of the heart increases during diastole and decreases during systole; therefore, the intensity of the incident x-rays on the fluoroscopic screen varies during the cardiac cycle, giving a record of the type illustrated in Figure 5–6. This record can be calibrated by placing a known thickness of x-ray opaque material in the beam during the course of measurement and recording the change in the record caused by the opaque material. This makes it possible to record in absolute units the pulsatile changes in thickness of the heart.

If it can be assumed that the changes in the other dimensions of the heart vary proportionately with the changes in A-P thickness, it should be possible to derive a reasonable formula for calculating cardiac output from the electrokymogram. Thus, Ring and his associates derived the following formula (1949):

$$\text{Stroke volume} = 12.2 \left(T^2_{\text{diastolic}} - T^2_{\text{systolic}} \right) \tag{5–20}$$

where T is the thickness of the heart.

Using this formula, Ring compared cardiac outputs measured by this procedure with cardiac outputs measured by the ballistocardiograph (1949), the Fick procedure (1950a), and the dye-dilution procedure (1950b). The comparative values were in almost all instance within 25 per cent of each other. This accuracy is probably not so satisfactory as that of the roentgen methods which measure the entire shadow of the heart. Nevertheless, the electrokymograph does provide a very simple procedure for estimating the cardiac output. Furthermore, it can be used without any inconvenience or pain to the patient, and there is reason to believe that it would have reasonable accuracy even in exercise and other types of physiological stress. In another laboratory, Greer (1958) demonstrated that Ring's electrokymographic method records changes in the A-P dimension of the heart quite satisfactorily when compared with measurements made by sonarcardiography.

Despite the relative simplicity of the electrokymographic and the roentgenkymographic techniques, these methods have almost completely disappeared from use. This can be attributed primarily to the increased popularity of other roentgenographic methods; namely, the serial x-ray exposure procedures described above, and the cinefluorographic methods to be described below, which have proven themselves to be more accurate and reliable.

CINEFLUOROGRAPHY AND CINEANGIOGRAPHY FOR ESTIMATING CARDIAC OUTPUT

Cinefluorography means making motion pictures of a fluoroscopic image, and cineangiography means making motion pictures of the fluoroscopic images of the cardiovascular system. The principles applied to the determination of cardiac output by cinefluorography are the same as those applied to the use of the serial x-ray exposure method, the only difference between the two methods being that with cinefluorography, as many as 60 or more x-ray frames are exposed each second.

There is no distinct advantage in making motion pictures of the heart rather than serial x-ray exposures for the determination of cardiac output. In using cinefluorography for this purpose, frames exposed during diastole and systole are selected, and the ventricular volumes during these two phases of the cardiac cycle are calculated by the same methods used to calculate ventricular volumes from serially exposed x-rays. However, the increasing popularity of cinefluorography is due to its ability to follow precisely the changes in other aspects of cardiac performance during the course of the cardiac cycle.

Satisfactory results have been obtained by using either single plane cinefluorography (Rushmer and Thal, 1951; Gribbe, 1959, 1960; Greene, 1967) or biplane cinefluorography (Chapman, 1958, 1966; Rackley, 1967; Tsakiris, 1968; Williams, 1968; Bove and Lynch, 1970a). Rackley (1967) compared the results of the direct Fick and the indicator-dilution methods with cardiac outputs determined by the cinefluorographic technique in a small number of patients with and without cardiovascular defects. In normal persons the mean cardiac output determined by the indicator-dilution method was 4.70 liters per minute, and by the cinefluorographic technique was 4.92 liters per minute, a difference of less than 5 per cent. In patients having a patent dutus arteriosus, mean cardiac output determined by the direct Fick principle was 7.00 liters per minute, and by the cinefluorographic method it was 6.84 liters per minute, a difference of less than 3 per cent. A good comparison between the results of indicator-dilution techniques and cinefluorography has been obtained in dogs by Tsakiris (1968).

A recent development which greatly facilitates the use of cinefluorography is the application of computer techniques to the analysis of the cinefluorographic data (Baker, 1961; Chapman, 1966; Bove and Lynch, 1970a). To do this, various methods have been devised by which the dimensions of the cardiac chambers may be obtained from the cinefilms and fed into an electronic computer. Using this information, the computer then calculates cardiac volume, and other cardiac parameters, by one of the conventional mathematical procedures.

SUMMARY

Since their origin more than 50 years ago, the roentgenographic methods for determining cardiac output have proven themselves to be reasonably accurate. The serial exposure of x-ray plates and the cinefluor-ographic method especially have provided good results, and these two techniques are becoming increasingly popular. However, both of these techniques have certain disadvantages: First, the equipment necessary to perform the procedures is expensive. Second, the necessity of exposing the subject to x-rays obviously limits its use. Finally, the uncertainty of the influence of contrast media on the factor being measured—cardiac output—casts a certain degree of doubt on the results obtained.

Chapter 6

DIRECT RECORDING OF CARDIAC OUTPUT USING FLOWMETERS

Though most of our knowledge of cardiac output *values* in the human being has been attained by use of one or more of the different cardiac output methods described in the preceding four chapters, direct measurement of cardiac output by inserting flowmeters into the circulatory system or by attaching a special flowmeter to the wall of a central vessel of the circulation has provided much of our information concerning cardiac output *regulation*.

The only place in the circulation that flowmeters can be inserted for measurement of cardiac output is some point in the large vessels of the central circulation in the thorax, namely, the aorta, the venae cavae, or the pulmonary artery. When one measures aortic flow or flow in the two venae cavae, the coronary blood flow is not included in the measurement, but measurements of pulmonary arterial flow do include the coronary flow along with the systemic flow. Later in the chapter we will describe methods for inserting flowmeters into the central circulation for recording the cardiac output, but first let us describe some of the different types of flowmeters which have been useful in studying cardiac output by this means.

FLOWMETERS THAT MEASURE MEAN FLOW

Some of the most valuable flowmeters, unfortunately, have a response time that is too long for them to measure pulsatile changes in flow but that nevertheless permit measurement of changes in mean flow over a period of a few seconds. Since it is usually mean flow that is important when measuring cardiac output, and because many of these flowmeters are very simple in design, they have played a very important role in elucidating the mechanisms of cardiac output regulation. Some of them are described below.

117

THE LUDWIG STROMUHR

Figure 6–1 illustrates a very simple flowmeter, the Ludwig stromuhr, which has been used for a century to measure blood flow. The basic parts of this flowmeter are two vertical chambers connected together by a wide-bore tube at the top. The lower portions of the chambers are filled with blood while the upper portions and the connecting tubes are filled with mineral oil. Normally blood flows through the flowmeter by two different pathways—up tube 1 and down tube 2 as well as up tube 3 and down tube 4. However, when tubes 2 and 3 are compressed so that no blood can flow through them, the blood then flows upward through tube 1 into the left-hand chamber. The rising level of blood in this chamber displaces the mineral oil upward, which pushes the blood downward in the right-hand chamber. By using a stopwatch, one can determine the rate of blood flow from the rate of movement of the blood-mineral oil meniscus. Once the blood has flowed upward in the left-hand chamber, tubes 2 and 3 are released, and tubes 1 and 4 are compressed. Now the blood flows upward through tube 3, displacing the mineral oil in the opposite direction in

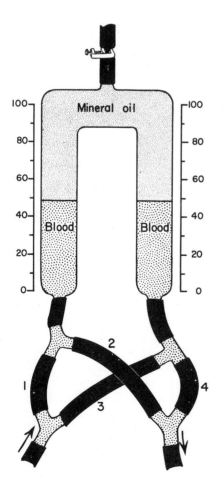

Figure 6–1. A Ludwig stromuhr.

the flowmeter. Here again, the rate of blood flow can be timed with a stop-watch.

The Ludwig stromuhr is described because of its simplicity and because of its inherent accuracy. In the present age of very sophisticated, expensive, and complex flowmeters, many researchers have forgotten how easy it is to make exceedingly accurate measurements of flow in this way. Also, in contrast to many other flowmeters, the Ludwig stromuhr has very little pressure drop, which is a real advantage when attempting to record cardiac output in the venae cavae where a significant pressure drop will cause a serious change in the cardiac output from the normal value. The principal disadvantage of this type of stromuhr is the length of time required to make a measurement.

THE ROTAMETER

Figure 6–2 illustrates a rotameter of the Shipley-Wilson type (Shipley, 1951) but slightly modified in our laboratory from the original design in the following ways: (1) increased size of the recording coil, which gives the rotameter considerably more sensitivity than that of the original type, and (2) use of a plastic float instead of a metal float to reduce blood clotting problems.

Blood flows upward into the rotameter and lifts the float. The space between the float and the conical wall of the flowmeter chamber starts at zero clearance but progressively increases as the float rises. This increase in flow cross-section allows an almost linear rise of the float in relation to the rate of flow.

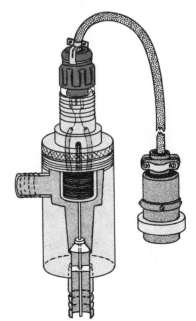

Figure 6–2. A modified Shipley-Wilson rotameter.

As the float rises in the rotameter, a stainless steel tube attached to the float moves upward through the recording coil. Inside the stainless tube is a core of soft iron. By appropriate shaping of the core, one can correct any slight deviations from linearity that might exist in the flowmeter calibration.

The coil of the rotameter forms one limb of an alternating current bridge circuit, and change in inductance of the coil as the float moves upward changes the output of the bridge circuit. This can then be recorded in terms of blood flow by any suitable electrical recorder.

The rotameter will respond to changes in blood flow within one-half to one second. This is not rapid enough to allow pulsatile changes in blood flow to be recorded with each heart beat. However, it is rapid enough to allow the recording of any significant changes in mean blood flow. The pressure drop across the flowmeter averages about 2 mm. Hg, which makes it a very suitable instrument for measuring most blood flows. Yet even this slight pressure drop can be severely detrimental to blood flow in the venae cavae, for, as we shall see in later chapters, a rise of only 7 mm. Hg in the venous circuit of a normal animal decreases the blood flow into the heart to zero. Thus, a 2 mm. pressure drop could decrease the cardiac output by approximately 28 per cent.

Other types of rotameters have been used for measuring cardiac output besides the one designed by Shipley and Wilson (Shipley, 1948; Eckstein, 1949a, 1949b; Hilger, 1956), but the Shipley-Wilson type has particular advantages in the large surface area of the float and its particular shape. These features cause the float to record mainly the momentum of blood flow rather than the resistance to flow. Since momentum is independent of viscosity, the calibration of this type of rotameter does not change greatly with changing hematocrit. On the other hand, the usual rotameters with bob-shaped floats do show considerable responsiveness to changes in viscosity as well as to changes in blood flow.

HEAT DISSIPATION METHODS FOR MEASURING MEAN FLOW

The Thermostromuhr

One of the most widely used heat dissipation methods for measuring blood flow has been the thermostromuhr, which was first introduced by Rein in 1928 (Rein, 1928; Baldes, 1937; Gregg, 1948; Wever, 1956a, 1956b; Aschoff, 1956). Among the best known of this type of flowmeter has been the Baldes thermostromuhr (Baldes, 1937), which was first introduced about 1932 and which is illustrated in Figure 6–3. This flowmeter consists of three essential parts. The figure shows a bakelite device with a slot along its length into which a blood vessel is placed. On the wall of the slot are three essential elements: (1) a thermocouple which lies adjacent to the upstream portion of the vessel, (2) a thermocouple which lies adjacent to the downstream portion of the vessel, and (3) a heater which lies against the vessel between the two thermocouples. As blood flows into the

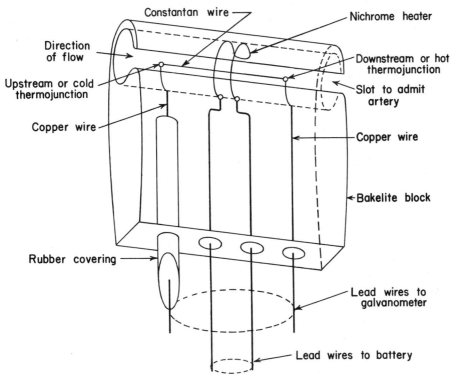

Figure 6–3. A thermostromuhr of the Baldes and Herrick type. [Redrawn from Gregg (1948).]

thermostromuhr, the first thermocouple measures the normal temperature of the blood. Immediately thereafter, the blood becomes heated by the heater, and by the time it reaches the second thermocouple its temperature will be somewhat increased. The second thermocouple then measures this higher temperature. The two thermocouples are connected together in such a way that their outputs oppose each other. Therefore, when the blood temperature is the same upstream and downstream there will be no electrical output. On the other hand, when the blood becomes heated as it passes through the thermostromuhr, a voltage difference will be recorded. If the blood flows very rapidly, there will be little time for it to become heated in the stromuhr. Consequently, the electrical output will be very low. On the other hand, if the blood flows slowly, it will become heated to a far greater extent, and the electrical output will also be very great. Thus, one can calibrate the rate of flow through the stromuhr in relation to the electrical output between the two thermocouples.

Various variations of the thermostromuhr have been devised (Gregg, 1948), including (a) a diathermy method for heating the blood rather than a nichrome wire, (b) a heater system protruding into the blood, (c) a cannulation type of thermostromuhr, which is inserted into the blood stream by cutting the blood vessel and cannulating it at both ends, and (d) various arrangements of thermocouples at different positions both upstream and downstream. Wever (1956a, 1956b) and Aschoff (1956) studied critically many difficult variations in thermostromuhr design and as a result have significantly improved the instrument.

Yet, despite all the different variations, the thermostromuhr is accurate only under special conditions. It is most accurate when the blood flow is completely nonpulsatile, and it is least accurate when marked changes in degree of pulsation occur in the flow. Indeed, under these conditions, the instrument can sometimes be in error more than 100 per cent.

Another problem with the thermostromuhr is that it must be calibrated under the experimental conditions in which it is to be used. For instance, when a change is made from one blood vessel to another, the cross-sectional area of the vessel can make a great difference in the calibration. Also the degree of pulsation can make much difference. Yet, if the thermostromuhr is used to measure blood flow under conditions in which the degree of pulsation is not changing greatly, and if calibration is performed under the precise conditions of the experiment, the flow measurements will be accurate within about 10 to 20 per cent.

The real advantages of the thermostromuhr are that it is inexpensive and that one need not open the blood vessel itself until the end of the experiment when the calibration is carried out. We shall see later that newer devices, which also do not require opening the vessel and have far greater accuracy, are now available for measuring blood flow. Yet the thermostromuhr is described because similar heat dissipation methods keep reappearing for the measurement of blood flow.

Other Heat Dissipation Types of Flowmeters

One of the earliest heat dissipation types of flowmeters was simply a resistance wire inserted down the length of a vessel. Electrical current was passed through the resistance wire, causing it to become heated. The greater the blood flow, the greater was the cooling effect of the blood and the less would the wire become heated. Appropriate electrical apparatus was used to measure the resistance changes of the heated wire. The slower the blood flow, the greater the change in resistance from normal, and the more rapid the flow, the less the change in resistance. By use of an appropriate calibration curve, the blood flow could be related to the resistance changes.

This same flowmeter principle has been applied to a catheter tip flowmeter, using a minute thermistor having a diameter of only approximately 0.5 mm. (Delaunois, 1958, 1961). The thermistor is placed in the wall of the catheter tip and then is inserted into a vessel, as into the root of the aorta. Electrical current passed through the two wires of the thermistor heats the thermistor junction. Because the flowing blood cools the junction, the more rapid the blood flow, the less is the heating of the thermistor, whereas the slower the blood flow, the greater is the heating. Even a change of a fraction of a degree in the temperature of the thermistor changes its resistance markedly, and this can be recorded with appropriate electrical instrumentation. Here again, the blood flow is calibrated against the change in resistance. Furthermore, because of the minute size of the thermistor, blood flow changes can be recorded within a fraction of a second so that the thermistor is capable of measuring extremely rapid changes in mean blood flow and can even record pulsatile changes in blood flow, though not with accuracy.

In more recent years many thermistor flow probes similar to that of Delaunois have been developed (Mellander, 1958, 1960; Suckling and Vogel, 1960; Van Der Werf, 1965; Grahn, 1968, 1969). Grahn and associates have made especially noteworthy improvements in the design of thermistor probes. Using more rapidly responding thermistors, these workers have been able to measure pulsatile aortic flow in dogs. Furthermore, they improved the design of the probe itself in such a manner that directional sensitivity was obtained, and forward flow could be distinguished from backward flow. This was not true of the thermistor probe of Delaunois.

One final point should be mentioned in respect to catheter tip heat dissipation flowmeter probes: these probes do not measure the volume flow of blood, but rather measure the velocity of blood flow. Velocity sensitivity is also a characteristic of other types of flowmeter probes to be discussed later in this chapter.

THE ELECTROMAGNETIC FLOWMETER

The electromagnetic flowmeter was first used in 1936 by Kolin and was independently developed by Wetterer in Germany in 1937. The essentials of this flowmeter are illustrated in Figure 6–4. Figure 6–4A illustrates the principle of electromotive induction in a wire that passes through a magnetic field. The arrows show the direction in which the wire is moving; the plus and minus signs show the polarity of the potential generated in the wire, and the deviation of the meter records the current flow from the two ends of the wire. Figure 6–4B illustrates the same principle, but shows how it applies to the generation of an electrical potential when blood flows between two magnetic poles. In this instance, it is not the wire that is moving but, instead, the blood inside the vessel. Blood, like the wire, is a conductor of electricity, and electrodes placed, as illustrated in the figure, on the surface of the vessel will record the electromotive force developed by the flowing blood. Here again, the plus and minus signs designate the development of electrical potential in the electrodes, and the meter records the current flow from the electrodes.

The earliest electromagnetic flowmeters utilized a large D.C. magnet (Kolin, 1936; Wetterer, 1937; Jochim, 1948), and the apparatus gave a direct relationship between electromotive force generated and the rate of blood flow. Furthermore, the instrument was capable of measuring instantaneous changes in blood flow so that all the minutest details of the pulse flow cycle could be recorded. Because of its linearity of calibration and its rapidity of response, and because it could be utilized without opening the blood vessel, this flowmeter seemed, in theory at least, to be

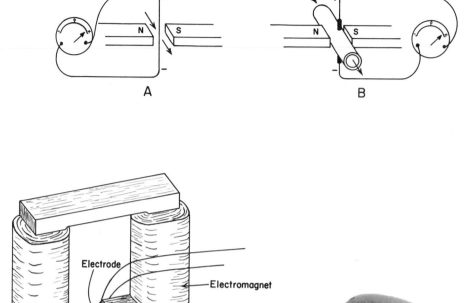

Figure 6–4. (A). Generation of an electromotive force in a wire as it passes through an electromagnetic field. (B). Generation of an electromotive force in two electrodes on a blood vessel when the vessel is placed in a strong magnetic field and blood flows through the vessel. (C). An early type of electromagnetic flowmeter probe. [Redrawn from Kolin (1960).] (D). A modern electromagnetic flowmeter probe for chronic implantation around blood vessels.

the ideal flowmeter. Yet, in practice, two major difficulties delayed widespread use of the instrument: First, to get sufficient electrical output, the size of the magnet had to be exceedingly large. Second, the baseline calibration for zero flow drifted continually because of electrode polarization. For 25 years progressive developments in the electromagnetic flowmeter have come nearer and nearer to solving these problems (Katz, 1938; Kolin, 1941a, 1941b, 1945, 1952, 1960; Richardson, 1952; Denison, 1955, 1960; Spencer, 1960b; Olmsted, 1961), which have now been minimized to an extent that the electromagnetic flowmeter is today one of the most valuable of all flowmeters.

The first major change in the electromagnetic flowmeter was to change from a permanent magnet to an alternating current magnet. A typical early arrangement is illustrated in Figure 6–4C, which shows a powerful alternating current magnet with its two poles applied to the sides of a blood vessel. Above and below the vessel are two minute pickup electrodes. By use of this arrangement, the output from the electrodes becomes alternating current, which prevents polarization of the electrodes and also allows easy amplification of the signal. This earlier form of electromagnetic pickup has been further refined (a) by use of higher and higher efficiency magnetic core materials, (b) by use of appropriate lamination of core materials, (c) by redesign of the shape of the magnet, and (d) by development of more and more sensitive electronic apparatus. Therefore, the modern counterpart of the electromagnetic flowmeter probe shown in Figure 6–4C is that illustrated in Figure 6–4D, in which the probe is entirely encased in plastic and has a size far smaller than that of the original probe; this probe can be implanted in tissues for long-term experiments. Probes are available for arteries as small as 1 mm. in diameter or for arteries as large as 30 mm. in diameter. By use of such implanted probes it is now possible to measure blood flow in animals under essentially normal physiological conditions—that is, assuming that implantation of the probe itself does not cause a change in the operation of the animal's circulation.

Figure 6–5 illustrates the electrical inputs and outputs from the electrodes of three different types of flowmeters, one using a permanent magnet or a D.C. magnet, one using a sine wave alternating current magnet, and one using a square wave alternating current magnet. Figure

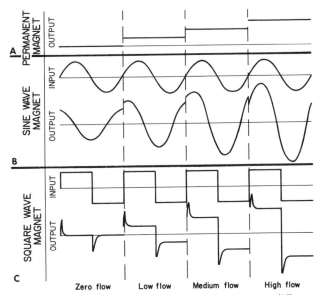

Figure 6–5. (A). Output of a permanent magnet flowmeter at different levels of flow. (B). Input to the electromagnet of a sine wave electromagnetic flowmeter, and output at the electrodes at different levels of flow. (C). Input to the electromagnet of a square wave electromagnetic flowmeter, and output at the electrodes at different levels of flow.

6–5A shows that when one uses the permanent magnet, which has no electrical input, the output increases proportionately as the flow increases. However, with this type of flowmeter, very special nonpolarizable electrodes must be used to prevent excessive drift.

In using the sine wave flowmeter, as shown in Figure 6–5B, there is usually an output from the probe even when the blood is not flowing. This is caused by the so-called "transformer effect"; that is, the alternating electromagnetic field directly induces electrical current in the pickup electrodes simply because of their proximity to the magnetic field and not because of flowing blood. Yet, as the blood flow increases, the electrical output also increases, as illustrated progressively to the right in Figure 6–5B. Also, there is a phase shift of the output from the probe caused by addition of the transformer current to the current resulting from blood flow. Two different types of electronic apparatus have been used to record blood flow from the sine wave output signal. One of these measures the change in amplitude of the output wave [called the "gated" sine wave electromagnetic flowmeter (Kolin, 1960] in which the flow is calibrated against the amplitude changes, and the other measures the phase shift of the output wave (Olmsted, 1961). Either of these types of electronic recording apparatus can give a linear relationship between flow and output.

The square wave electromagnetic flowmeter combines many of the advantages of the D.C. and sine wave types. Each time the square wave current to the magnet reverses polarity, a transformer effect occurs, causing the spikes illustrated in the output signal in Figure 6–5C; these spikes have nothing to do with flow. However, after the spikes are over, flat segments occur in the output recording which do vary with flow. At zero flow, the flat segments are exactly on the zero line. However, they deviate further and further from the zero line as the flow becomes greater and greater. The electronic apparatus for this type of flowmeter "blanks out" the transformer effect and records only the flat portions of the recordings which are then rectified to give a recording that is directly proportional to the rate of blood flow.

Nevertheless, there remains one major difficulty with the electromagnetic flowmeter, and this is the difficulty in determining the zero flow level when the probe is implanted in the tissues. Changes in angulation of the probe on the vessel, changes in electrolytic conditions around the probe, and so forth can all alter this zero over a period of time, and the only way that has proved to be completely satisfactory under all conditions for determining the zero level has been to stop blood flow through the vessel momentarily. Unfortunately, occlusion of the vessel cannot be accomplished with ease in internal vessels, although various devices have been constructed to facilitate this procedure (Khouri and Gregg, 1967; Nelson, 1967; Henry, 1968). Several electronic methods are now available for finding the zero (Denison, 1955, 1960; Kolin, 1960; Olmsted, 1961; Westersten, 1969; Folts, 1970), but it is doubtful that these work under all conditions.

A recent development which makes the use of the electromagnetic flowmeter more applicable to the determination of cardiac output in human subjects is the catheter tip electromagnetic flow probe (Mills, 1966,

1967; Bond and Barefoot, 1967; Wexler, 1968; Braunwald, 1969; Gabe, 1969). In essence, this device consists of an alternating current magnet constructed within the tip of an especially designed catheter, which, when inserted into a blood vessel, permits the blood to flow through the catheter tip probe. Thus, the principle of this catheter tip electromagnetic flow probe is that of electromotive induction as described above. However, an important difference between the catheter tip probe and the type of probe designed to fit around a vessel is that the signal provided by the catheter tip probe is proportional to the flow velocity of blood rather than the volume of flow. This point can be clarified by recalling that the volume flow of blood through a vessel is equal to its flow velocity times the cross sectional area of the vessel, or:

$$\text{Flow} = \text{Velocity} \times \text{Cross sectional area} \qquad (6-1)$$

In the cuff type of electromagnetic probe discussed above, the cross sectional area is constant, and the signal provided by these probes is, consequently, proportional to the volume flow of blood as well as its flow velocity. When using the catheter tip probe, on the other hand, the cross sectional area of the vessel at the tip of the probe is not necessarily constant. Thus, in order to obtain maximum accuracy in determining flow through a vessel with the catheter tip probe, the cross sectional area of the vessel should be determined simultaneously with the velocity signal from the probe. To do this, the diameter of the vessel may be obtained from simultaneous radiographic measurements, and the cross sectional area calculated.

Gabe (1969) used this method to determine aortic flow in human subjects and compared the results with those obtained by a standard indicator-dilution technique. The two methods provided nearly the same mean results, but there was a substantial variation, which was attributed, first, to the difficulty in placing the catheter tip probe correctly within the aorta and, second, to the errors associated with the calculation of aortic cross sectional area. It should be noted, however, that the cross sectional area of the ascending aorta normally changes only about 5 per cent during the course of a cardiac cycle (Greenfield and Patel, 1962). Therefore, the error introduced by assuming a constant area in the ascending aorta would probably be small, and the simultaneous determination of aortic diameter is most likely unnecessary.

THE ULTRASONIC FLOWMETER

In the past few years, another type of flowmeter, the ultrasonic flowmeter, that might prove to be as valuable as the electromagnetic flowmeter has been developed (Kalmus, 1954; Franklin, 1958, 1959; Herrick, 1960). The essentials of such a flowmeter are illustrated in Figure 6-6A, which shows a device that clamps on a blood vessel. A small piezoelectric crystal is mounted in the wall of each half of the device; one of these crystals transmits sound diagonally across the vessel and the other receives

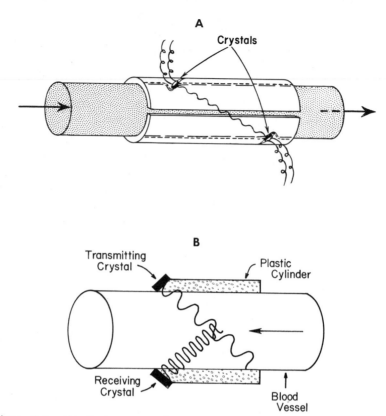

Figure 6-6. (A). Basic construction of the ultrasonic flowmeter probe. (B). Basic essentials of the Doppler ultrasonic flowmeter probe. [Modified from Franklin (1963).]

the sound. The electronic apparatus alternates the direction of sound transmission several hundred times per second, transmitting the sound first downstream and then upstream. The sound frequency can be anywhere between 100,000 cycles and 5,000,000 cycles. When the blood is flowing very rapidly, sound waves travel downstream with considerably greater velocity than upstream. Therefore, the difference between these two velocities is a measure of the rate of blood flow.

Thus, the theory of the ultrasonic flowmeter is very simple, but the electronic instrumentation that goes with it has been difficult to develop for the following reason: The velocity of sound transmission in blood is 1575 meters per second, whereas the normal mean velocity of blood flow in even the most rapidly flowing arteries is normally only ⅓ meter per second. A blood velocity of this value changes the time interval for sound transmission between the two crystals only 0.02 per cent. To devise an electronic apparatus which can detect this slight change in time interval has been a very difficult problem. However, it has been solved by the alternate transmission of sound first down the vessel and then up the vessel. The various extraneous factors besides blood velocity that affect sound transmission in the vessel, such as changes in the physical dimensions of the apparatus, changes in blood temperature, changes in blood density, and others, all alter the velocity of downstream and upstream sound transmission equally. Therefore, these factors can be electronically neutralized. On the other hand, when the blood velocity changes, the velocity of downstream transmission of sound increases while the upstream velocity of transmission decreases. Therefore, while the extraneous factors are neutralized, the blood flow effect actually becomes doubled.

Basically, three types of ultrasonic flowmeters have been developed. The first to be developed depended upon measurement of phase shift of the sound wave picked up by the receiver (Kalmus, 1954; Herrick, 1960). Let us assume that when there is zero flow, the sound wave reaches the downstream crystal pickup exactly in phase with the upstream transmitter. As the flow increases, the phase of the picked-up wave shifts progressively further and further ahead of that of the transmitted wave. By utilizing appropriate electronic apparatus to detect this phase shift, one can record the blood flow.

The second type of ultrasonic flowmeter is the pulsed flowmeter (Franklin, 1958, 1959), which transmits a very short pulse of about 10 sound waves in one direction, then delays for a period of time, transmits an equally short pulse in the other direction, and then delays for another period. This apparatus does not measure phase shift but instead measures the duration of time between transmission of the pulse by the transmitter and reception of the pulse at the receiver. The more rapid the flow, the shorter the time interval for downstream transmission and the longer the time interval for upstream transmission. Thus, except for the manner of transmission and reception of the signal, the pulsed flowmeter records flow in the same way as the phase shift type of meter.

The third and most recent type of ultrasonic flowmeter is the Doppler flowmeter, which is based on the measurement of a frequency shift between the transmitting and the receiving crystals (Franklin, 1961, 1963, 1964, 1966; Benchimol, 1968; Van Citters, 1969; Vatner, 1970). The essentials of this flowmeter are illustrated in Figure 6–6B. The probe consists of two halves of a plastic cylinder which are clamped around a blood vessel as illustrated. A piezoelectric crystal is mounted in each half of the plastic cylinder and faces diagonally into the lumen of the cylinder at an angle of approximately 45 degrees. One of these crystals transmits ultrasound at a frequency of 5,000,000 cycles diagonally across the blood vessel. Some of the transmitted ultrasound is reflected by particulate matter within the blood, and this reflected ultrasound is detected by the second crystal. If the blood is not moving, the transmitted and reflected ultrasound will have the same frequency. However, when the blood is flowing along the cylinder, the frequency of the reflected ultrasound is altered by virtue of the Doppler shift, and the difference in the frequencies of the transmitted and received signals is proportional to the velocity of blood flow. An associated electrical circuit detects and amplifies the frequency shift between the two crystals.

A particular attraction of the Doppler ultrasonic flowmeter is that it offers a good means for radio telemetry of flow signals. Indeed, Franklin and associates (Franklin, 1961, 1963, 1964, 1966; Van Citters, 1969) have used this system for radio telemetry of flow in major vessels of free roving baboons, running horses and dogs, diving elephant seals, swimming sharks, and alligators. And Benchimol (1968) used this system to measure and telemeter blood flow in man.

A particular disadvantage of the Doppler flowmeter is that it cannot distinguish between forward and backward flow. Thus, in cases where backward flow is significant, this system cannot be used accurately. Another disadvantage of the Doppler flowmeter, as well as the other ultrasonic flowmeters, is that it measures the velocity of flow rather than the volume of flow.

METHODS FOR INSERTING FLOWMETERS INTO THE CIRCULATION TO MEASURE CARDIAC OUTPUT

At the beginning of this chapter it was pointed out that to measure cardiac output, a flowmeter must be inserted in or applied to some central part of the circulation, such as the aorta, the pulmonary artery, or the venae cavae. Furthermore, when the aorta or the venae cavae are used, the coronary blood flow is excluded so that, in reality, only in the pulmonary artery can one measure the true cardiac output. In this present section we will describe procedures for recording cardiac output from all these points and then will describe still an additional procedure for bypassing the right heart which also allows recording of total cardiac output and which has been exceedingly useful in studying the effects of systemic circulatory factors on cardiac output regulation.

INSERTION OF FLOWMETERS INTO THE AORTA

Figure 6–7 illustrates a method which may be used for inserting a flowmeter probe, such as the rotameter, into the aorta for measuring cardiac output (minus the coronary flow). The surgical sequence for inserting the flowmeter is the following: The descending aorta is cut and cannulae are inserted into each of the two stalks. These are connected to the two ends of the flowmeter probe. Then blood flow is reestablished through the descending aorta. Now the subclavian and innominate arteries are divided and additional cannulae leading from the output side of the flowmeter are inserted into the peripheral stumps of these arteries. Then blood flow is then reestablished through these arteries also. Thus, the preparation now records total systemic blood flow, which is equal to cardiac output minus the coronary flow. In order to determine total cardiac output, coronary blood flow must be measured simultaneously. Eckstein (1949a, 1949b), Sarnoff (1952), and Herndon (1969) have used procedures similar to this for measuring systemic flow. Eckstein and Sarnoff also cannulated the coronary vessels and obtained total cardiac output rather than simply systemic flow. These techniques for cannulating the aorta to measure cardiac output have been exceedingly useful

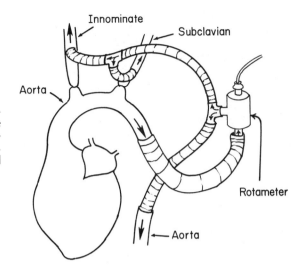

Figure 6-7. Method for inserting a flowmeter into the aorta for measuring cardiac output (minus coronary flow). [Modified from Sarnoff (1952).]

in the hands of Eckstein and Sarnoff in studying the dynamics of cardiac function, and especially the relationship between coronary blood flow and cardiac function.

In recent years the electromagnetic flowmeter (Schenk, 1958; Spencer, 1958; Sugimoto, 1966; Bishop, 1964), the ultrasonic flowmeter (Franklin, 1959), and various types of catheter tip flowmeters (Fry, 1956; Delaunois, 1958; Gabe, 1969) have been used to measure blood flow in the root of the aorta. The procedure for using these instruments is much simpler than that described above, since with these instruments blood flow in the aorta does not have to be interrupted.

The principle advantage of measuring cardiac output in the aorta is that a reasonable pressure drop in the flowmeter usually does not cause significant alteration in cardiovascular dynamics. The reason for this is that the pressure in the aorta is so great that a pressure change of only a few millimeters of mercury has almost no effect.

INSERTION OF FLOWMETERS INTO THE VENAE CAVAE

Several different investigators (Wegria, 1943; Gregg, 1944; Huggins, 1949; Guyton, 1952c; Elliot, 1961a, 1961b) have cannulated the two venae cavae and then inserted a flowmeter from these back to the right atrium for measurement of cardiac output. When this procedure is used, the azygos vein is always ligated. Unfortunately, as will be discussed in far greater detail in Chapter 11, a 7 mm. back pressure on the venae cavae, when the circulation is devoid of compensatory reflexes, will completely stop blood flow around the circulation. Therefore, cannulating the venae cavae can alter circulatory function very dramatically.

At least two different procedures have been used to prevent the alteration in circulatory function when the venous system is cannulated. A method used in Wigger's laboratory (Wegria, 1943) was to allow the

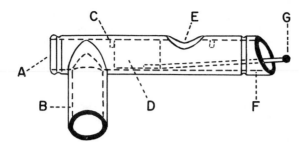

Figure 6-8. Cannula devised by Gregg and Shipley for rapid cannulation of the venae cavae. [Redrawn from Gregg and Shipley (1944).]

blood to drain from the venous cannulae into a reservoir placed below the level of the animal. This caused suction of blood out of the venae cavae. Then the blood was pumped to a high reservoir from which is was allowed to run back into the right atrium. In our laboratory (Guyton, 1952c) we simply used a pump in series with the flowmeter so that the resistance drop in the flowmeter and cannulae was nullified by the pumping action. In both these procedures, the circulation is very nearly normal in contrast to a greatly reduced cardiac output in the animal when a flowmeter is inserted directly between the venae cavae and the right atrium.

Cannulation of the venae cavae is a difficult surgical procedure, because blocking the flow from the veins to the heart for any prolonged period of time damages the circulatory system beyond repair. For this reason, the dexterity of the operator determines whether a successful preparation can be made. Ordinarily, inferior vena caval flow cannot be stopped for more than 30 to 45 seconds, or otherwise it will be impossible to maintain normal blood volume in the animal thereafter. Blood flow in the superior vena cava, however, can be stopped for as long as 1 to 2 minutes without noticeable damage to the preparation.

To prevent prolonged delays in cannulating the venae cavae, Gregg and Shipley (1944) devised the cannula illustrated in Figure 6-8. This cannula has four openings: opening A which goes to the superior vena cava, opening E which goes to the right atrium, opening F which goes to the inferior vena cava, and opening B which goes to the rotameter. The azygos vein is tied, the superior vena cava is opened, and the cannula is slipped down through the right atrium into the inferior vena cava. Immediately thereafter, the superior vena cava is pulled over opening A and ligatures are tied around openings A and F. Blood flows from both the superior vena cava and inferior vena cava through opening E into the right atrium. Opening B is then connected to a flowmeter, the other end of which is connected to the auricular appendage of the right atrium. Now a thin walled cylinder, D, which is located inside the cannula, is pulled downward by knob G to cover opening E. After this, no blood can flow directly from the cannula into the right atrium, but instead the blood can flow only through the flowmeter into the auricular appendage. Here again, however, to allow normal operation of the circulation (that is, to neutralize the effects of the resistance in the external circuit) a pump must be in series with the flowmeter.

INSERTION OF A FLOWMETER INTO THE PULMONARY ARTERY

The pulmonary artery is the only place in the circulation where the total cardiac output can be measured by cannulating a single vessel. However, it is technically difficult to place a flowmeter in the pulmonary artery because of the short length of the vessel. Nevertheless, flowmeters of several different types, including the electromagnetic flowmeters (Spencer, 1958), the ultrasonic flowmeter (Franklin, 1962), and the rotameter (Seely, 1950a, 1950b), have been successfully applied to this vessel. Indeed, electromagnetic and ultrasonic flowmeters, have been implanted in the chest and utilized for recording cardiac output over a period of weeks or months.

A pressure drop of a few millimeters of mercury in a flowmeter in the pulmonary artery will usually be compensated for by increased force of contraction of the right ventricle, and the cardiac output will hardly be altered. This is in marked contrast to the effect of even the slightest pressure drop in the venae cavae where such a pressure drop will cause a serious decrease in cardiac output.

RECORDING BLOOD FLOW FROM A RIGHT HEART BYPASS SYSTEM

Figure 6-9 illustrates a system that we have used in our laboratory to great advantage for recording pulmomonary arterial blood flow continuously, using a right heart bypass system (Guyton, 1955b, 1957b, 1957c, 1958c, 1958d). The special advantage of this system is that in using it one can control cardiac function almost exactly while studying the many different noncardiac factors that can alter cardiac output. The essentials of the procedure are the following:

A cannula is tied into the wall of the right atrium, and blood then passes through the cannula and through a thin segment of tube that can be raised or lowered to any specified height. On the distal side of this thin segment of tube is a pump that is always adjusted to keep the thin segment sucked to a semicollapsed state. Blood passes from the pump through a flowmeter, through a heater circuit, and finally into the pulmonary artery. The only time that the circulatory system is interrupted during the establishment of this right ventricular bypass system is for approximately 30 seconds while the pulmonary artery is cannulated.

This system can be used to regulate cardiac function by elevating or lowering the thin segment of tube in the flow system. Because this tube is constantly sucked to a semicollapsed state, the pressure inside it is equal to atmospheric pressure at the hydrostatic level of the tube. By elevating the tube one can raise the right atrial pressure to any set value. By lowering the tube, one can lower the pressure in the right atrium to any desired level. Thus, one can set the right atrial pressure to any predetermined value between the limits of −50 mm. or more of mercury up to equally as positive a pressure. Within physiological limits the left ventricle auto-

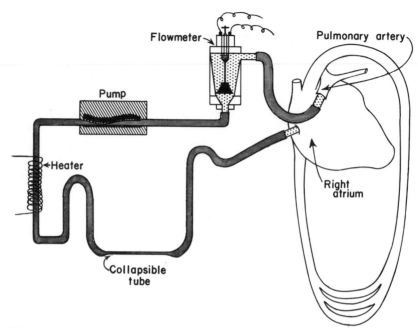

Figure 6–9. Right heart bypass system for measuring total cardiac output and for controlling cardiac function while studying noncardiac factors that affect cardiac output.

matically pumps whatever amount of blood that flows into it from the bypass system. Therefore, in effect, the bypass system controls the function of the entire heart. We shall see in Chapters 11 through 13 that the effect on cardiac output of many noncardiac factors, such as changes in blood volume, changes in peripheral resistance, changes in relative resistance of different vascular segments, and so forth, can all be studied to very great advantage using this system. This would not be possible if the function of the heart were not controlled during the course of the studies.

Obviously, the right heart bypass method records the total cardiac output because the coronary venous return flows along with the other venous return from the right atrium into the external pump.

II

REGULATION OF CARDIAC PUMPING ACTION

Chapter 7

INTRODUCTION TO THE REGULATION OF CARDIAC OUTPUT

One of the real enigmas of circulatory research has been the complete understanding of cardiac output regulation. The cause of this is that literally hundreds of different individual factors contribute to this regulation. For instance, dilatation of a single vessel in the periphery, however small this vessel might be, affects the cardiac output in its own minute way. Most investigators who have studied cardiac output regulation have dealt with only one or a few of the many factors that enter into cardiac output regulation rather than synthesizing these into a composite control system. For this reason, almost as many explanations for the regulation of cardiac output have been offered as there have been research workers in the field. In general, however, these explanations can be classified in two major categories: regulation of cardiac output by the heart and regulation of cardiac output by the peripheral circulation.

REGULATION OF CARDIAC OUTPUT BY THE HEART

Because the heart is the organ that provides the motive force for cardiac output, it is only natural, on first thought, to assume that the heart itself is the prime regulation of cardiac output. Therefore, the earliest theories for the regulation of cardiac output were built almost entirely around the heart itself. Furthermore, when it was discovered that cardiac activity can be increased and decreased by sympathetic and parasympathetic stimulation, it was immediately assumed that the activity of the heart and, consequently, the level of cardiac output are regulated by the nerves to the heart.

If the heart alone is thought of as the regulator of cardiac output, then we must assume that at the input side of the heart a ready supply of blood is always available to the pumped. Then, when the activity of the heart increases, this blood is pumped into the arteries, and the supply is replenished as rapidly as the heart pumps the blood. This concept is

137

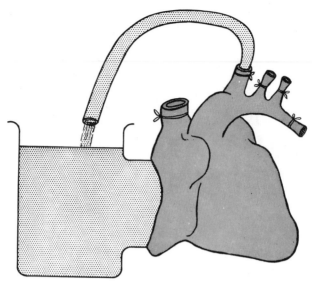

Figure 7–1. The "cardiac concept" of cardiac output regulation, showing a central reservoir with blood always available to the right atrium.

illustrated by Figure 7–1, which shows a large reservoir connecting directly with the right atrium of the heart in such a way that there is essentially no resistance between the reservoir and the right atrium. *Under such conditions,* just as soon as the activity of the heart is increased, the cardiac output obviously also increases, and sufficient blood returns to the reservoir to keep it full all the time. It is immediately evident that the heart alone would be the controller of cardiac output, and different factors in the periphery, such as storage capacity of the vascular system, amount of blood volume, and resistance in the vessels, would have little to do with the regulation of cardiac output.

A few very simple experiments, however, have disproved this concept that the heart alone is the regulator of cardiac output. Some of these may be listed as follow:

1. Increasing the activity of the heart by stimulating the cardiac sympathetic nerves (Carrier, unpublished observations) or by increasing the heart rate using an electrical pacemaker (Miller, 1962; Snyder, 1962) increases the cardiac output only a very slight amount if at all, even though cardiac activity itself is greatly enhanced.

2. Replacing the heart by a pump that is capable of pumping *infinite* amounts of blood causes only normal amounts of cardiac output despite very intense activity of the pump (Guyton, 1957b). This indicates that there is not an excess of blood at the input side of the heart always available to be pumped.

3. Increasing the blood volume increases the cardiac output instantaneously, and, conversely, decreasing the blood volume instantaneously decreases the cardiac output (Guyton, 1957c). Even a few milliliters' alteration of the blood volume in a dog will cause these instantaneous

effects if the cardiac output is being recorded continuously with a rapidly responding recorder.

4. Alterations in peripheral resistance, whether caused by opening an A-V fistula (Guyton, 1961b), by vasodilatation in response to diminished oxygen supply to the tissues (Öberg, 1961; Gorlin, 1954; Huckabee, 1960), by vasoconstriction resulting from vasoactive drugs (Guyton, 1958c), or by occlusion of blood vessels with microspheres or ligature (Guyton, 1959b), always have inverse and immediate effects on the cardiac output, indicating very strongly that the regulation of cardiac output is directly dependent upon changes that occur in the peripheral circulation as well as on cardiac activity itself.

From the above experiments it is evident that many noncardiac factors play major roles in the regulation of cardiac output in addition to the effect of changes in activity of the heart itself.

Fifty years ago Starling and his contemporaries recognized these interrelationships between cardiac activity and the peripheral circulatory system in the regulation of cardiac output (Starling, 1918; Patterson, 1914b; Straub, 1914). Despite this, some recent investigators, who have mainly studied the role of the heart in the circulation without delving deeply into the peripheral circulatory system, have come back to the concept that the heart itself is the primary regulator of cardiac output under normal conditions (Stead, 1947a, 1947b; Warren, 1945, 1948b, 1957; Rushmer, 1961). This has not been the experience of others (Chapman, 1960; Wang, 1960; Frye, 1960). Also it is not supported by modern control theory analyses of cardiac output regulation, using the accumulated mass of isolated circulatory measurements that are available from hundreds of laboratories (Guyton, 1955a; Grodins, 1959; Warner, 1959).

REGULATION OF CARDIAC OUTPUT BY PERIPHERAL CIRCULATION

Another theory of the regulation of cardiac output that is almost diametrically opposed to the concept that the heart alone regulates cardiac output is that cardiac output is controlled almost entirely by "venous return" to the heart. This concept is illustrated by Figure 7–2, which shows a reservoir of blood elevated above the level of the heart. Between this reservoir and the heart is considerable resistance, and the blood flows through a thin walled tube that will collapse if one attempts to suck blood through it. The hydrostatic pressure in the reservoir forces blood through the resistance. The heart is assumed to have enough reserve pumping capacity to keep the thin walled tube partially collapsed all the time, and it is assumed to pump any blood that enters the right atrium on through the heart automatically, whatever the amount of blood entering. Furthermore, an increase in heart activity simply collapses the thin walled tube more rather than increasing the flow. Therefore, the amount of blood pumped by the heart is determined by the amount of blood that is capable of flowing from the reservoir into the right atrium and not by the activity of the heart. *Under these conditions,* the heart itself would have little to do with the regulation of cardiac output but would simply function as a

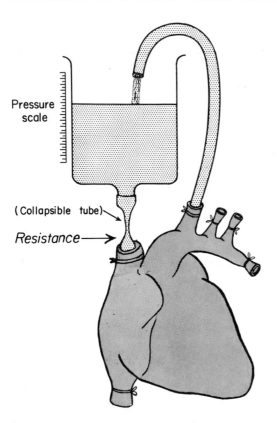

Pressure scale

(Collapsible tube)

Resistance

Figure 7-2. The "peripheral concept" of cardiac output regulation, showing a head of pressure in the periphery with a collapsible resistance tube between this head of pressure and the heart. The heart is capable of pumping any amount of blood that flows into the right atrium.

sump pump, always pumping whatever amount of blood flows into the right atrium. This theory originated principally with the advent of the heart-lung preparation (Patterson, 1914b), because it was found that, true enough, within physiological limits, the amount of blood pumped by the heart-lung preparation is determined almost entirely by the pressure head in the venous reservoir and the resistance between the reservoir and the right atrium. That is, the heart has a tremendous capability of adapting automatically to increasing loads of inflowing blood.

Yet under many different conditions this theory also fails to explain the regulation of cardiac output. Some of these conditions are the following:

1. When tremendous amounts of blood are allowed to flow into the heart from a reservoir, as shown in Figure 7-2, a limit is finally reached above which the heart cannot pump extra quantities of blood (Sarnoff, 1955). Once this point is reached, it is then very evident that the limiting factor in cardiac output regulation is primarily the heart itself and not the rate at which blood can flow from the reservoir into the right atrium.

2. When the effectiveness of the heart as a pump is severely compromised, such as by myocardial failure, valvular heart disease, or other similar conditions, the cardiac output always decreases (see Chapters 1, 26, and 27). The "cardiac reserve" must be used up before this occurs, but eventually it does occur.

3. In severe cardiac failure, any recovery of cardiac effectiveness always increases the cardiac output (see Chapter 26). This is different from the effect that occurs in the normal circulation where an increase in cardiac effectiveness hardly affects the output (Snyder, 1962). Nevertheless, it does illustrate that under special conditions, the heart plays a major role in cardiac regulation.

CARDIAC REGULATION OF THE "PERMISSIBLE" LEVEL OF CARDIAC OUTPUT

A way to express the role of the heart in cardiac output regulation is to state that the heart, in general, controls the *permissible* amount of output that can be pumped per minute, but not necessarily the *actual* amount. But why the discrepancy between these two? To answer this, let us take the example of the normal person. The actual cardiac output is about 5 liters per minute, while the heart is capable of pumping 12 to 15 liters per minute. The only condition required to cause increased pumping up to the limit of 12 to 15 liters per minute is sudden inflow of blood into the right atrium. Thus, the heart has a permissible level of pumping almost three times the actual level of pumping.

The permissible level of cardiac pumping can be changed in many different ways. Sympathetic stimulation of the heart increases the permissible level 70 to 100 per cent, as will be discussed in Chapter 8. Likewise, hypertrophy of the heart can increase the level perhaps equally as much (Chapter 8). On the other hand, abnormalities of heart function— myocardial infarction, valvular disease, and so forth—will decrease the permissible level of cardiac pumping to any value between normal and zero, depending on the severity of the abnormality.

REGULATION OF ACTUAL CARDIAC OUTPUT BY PERIPHERAL FACTORS

Even though the normal heart, under resting conditions, is capable of pumping 12 to 15 liters per minute, it obviously cannot pump this amount if inflow of blood from the veins is less than this, which is the normal condition. Therefore, cardiac output is most often limited not by the heart itself but, instead, by factors that determine venous inflow of blood to the heart.

The factors that control return of blood to the heart from the peripheral circulation can be divided into two major categories: first, the *degree of dilatation of the peripheral blood vessels*—that is, the resistance to blood flow through the systemic circulation—and, second, the *degree of filling of the vasculature with blood*. The second of these factors plays a major role in cardiac output regulation under special conditions, such as following hemorrhage, following overfilling of the circulatory system by transfusion, or following massive changes in capacitance of the circulatory system itself.

Regulation of Venous Return by Local Tissue Vasodilatation

In general, blood flow through each local tissue is automatically adjusted by increase or decrease in the degree of vasodilatation in proportion to the need of the respective tissue for flow. In most tissues the important tissue need related to flow is the need of the cells for oxygen. However, in a few areas, the greatest need is for removal of carbon dioxide; this occurs most importantly in the brain and perhaps in the liver. Regarding the kidneys, the primary need is to deliver end-products of metabolism to the kidneys for excretion, and, in ways not presently understood, the blood concentrations of these substances seem to be the primary regulator of renal vascular resistance. Blood flow to the skin, on the other hand, is controlled almost entirely by the nervous thermoregulatory system of the body, the primary center for which is located in the hypothalamus; signals to the skin vessels are mediated through the sympathetic nervous system. Probably, specific local regulatory factors control blood flow in other tissues.

Venous Return as the Sum of Local Blood Flows

An axiomatic fact often forgotten is that the total quantity of blood flowing to the heart each minute is equal to the sum of the blood flows through the individual tissues. Therefore, if each individual tissue has its own specific mechanism for local control of blood flow, it follows that venous return is controlled not by one, single factor but, instead, by great numbers of individual factors affecting the respective individual tissues. Over any prolonged period of time, the blood flow to each tissue seems to obey the basic principle that it is adjusted to the need of the tissue—no more, no less—and this readjustment may take place as a result of changes in the degree of vasomotor tone in the vessel walls themselves, changes in sizes of the blood vessels, or changes in the numbers of blood vessels (called *vascularity* changes). For instance, after blockage of a major blood vessel, collateral vessels enlarge, and new vessels sometimes sprout. These effects tend to return blood flow to its normal value, and they are all part of the overall venous return control mechanism—therefore, also part of the cardiac output control mechanism. These local mechanisms of blood flow control and their effects on cardiac output regulation will be discussed in more detail in future chapters.

Role of Vascular Filling Pressure (Mean Systemic Pressure) in Cardiac Output Regulation

The degree of filling of the circulation with blood can be measured by stopping cardiac output and measuring the circulatory filling pressure when all pressures come to equilibrium. This filling pressure is called "mean circulatory pressure" when the entire circulation is considered, or "mean systemic pressure" when only the systemic portion is considered. Even under normal conditions, changes in this filling pressure are important in the rapid control of venous return and cardiac output. For instance, if all blood vessels of the circulatory system are nervously excited simultaneously but the blood volume remains constant, the pressure of the blood in each of the vessels will rise. Therefore, filling pressure of the system increases. Let us assume, for instance, that the large veins contract, building up pressure in these veins. This immediately causes large quantities of blood to be pushed from the veins toward the right heart. Since the heart pumps this extra amount of blood with essentially no increase in right atrial pressure, the pressure gradients from the veins to the heart becomes a major determinant of cardiac output. If at the same time the arteries also contract, thereby raising the pressure in the arteries, the flow of blood from the arteries to the veins likewise is increased.

Thus, one can see that the simple expedient of contracting all the large blood vessels of the systemic circulation (but not contracting the small resistance vessels) can increase cardiac output, indeed, as much as two to three fold. Within a minute or more, however, the cardiac output begins to return toward normal because of readjustment of the vasodilator mechanisms that control local blood flow in each of the tissues. Nevertheless, the overall acute control of cardiac output is vested in an interplay between these two respective mechanisms: the filling pressure of the peripheral circulation, and the degree of vasodilatation in each of the local tissues throughout the circulation. These interrelationships will be discussed in much more quantitative detail in future chapters.

RELATION OF PERMISSIBLE LEVEL OF CARDIAC PUMPING TO VENOUS RETURN

If a heart has a permissible level of cardiac pumping greater than the return of blood to the heart, then the cardiac output obviously will equal the inflow into the heart and not the permissible level of pumping. Therefore, under normal resting conditions, the cardiac output is controlled almost entirely by the peripheral factors governing return of blood to the heart.

On the other hand, at times, the peripheral circulation attempts to return a quantity of blood to the heart that is greater than the permissible level of cardiac pumping. This can occur either when the peripheral tissues become more demanding for blood flow, such as during very heavy exercise, or when the permissible level of cardiac pumping becomes greatly decreased, as occurs following a serious myocardial infarction. Therefore, it is equally obvious that when greater amounts of blood attempt to enter the heart than can be pumped, the limiting factor to cardiac output then becomes the heart and not the peripheral factors.

These interrelationships between the permissible level of cardiac pumping and the tendency for venous return are not quite as "all or none" as the above discussion might indicate. This is particularly true when the maximum permissible level of cardiac pumping is only slightly greater than venous return. It is not possible to express in words the details of the interplay that occurs under this condition. However, in quantitative analyses of this problem, even the minute detail of this interplay become apparent. These will be presented in both algebraic and graphical analyses of cardiac output regulation in subsequent chapters.

THE CONCEPT OF CARDIAC RESERVE

Clinicians have long recognized the difference between the permissible level of cardiac output and the actual cardiac output. They have termed this difference *cardiac reserve*. That is, if the permissible level of cardiac pumping is 15 liters per minute but the inflow of blood to the heart, and therefore the cardiac output, is only 5 liters per minute, then the cardiac reserve is 10 liters per minute, or 200 per cent. It has also been known for many years that progressive cardiac debility at first reduces this cardiac reserve while the cardiac output itself remains essentially normal. It is only when the pumping capability of the heart becomes severely depressed that the cardiac output itself begins to be compromised. Many clinical tests have been designed specifically to estimate cardiac reserve, such as the step test, running on treadmills, and so forth, all of which increase venous return to the heart and thereby test endurance or other factors related to circulatory function, thus effecting crude estimates of cardiac reserve.

A person with a cardiac reserve that is depressed as much as 50 per cent might easily have a normal cardiac output under resting conditions; depression of cardiac function becomes evident only when he exercises, because his peripheral tissues then demand more blood flow than the heart is capable of supplying.

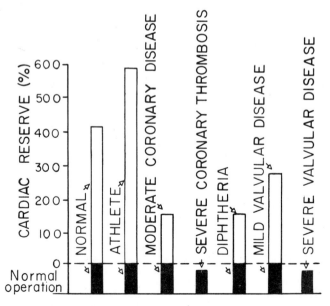

Figure 7–3. Cardiac reserve in different conditions.

The term cardiac reserve, as most often used, also includes the additional reserve that can be attained by autonomic stimulation of the heart — that is, by decreased parasympathetic stimulation and by increased sympathetic stimulation, the two of which together increase both heart rate and strength of heart contraction. Therefore, one should perhaps differentiate between what might be called "instantaneous cardiac reserve" and "total cardiac reserve." Instantaneous reserve is the momentary reserve capability of the heart to pump increased amounts of blood without any change in its autonomic stimulation. On the other hand, total cardiac reserve includes both the instantaneous reserve and the additional increase in output that can be achieved by autonomic adjustment. The instantaneous cardiac reserve in the human being has never been measured, but in the dog it is between 150 and 200 per cent. The total cardiac reserve in a young untrained human being, and likewise in the dog, is about 300 to 400 per cent. Following athletic training, the total cardiac reserve can increase to as high as 600 per cent. Some of the total cardiac reserves under different conditions are illustrated in Figure 7–3.

ROLE OF ARTERIAL PRESSURE REGULATION IN CONTROL OF CARDIAC OUTPUT

If each local tissue is to control its own blood flow by dilating or constricting its blood vessels, then it is essential that the arterial pressure be maintained at a pressure high enough to supply the blood demanded by the tissues. Furthermore, for the tissues to be precise in their regulation of blood flow, the arterial pressure also needs to be held at a reasonably constant level despite changes in blood flow demand by the tissues. Therefore, one of the most essential features of overall cardiac output regulation is that there be concomitant background regulation of arterial pressure (Banet and Guyton, 1971).

Over short periods of time, arterial pressure is regulated almost entirely by circulatory nervous reflexes that are capable of reacting with half-times of only a few seconds to raise arterial pressure whenever it attempts to fall, or to lower arterial pressure whenever it attempts to rise. Recent measurements of feedback gain in the nervous pressure feedback control system, including the gains of both the baroreceptor and the chemoreceptor systems, indicate this to be about 6. This means that an initial instantaneous change in pressure will be returned within a few seconds about six-sevenths of the way back toward normal pressure. Thus, the overall nervous control system plays an extremely important role in maintaining a reasonably constant arterial pressure level despite variable demands of blood flow by the tissues.

As an example, during heavy exercise in a sympathectomized animal, the local vasodilating effect of the muscle activity decreases the arterial pressure to 40 to 50 mm. Hg (Ashkar and Hamilton, 1963). However, in a normal animal with normally functioning sympathetic reflexes, the same degree of heavy exercise causes the arterial pressure to rise to about 130 mm. Hg. This occurs despite the fact that the total peripheral resistance decreases to about one-third normal. The reason for this obviously is not an effect of sympathetic signals to increase peripheral resistance but, instead, an effect of the signals to constrict the reservoir vessels of the peripheral circulation, especially the veins. Constriction of these vessels translocates large quantities of blood from the peripheral circulation to the heart, thus increasing the venous return, increasing cardiac output, and thereby returning the arterial pressure not only to its normal level but also to a slightly elevated level during exercise.

It is clear, therefore, that arterial pressure regulation is an essential ingredient in cardiac output regulation. And it is also clear that this regulation occurs not through increases in peripheral resistance but, instead, through changes in contraction of the peripheral reservoir.

The Mechanism of Pressure Control

It is often thought that nervous control of arterial pressure is effected almost entirely by changing the resistance to blood flow through the small, tissue blood vessels. However, an increase in resistance would decrease blood flow through the tissues. Therefore, when a tissue demands additional quantities of blood flow because of its local needs, vasoconstriction of its arterioles to maintain the arterial pressure would be very detrimental to the tissue's own needs. Fortunately, the local vasodilating effect caused by increased metabolism usually prevails over the vasoconstricting effect of the nervous signals, and the net result is decreased vascular resistance rather than increased resistance. Yet, how can the nervous system maintain arterial pressure in the face of the decreasing vascular resistance? The answer is: by increasing the filling pressure of the circulation. Strong sympathetic stimulation of the large vessels, particularly the veins, can increase this pressure, called the *mean systemic pressure,* from a normal value of 7 mm. Hg up to 18 to 21 mm. Hg, almost a three fold increase. This is essentially the same effect as increasing the pressures in all the peripheral vascular reservoirs by an average of three fold, which greatly increases venous return and cardiac output. Therefore, the arterial pressure is maintained by an increase in cardiac output and not by an increase in peripheral resistance.

Chapter 8

THE PUMPING ABILITY OF THE HEART AS EXPRESSED BY CARDIAC FUNCTION CURVES

METHODS FOR QUANTITATING THE HEART'S PUMPING ABILITY

The amount of blood actually pumped by the heart and the *ability of the heart to pump blood* are two entirely different things. For instance, the heart may have the ability to pump tremendous quantities of blood and, yet, without blood available at the input side of the heart, the cardiac output will still be zero. Therefore, our first problem in discussing the pumping ability of the heart is to decide upon some means for quantitating the heart's pumping ability.

First, let us list some of the ways in which the pumping ability of the heart *cannot* be expressed. It cannot be expressed in terms of cardiac pressure output alone; it cannot be expressed in terms of cardiac output alone; it cannot be expressed in terms of stroke work output alone, minute work output alone, or any other single parameter of heart function, because all these parameters are dependent upon additional variables besides the ability of the heart to pump blood.

On the other hand, the heart's ability to pump blood *can* be expressed in a quantitative way by use of *function curves*, many different kinds of which have been utilized for this purpose, including:

1. Cardiac output plotted as a function of mean right atrial pressure when the systemic resistance remains constant.

2. Cardiac output plotted as a function of mean right atrial pressure when the systemic arterial pressure remains constant.

3. Cardiac output plotted as a function of right ventricular end-diastolic pressure (a) when the systemic resistance or (b) when the systemic arterial pressure remains constant.

4. Cardiac output plotted as a function of end-diastolic volume of

147

the right ventricle or the left ventricle when the systemic resistance or the systemic arterial pressure remains constant.

5. Minute work output of the heart plotted as a function of mean right atrial pressure or end-diastolic volume of one of the ventricles when the systemic resistance or systemic pressure remains constant.

6. Curves similar to any of the above but expressed in terms of stroke volume output, stroke work output, or systemic arterial pressure instead of cardiac output or minute work output.

7. Curves similar to any of the above but for each ventricle instead of for the entire heart.

The above list actually includes some 50 or more different types of function curves, each of which is slightly different from the others and actually has a different meaning. If we are interested in the ability of the heart to supply blood to the systemic arterial system, we need to express the pumping of blood by the heart in terms of one of the cardiac output curves. If we are interested in the quantity of blood pumped during each heart beat rather than the integrated amount over a period of time, we would use one of the stroke volume output curves. Or, if we are interested in the amount of work the heart can perform, we would use one of the work output curves.

Three types of these cardiac function curves have been used most often in quantitating the heart's ability to pump. These are (a) cardiac output plotted as a function of mean right atrial pressure (Patterson, 1914b; Wiggers, 1922b; McMichael, 1944; Wang, 1960; Frye, 1960; Chapman, 1960; Crowell, 1962; Stone, 1963); (b) pressure output of each ventricle plotted as a function of the ventricular end-diastolic volume (Patterson, 1914a); and (c) ventricular work output plotted as a function of atrial pressure (Ferguson, 1953, 1954; Sarnoff, 1955; Berglund, 1955a; Hawthorne, 1958). Each of these different types of curves supplies a different type of information about the pumping ability of the heart and therefore is important in its own right. To aid in understanding the importance of these function curves, each will be explained in detail.

Cardiac Output Plotted as a Function of Mean Right Atrial Pressure

One of the earliest types of cardiac function curves to be used was cardiac output plotted as a function of mean right atrial pressure. Figure 8-1 illustrates eight such function curves measured by Patterson and Starling (1914b) in heart-lung experiments in their original studies with this preparation. These curves show that at a right atrial pressure of zero, none of the hearts pumped any blood. However, as the right atrial pressure approached 5 to 10 mm. Hg the cardiac output reached a maximum and then, at still higher pressures, the output often decreased.

One can see from the curves in this figure that it would be impossible to compare the pumping abilities of the different hearts without using the entire function curves. For instance, at 5 mm. Hg right atrial pressure the heart represented by the heavy solid line has a cardiac output twice

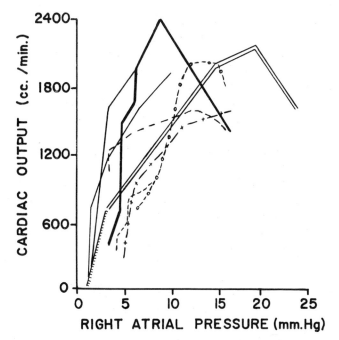

Figure 8–1. Cardiac function curves obtained in eight heart-lung preparations by Patterson and Starling, depicting cardiac output as a function of mean right atrial pressure. [Redrawn and axes transposed from Patterson and Starling (1914b).]

as great as the output of the heart represented by the double parallel lines. However, at a right atrial pressure of 17 mm. Hg, the converse is true. Therefore, to express the relative pumping abilities of these two respective hearts, the entire curves are needed. Yet, although the patterns of function curves for individual hearts are different from each other, nevertheless a general average trend of the curves in Figure 8–1 can be observed.

The function curves obtained in these heart-lung preparations are applicable to the intact heart only in their general form, but certainly not in detail, for several different reasons. First, the curves of Figure 1 were measured in a preparation in which the arterial pressure against which the hearts pumped blood was automatically controlled at a constant level. In the intact animal the arterial pressure is not constant but, instead, rises as the cardiac output increases. Second, the quantitative values for the curves change considerably when the heart is in the closed chest in contrast to the open chest. These differences will be discussed at further length in this and the following chapter.

Left Ventricular Systolic Pressure Output as a Function of Left Ventricular End-Diastolic Volume

Figure 8–2 illustrates the pressure generated during systole by the left ventricle of a dog when the left ventricular end-diastolic volume was progressively increased from 0 up to 60 ml. [This curve was extrapolated

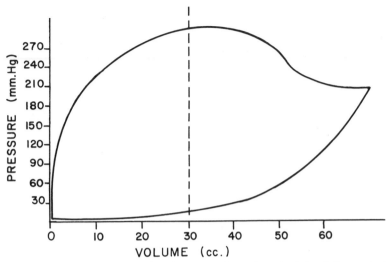

Figure 8–2. Left ventricular function curve for a dog, depicting left ventricular systolic pressure by the upper curve and left ventricular diastolic pressure by the lower curve as a function of different degrees of end-diastolic filling of the ventricle. [Modified from Patterson, Piper, and Starling (1914a).]

to the dog by Patterson, Patterson, and Starling from data obtained by O. Frank in the frog heart (Patterson, 1914a).] The lower curve represents the pressure in the ventricle before contraction of the heart, while the upper curve represents the pressure at the height of contraction with the aorta completely occluded so that no blood could leave the ventricle.

The diagram in Figure 8–2 depicts the cardiac pressure generated by *isometric* contraction of the heart. That is, since the heart muscle fibers are prevented from shortening, or at least from shortening more than a very slight amount, this curve is actually an isometric contractile tension curve, which is almost identical, even quantitatively, with curves of this type obtained from skeletal muscle. If one is particularly interested in the contractile ability of the cardiac muscle or in the pressures that can be generated by the ventricles, this type of curve can convey tremendous amounts of information. Similar curves relating end-diastolic volume to ventricular work output (Kozawa, 1915; Starling, 1927; Katz, 1928) are equally valuable in understanding ventricular contractility.

Ventricular Work Output Plotted as a Function of Mean Atrial Pressure

Figure 8–3 illustrates studies by Sarnoff and his colleagues (1955) depicting left and right ventricular stroke work outputs plotted as functions of the respective left and right mean atrial pressures. These two curves illustrate that ventricular stroke work output increases as the atrial pressure increases. Furthermore, Sarnoff has shown that, within reasonable physiological ranges, the amount of work output of each ventricle at a given mean atrial pressure remains almost the same, regardless of the

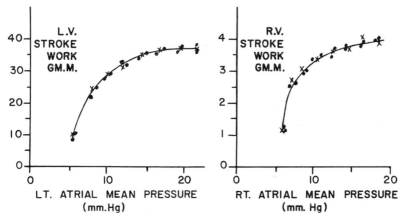

Figure 8–3. Right and left ventricular function curves in a dog, depicting ventricular stroke work output as a function of the respective right and left mean atrial pressures. [Curves reconstructed from data in Sarnoff (1955).]

type of work load against which the ventricle must work, that is, whether this load be a high arterial pressure and low ventricular output or a low pressure and high output. Though this relationship is not exact, nevertheless it does show that the heart increases its *energy* output as the atrial pressure increases, this representing an automatic mechanism by which the heart adapts its pumping activity to a load of blood that must be pumped.

These curves, like the curves discussed above, are not very useful in predicting cardiac output, because it is difficult to translate stroke work into cardiac output for two different reasons: First, these curves do not take heart rate into consideration. Second, before one can translate work output into cardiac output he also needs to know the arterial pressure at each point on the curve.

SUMMARY OF METHODS FOR QUANTITATING THE PUMPING ABILITY OF THE HEART

From the foregoing discussion it becomes apparent that each type of function curve has its own value, but it also is equally apparent that, when we are attempting to predict cardiac output, the function curve must be expressed in terms of cardiac output before it is meaningful. Stroke work output curves can be reduced to cardiac output curves if the respective arterial pressures and heart rates are known for each point on the curve. A left ventricular pressure output curve can be reduced to a cardiac output curve provided the systemic resistance is known during the measurement of the pressure curve. However, for ease of analysis, it is far better to represent cardiac or ventricular function curves directly in terms of output.

CARDIAC OUTPUT CURVES

In this book the terms *cardiac function curve* and *cardiac output curve* will be used interchangeably and will always refer to the relationship between cardiac output and mean right atrial pressure when the systemic resistive load remains constant. Similarly, the terms *ventricular output curve* and *ventricular function curve* will refer to the output of each separate side of the heart as a function of the respective mean atrial pressure.

The reason for choosing this type of curve over all other function curves is the following: It is expressed in terms of mean right atrial pressure and in terms of blood flow in the circulation per minute. These same two parameters can be used to describe function in the systemic circulation, which will be discussed in detail in Chapters 10 through 13. And, when the functions of both the heart and the systemic circulation are expressed in the same parameters, they can be equated together to give a prediction of cardiac output (Guyton, 1955; Grodins, 1959; Warner, 1959). Since this is our goal, this type of curve is ideal for our purposes.

The Heart and Pulmonary Circulation Considered as a Unit When Determining Cardiac Output Curves

Since the cardiac output curve expresses the output of the heart in relation to the input pressure at the right atrium, this curve is a composite function curve for the entire segment of the circulatory system between the input of the heart and its output, including, of course, both sides of the heart as well as the pulmonary circulatory system.

Obviously, in many conditions of circulatory function it will not be satisfactory to consider both sides of the heart and the lung as a single unit in analyzing cardiac output. However, we shall see that *except in those conditions involving imbalance between the two sides of the heart,* this is a quantitatively accurate procedure which greatly simplifies the analysis (Guyton, 1962c). Therefore, in the earlier portions of our discussions on the regulation of cardiac output, we will use this simplified procedure — that is, we will utilize cardiac output curves — for analyzing the regulation of cardiac output. However, in Chapter 14 we will go to the more complex analysis of cardiac output regulation in which it is necessary to use individual ventricular output curves for each of the two ventricles instead of cardiac output curves.

Methods for Determining Cardiac Output Curves

Cardiac output curves can be determined very readily in the heart-lung preparation or in the open-chest experimental animal. In either of these two cases, one of the flowmeters described in Chapter 6 is used to measure the output while the right atrial pressure is elevated or lowered by raising or lowering a large reservoir of blood connected directly to the right atrium (Patterson, 1914a, 1914b; Sarnoff, 1954a, 1955; Isaacs, 1954; Case, 1955). Typical curves of this type were illustrated in Figure 8–1.

It was pointed out earlier in the chapter that curves obtained in the open-chest animal are quantitatively different from those obtained in the closed-chest animal because of loss of the negative intrathoracic pressure when the chest is opened. Therefore, we in our laboratory (Crowell, 1962; Fermoso, 1964; Stone, 1963) as well as Sarnoff and his colleagues (Sarnoff, 1955) have measured these curves in the closed-chest animal. In our procedure: (a) the cardiac output is recorded continuously using the continuous Fick output recorder described in Chapter 2; (b) a very large catheter is inserted down the external jugular vein to the right atrium; (c) the right atrial pressure is raised or lowered by transfusing or bleeding the animal while the cardiac output is recorded; and (d) the right atrial pressure is then plotted against cardiac output to obtain the cardiac output curve. In some of our experiments, an X-Y recorder has been used to record the curves continuously as the right atrial pressure is altered.

Extrapolation of Cardiac Output Curves to the Human Being

Most of the cardiac output curves to be used in this book have been extrapolated from animals to human beings even though complete cardiac output curves have never been determined in man. This extrapolation can be questioned, but in the clinical research literature one can find measurements of literally hundreds of individual points on different cardiac output curves, and in a few instances large segments of complete cardiac output curves have even been determined in the human being (McMichael, 1944; Frye, 1960; Wang, 1960). All these data show these curves to have almost identically the same contours as those derived from experimental animals. Furthermore, the ratios of the values determined in animals versus human beings give a reasonably accurate basis for making the extrapolation.

The extrapolations to be used are generally based on the following facts: (1) that the normal cardiac output of an adult human being is 5.0 liters per minute (see Chapter 1 for a review), (2) that the normal right atrial pressure under resting conditions in the human being is 0 mm. Hg; (3) that the maximum cardiac output for a young healthy human heart after reasonable athletic training can be as great as 24 liters per minute during maximal muscular exercise (Christensen, 1931; Wang, 1960; Chapman, 1960); (4) that in moderately severe exercise the right atrial pressure ordinarily does not rise significantly (Chapman, 1960; Rushmer, 1959) but in severe exercise does rise slightly; and (5) that the cardiac output can change instantaneously as much as 100 per cent on opening large A-V fistulae (Harrison, 1924; Warren, 1951b; Guyton, 1961b). These types of data, plus many thousands of clinical measurements of cardiac output made simultaneously with measurements of right atrial pressure, can be used to give one an almost exact plot of cardiac output curves in almost all circulatory conditions, even in human beings.

Time-Dependent Factors in Cardiac Output Curves

The ideal cardiac output curve would be one in which all points on the curve could be obtained instantaneously without any lapse of time

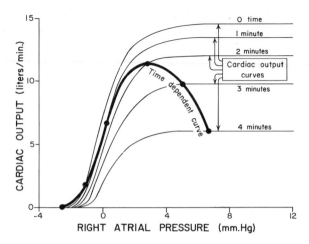

Figure 8–4. A time-dependent curve recorded during the course of an experiment in which the heart was becoming progressively weaker. The light curves represent the true cardiac output curves, which are changing with time. The dark points represent individual points recorded as the right atrial pressure was being increased and the heart was deteriorating. The dark curve drawn through the points represents the resulting time-dependent curve.

between the separate points of measurement, for what we actually wish to depict by the cardiac output curve is not the real cardiac output at any given instant, but, instead, the *ability* of the heart to pump different cardiac outputs at different right atrial pressures at any given instant. If the heart's ability to pump is changing while the curve is being recorded, the recorded curve will not represent the true cardiac output curve, but instead will be a *time-dependent curve.* Many instances of time-dependent curves have appeared in the literature and have led to serious error. Some of these are the following:

TIME-DEPENDENT CURVES RECORDED WHILE THE HEART IS BECOMING PROGRESSIVELY WEAKER. Let us assume that the cardiac output curve is determined while the heart is becoming progressively weaker. Figure 8–4 illustrates a series of cardiac output curves (the light curves) which represent the true changing functional state of a rapidly deteriorating heart at one minute intervals. Now let us suppose that the right atrial pressure is raised slowly over a period of several minutes in order to determine the cardiac output curve. The solid points shown in the figure would be the actual points that would be determined. On drawing a curve through these points (the dark curve) we find a peculiar, peaked curve. This curve does not represent a cardiac output curve at all but instead represents a time-dependent curve based on far more factors than the true cardiac output curve itself. Obviously such a curve as this could not be used in any possible way in analyzing cardiac output dynamics.

There is much reason to believe that many of the so-called classic "cardiac function curves" have actually been time-dependent. For instance, if we refer back to Figure 8–1, we see typical peaks in many of the curves of this figure but not in all of them. On the other hand, our experience with the X-Y recorder in recording cardiac output curves, and also Sarnoff's experience in recording cardiac function curves in the normal heart (Sarnoff, 1954a), shows that these curves usually come to a plateau rather than to a peak, provided the curves are run rapidly to avoid time-dependent factors.

Even when studying extremely weak hearts, we have found in our laboratory that a sudden positive increment in right atrial pressure, at least up to +15 to 20 mm. Hg, always either increases the cardiac output still further or at least does not cause the cardiac output to fall, and this is the same experience of Schnabel (1959) in similar studies on patients with serious mitral valvular disease. Therefore, even for a very weak heart, we do not find a "descending limb" in the true cardiac output curve. Yet if the elevated right atrial pressure is maintained for even a few moments' time, the cardiac output does not fall. For this reason, we have come to believe that the classic humped cardiac output curve, which is often used to explain cardiac failure, may indeed be a time-dependent curve rather than a true cardiac output curve. [If one thinks for a moment about the differences between cardiac output curves and work output curves, he will see that anytime a plateau occurs in the cardiac output curve, there will be a descending limb in the work output curve. The reason for this is that as the atrial pressure rises, the work output decreases because atrial pressure must be subtracted from the output pressure. Thus, the work output falls even though the cardiac output remains constant. Furthermore, the weaker the heart, the greater will this effect be because the atrial pressure then nearly approaches the output pressure. Therefore, Sarnoff's (1955) finding of a descending limb in the work output curve of the weak heart is in complete accord with our findings of a plateau in the cardiac output curve. Furthermore, we will see in Chapter 26 that it is not necessary to assume a descending limb in the output curve to explain cardiac output dynamics in cardiac failure.]

TIME-DEPENDENT CURVES CAUSED BY AUTONOMIC STIMULATION. Figure 8–5 illustrates another type of time-dependent curve which we have recorded in our laboratory during parasympathetic and sympathetic stimulation. When the parasympathetic nerves are stimulated, the cardiac output curve falls, as illustrated in the figure, the degree of fall depending upon the degree of parasympathetic stimulation. Conversely, sympathetic stimulation increases the cardiac output curve. However, if during the course of the experiment the right atrial pressure is decreased at the same time that we change from full parasympathetic stimulation to full sympathetic stimulation, the large black dots of the figure will represent the individual points recorded. Now if we draw a curve through these points, we find a curve that has a contour almost at right angles to the true cardiac output curves. This is indeed a time-dependent curve, which can make one believe the oddest things about the circulatory system. Such a time-dependent effect as that illustrated in Figure 8–5 was actually derived by Rushmer (1959) (though he did not actually plot the data in the form of a curve) in his efforts to show that cardiac function curves of the Starling type are of little value in predicting cardiac output responses to exercise. He pointed out that, when an animal exercises, the cardiac output rises

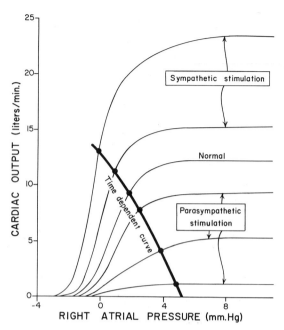

Figure 8-5. A time-dependent curve resulting from changes in parasympathetic and sympathetic stimulation of the heart during measurement of the curve. The light curves in the figure represent the true cardiac output curves. The dots represent individual points determined during the experiment as the right atrial pressure decreased but with the degree of autonomic stimulation of the heart also changing simultaneously. The very dark curve illustrates the resulting time-dependent curve.

while right atrial pressure often falls; he came to the conclusion that this effect was opposite to that which would be predicted by cardiac function curves. Figure 8–5 illustrates what was actually happening in his experiments, showing that as he changed from the resting state to the exercise state, the cardiac output curve was also changing from the normal to the sympathetically stimulated curve. Therefore, the effect was so time-dependent that it was not a cardiac output curve of the Starling type at all.

In conclusion, therefore, anyone using cardiac output curves to analyze cardiac output dynamics must always be extremely careful that his curves are not time-dependent. Because of this possible error in the determination of cardiac output curves, I have made special attempts to remove all time-dependent factors in the construction of the curves in this book. In making our measurements, we have always attempted to keep the pumping ability of the heart from changing while determining the curves and checked our determinations by increasing the right atrial pressure to a high level to obtain a point on the curve and then lowering this pressure rapidly back to its original level to see whether the heart still has the same output that it had had previously. Fortunately, when cardiac conditions are well controlled and the complete curves are measured within a few minutes, the curves will usually be almost entirely non-time-dependent. Sarnoff and his associates (1954a, 1955; Isaacs, 1954) had this same experience, having shown that the curves can be repeated over and over again as long as rigid control is maintained over other circulatory conditions.

SIGNIFICANCE OF CARDIAC "SUCTION"

Many different investigators, foremost among whom perhaps has been Brecher (1954a, 1956a, 1956b; also, Katz, 1930; Cotton, 1934; Böhme, 1936; Altman, 1954; O'Brien, 1960), have pointed out that under some conditions the heart actually sucks blood from the veins into its chambers. For instance, after contraction of the left ventricle, the turgor of the ventricular wall is great enough that during diastole blood is pulled from the left atrium into the ventricle.

Brecher has also pointed out still another type of suction into the heart: When the ventricles contract, the atrial attachments to the ventricles are also pulled downward and to the left by the ventricles; this actually tends to pull the atria open and thereby enlarges the volumes of the atria. Obviously such an effect promotes a negative pressure in the atria during ventricular systole and thereby pulls blood from the central veins.

Both these types of suction contribute to the pumping effectiveness of the heart. Cardiac suction reduces the mean right atrial pressure, and, were it not for this suction phenomenon, the mean atrial pressure would have to rise to higher values to make the heart fill adequately between each pair of heartbeats. Therefore, cardiac suction plays an important role in the overall effectiveness of the heart as a pump. Fortunately, the cardiac output curve depicts not only the propulsive characteristics of the heart but also its suction effects, for this curve represents the overall relationships between right atrial pressure and cardiac output, whether these relationships are established as a result of cardiac propulsion of blood, cardiac suction, or both these effects together (Guyton, 1962a).

Chapter 9

PATTERNS OF CARDIAC OUTPUT CURVES

Because the cardiac output curve is different from one heart to another and even from moment to moment for the same heart, we will in the present chapter characterize the different patterns which the cardiac output curve can assume and the manner in which it can change from time to time. Fortunately, there are only a few fundamental patterns of cardiac output curves (Patterson, 1914b; Sarnoff, 1954a, 1955; Case, 1954; Stone, 1963). Representative curves will be shown in the figures of this chapter, and these can then be used in subsequent chapters along with venous return curves to analyze the alterations in cardiac output under different circulatory conditions.

EFFECT ON THE CARDIAC OUTPUT CURVE OF CHANGING THE CARDIAC LOAD

Obviously, the greater the load against which the heart pumps blood, the less will be the amount of blood pumped. However, under most physiological conditions this factor is not as important as one might expect it to be, because each ventricle has the capability of adapting to different loads in accordance with Starling's law of the heart (Patterson, 1914b; Straub, 1914; Starling, 1918), which may be explained as follows: When the load on the heart becomes increased, either by an increased quantity of blood to be pumped or an increased resistance in the arterial tree, the volume of blood remaining in the ventricle at the end of systole also increases (Nylin, 1943; Bing, 1951; Holt, 1956, 1957; Gribbe, 1959). Therefore, the ventricular musculature is stretched more than previously, resulting in an increased force of contraction (Linden, 1960) and, consequently, automatic adjustment of cardiac contraction to the increased load. Furthermore, each ventricle is capable of adapting in this way to the increased load (Knowlton, 1912; Markwalder, 1914; Patterson, 1914b; Sagawa, 1967a).

158   Yet there is a limit to this adaptation process in each ventricle, for

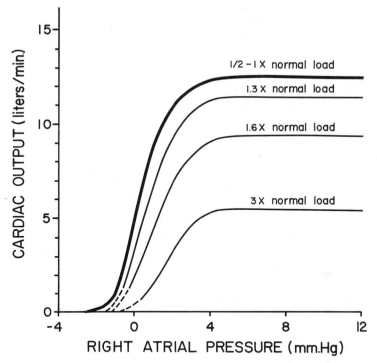

Figure 9–1. Effect on the cardiac output curve of changing the resistive load.

eventually the ventricle reaches its load limit. This fact has much significance in determining the characteristics of the output curves at different systemic resistive loads. Let us analyze the curves of Figure 9–1. The very dark curve is approximately that to be expected for a normal resistive load in the systemic circulation and for a load which is one-half the normal load. Why does the cardiac output not increase appreciably when the resistive load is decreased to one-half normal? The answer to this is that once we have reached the plateau of the curve, both ventricles are normally working near their fullest capacity. Decreasing the systemic resistive load would allow the left ventricle to pump far greater quantities of blood than normally but would have only a slight effect on the load of the right heart. Therefore, the right heart becomes the major limiting factor in determining the characteristics of the cardiac output curve and prevents its rising significantly above the normal level.

On the other hand, when the systemic resistive load is increased above normal, the left heart becomes the limiting factor in determining the characteristics of the cardiac output curve. Sarnoff (1955) has pointed out that for any given atrial pressure the output of a ventricle is almost inversely proportional to the resistive load. Therefore, as the systemic resistive load is progressively increased, the left ventricle output curve, and therefore the total cardiac output curve as illustrated in Figure 9–1, decreases almost inversely with the increase in load. It will be noted in the figure that the decrease is not quite as great as the increase in load, because this relationship between load and resistance is only "almost" proportional but not quite entirely so.

Constant Resistive Load Versus Constant Pressure Load

We need to distinguish between resistive load and pressure load. The term "resistive load" applies to the resistance of the circuit through which the blood will be pumped, while "pressure load" refers to the pressure in the arterial tree into which the heart must pump the blood. One of the reasons for making this distinction is that most cardiac output curves have been determined in heart-lung preparations using a so-called Starling's resistance (Patterson, 1914a, 1914b) to maintain a constant arterial pressure instead of a constant systemic resistance. Figure 9–2 illustrates the difference between the two types of curves. When the resistance remains constant, the arterial pressure rises progressively along with the rise in cardiac output so that at very high outputs the pressure is also very high. Therefore, the maximal amount of blood that can be pumped is less than that which can be pumped when the pressure remains at a normal level. On the other hand, when the pressure is kept at a constant level, the cardiac output curve is somewhat steeper and rises to a higher level, as can be seen by the dashed curve of Figure 9–2.

Sagawa has studied the effect of changing the pressure load on both the output curve on the isolated left ventricle (Sagawa, 1961a) and the total cardiac output curve (Herndon and Sagawa, 1969). The results of these two studies are illustrated in Figure 9–3, which shows mean left ventricular output curves determined in dogs under various constant pressure loads (graph A), and mean cardiac output curves determined in dogs under various constant pressure loads (graph B). It may be seen that at high left atrial pressures, the output of the left ventricle increases substantially when the pressure load is reduced below normal; that is, the plateau of the left ventricular output curve increases significantly when the pressure load is decreased. On the other hand, the plateau of the

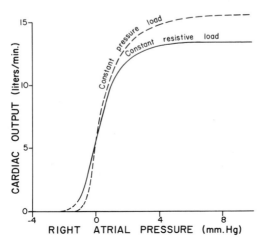

Figure 9–2. Difference between the cardiac output curves (1) when there is a constant pressure load and (2) when there is a constant resistive load.

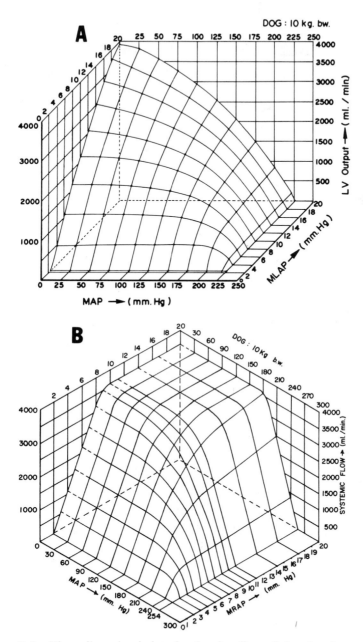

Figure 9–3. Three dimensional plots showing the effects of changing the arterial pressure load on the left ventricular output curve and on the cardiac output curve. Plot A shows the relationship between left ventricular (LV) output and mean left atrial pressure (MLAP) when mean arterial pressure (MAP) remains constant at various levels. [From Sagawa (1967a).] Plot B shows the relationship between cardiac output (aortic flow) and mean right atrial pressure (MRAP) at various constant pressure loads. [From Herndon and Sagawa (1969).]

total cardiac output curve does not rise when the pressure load is reduced below its normal level. The reason for this was explained earlier in regard to the effect of changes in the resistive load on the cardiac output curve. That is, lowering the systemic load does not appreciably alter the load on the right ventricle. Therefore, although the left ventricle has the capacity to pump greater quantities of blood when the systemic load is reduced, the right ventricle becomes the limiting factor that prevents a rise in the cardiac output curve.

Note also in Figure 9–3 that when the pressure load is increased to extremely high levels, both the left ventricular output curve and the cardiac output curve are reduced to zero, since the ventricles simply cannot pump against this high pressure.

When one determines the cardiac output curve in the intact animal, the curve is mainly that of the constant resistive load type rather than of the constant pressure load type. Actually the resistance decreases somewhat as the cardiac output increases because the increasing arterial pressure expands the arterioles and other systemic vessels, thereby decreasing the resistance. Therefore, when we use the term "normal resistive load" in the context of the present discussion, it is meant that the resistive load stays constant except for the decrease in resistance which automatically results from the rising arterial pressure. That is, the resistance is normal for each given arterial pressure even though it is not precisely constant.

The cardiac output curves of this chapter and subsequent chapters are based on the "normal resistive load." In Figure 9–1 the normal cardiac output curve for a normal resistive load is shown. Then, as the systemic resistance increases to 1.6 times normal, the curve decreases about 30 per cent. On the other hand, as the systemic resistance decreases to about one-half normal, the curve does not rise noticeably. It is within these narrow limits that most circulatory function occurs.

EFFECT OF SYMPATHETIC AND PARASYMPATHETIC STIMULATION ON THE CARDIAC OUTPUT CURVE

Figure 9–4 illustrates the effects on the cardiac output curve of stimulating the sympathetic or the parasympathetic nerves (see Sarnoff, 1955; Peterson, 1950). The normal curve of the figure is the same as the normal resistive load curve of Figure 9–1; that is, this is the cardiac output curve found under average normal conditions. When the sympathetic nervous system is stimulated maximally, the plateau of the cardiac output curve rises to about 67 per cent above the plateau of the normal curve. For instance, in the young adult human being, this plateau rises during maximal sympathetic stimulation, such as during very heavy exercise, to 20 to 25 liters per minute.

When the sympathetic nerves to the heart are blocked, the heart loses its tonic stimulation by the naturally occurring sympathetic impulses

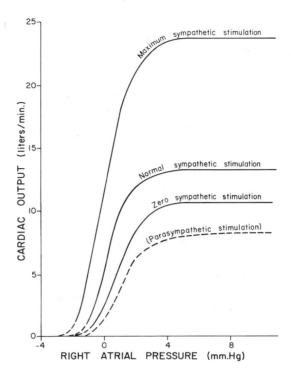

Figure 9–4. Effect on the cardiac output curve of different degrees of sympathetic and parasympathetic stimulation.

(Bronk, 1936). Therefore, the cardiac output curve decreases as shown by the lower solid curve of Figure 9–4. (This fall in cardiac output curve from the normal level to the zero sympathetic stimulation level has been demonstrated in our laboratory by giving total spinal anesthesia to an animal. The maximal output of the heart normally falls about 20 per cent under these conditions. A slow infusion of a sympathomimetic drug will bring the cardiac output curve back up to normal.)

To summarize the upper three curves of Figure 9–4, the normal cardiac output curve can be increased about 60 to 70 per cent by maximal sympathetic stimulation or can be decreased about 20 per cent by complete sympathetic inhibition. Obviously, intermediate degrees of sympathetic stimulation can result in cardiac output curves that lie anywhere between the zero sympathetic stimulation level and the maximal sympathetic stimulation level. Such a series of curves is called a "family of curves," and the actual curve on which the heart is momentarily operating depends upon the momentary degree of sympathetic stimulation.

Parasympathetic Stimulation

Parasympathetic stimulation causes opposite effects to sympathetic stimulation, but unlike sympathetic stimulation it does not affect the strength of ventricular contraction (Carstein, 1958). Instead it affects cardiac output by altering the heart rate and to some extent by altering the strength of atrial contraction. Any factor that reduces the heart rate, even though it does not affect stroke volume output, still reduces cardiac output. Therefore, the cardiac output curve is reduced by parasympathetic stimulation; furthermore, all levels of reduction can be achieved, even down to zero if the parasympathetic stimulation is great enough to stop the heart. Ordinarily, when parasympathetic stimulation causes the heart to stop, the ventricles will "escape" within 7 to 10 seconds and will then beat at their own intrinsic rate of rhythm. Under these conditions, the cardiac output curve will return part way toward normal. Figure 9–4 illustrates by the dashed cardiac output curve approximately the level of output that might be observed after ventricular escape.

To summarize the effect of parasympathetic stimulation on the cardiac output curve, mild degrees of parasympathetic stimulation will reduce the level of the curve slightly and shift the lower margins of the curve to the right. Intense parasympathetic stimulation can reduce the curve to zero for as long as 7 to 10 seconds, but the ventricles then escape, and the level of the curve is thereafter approximately that represented by the dashed curve of Figure 9–4.

EFFECT OF HEART RATE ON THE CARDIAC OUTPUT CURVE

In the above discussions of sympathetic and parasympathetic stimulation of the heart, we noted that heart rate plays a significant role in determining the characteristics of the cardiac output curve. Following sympathetic stimulation the increase in the cardiac output curve is caused partly by an increase in heart rate (Rushmer, 1959) and partly by an increase in strength of ventricular contraction, an effect called "increased contractility" of the ventricles (Sarnoff, 1955). Following parasympathetic stimulation, the decrease in the cardiac output curve is caused almost entirely by a decrease in heart rate.

When other factors besides autonomic stimulation affect the heart rate, the cardiac output curve reaches its highest level at an optimum heart rate, as shown both in heart-lung preparations (Krayer, 1930, 1931) and in the intact dog (Miller, 1962; Snyder, 1962), but it falls to a lower level when the rate either falls below this optimum range or rises above it. In intact dogs this optimum rate is between 100 to 150 beats per minute, as is illustrated by Figure 9–5. The reason for the decreased output at the higher rates is supposedly inability of the heart to fill adequately during diastole.

This figure is important simply to point out that heart rate *per se* can change the cardiac output curve and, therefore, can have much to do with the regulation of cardiac output, a fact that has been pointed out by many different investigators (Meek, 1923; Henderson, 1923, 1927b; Anzola, 1956b; Rushmer, 1959; Gorten, 1961, and many others). If one were dealing strictly with stroke volume output or stroke work output curves, he might easily be led to believe that heart rate is unimportant in the control of cardiac output, for when the heart rate changes, the stroke

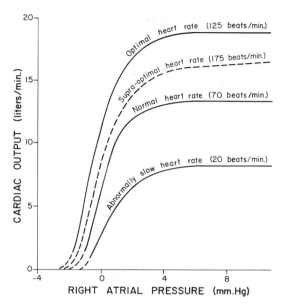

Figure 9-5. Effect on the cardiac output curve of different heart rates, showing that when the heart is driven electrically, the output becomes optimal at about 125 beats per minute.

volume or work output might still remain the same while the cardiac output curve changes along with the change in heart rate.

One feature which must be noted in relation to Figure 9-5 is that the maximal cardiac output curve at optimal heart rate but normal sympathetic stimulation is not as great as the maximal cardiac output curve caused by maximal sympathetic stimulation. The reason for this difference is that sympathetic stimulation not only increases the heart rate but also increases the strength of the heart as well.

EFFECT OF CARDIAC HYPERTROPHY ON CARDIAC OUTPUT CURVES

Almost no precise information is available on the effects of cardiac hypertrophy on cardiac function curves. However, spot checks of cardiac outputs, right atrial pressures, and other parameters of heart function have demonstrated that the hypertrophied heart, such as found in a well trained marathon runner, can pump as much as 50 per cent or more blood than can the average heart (Christensen, 1931). Therefore, we can assume that hypertrophy can increase the cardiac output curve in exactly the same way that sympathetic stimulation increases it.

It must be emphasized that the hypertrophied heart, which is already capable of pumping 50 per cent above normal cardiac output, can still increase its upper limit for cardiac output another 50 to 70 per cent as a result of maximal sympathetic stimulation. Thus, hypertrophy and sympathetic stimulation can summate to cause an even higher cardiac output curve than that which would develop with one of these conditions alone.

EFFECT OF CORONARY FLOW ON THE CARDIAC OUTPUT CURVE

One of the best studied factors affecting cardiac function curves is the effect of coronary flow and oxygen concentration in the coronary blood (Case, 1954, 1955; Rosenbleuth, 1961; Stone, 1963). Figure 9–6 illustrates a typical effect of gradual obstruction of the coronary flow, showing progressive reduction in the cardiac output curve. The coronary constriction curves of this figure have been drawn to peak at an optimal right atrial pressure instead of plateauing as is the usual case. This type of curve is frequently called a "humped curve" in contradistinction to the curve of the normal heart, which reaches a plateau and remains on this plateau. However, it is quite possible that the humped curves that have been reported to severe coronary constriction (Howarth, 1948; Judson, 1955; Taquini, 1961) are time-dependent curves rather than true cardiac output curves (see the previous chapter for discussion). The reason for this is that in the process of determining most cardiac output curves, the right atrial pressure is gradually increased from some lower value to a higher value. If the heart should progressively weaken as the atrial pressure rises, a time-dependent curve would be measured instead of a true cardiac output curve. Indeed, in dog hearts with severe coronary occlusion caused by injecting microspheres (Stone, 1963) a rapid increase in atrial pressure to very high levels does not cause a humped curve at all but instead the typical plateaued curve; this was the same effect found by Schnabel (1959) in patients with severe mitral stenosis. These results indicate that, if we measure the entire curve rapidly enough, it will perhaps display a plateau, as is characteristic of almost all other cardiac output curves.

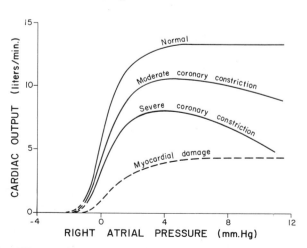

Figure 9–6. Effect on the cardiac output curve of different degrees of coronary constriction, and also the effect of myocardial damage.

EFFECT OF MYOCARDIAL AND OTHER TYPES OF CARDIAC DAMAGE ON THE CARDIAC OUTPUT CURVE

Obviously, many different conditions can reduce the effectiveness of the heart as a pump, including such effects as myocardial infarction, cardiac trauma, valvular heart disease, myocarditis, and others. Since no true cardiac output curves have ever been determined in these different conditions in human beings, or even satisfactorily in animals, it is necessary to deduce these curves from spot measurements of cardiac outputs and right atrial pressures. A typical deduced curve is shown by the dashed curve in Figure 9–6. We have recorded such a curve in the dog under all the following different conditions: (a) at the termination of a long cardiac experiment in which the heart has received much abuse, (b) in hearts that have been damaged by injecting microspheres into the coronaries (Stone, 1963), and (c) in hearts that have been weakened by anoxia resulting from cyanide poisoning (Öberg, 1961). Note particularly that the dashed curve of Figure 9–6 does not have a hump. This curve is based on measurements which were made by rapidly increasing the right atrial pressure to a higher value, then measuring the cardiac output, and returning the right atrial pressure back to a normal level; after making many such successive spot measurements at different atrial pressures, the curve was drawn. In none of these curves have we observed a hump, which is another of the reasons for our belief that the humped curve of severe coronary constriction might well be time-dependent rather than a true cardiac output curve.

Obviously, the greater the degree of myocardial damage, the lower becomes the level of the curve. Therefore, cardiac output curves representing myocardial damage form an infinite family of curves between the normal level and the zero cardiac output axis.

EFFECT OF OPENING THE CHEST AND OF PRESSURE BREATHING ON THE CARDIAC OUTPUT CURVE

Since the heart is located in the thoracic cavity, the effective filling pressures of the heart is determined not only by the intra-atrial pressure but also by the intrapleural pressure; that is, it is determined by the *transmural pressure*, which is equal to intra-atrial pressure minus intrapleural pressure. Therefore, any factor which changes the intrapleural pressure also changes the entire cardiac output curve at the same time. This effect is illustrated in Figure 9–7, which shows (a) the normal cardiac output curve, (b) the effect of opening the chest or of positive pressure breathing, either of which increases the intrapleural pressure, and (c) the effect of negative pressure breathing, which reduces the intrapleural pressure. Note that changing the intrapleural pressure does not alter

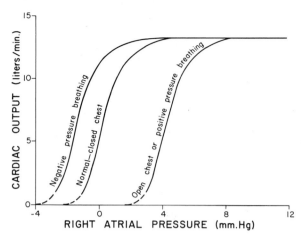

Figure 9–7. Effect on the cardiac output curve of negative pressure breathing, positive pressure breathing, and opening the chest to atmospheric pressure.

the level of the plateau but only shifts the curve horizontally. Thus, when the chest is opened, the right atrial pressure must rise approximately 4 mm. Hg to cause the heart to pump the same output as it had been pumping before the chest was opened (Fermoso, 1964.) On the other hand, during negative pressure breathing, the right atrial pressure can actually fall along with a decrease in intrapleural pressure to lower values while the heart continues to pump the same quantity of blood, because the transmural pressure remains constant. The curves in Figure 9–7 obviously are of extreme importance in analyzing the effects of pressure breathing, either negative or positive, and of opening the chest on cardiac output dynamics, as will be explained in detail in Chapter 24.

At first thought, one might wonder why we do not simply plot all the cardiac output curves in terms of the "effective atrial filling pressure" rather than right atrial pressure referred to atmospheric pressure. The reason for this is that the entire peripheral circulatory system is exposed to atmospheric pressure transmitted from the air to the tissues. For this reason, pressures in the peripheral circulation must be related to atmospheric pressure to be meaningful. Therefore, as we will see in Chapters 14 to 17, cardiac pressures must also be referred to this same pressure level if we are to be able to analyze the function of the entire circulation for the control of cardiac output.

Effect of Cardiac Tamponade on the Cardiac Output Curve

Cardiac tamponade causes very much the same effect on the cardiac output curve as opening the chest (Nerlich, 1951; Metcalfe, 1952; Isaacs, 1954) except for the following difference: In opening the chest, the pressure surrounding the heart increases a fixed amount equal to the difference between the atmospheric and intrapleural pressures, whereas in cardiac tamponade the pressure surrounding the heart depends not only upon the amount of fluid in the pericardial cavity but also upon the volume

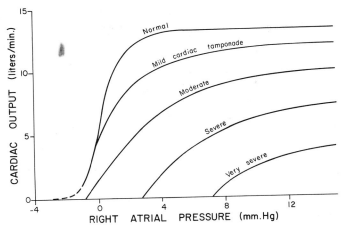

Figure 9–8. Effect on the cardiac output curve of different degrees of cardiac tamponade.

of the heart itself. Therefore, as illustrated in Figure 9–8, when only a small amount of fluid is in the pericardial cavity, there may be no tamponade at all at low cardiac volumes, while at large cardiac volumes the heart may be compressed, causing the cardiac output to be correspondingly reduced. When the amount of fluid in the pericardial cavity increases still further, there may then be slight tamponade when the heart is small and very severe tamponade when the heart becomes enlarged. Therefore, the lower portion of each curve in Figure 9–8 is shifted to the right much less than the upper portion. In very severe cardiac tamponade, the right atrial pressure must ·rise to a value greater than the pressure in the pericardial cavity before the heart can fill at all (Landis, 1946; Isaacs, 1954). Some of the curves in Figure 9–8 do not have a plateau because the output of the heart under these conditions is limited by the filling of the heart and not by the contractility of the heart. Within the physiological right atrial pressure range, the normal plateau is not reached, though at very high right atrial pressures it might eventually be reached.

SUMMARY

One can readily observe from the figures of this chapter that several different factors can either increase or decrease the cardiac output curves. For instance, hypertrophy of the heart, sympathetic stimulation, or reduced load on the heart can all increase the cardiac output curves in almost identically the same manner. Likewise, parasympathetic stimulation, reduced heart rate, and myocardial damage of almost any type can all reduce the cardiac output curves in very much the same way.

Another general pattern of cardiac output curves is caused by those factors that affect the pressure surrounding the heart—such factors as positive pressure breathing, opening the chest, cardiac tamponade, or constrictive pericarditis—all of which shift the cardiac output curves to the right. In cardiac tamponade and constrictive pericarditis, the upper plateau of the curve may not be reached within the physiological right atrial pressure range because of limited filling of the heart. Negative pressure breathing shifts the cardiac output curve to the left. Indeed the cardiac output curve actually shifts back and forth during respiration, shifting to the right during expiration and to the left during inspiration. As we shall see in Chapter 24, this explains why blood flows into the heart from the veins far more rapidly during inspiration than during expiration.

III

REGULATION OF VENOUS RETURN

Chapter 10

PERIPHERAL VASCULAR CONTRIBUTION TO CARDIAC OUTPUT REGULATION – THE CONCEPT OF "VENOUS RETURN"

Throughout the years of cardiovascular research many different circulatory physiologists, including especially Henderson (1923), Warren (1945, 1948b, 1957), Stead (1947a, 1947b), Weissler (1957a), Rushmer (1959), and their colleagues, have believed that cardiac output is regulated mainly by cardiac factors. However, another group of investigators, including Starling (1897), Starr (1940a, 1940b), Anderson (1954), and workers in our own laboratory (Guyton, 1952c, 1955a, 1955b, 1962c), have believed very strongly that peripheral vascular factors are equally as important as cardiac factors in the regulation of cardiac output and, indeed, sometimes even more important.

To emphasize the importance of peripheral vascular factors in the regulation of cardiac output we need only to consider two possible extremes: infinite resistance in the systemic circulation, and zero resistance in the systemic circulation. When infinite resistance occurs, obviously no blood at all can be pumped through the circulation. Under these conditions the heart is still the same heart and the basic cardiac pumping ability has not been changed. In life, infinite resistance in the systemic circulation does not occur, but increases in systemic resistance of as much as four, five, and rarely six fold do occur in abnormal states, and this much increase in resistance can have very great effects on the cardiac output, as will become apparent from quantitative studies to be discussed in Chapter 13 and 22.

At the other extreme, zero resistance would allow blood to flow instantaneously from the aorta into the venae cavae and thence into the right atrium. As a result, the right atrial pressure would be equal to the aortic pressure, and there would be essentially no load on the left ventricle. As a consequence, the heart might easily pump four, five, or six times as

173

much as normal amounts of blood around the circulation in a minute. Indeed quantitative studies on the instantaneous opening of A-V fistulae demonstrate precisely this effect, as will be discussed in detail in Chapters 13 and 23. During normal operation of the circulation, absolute zero resistance, like infinite resistance, never occurs, but the peripheral resistance does sometimes decrease to values as low as one-fourth to one-sixth normal in abnormal states, and even in very heavy exercise the total peripheral resistance can decrease to as little as one-third normal. These marked changes in peripheral resistance are sufficient to cause extreme effects on cardiac output. Therefore, it is obvious that peripheral factors as well as cardiac factors affect cardiac output.

In addition to alterations in resistance, it has also been learned that other factors such as changes in blood volume (De Burgh Daly, 1925; Eckstein, 1947a; Fitzhugh, 1953; Judson, 1955; Guyton, 1958d; Schnabel, 1959; Richardson, 1961), changes in peripheral vascular capacitance (Guyton, unpublished results), alterations in the ratio of arterial to venous resistance (Guyton, 1959b), and still a number of other factors, all primarily operating in the peripheral vascular tree rather than in the heart, have very significant effects on the control of cardiac output.

THE CONCEPT OF "VENOUS RETURN"

When one uses the term "venous return," he almost invariably means the flow of blood into the heart from the peripheral circulation, though occasionally one also speaks of venous return to the left heart. In many ways the term "venous return" is very unfortunate, because under most circulatory conditions the venous return is almost exactly equal to the cardiac output. That is, the amount of blood flowing into the right atrium over any prolonged period of time must equal the amount of blood pumped out of the left ventricle except for a minute amount of blood that flows from the bronchial arteries directly into the pulmonary circulation, an amount estimated to be about 1 to 3 per cent of the total cardiac output (Aviado, 1961).

The justification for using the term "venous return" in addition to the term "cardiac output" is that during transient changes in circulatory function the venous return can be markedly different from the cardiac output. For instance, if one suddenly compresses the aorta, thereby shutting off most outflow from the left ventricle, the venous return will be greater than the cardiac output for a few heart beats, causing blood to dam up in the heart and lungs. Conversely, if the veins leading to the heart are suddenly compressed, blood continues to be pumped out of the cardiac chambers and lungs into the aorta for a few beats of the heart even though essentially no blood may be flowing into the right atrium. Thus, for short, transient periods of time, the cardiac output can be far greater or far less than the venous return.

Yet despite this justification for the use of the term "venous return," simple logic demands that under steady state conditions we consider venous return to be equal to the cardiac output; therefore, any factor which affects venous return will, in the steady state condition, also affect cardiac output, or, conversely, any factor that affects the cardiac output in the steady state condition will also affect venous return. Thus, we would be arguing in circles to say which is more important, venous return or cardiac output. They are interdependent and, except transiently, are equal to each other.

Nevertheless, when the venous return changes before the cardiac output changes, physiologists often say that the change in venous return changes the cardiac output. When the cardiac output increases before the venous return changes, it is often said that the increase in cardiac output cause an increase in venous return. It is mainly factors in the peripheral circulation that cause the venous return to change ahead of cardiac output, and it is mainly cardiac factors that cause the cardiac output to change ahead of venous return. Yet in making this distinction, one must always be cautious to recognize that he is speaking only about transient states that last for a maximum period of a few heart beats, because venous return and cardiac output almost never remain different from each other for more than 5 to 10 seconds (Buckley, 1955; Berglund, 1954).

In the present chapter, we shall describe the peripheral vascular contribution to cardiac output regulation in the usual classic way. Unfortunately, this method of presentation does not lend itself well to the quantitation of venous return, but the logic and philosophy of venous return as presented in this way does give one a very satisfactory introduction to the problems which will be considered more quantitatively later when we combine peripheral and cardiac factors in a composite analysis of cardiac output regulation.

FORCES THAT MOVE BLOOD THROUGH THE SYSTEMIC CIRCULATION

The Classic Concept of Vis a Tergo

The term vis a tergo means "force from behind." At each point in the peripheral circulation a force exists which is pushing blood toward the venous input to the heart, as illustrated in Figure 10–1. This force is called vis a tergo (Landis, 1950; Franklin, 1937; Brecher, 1956b), and its value at any given point in the circulation can be expressed quantitatively as the pressure gradient from the respective point to the right atrium. Its mean value is approximately 100 mm. Hg in the arterial tree, 25 mm. Hg in the capillaries, 15 mm. Hg at the beginning of the venules, and so forth.

Vis a tergo is also sometimes expressed in terms of energy gradient (Duomarco, 1954). The total amount of energy contributed each minute by the heart to the blood as it is pumped into the arterial tree is equal to the quantity of blood pumped times the increase in pressure. Thus, if 5000 ml. of blood is pumped per minute and the pressure increase is 100

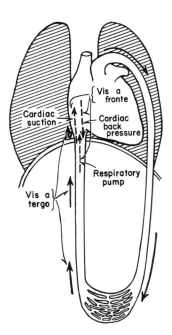

Figure 10-1. Vis a tergo and vis a fronte.

mm. Hg (133,280 dynes), then the total amount of energy contributed each minute to the blood entering the aorta will be 666,400,000 ergs. By the time the blood has flowed through the arterial tree and reached the capillaries, approximately three-fourths of this energy has been dissipated in the form of heat produced by resistance in the vessels. Therefore, the total amount of energy remaining to cause venous return will be 141,350,000 ergs. Likewise, the total amount of energy remaining at the beginning of the venules will be approximately 84,810,000 ergs, and at the point at which the blood returns to the heart all the energy which originally constituted the vis a tergo is then considered to have been expended. In this concept, the vis a tergo is the energy available at each particular point in the circulation to propel blood the rest of the way back to the heart.

The Classic Concept of Vis a Fronte

Very early in the study of venous return it became evident that slight changes in the dynamics of the venous system at the input side of the heart can have a tremendous effect on cardiac output (Franklin, 1937; Brecher, 1956b; Morhardt, 1935; Smith, 1952; Ohara, 1957). For instance, compression of the inferior vena cava to an extent that the total peripheral resistance increases only a few per cent can decrease venous return by as much as 50 per cent (Guyton, 1952c, 1957b). Likewise, suddenly opening the thoracic cavity can decrease the venous return as much as 20 per cent (Fermoso, 1964), particularly when compensatory reflex mechanisms have been blocked.

Because of these very marked effects on cardiac output of hemodynamic changes at the input side of the heart, another term came into usage, vis a fronte, which means "force from in front." Unfortunately, this form has included almost any factor acting on the veins in the near vicinity of the heart that affects the flow of blood into the right atrium (Franklin, 1937; Brecher, 1956b). For instance, as illustrated in Figure 10–1, vis a fronte has been used to mean (a) the back pressure from the right atrium which impedes blood flow from the veins into the heart, (b) cardiac suction of blood from the central veins into the chambers of the heart, (c) suction of blood from the peripheral veins into the thoracic veins because of negative intrathoracic pressure, and (d) impediment of blood flow into the central veins by positive intrathoracic pressure, compression of veins by mediastinal masses, and so forth.

Therefore, it is evident that the term vis a fronte is so all-inclusive that it has almost no quantitative importance; instead it is merely a qualitative descriptive term. Nevertheless, a few of the factors that have been included in vis a fronte require description because of their very important effects on venous return.

EFFECT ON VENOUS RETURN OF INCREASING THE RIGHT ATRIAL PRESSURE. When the heart suddenly becomes weakened and causes the right atrial pressure to increase from its normal value of about zero up to a positive value of only 3 to 4 mm. Hg, the back pressure on the veins causes the venous return to become instantly reduced to about one-half normal (Guyton, 1957b). If the cardiovascular reflexes are intact, reflex adjustments can develop within the next 15 to 30 seconds to overcome much of this reduction in venous return, but, if the reflexes are not intact, this rise in right atrial pressure will depress the venous return for prolonged periods of time.

Quantitatively, in a normal dog in which all cardiovascular reflexes have been blocked, a rise of 1 mm. Hg in the right atrial pressure decreases the venous return (and cardiac output) an average of 14 per cent; a 3.5 mm. rise decreases venous return 50 per cent; and a 7 mm. rise stops all venous return (Guyton, 1957b). Therefore, it immediately becomes evident that conditions at the input side of the heart are exceedingly important in determining how much blood can flow per minute from the peripheral circulation back into the heart and, therefore, also in determining the cardiac output.

However, one must also note that under certain conditions the right atrial pressure can be greatly elevated and yet the venous return will be completely normal. There are two principal conditions in which this can occur: The first of these is strong activation of the cardiovascular reflexes, which cause a high degree of sympathetic tone and thereby constrict all the peripheral vessels. The vascular compression elevates the pressures throughout the systemic circulation, thereby overcoming the elevation in right atrial pressure and allowing normal quantities of blood to flow into the right heart (Guyton, 1958c). The second condition is an increase in blood volume; this overfills the vascular tree and elevates most of the peripheral pressures. Here again, the increase in right atrial pressure is overcome by the elevated peripheral pressures (De Burgh Daly, 1925; Guyton, 1958d) and blood continues to flow into the heart with ease.

The quantitative effects of the elevated right atrial pressure on venous return will be considered in detail in the following chapter, because this is one of the most important of all the factors that determine blood flow from the peripheral circulation into the heart.

CARDIAC SUCTION. In Chapter 8 it was pointed out that the heart actually has the ability to suck blood from the veins, or at least this is true under certain circumstances (Katz, 1930; Cotton, 1934; Böhme, 1936; Blair, 1946; Altman, 1954; Brecher, 1954a, 1956a, 1956b; Fowler, 1958; O'Brien, 1960). The causes of this are two fold: First, when the ventricles relax, the turgor of the ventricular walls often causes the ventricles to round up and thereby suck blood from the atria into the ventricles, this in turn reducing the atrial pressure and aiding blood flow from the peripheral veins into the atria. But more important than this is a second effect: During ventricular systole the atrioventricular rings of the heart thrust downward and to the left as the ventricles contract. This downward thrust pulls the lower borders of the atria in such a way that the atria tend to enlarge, thereby causing negative pressure to develop in the atria, which in turn sucks blood from the central veins into the heart.

These cardiac suction factors, particularly the latter one, have been considered by many investigators to be a major aid to venous return, but in attempting to prove this concept, one is caught in a discussion that can proceed in a circle. Is cardiac suction one of the factors that enhances the ability of the heart to pump blood, or is it one of the factors concerned with the flow of blood along the veins? Cardiac suction certainly increases the effectiveness of the heart as a pump and in so doing reduces the mean right atrial pressure. If we refer to the discussion above that pointed out the extreme dependence of venous return on very slight changes in right atrial pressure, it becomes evident that cardiac suction, by virtue of reducing the mean right atrial pressure, can greatly increase the venous return (Guyton, 1962a).

Some physiologists have postulated that cardiac suction aids venous return also because of the pulsating nature of the suction (Brecher, 1956b; Krug, 1960). That is, it has been postulated that the resulting pulsatile waves transmitted into the veins actually help to propel blood toward the heart. To test this thesis, we developed a technique for introducing artificial pulsations into the right atrium to determine the effect of pulsations *per se* on venous return. This will be discussed more fully in the following chapter, but, briefly, our results showed that pulsations *per se* had either no effect or a detrimental effect on venous return but never a helpful effect (Guyton, 1962a). Therefore, our conclusion was, very simply, that cardiac suction benefits venous return by decreasing the mean right atrial pressure and not by virtue of the pulsations.

RESPIRATORY SUCTION. During each inspiration, the intrapleural pressure falls to a more negative value than usual. This increased negativity is transmitted into the atria and intrathoracic veins to cause a decrease in their intraluminal pressures. As a result, blood now flows easily and rapidly from the peripheral veins into the thoracic veins and right atrium. Measurements of blood flow during respiration, as illustrated in Figure 10–2, therefore show marked increase in venous return during

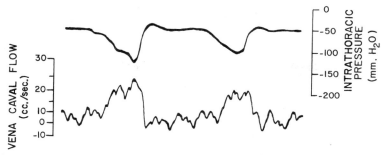

Figure 10–2.   Relationship of intrapleural pressure (upper record) to venous return (lower record) during respiration, showing an increase in venous return when the intrapleural pressure decreases, and a decrease in venous return when the intrapleural pressure increases. [Redrawn from Brecher (1956b).]

inspiration and, conversely, marked decrease during expiration (Brecher, 1956a).

Respiration also compresses the abdominal contents during inspiration because of the downward movement of the diaphragm. This tends to squeeze blood out of the abdomen and into the thoracic veins (Alexander, 1951; Eckstein, 1947b; Krug, 1960). However, it is unfortunate that these same movements increase the resistance to blood flow through the liver (Franklin, 1934; Alexander, 1951; Krug, 1960) so that the net effect of abdominal compression on venous return is very slight during normal respiration. Only during hyperpnea is the effect quantitatively significant (Alexander, 1951).

PARTIAL COLLAPSE OF THE CENTRAL VEINS WHEN THE RIGHT ATRIAL PRESSURE BECOMES NEGATIVE.   When the right atrial pressure becomes negative, the veins immediately outside the thorax become partially collapsed. This effect is the same as that observed when one attempts to suck through a thin-walled tube. It is caused by the atmospheric pressure compressing the veins; this pressure is transmitted to the veins through the soft tissues of the body (Holt, 1941, 1943, 1944a; Duomarco, 1945, 1946, 1950a, 1950b, 1950c; Brecher, 1952a, 1952b; Guyton, 1952a; Ryder, 1944). Because of this effect, pressure inside the veins remains almost exactly equal to the atmospheric pressure as long as the right atrial comes even more negative, the veins collapse still more, but their intraluminal pressures still remain approximately zero with respect to atmospheric pressure. For this reason, once the right atrial pressure has fallen a few millimeters of mercury below zero, a greater decrease in pressure does not further enhance venous return (Guyton, 1957b).

However, the veins do not collapse suddenly at a sharp pressure point for two different reasons: First, the walls of the veins themselves have a certain amount of turgor, which prevents their collapse until the pressure becomes 1 mm. Hg or so negative (Holt, 1959). This is especially true of the veins passing through the liver, which are held open by the structure of the liver itself (Guyton, 1952a). Second, different veins enter the thorax at different hydrostatic levels. That is, some veins lie at higher levels above or below the heart than others, which makes a difference in the pressure at which each vein will collapse (Guyton, 1962a). Because of these two factors, the veins in an animal lying in the horizontal position begin to collapse at approximately +1 mm. Hg and reach total collapse when the right atrial pressure falls to approximately 2 to 4 mm. Hg below atmospheric pressure. For this reason, cardiac or respiratory factors that reduce the right atrial pressure into the negative range can enhance venous return a little at first, but once all the veins have reached their individual collapse pressures, further enhancement of venous return will not occur. The problem of venous collapse will be discussed more quantitatively in relation to the venous return curve in the following chapter.

EFFECT OF PERIPHERAL VASCULAR FILLING ON VENOUS RETURN

It is immediately obvious that if no blood is in the peripheral circulation, no blood can flow into the heart, and the cardiac output likewise becomes zero. If one begins to fill the vascular system, a point is finally reached at which some of the blood will flow into the heart and begin to be pumped around the circuit. As the degree of filling becomes greater and greater, the amount of blood pumped around the circuit also becomes greater and greater. To express this another way, the greater the volume of blood in relation to the "capacitance" of the vascular system, the more rapidly blood will flow into the heart to be pumped.

The "Capacity" or "Capacitance" Vessels

The term "capacity" or "capacitance" vessels has been used for many years to mean the highly distensible vessels of the circulatory system, which are mainly the veins (Franklin, 1937; Alexander, 1948, 1953; Eckstein, 1957; Connolly, 1954; Kidd, 1958). The term "capacitance" is derived from a similar term used in electrical terminology to mean the increase in quantity of electrical charge held in a condenser for a given increase in electrical potential. The analogous function of the veins—their ability to hold progressively larger and larger quantities of blood as the pressure increases—is particularly important in relation to venous return. Mathematically, capacitance can be expressed as dV/dP, meaning the change in volume per unit change in pressure. Other terms that have been used instead of capacitance have been *distensibility, overall distensibility, volume distensibility,* and *compliance.* The reason for our not using the term "distensibility," which has been more often used than "capacitance," is that this term is often also used to mean dV/(dP · V), which causes constant confusion.

The veins are not the only capacitance vessels of the circulation, because the arteries are also capable of holding small amounts of additional blood with increasing pressure. The ratio of the capacitance of the entire arterial tree to that of the entire venous tree is about 1 to 18 (Guyton,

1956b), which illustrates that for many practical purposes the arteries are hardly worth considering as capacitance vessels. However, if one recognizes that the pressures in the arteries are also very high in comparison with those in the veins, he then sees that the arteries can still be a major storage area for blood despite their low capacitances. For instance, assuming the mean pressure in the arteries to be six times as great as the mean pressure in the veins, one finds that the amount of blood stored in the arteries is equal to one-fourth the amount of blood stored in the veins. Yet even in this example, the veins are still the major storage areas for blood. However, included in the venous system are such large storage areas as the spleen, the liver sinuses, and the venous plexuses of the skin.

When the venous tree is inadequately filled with blood, the blood obviously will not flow the rest of the way into the heart. If, on the other hand, the capacitance vessels become well filled, their pressures will rise high, and blood will flow into the heart with great ease. Clearly, therefore, the degree of filling of the vessels is one of the major factors affecting blood flow from the peripheral circulation into the heart. To express this another way, it is the *ratio* of the *blood volume* to the *capacitance* of the systemic circulation that determines how high the average peripheral pressures (mainly the venous pressure) will be and, therefore, that also determines the ease with which blood can flow around the circulation. This ratio of blood volume to the capacitance of the systemic circulation has been unified in the concept of *mean systemic pressure* (Starling, 1897; Guyton, 1962c), which will be discussed in detail in Chapter 12. In essence, it has been shown both mathematically and experimentally that the venous return to the heart is almost directly proportional to the mean systemic pressure (Guyton, 1955b).

Venous Pressure Gradient

Another concept closely allied to the concept of capacitance vessels is the relationship between venous pressure gradient and venous return. Venous return is directly related to this pressure gradient for the following reason: the veins are the principal capacitance vessels of the body, in which most of the blood is stored, and because the blood is attempting to flow from this storage area to the right atrium, the pressure gradient between the veins and the right atrium should, theoretically, be a major determinant of the rate at which blood will flow into the heart. This concept is illustrated in Figure 10–3. Using this logic, one can easily explain how factors such as increased blood volume and increased tone in the capacitance vessels can increase the venous return for, obviously, either an increased blood volume or an increased tone will increase the mean pressure in the capacitance vessels, thereby increasing the venous pressure gradient. Likewise, this concept helps to explain why an increase in right atrial pressure will reduce venous return, because an increase in right atrial pressure will obviously decrease the venous pressure gradient.

Even though the concept of venous pressure gradient for blood flow is valuable in explaining many of the factors related to venous return, it

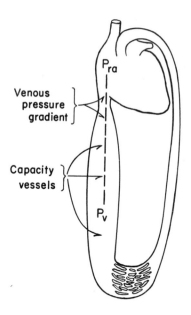

Figure 10-3. Concept of "capacity" vessels.

still is not a highly quantitative way to analyze venous return because it fails to consider the arteries as well as the veins as capacitance vessels; as noted above, even under normal circumstances, the blood stored in the arteries as a result of their high filling pressures may be as great as one-fourth of the total blood stored in the veins. For this reason a much more quantitative analysis can be based on the concepts of *mean systemic pressure* and the so-called *pressure gradient for venous return,* which will be discussed mathematically in Chapter 15.

EFFECT OF HYDROSTATIC FACTORS ON VENOUS RETURN

Too frequently in discussing venous return one considers the entire vascular tree to lie at the same hydrostatic level as the heart. In the lying position, this is almost true, and the hydrostatic factors can then, in general, be neglected, but in the standing position tremendous hydrostatic pressure differences result between the vessels of different parts of the body, these pressure differences resulting very simply from the weight of the blood itself. Figure 10-4 illustrates the pressures developing in different venous areas of the body on quiet standing, showing that pressures as great as 90 mm. Hg can occur in the ankle veins. If we assume that there is negligible resistance to blood flow in the veins and that the heart is pumping adequately to maintain a right atrial pressure of zero mm. Hg, then the hydrostatic pressure in the ankle veins will be equal to the pressure at the bottom of a column of blood open at the top to the air and the same height as the distance from the ankle to the right atrium.

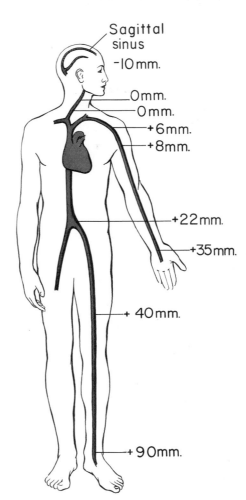

Sagittal sinus
-10 mm.
0 mm.
0 mm.
+6 mm.
+8 mm.
+22 mm.
+35 mm.
+40 mm.
+90 mm.

Figure 10-4. Effect of hydrostatic forces on the venous pressures throughout the body.

Above heart level, hydrostatic forces can cause *negative* pressure in the veins, which effect is illustrated in the sagittal sinus of the brain shown in Figure 10-4. This figure also shows that the pressure in the veins at different points in the neck remains almost exactly zero mm. Hg at all levels. The cause of this is that atmospheric pressure compresses the veins whenever the pressure at any point in these veins tend to fall below zero, which impedes blood flow sufficiently to keep the pressure from falling further. Yet, in the cranium, the dural attachments prevent the veins from collapsing, thus allowing hydrostatic factors there to develop true negative pressures in the dural sinuses.

The major problem in the present discussion, however, is not to point out all the peculiarities of hydrostatic factors, but instead to discuss the effect of these on venous return. When one stands quietly, the arterial pressure in the foot becomes equal to the pressure in the thoracic aorta plus the hydrostatic pressure, that is, 100 mm. Hg + 90 mm. Hg, or 190 mm. Hg. At the same time, the pressure in the foot veins rises from 0 to

90 mm. Hg. The increase in pressure in the arteries equals the increase in the veins so that no net change occurs in the force to propel blood from the aorta back to the right heart. Yet another effect has occurred which can alter venous return to a major extent. That is, the capacitance of the veins (and, to a much smaller extent, of the arteries) is great enough that an increase in pressure of 90 mm. Hg causes far more blood to be stored in the vessels of the lower body than usual, which means that an increase in total blood volume is needed immediately to keep the vascular tree adequately filled. Fortunately, immediately upon standing, one initiates a series of compensatory measures that prevent the detrimental effects of hydrostatic pressures. These include (a) tensing one's abdominal and leg muscles, both of which actions compress the vessels within their boundaries and often totally nullify the detrimental effects of the high hydrostatic pressure; (b) initiation of autonomic reflexes, which increases vascular tone, including an increase in venous tone as well as arteriolar tone (Ralston, 1946; Peterson, 1951, 1952; Rashkind, 1953; Alexander, 1954, 1955, 1956; Page, 1955; Merritt, 1959); and (c) activation of the venous pump, which will be described below.

"Pooling" of Blood Resulting from High Hydrostatic Pressure

At times, the detrimental effects of high hydrostatic pressures in the lower body are not compensated by the above factors. For instance, if a person is placed comfortably on a tilt table and tilted to the vertical position without excitement and without the necessity for contracting his muscles to hold himself on the table, the hydrostatic factors do then affect venous

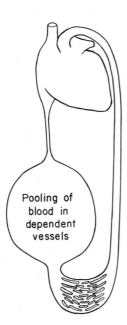

Pooling of blood in dependent vessels

Figure 10–5. Pooling of blood in the dependent vessels of the body.

return very greatly, for now the lack of abdominal and leg muscle contraction allows the vessels of the lower body to become markedly distended (Allen, 1945; Hickman, 1951). Under these conditions, the blood volume simply is not sufficient to fill the dependent vessels, as well as all the other vessels in the body, at the same time. Consequently, venous return to the heart becomes greatly impeded and sometimes ceases. This phenomenon, called "pooling of blood," is illustrated diagramatically in Figure 10–5, which shows distention of the lower vessels and actual collapse of the vessels near the heart.

Pooling of blood in the peripheral vasculature is also likely to occur in persons whose circulatory reflexes have been blocked by spinal anesthesia or after administration of drugs such as hexamethonium that block the sympathetic reflexes (see Chapter 20). Particularly is this true when the person is placed in the upright position at the same time, though in these same states venous return may be completely satisfactory when the person is in the lying position.

Effect of Venous Valves and of the Venous Pump on Venous Return

It is mainly because of the venous valves and the "venous pump" that our circulatory system is able to resist pooling of blood in the lower body in the standing position. Almost no one stands completely still for any significant period of time, but instead each person moves almost continually, the muscular movements intermittently compressing the veins both within the muscles and adjacent to them. Furthermore, movement of the joints compresses, stretches, or bends the veins in the near vicinity. Each time a vein is compressed, blood must flow out of the compressed segment, and, because the valves are all oriented toward the heart, blood can be forced only in that direction. Obviously, therefore, our intermittent muscular movement causes a pumping action in the veins which is called the *"venous pump"* or sometimes the "muscle pump" (Pollack, 1949a, 1949b; Hickam, 1949; Walker, 1950; Hojensgard, 1952). The present concern, however, is not to describe the venous pump itself but to analyze its importance in maintaining adequate venous return and the conditions under which it operates.

Figure 10–6 illustrates the average effect of the venous pump on the venous pressures at the ankle when a person begins to walk after a period of very quiet standing (Pollack, 1949b). During quiet standing, the venous pressure was 87 mm. Hg. Then walking began at a velocity of 1.7 miles per hour. Immediately the venous pressure fell to 15 to 35 mm. Hg and remained at this level during the walking. At the end of walking, about 35 seconds was required for the pressure to return to its previous resting level. Since almost no one in the standing position fails to make some reasonable movement in his lower limbs for more than a few seconds at a time, venous pressure at ankle level normally ranges in the order of 20 to 30 mm. Hg rather than at the level of 90 mm. Hg which would be true without the venous pump. To express this another way, the venous pump prevents the veins from "pooling" more than a small fraction of the blood which they

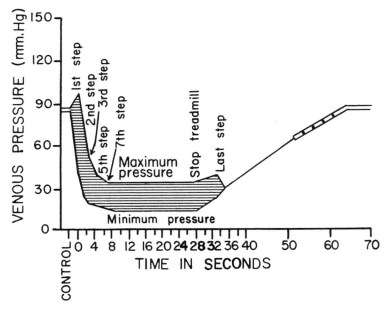

Figure 10–6. Average change in venous pressure at the ankle produced by walking at a speed of 1.7 miles per hour (average of 10 subjects). [Redrawn from Pollack and Wood (1949b).]

would pool were it not for the pump. Therefore, the pooling effect in the dependent vessels of the body is greatly reduced.

A word of caution, however: The venous valves normally affect venous return only from the limbs, because valves are not present in the venae cavae. Unfortunately, vascular pooling can occur also in the abdominal vascular tree as well as in the legs. Indeed, from a quantitative point of view, even though the abdomen is far less dependent than the legs, nevertheless, because of the very great capacitance of the abdominal vascular tree, the overall pooling effect here is often even greater than in the limbs, a type of pooling that unfortunately is not overcome by the venous valves and venous pumps. The only mechanism for overcoming this pooling is contraction of the entire abdominal musculature with consequent elevation of the intra-abdominal pressure.

EFFECT OF INCOMPETENT VALVES AND OF VARICOSE VEINS. A person who has incompetent valves does not have the benefit of the venous pump, in which case the venous pressure in the lower legs as well as the amount of stored blood becomes tremendously increased on standing. Furthermore, if the veins have become stretched until they have reached the state of varicose veins, which often have tremendous capacitance, the pooling effect becomes even more serious. Thus, incompetent valves complicated by varicose veins can sometimes affect venous return so greatly that a person so afflicted faints when he simply stands up (Krug, 1960), this resulting from failure of blood to return to the heart.

PROBLEMS NOT EXPLAINED WELL BY THE CLASSIC ANALYSIS OF VENOUS RETURN

Perhaps the greatest criticism of the classic method for analyzing venous return is that it is almost entirely nonquantitative. For instance, how do peripheral factors that we have discussed in this chapter relate to the cardiac factors discussed in earlier chapters? How does venous resistance relate to arterial resistance in the regulation of cardiac output? How does respiration affect the overall control of cardiac output, and so forth? Until quantitative answers to these questions are available, one can never assess the relative importance of the different factors that affect venous return. Oftentimes a qualitative point of view is adequate, but, on the other hand, in certain problems of circulatory function, the qualitative point of view is not only qualitative but actually misleading. For instance, qualitative analyses have led to widely conflicting views on the regulation of cardiac output in muscular exercise (see Chapter 25), cardiac failure (Chapter 26), the opening of A-V fistulae (Chapter 23), anemia (Chapter 22), and many other conditions.

Therefore, in the following chapters we will attempt to reduce the factors that affect venous return to quantitative concepts in such a way that they can be equated with cardiac factors to provide an overall analysis of cardiac output regulation.

Chapter 11

EFFECT OF RIGHT ATRIAL PRESSURE ON VENOUS RETURN – THE NORMAL VENOUS RETURN CURVE

The very marked effect on venous return caused by changing the right atrial pressure was emphasized in the previous chapter. The purpose of the present chapter will be to quantitate the relationship between right atrial pressure and venous return. However, before describing these quantitative relationships, the methods for studying them will first be discussed.

METHODS FOR STUDYING THE EFFECT OF RIGHT ATRIAL PRESSURE ON VENOUS RETURN

In studying the effect of right atrial pressure on venous return it is desirable to change only the right atrial pressure without changing any other peripheral circulatory characteristics. By progressively weakening the heart, one can raise the right atrial pressure to any desired value, while recording the venous return (Guyton, 1957b). To decrease the right atrial pressure, on the other hand, one can have the animal breathe against negative pressure (Holt, 1943, 1944a; Fermoso, 1964).

A far better method in the experimental animal, however, is to substitute a pump either for the entire heart or for part of the heart in such a way that the degree of pumping can be controlled by the external pump instead of by the heart (Guyton, 1955b). In this way, the effectiveness of pumping can be either decreased to no pumping at all or increased to values well above the pumping effectiveness of the normal heart. We have studied the effect of right atrial pressure on venous return in this manner by two different experimental procedures. First, we have replaced the entire heart and lungs with a cardiac bypass system. However, much more useful has been the method illustrated in Figure 11–1, which can be described as follows:

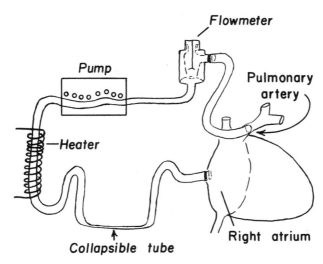

Figure 11–1. System used for controlling the right atrial pressure while studying the effect of right atrial pressure on venous return.

Figure 11–1 illustrates a bypass sytem composed of a pump, a flowmeter, a heater circuit, and a collapsible tube segment, which can be raised or lowered. Blood is sucked into the system from the right atrium, and it eventually returns to the pulmonary artery. Thus, the system allows the blood to bypass the right ventricle; fortunately, the left ventricle will always pump however much blood passes through the external pump system, and within physiological limits this occurs with so little change in pulmonary blood volume that we have been able to detect no difference between the results when using this system and when using the complete cardiac bypass. If the pumping of the external pump is reduced to zero, the pumping of the entire heart is also reduced to zero, and as a result the right atrial pressure rises. Conversely, if the pumping of the external pump is increased above that of the normal right heart, extra quantities of blood are pumped into the lungs and left ventricle, and the left ventricle automatically follows along and pumps the same quantity of blood.

The collapsible tube segment of the system permits very exact control of the right atrial pressure. The pump itself is always adjusted to keep the pressure on the left-hand side of the collapsible tube about −10 to −20 mm. Hg, but since the outside of the collapsible tube is exposed to the air, the pressure at the right-hand end is always exactly zero mm. Hg at the hydrostatic level of the tube itself. By raising and lowering the collapsible tube, the hydrostatic pressure difference between the zero pressure in the tube and the pressure in the right atrium can be altered. When the collapsible tube is below the right atrium, the hydrostatic column from the right atrium to the tube causes a negative pressure in the right atrium. However, when the collapsible tube is above the right atrium, the hydrostatic column affects the right atrial pressure oppositely, causing it to rise. Thus, by raising and lowering the collapsible segment, the right atrial pressure can be adjusted to any desired value. In this way, we have studied the effect of right atrial pressure on the flow of blood from the peripheral vascular tree into the right atrium under many different circulatory conditions.

Study of the Effect of Right Atrial Pressure on Venous Return in the Closed Chest Animal

Obviously, the method illustrated in Figure 11–1 must be used in an opened chest animal. Unfortunately, there is often doubt that results obtained in the open chest animal can be applied precisely to animals with closed chests. Therefore, to determine whether our results obtained in this way apply equally as well to animals with closed chests, we developed another preparation in which a balloon tipped catheter is inserted into the pulmonary artery. The animal is made to breathe against -10 mm. Hg negative pressure, which lowers the control right atrial pressure down to about -11 mm. Hg. Then the balloon in the pulmonary artery is progressively inflated, thereby causing the right atrial pressure to rise to any desired value between -11 mm. Hg and the level at which all cardiac output ceases — usually about $+7$ to $+14$ mm. Hg. The cardiac output, which is equal to venous return, is then recorded by use of the continuous Fick recorder described in Chapter 2. Using this system, we were able to determine in the closed chest animal the effect on venous return of raising the right atrial pressure (Fermoso, 1964). Then the chest was opened and the same study was made again.

To make a long story short, the venous returns obtained in the opened chest animal were the same as those obtained in the closed chest animal (quantitatively within less than 3 per cent). Since this was well within the limits of experimental error, the results obtained in the opened chest dog seem to be entirely applicable to the closed chest dog. It will be recalled that this is not true of the effect of right atrial pressure on the cardiac output curve, because opening the chest alters the external pressure on the heart and thereby markedly changes the heart's function, as was pointed out in Chapter 9.

HYDROSTATIC PRESSURE LEVEL TO WHICH VENOUS PRESSURES ARE REFERRED

The Physiologic Reference Point

It will be evident from the dicussions in this chapter that very slight changes in right atrial pressure can cause marked alterations in venous return. Therefore, it is extremely important to have a precisely defined hydrostatic reference level to which all venous pressures can be referred. For instance, if we use the back of a supine animal as a reference point, the normal right atrial pressure would be about $+6$ to $+8$ mm. Hg. If we should use the anterior of the chest, it would be -4 to -5 mm. Hg. Often one also refers pressure measurements to the level of the right atrium, but unfortunately the right atrium lies in a fairly large area in space.

For these reasons, we concluded early in our studies that the best point to which we could refer all our pressure measurements would be that point in the venous circulation at which the central venous pressure changes least when the animal is rotated through all positions in space. To find this point, a special rotational device was devised in which an animal could be rotated along either the longitudinal axis or horizontal axis or both and, therefore, could be changed to any position in space (Greganti, 1955; Guyton, 1956c). Furthermore, these axes could be moved forward or backward or cephalad or caudad on the animal's body. A catheter was inserted into the right atrium, and the animal was rotated in space while the axes were moved progressively from point to point until the most precise axes could be determined at which the right atrial pressure varied the least amount.

In a study of 25 normal dogs, we found a very precise point at the intersection of the three axes—longitudinal, transverse, and anteroposterior—at which the right atrial pressure did not vary more than 1 mm. Hg regardless of the position of the animal. Futhermore, this point was also very precise from animal to animal, especially in the anteroposterior direction. The coordinates for this minimal pressure change during rotation in all planes of space averaged as follows:

TRANSVERSELY: Precisely midway between the two sides of the chest.

ANTEROPOSTERIORLY: 61.4 (±1.7 S.D.) per cent of the thickest part of the chest, anterior to the back.

LONGITUDINALLY: 76.7 (±5.3 S.D.) per cent of the distance from the suprasternal notch to the tip of the xiphoid process.

Since almost all experimental studies are performed with an animal lying on its back, all the pressures dicussed in this chapter and other chapters of this book will be referred to a level 61 per cent of the thickness of the chest anterior to the back, which coincides with the coordinates given above. At this hydrostatic level the animal can be turned from a prone to a supine position or back again, and still the right atrial pressure, as measured by a catheter, remains almost precisely constant.

After determining the normal coordinates to which right atrial pressures should be referred, we made the animals' circulatory systems abnormal in many different ways, such as by continuous infusion of epinephrine, bleeding the animals, and excessive transfusion of the animals. Then on rotating the animals in space it was found that the axes for least variation in right atrial pressure were exactly the same as the axes in the normal animal (Guyton, 1956c). Furthermore, on plotting these axes on x-ray pictures of the heart filled with a contrast medium, we found the axes to intersect in the heart just at the opening of the A-V valve into the right ventricle, as illustrated in Figure 11–2. Upon finding this, it became evident why the venous pressure at this level remains precisely constant; this can be explained as follows:

If the pressure at the point at which blood flows from the right atrium into the right ventricle rises to a higher than normal value, the filling of the right ventricle becomes increased, and the strength of contraction increases in accordance with Starling's law of the heart (Patterson, 1914b; Starling,

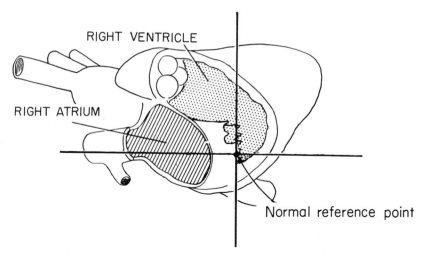

Figure 11–2. Location at the tricuspid valve of the "physiologic reference point" for venous pressure measurements (explained in the text). [Modified from Guyton and Greganti (1956c).]

1918), thereby enhancing the cardiac output. Enhancement of the output in turn reduces the right atrial pressure back toward normal. Conversely, if the pressure at the input point to the right ventricle falls below normal, the filling of the ventricle decreases, and the cardiac output falls. This effect causes blood to dam up in the right atrium, thus increasing the right atrial pressure again back toward normal.

In effect, then, the right ventricle acts as a servo feedback mechanism for regulation of its own input pressure at the point of entry of blood from the right atrium. For this reason, we have called this point in the venous system the *physiologic pressure reference point* (Guyton, 1956c).

Significance of the Physiologic Pressure Reference Point in Venous Studies

Many investigators have referred right atrial pressure measurements to arbitrary levels, such as "the level of the right atrium," "a level 10 cm. in front of the back of the animal," "a level 2/3 the chest thickness in front of the back," and so forth. In the subsequent portions of this chapter it will be explained that even in a normal animal, a change in right atrial pressure of 1 mm. Hg ordinarily causes a 14 per cent change in venous return. Therefore, if the pressure reference level is as much as 1.36 cm. away from the physiologic pressure reference level, one would expect a 14 per cent error in the estimation of the effect of right atrial pressure on venous return.

One could readily argue that if he always uses the same reference level, this would be adequate. However, in using certain reference levels, such as so many centimeters in front of the back of the animal, this can cause very significant errors simply because the thickness of the animals differ; when one uses some ratio of chest thickness for the reference level, a similar though not so drastic error can result. Fortunately, most studies on venous pressure have been referred to half the thickness of the chest, two-thirds the thickness of the chest, or to the "level of the right atrium," all of which give errors of not more than 2 to 3 mm. Hg. Yet, since 2 to 3 mm. Hg can cause as much as a 20 to 40 per cent change in normal venous return, it becomes extremely important that we use in our present discussion a reference level that has real physiologic significance, such as the axes described above for the physiologic pressure reference level. Were it not for the extreme dependence of venous return on right atrial pressure, such precision in the pressure reference level would not be of any real significance.

EFFECT OF POSITIVE RIGHT ATRIAL PRESSURES ON VENOUS RETURN

Figure 11–3 illustrates the average results of increasing the right atrial pressure from 0 to 7 mm. Hg in 14 separate dogs whose reflexes had been blocked by total spinal anesthesia but whose vasomotor tone was maintained at a normal value with an epinephrine drip (Guyton, 1957b). Note that the venous return at 0 mm. Hg was approximately 1200 cc./min. Then, as the right atrial pressure rose, the venous return fell progressively and almost linearly. This figure demonstrates dramatically how severe an effect elevating the right atrial pressure has on venous return. To express this mathematically, a 1 mm. Hg rise in right atrial pressure causes, on the average, a 14 per cent decrease in venous return. Furthermore, by the time the right atrial pressure has risen to approximately 7 mm. Hg, the venous return in the normal dog whose reflexes have been blocked will have decreased to zero. This means that a back pressure of only 7 mm. Hg in the veins is sufficient to prevent all inflow of blood from the systemic circulation to the heart. Note again, however, that in obtaining these results the circulatory reflexes were prevented beforehand from compensating for the depressed venous return. This factor will be discussed in detail later in the chapter.

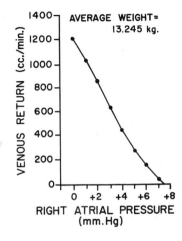

Figure 11–3. Average effect of positive right atrial pressures on venous return in 14 normal dogs. [Modified from Guyton, Lindsey, Abernathy, and Richardson (1957b).]

Explanation of the Marked Depression of Venous Return

Figure 11–4 gives an explanation of the marked depressant effect on venous return of increasing the right atrial pressure. This figure shows that as cardiac pumping falls toward zero, the right atrial pressure rises progressively. However, the arterial pressure falls simultaneously, and in the dog the point at which the arterial pressure equilibrates with the right atrial pressure when the reflexes are blocked is approximately 7 mm. Hg; this value is called the *mean systemic pressure* and is discussed in detail in the following chapter. Measurements of the mean systemic pressure have been made in several hundred intact dogs in our laboratory, and this value averages 6.9 mm. Hg with a standard deviation of only ±0.9 mm. Hg *when referred to the physiologic pressure reference level* (Guyton, 1952c, 1954c; Richardson, unpublished results). Here again, it must be noted that these measurements were made extremely rapidly before sympathetic reflexes could take place. The importance of making such measurements before reflex compensations can take place is discussed both later in this chapter in relation to the normal venous return curve and in the following chapter in relation to the significance of the mean systemic pressure.

Note especially in Figure 11–4 that as cardiac output decreases, the pressure gradient from the aorta to the right atrium falls progressively, and when the right atrial pressure reaches the level of the mean systemic pressure, 7 mm. Hg, no pressure gradient at all exists to cause any blood flow through the peripheral vessels.

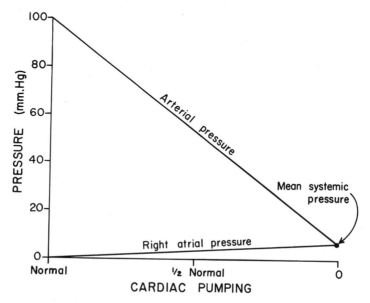

Figure 11–4. Schematic effect on right atrial pressure and arterial pressure of progressively depressing the cardiac output, showing that when the heart stops pumping entirely, the arterial and right atrial pressures become equal to each other at the level of the mean systemic pressure.

Another way of explaining the very marked effect of right atrial pressure on venous return is based on the extreme difference between the capacitance of the arterial tree and that of the venous tree. In studies in our laboratory on live dogs, we pumped blood rapidly from the arteries to the veins through an external circuit immediately after the heart was fibrillated. As the blood was transferred from the arterial tree to the venous tree, the arterial pressure fell 18 times as much as the venous pressure rose (Armstrong, 1954; Guyton, 1956b). Therefore, when the right atrial pressure rises, as occurs for instance when the heart becomes progressively weakened, blood dams up in the venous tree but is removed from the arterial tree. In other words, weakening of the heart acts to *translocate blood from the arterial to the venous tree.* Since the arterial pressure falls 18 times as much as the venous pressure rises, we find that the systemic pressure gradient becomes progressively less and less as cardiac pumping becomes weaker and weaker until finally, there remains no pressure gradient at all. The right atrial pressure at this point averages 7 mm. Hg.

EFFECT OF NEGATIVE RIGHT ATRIAL PRESSURES ON VENOUS RETURN

Figure 11–5 illustrates studies in which the right atrial pressure was made progressively more and more negative in the same animals from which the curve in Figure 11–3 was determined (Guyton, 1957b). Note that venous return rises about 10 per cent as right atrial pressure falls from 0 mm. Hg to −1 mm. Hg, then another 6 per cent from −1 to −2 mm. Hg, and another 4 per cent from −2 to −4 mm. Hg. From there on, the curve is entirely flat without any further increase in venous return even though the right atrial pressure was decreased to as low as −20 to −30 mm. Hg. To express this another way, negative right atrial pressures from 0 mm. Hg down to −4 mm. Hg can increase venous return about

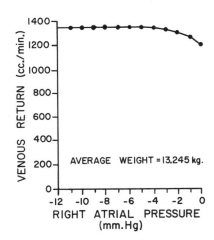

Figure 11–5. Average effect of negative pressures on venous return in 14 normal dogs. [Modified from Guyton, Lindsey, Abernathy, and Richardson (1957b).]

20 per cent, the range varying between 10 and 30 per cent, but beyond -4 mm. Hg, further increase in the negative pressure causes no increase at all in the venous return. This failure of very negative right atrial pressures to continue increasing venous return is explained by collapse of the veins entering the thorax when the central venous pressure becomes sufficiently negative, an effect so important in relation to venous return that it deserves special comment in the following section.

COLLAPSE OF THE CENTRAL VEINS AS A LIMITING FACTOR TO VENOUS RETURN

In all the experiments from which the graph of Figure 11–5 was derived one could observe visually the collapse of the veins leading into the heart as the right atrial pressure became progressively more and more negative. In these opened chest animals, venous collapse occurred in the veins immediately adjacent to the heart. In the closed chest animals, on the other hand, the negative intrathoracic pressure keeps the intrathoracic veins open and transmits the negative pressure to the points at which the veins enter the thorax (Holt, 1941, 1943, 1944a, 1959; Duomarco, 1945, 1946, 1950a, 1950b, 1950c, 1954; Brecher, 1952a, 1952b; Guyton, 1954a). In these animals, therefore, the veins collapse immediately outside the thorax rather than inside the thorax. This effect is illustrated in Figure 11–6, which shows open veins in the thorax but collapsed veins in the neck and in the abdominal region. The veins in the liver region do not collapse so easily as those distal to the liver; this has been demonstrated by catheter studies in the inferior vena cava (Guyton, 1954a).

Not all the veins collapsed simultaneously, nor did each vein collapse instantly and suddenly at a critical pressure. Instead, the veins collapsed gradually through a range of pressures because of the combined effect of three different phenomena. First, atrial pressure pulsations are transmitted

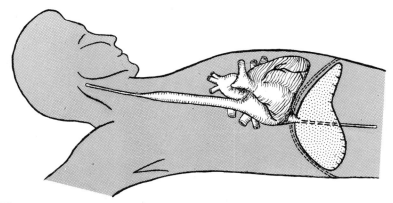

Figure 11–6. Collapse of the veins entering the thoracic cavity when the right atrial pressure is negative; the veins in the liver region do not collapse as readily as the other veins.

backward into the veins. Once the mean right atrial pressure falls below the zero level, most of the veins collapse during part of the pulsating pressure cycle. Then, as the right atrial pressure becomes more and more negative, the duration of collapse during each pressure cycle becomes progressively greater and greater until finally the veins remain collapsed during the entire pressure cycle (Guyton, 1962a).

Second, the hydrostatic levels of the veins entering the thorax are different. For instance, in the supine position, the inferior vena cava lies slightly posterior to the innominate veins. Therefore, collapse of the innominate veins will begin slightly ahead of collapse of the inferior vena cava. Thus, this hydrostatic pressure difference between different veins is another factor that prevents sudden and complete collapse of all the veins simultaneously.

Still a third factor that prevents simultaneous collapse of all the central veins is turgor of the veins themselves. The veins lying free in the thorax have very little turgor, but in the living closed chest animal, tissues adjacent to the veins must be displaced in order for the veins to collapse. Catheter studies of pressures in the central veins indicate that this turgor allows some of the central veins to transmit negative pressures at least as low as -2 to -3 mm. Hg. This is especially true of the veins passing through the liver where the venous walls are held open by the connections to the septa of the liver (Guyton, 1954a).

To summarize, therefore, collapse of the veins entering the thorax is not a sudden phenomenon but occurs (in the horizontal animal) gradually and slowly between the limits of 0 and -4 mm. Hg mean right atrial pressure. In an occasional animal, the level goes as low as -6 mm. Hg, while in other animals collapse is relatively complete at -2 mm. Hg.

THE NORMAL VENOUS RETURN CURVE

If we now take the results of the experiments illustrated in Figure 11-3 and put them together with the results illustrated in Figure 11-5, we obtain

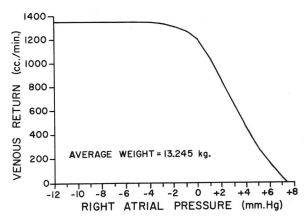

Figure 11-7. The normal venous return curve for the dog. [Reprinted from Guyton, Lindsey, Abernathy, and Richardson (1957b).]

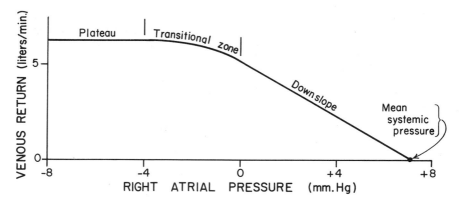

Figure 11–8. A normal venous return curve extrapolated to the human being.

an average normal *venous return curve* for the 14 animals studied in these experiments (Guyton, 1957b). The composite curve is illustrated in Figure 11–7, which shows the effect on venous return of progressively increasing the right atrial pressure from -12 mm. Hg up to $+7$ mm. Hg.

Figure 11–8 gives an extrapolation to the human being of the normal venous return curve. This extrapolation is based on the fact that man's normal venous return averages 5 liters per minute and that essentially all pressures in all segments of the systemic circulation are the same in man as in the dog. Unfortunately, venous return curves have never been measured in the human being. However, experience with cardiac bypass machines at the surgical operating table has definitely demonstrated that very slight elevations in right atrial pressure decrease venous return in precisely the same way as in the experimental animal. These results, therefore, demonstrate very forcefully that the human being is not different from the dog in relation to venous return.

Importance of the Venous Return Curve

The venous return curve is important for several different reasons: First, it demonstrates very forcefully the disastrous effect that elevating the right atrial pressure has on venous return.

Second, it illustrates the fact that negative pressures beyond a limit of negativity cannot further enhance venous return.

Third, and most important of all, the venous return curve can be used with the cardiac output curves of Chapter 9 to analyze the regulation of cardiac output (Guyton, 1955a, 1963a). Note that the venous return curve is expressed in terms of *flow* around the circulation (called, in this instance, *venous return*) and right atrial pressure. If we refer back to Chapter 9, we will see that the cardiac output curve is also expressed in terms of *flow* around the circulation (expressed in these curves as *cardiac output*) and right atrial pressure. But why is it important that the venous return curve have the same coordinates as the cardiac output curve? The answer to this question is that the venous return curve is a *function curve* that depicts the ability of blood to flow through the systemic circulation, while the cardiac output curve is a *function curve* that denotes the ability of the heart to pump the blood. Since these two parts of the circulation must work together in the total circulation, we can utilize the two curves together in a simple graphical analysis to assess the relative importance of the peripheral factors versus the cardiac factors in cardiac output regulation. This method of analysis will be explained in detail in Chapter 14. However, this introduction explains why we are placing so much stress on the venous return curve.

Factors That Can Affect the Venous Return Curve

In the following two chapters the different factors that can affect the venous return curve will be discussed in detail. However, for the present, we need to remark that the venous return curve, like the cardiac output curve, can change from second to second, from minute to minute, or from one physiological state to another. For instance, circulatory reflexes or autonomic drugs can shift the entire venous return curve upward or downward (Guyton, 1958c; Richardson, 1964), or changes in blood volume can do the same thing (Guyton, 1958d). Also, alterations in peripheral vascular resistance can cause the downslope of the curve to change markedly, decreased resistance causing the slope to become greater and increased resistance causing the slope to become less (Guyton, 1959b). These are a few of the changes that can occur. Others will be discussed at later points in the book.

Mean Systemic Pressure as the Upper Limit of Right Atrial Pressure

The pressure level at which the downslope of the venous return curve crosses the zero venous return axis is equal to the *mean systemic pressure,* which is the pressure in all parts of the systemic circulation when all blood flow ceases. Therefore, the mean systemic pressure has special importance in that it is the upper limit to which the right atrial pressure can rise. It also follows that *the venous return approaches zero as the right atrial pressure approaches the mean systemic pressure.* The quantitative aspects of the mean systemic pressure as it affects venous return and the venous return curve will be discussed in the following two chapters. However, briefly, the mean systemic pressure rises (a) when the blood volume increases, (b) when the vascular tone increases, or (c) when the vasculature is compressed externally, such as during muscular contraction or abdominal compression. Conversely, this pressure decreases (a) when the vascular tone decreases or (b) when the blood volume decreases (Guyton, 1954c, 1963; Richardson, 1961).

Time-Dependent Curves Caused by Circulatory Reflexes

A word of explanation must be given at this point because many investigators have already perceived as they have read this chapter that in some of their own experiments, progressive weakening of the heart

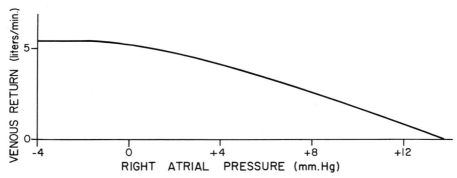

Figure 11–9. A time-dependent venous return curve, illustrating the error that can be made in determining the curve when the right atrial pressure is elevated very slowly while reflex compensations are taking place.

often does not cause complete cessation of venous return until the right atrial pressure has risen well above 7 mm. Hg, more likely to a value of 12 to 14 mm. Hg. Indeed, if one increases the right atrial pressure very slowly, the recorded venous return curve will be essentially that illustrated in Figure 11–9 (Fermoso, 1964). However, this is a *time-dependent curve* because, as the rising right atrial pressure causes venous return to decrease, compensatory reflexes become more and more active. For example, the pressoreceptor reflexes and the central nervous system ischemic response cause a barrage of sympathetic impulses to the peripheral vascular tree, which decreases the "capacitance" of the peripheral vasculature and thereby progressively elevates the mean systemic pressure while the venous return curve is being measured. Thus, the upper portion of the venous return curve in Figure 11–9, in the range of zero mm. Hg, is perfectly normal, but, as the right atrial pressure rises to positive values, powerful sympathetic reflexes set in so that now we are no longer measuring portions of the original venous return curve but instead are measuring points on successive venous return curves that represent a progressively more highly stimulated sympathetic nervous system.

In using venous return and cardiac output curves to analyze circulatory phenomena, it is essential never to use a time-dependent curve but instead to use a curve that tells one precisely what the venous return would be at a given instant at any given right atrial pressure.

One method for determining a non-time-dependent curve is to increase the right atrial pressure very rapidly from its normal level up to a high level and then determine the venous return before compensatory reactions can set in. Then the right atrial pressure is returned once again to the zero level, and the same process is repeated for another pressure level again and again until the entire curve is determined.

Another method for determining non-time-dependent venous return curves is to eliminate the sympathetic reflexes before determining the curve. We have done this in our laboratory in the following way (Guyton, 1957b): A total spinal anesthesia is given to the animal by injecting into the lower spinal canal 20 ml. or more of solution containing 150 mg. of

Metycaine. This results in immediate and total anesthetization of the entire spinal cord and even of the basal regions of the brain, thus eliminating the efferent limbs of all the cardiovascular reflexes. However, this procedure also decreases the vasomotor tone throughout the body. Therefore, a very slow, continuous infusion of norepinephrine is given to the animal to return the animal's arterial pressure to its normal level. The animal can be maintained in this state for hours with no functional circulatory reflexes and yet with normal vasomotor tone. The normal venous return curve of Figures 11–3, 11–5, and 11–7 of this chapter was determined in this manner.

EFFECT OF RIGHT ATRIAL PULSATION ON VENOUS RETURN – A RECTIFICATION PHENOMENON

In the discussion of the collapse factor earlier in the chapter it was pointed out that pulsation in the central venous pressures is one of the factors that prevents venous collapse at a single critical right atrial pressure. The effect of right atrial pulsation on venous return requires additional discussion before leaving this chapter, because considerable emphasis has been placed by different research workers on the importance of venous pulsation to venous return (Brecher, 1956; Krug, 1960). The present section, therefore, will attempt to analyze the part that right atrial pulsation plays in promoting venous return, especially the question whether right atrial pulsation *per se* has a beneficial effect or a harmful effect on venous return.

First, it cannot be denied that right atrial pulsation resulting from atrial contraction is beneficial to cardiac output and, therefore, also beneficial to venous return. Atrial contraction causes the atrial pressure to rise just when extra filling of the ventricles will make the heart a stronger pump. Therefore, atrial contraction increases the efficacy of the heart as a pump (Linden, 1960), which in turn decreases the mean right atrial pressure and increases the venous return. In this instance, the venous return is truly enhanced as a result of atrial pulsation. Yet it is not the pulsation *per se* that enhances the venous return, but instead the *reduction in mean right atrial pressure* caused by increased effectiveness of the pumping action of the heart.

Another condition in which atrial pulsation has been considered to increase venous return has been the pulsatile suction of blood by the heart from the central veins during cardiac systole, which was discussed in Chapter 8. Both Brecher (1956b) and Krug (1960) have postulated that the pulsations transmitted down the veins in some way enhance venous return. However, this pulsatile suction, like atrial contraction, decreases the mean right atrial pressure, and here again one can ascribe the beneficial effect of the phenomenon to the decrease in mean right atrial pressure without having to assume that it is the pulsations *per se* that are causing the increase in venous return. Indeed, in the subsequent paragraphs we will show that the pulsations themselves are probably harmful rather than beneficial to venous return.

Rectification of Right Atrial Pressure by the Collapse Phenomena

Figure 11–10 illustrates on one axis the right atrial pressure and on the other axis the venous pressure outside the thoracic cavity. The heavy black line denotes the relationship between right atrial pressure and the pressure in the veins outside the thorax. Note that when the right atrial pressure is in the positive range, all the veins are filled with blood, and the venous pressure is essentially equal to the right atrial pressure. However, when the right atrial pressure becomes slightly negative, all the veins leading into the thoracic cavity collapse so that the right atrial pressure is then no longer transmitted to the peripheral veins. As a result, the venous pressure a few centimeters away from the thorax will be either 0 mm. Hg or at most a few millimeters less than atmospheric pressure.

In the lower part of Figure 11–10, a horizontal sine wave denotes pulsation of the right atrial pressure between the limits of -20 mm. Hg and $+20$ mm. Hg. The dashed lines illustrate corresponding points between the pulsatile right atrial pressure and the pressure changes in the peripheral veins. Note that when the right atrial pressure rises into the positive range, the venous pressure also rises in an equally positive fashion. However, when the right atrial pressure falls into the negative range, the venous pressure fails to fall to equally negative pressures. If we now average the venous pressures, as illustrated by the arrow, we find that the mean venous pressure is a positive value of approximately $+6$ mm. Hg, whereas the mean right atrial pressure is 0 mm. Hg.

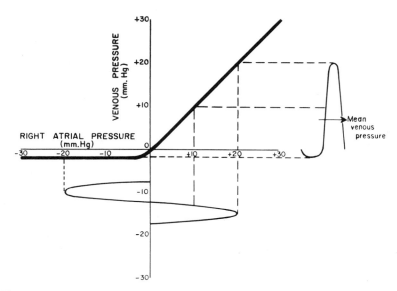

Figure 11–10. A rectification diagram, showing the resultant pressure changes in the extrathoracic veins when the right atrial pressure is pulsating negatively and positively (explained in the text). [Reprinted from Guyton, Langston, and Carrier (1962a).]

To summarize the concept presented in Figure 11–10, a pulsatile right atrial pressure causes the mean venous pressure to be greater than the mean right atrial pressure. Now, if we study again Figure 11–7, which shows the normal venous return curve, it becomes evident that right atrial pressure pulsation, by increasing the mean pressure in the veins entering the thorax, should have an extraordinary depressant effect on venous return.

Proof of the Depressant Effect of Right Atrial Pulsation on Venous Return

To prove that this rectification phenomenon does indeed exist when pulsations occur in the right atrium, we developed a method for sinusoidally injecting and removing blood from the right atrium (Guyton, 1962a). The pulse volumes were changed from 0 to 68 ml. per pulse, and the frequency of pulsations was altered from 60 cycles/minute to 240 cycles/minute. Figure 11–11 illustrates the results of a study accomplished by this procedure. The dark curve shows a venous return curve determined in a single animal prior to instituting the artificial right atrial pulsation. Then artificial right atrial pulsations were instituted with pulse volumes of 4 cc./pulse, 8 cc./pulse, and 22 cc./pulse. Note that the pulsations caused the venous return curves to decrease markedly in certain ranges of mean right atrial pressures. Particularly was this true when the mean right atrial pressure was near zero mm. Hg and the veins were alternately opening and collapsing with each pulsation. However, when the mean right atrial pressure was set at a very negative value, below −20 mm. Hg, the pulsations had no effect on venous return. In this range, even the positive peaks of the pressure pulsations did not rise above the zero level. In other words, the veins were always in the collapsed state, and no rectification could occur. Likewise, when the mean right atrial pressure was elevated to higher values, to about +8 mm. Hg, the curves

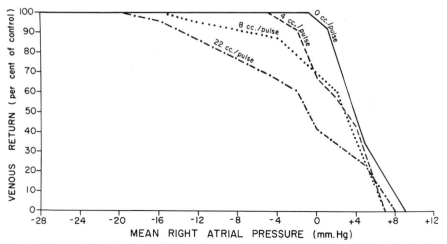

Figure 11–11. Effect of right atrial pulsations on venous return, illustrating that in the normal right atrial pressure range, pulsations are detrimental to venous return. [Reprinted from Guyton, Langston, and Carrier (1962a).]

again came very close to each other. In this range, the negative peaks of the pulsations never fell low enough to cause collapse of the veins so that rectification could not occur here either. Yet in the normal physiological range of −4 to +2 mm. Hg, pulsations caused a very detrimental effect on venous return.

From this study, then, we can conclude that right atrial pulsations *per se* cause only a detrimental effect on venous return unless they are synchronized with cardiac action in such a way that they increase the effectiveness of the heart as a pump. If the effectiveness of the heart as a pump is increased, this can often decrease the mean right atrial pressure sufficiently to overcome the detrimental effect of the pulsations themselves on venous return and, indeed, can often even enhance venous return, an effect that has been demonstrated especially by the research work of Brecher (1956b).

Chapter 12

MEAN CIRCULATORY PRESSURE, MEAN SYSTEMIC PRESSURE, AND MEAN PULMONARY PRESSURE AND THEIR EFFECT ON VENOUS RETURN

The subject of this chapter was introduced in the previous chapter when it was pointed out that the mean systemic pressure is the upper limit to which the right atrial pressure can rise. The purposes of the present discussion are, first, to explain what is meant by the *mean circulatory pressure,* the *mean systemic pressure,* and the *mean pulmonary pressure;* second, to explain quantitatively how the mean systemic pressure affects venous return; third, to delineate the factors that can alter the mean systemic pressure; and, fourth, to explain the interrelationships between the mean systemic pressure, the mean pulmonary pressure, and the mean circulatory pressure.

MEAN SYSTEMIC PRESSURE, MEAN PULMONARY PRESSURE, AND MEAN CIRCULATORY PRESSURE

DEFINITIONS

The *mean circulatory pressure* is the pressure that would be measured at all points in the entire circulatory system if the heart were stopped suddenly and the blood were redistributed instantaneously in such a manner that all pressures were equal.

The *mean systemic presure* is the pressure that would be measured at any given instant anywhere in the systemic circulation if all inflow and all outflow from the systemic circulation were to cease suddenly and

205

the blood were redistributed in such a manner that the pressure would be the same in each part of the systemic circulation.

The *mean pulmonary pressure* is the same measurement in the pulmonary circulation.

The concepts of mean pulmonary and mean systemic pressures have received almost no attention in the literature, but the importance of the mean circulatory pressure in circulatory dynamics has been recognized for over half a century. It has been called by a number of different names such as "mean systemic pressure" by Starling (1897), then later "hydrostatic mean pressure" and "hydrokinetic mean pressure" by Bolton (1903), "static pressure" by Starr (1940a, 1940b), "mean circulatory filling pressure" by ourselves in earlier publications (Guyton, 1954c, 1955b), and "mean filling pressure" by Krug (1960). One immediately notes the confusion between Starling's use of the term "mean systemic pressure" and our present usage as defined above. However, Starling's description of his actual measurements shows that he was measuring the mean pressure in the entire circulatory system and not simply that in the systemic circulation. He realized, however, that the mean circulatory pressure and the mean systemic pressure are almost equal to each other (as will be pointed out later in this chapter), which undoubtedly explains his usage of this term.

Significance of the Mean Pressures

The *mean circulatory pressure* is actually a measure of the degree of filling of the systemic circulation with blood (Guyton, 1954c; Richardson, 1961). If the holding capacity of the circulatory system is very great but the blood volume is very low, the mean circulatory pressure will be very low. On the other hand, if the holding capacity of the circulation is low but the volume is great, the mean circulatory pressure will be high.

Likewise, the *mean systemic pressure* is a measure of the degree of filling of the systemic circulation at any given time, and the *mean pulmonary pressure* is a measure of the degree of filling of the pulmonary circulation.

One might wonder why it is important to determine the degree of filling of the entire circulation or of the systemic or pulmonary system, but if he will think for a moment of a circulatory system filled only slightly with blood, not enough to stretch the vessels at all, he will see that no pressure will develop in the peripheral vessels, and without pressure there will be no force to move blood toward the heart. As a consequence, the cardiac output will be zero however actively the heart might pump. Therefore, to explain the importance of these mean pressures, we need only to point out that both experimentally and mathematically these mean pressures have been shown to be among the most important of all factors that determine the rates at which blood can flow from the peripheral vessels into the chambers of the heart (Starr, 1940a, 1940b; Guyton, 1955a, 1955b, 1963a). The mathematical proof of the direct relationship between these pressures and blood flow to the heart will be given in Chapter 14.

The Dynamic Nature of the Mean Pressures

The mean circulatory pressure can be determined only by stopping the circulation and bringing the different pressures to equilibrium, the method for which will be described later in the chapter. In the human being this pressure has been measured only after death (Starr, 1940b), and this has led some persons to call the pressure "dead pressure." Unfortunately, this has made many investigators believe that these mean pressures have no significance in the living animal. However, this is farthest from the truth, because all the pressures throughout the different parts of the circulation are quantitatively dependent upon these mean pressures. Indeed, the quantitative value of the mean circulatory pressure is the weighted average of the pressures in all segments of the circulation when each of these pressures is weighted in proportion to the capacitance of each segment (Guyton, 1954c). Likewise, the mean systemic and mean pulmonary pressures are weighted averages for the systemic and pulmonary circulations respectively. Therefore, these mean pressures are actually dynamic quantities, so much so indeed that Bolton (1903) actually called the mean circulatory pressure the "hydrokinetic mean pressure" of the circulation.

METHODS FOR DETERMINING THE MEAN PRESSURES

Determination of Mean Circulatory Pressure

Determination of mean systemic and mean pulmonary pressures is a difficult experimental procedure, but determination of the mean circula-

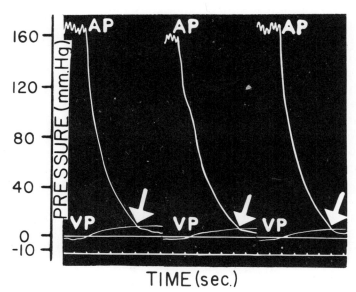

Figure 12-1. Repeated measurement of the mean circulatory pressure. The pressure at the point of crossing is the mean circulatory pressure. [Reprinted from Guyton, Polizo, and Armstrong (1954c).]

tory pressure is relatively easy and has been accomplished several thousand times in our laboratory (Guyton, 1954c; Richardson, 1961) in the following manner:

First, a catheter is inserted through one of the arteries into the arch of the aorta and another into the right atrium to measure pressures from these two points. Still another catheter is inserted upward through the femoral artery into the aorta with the tip of the catheter lying almost exactly at the point where the aorta passes the liver. A final catheter is inserted upward through a femoral vein into the inferior vena cava. Once these preparations have been made, an alternating current of 110 volts is applied to two syringe needle electrodes inserted beneath the skin of the anterior chest, one immediately cephalad and one immediately caudad to the heart. This causes the heart to fibrillate. Within one second after fibrillation ensues, a pump is started which pumps blood from the aortic catheter into the catheter in the inferior vena cava. This causes immediate translocation of blood from the arterial tree to the venous tree, bringing the pressures of these two major portions of the systemic circulation to equilibrium within two to seven seconds, as illustrated in Figure 12–1. The point of crossing of the two pressure recordings is equal to the mean circulatory pressure. The reason for placing the tip of the catheter at the level of the liver is that the aorta will not collapse completely at this point, thus preventing occlusion of the tip of the catheter while blood is being pumped rapidly from the aorta into the vena cava.

Immediately after the pressures have been brought to equilibrium, the heart is defibrillated by passing 440 volt current at approximately 10 amperes for 1/10 second anteroposteriorly through the chest (for method, see Guyton, 1951). To accomplish satisfactory defibrillation in this manner, the electrodes used on the chest must be larger than the size of the heart and must make excellent contact with the anterior and posterior surfaces of the chest. To achieve adequate contact, the skin is shaved, and a copper sponge soaked in saturated sodium chloride solution is placed between the electrodes and the chest wall. Also the electrodes are pressed tightly against the chest immediately before application of the current.

One might wonder why the elaborate procedure is used for pumping blood from the arteries to the veins to establish equilibrium, or he might also wonder why equilibrium must be established rapidly. The answer to these questions is that immediately after the heart begins to fibrillate, which causes a resultant fall in arterial pressure, intense sympathetic reflexes begin to develop. These cause no significant effect on the peripheral vasculature within the first 7 seconds, but after 7 seconds, one finds a progressive rise in mean circulatory pressure as shown in Figure 12–2 (Guyton, 1954c), this rising to a maximum at 1 minute and 45 seconds after fibrillation and then falling off to a minimum about 14 minutes later. Therefore, if the mean circulatory pressure is not measured within the first 7 seconds after fibrillation of the heart, it is likely to be in serious error.

Another question that will immediately enter one's mind is whether the equilibrium pressure measured in this manner is the true mean circulatory pressure. To test this, we measured the mean circulatory

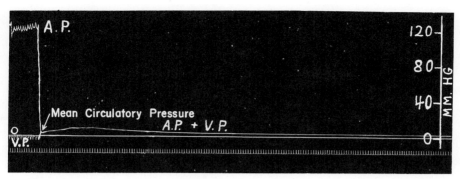

Figure 12–2. Measurement of mean circulatory pressure. The heart was not defibrillated after the initial measurement was made; therefore, the mean circulatory pressure rose to double the normal and then fell gradually over a period of 15 minutes. (Time mark every 5 seconds.) [Reprinted from Guyton, Polizo, and Armstrong (1954c).]

pressure in dogs in which all circulatory reflexes had been abrogated by total spinal anesthesia (Guyton, 1954c) in the following manner: The heart was fibrillated, and the pressures were brought rapidly to equilibrium. Then the pump between the aorta and vena cava was stopped, and equilibrium pressure was recorded continuously for 10 minutes. The mean circulatory pressure established in this way only 3 seconds after fibrillation was precisely the same as that maintained throughout the following 10 minute period. This result demonstrated that additional blood besides that pumped from the arterial tree to the venous tree did not need to be translocated in order to obtain a satisfactory measurement of mean circulatory pressure.

Another feature of this measurement of mean circulatory pressure is that it can be repeated again and again. Figure 12–1 illustrates three such measurements in the same animal that were repeated approximately 15 minutes apart. Such measurements have been made as many as 30 times in the same animal. To obtain accurate measurements, the only serious precaution is not to make a second measurement less than 2 minutes after the first measurement. Otherwise, autonomic reflexes initiated by the first measurement will still be effective in the circulation and the measurement will be too high.

The mean circulatory pressure measured in this manner in several hundred animals has been almost exactly 7 mm. Hg with a standard deviation of less than 1 mm. Hg (actually 6.9 mm. Hg ± 0.9 mm. Hg). Therefore, it is evident that the mean circulatory pressure in the normal dog is a very exactly controlled value. We shall see later that the mean circulatory pressure can fall as low as zero, or it can rise as high as 30 to 40 mm. Hg under special conditions.

Measurements of Mean Systemic Pressure and Mean Pulmonary Pressure

We have made several hundred measurements of mean systemic and mean pulmonary pressures using dogs prepared two weeks ahead of time with plastic loops placed around both the pulmonary artery and the aorta, with one end of each loop attached to an anterior rib and the other end brought out on the back of the animal; when the end was pulled, the loop would occlude the artery. (See Lindsey, 1957, 1959, for original method.) Then catheters were placed at appropriate points in the circulation, including the pulmonary artery beyond the constrictive loop. The loops were suddenly occluded, pressures brought to equilibrium, and mean systemic and mean pulmonary pressures measured.

The values for mean systemic pressure determined in this way were so nearly identical to the mean circulatory pressure measured as described above that we could not distinguish the difference, both of these pressures averaging almost exactly 7 mm. Hg. The values determined for mean pulmonary pressure averaged 5 mm. Hg.

In summary, measurements of mean systemic pressure and mean pulmonary pressure in the normal dog have been, respectively, 7 and 5 mm. Hg.

Interrelationships Between Mean Systemic, Mean Pulmonary, and Mean Circulatory Pressures

In the same experiments in which the mean systemic and mean pulmonary pressures were measured, we also determined the relative capacitances of the systemic and pulmonary circulations. To determine these, one of the plastic loops was occluded ahead of the other, permitting translocation of blood from one of the circulations to the other; then, suddenly, the second plastic loop was occluded. In this way the mean pulmonary pressure and mean systemic pressure could be measured after translocation of blood. These studies showed that the mean pulmonary pressure changed seven times as much as the mean systemic pressure when blood was translocated (calculated from data in Lindsey, 1957, 1959), illustrating that the capacitance of the systemic circulation is about seven times as great as that of the pulmonary circulation.

From these translocation measurements, it was possible to work out the interrelationships between mean circulatory pressure, mean systemic pressure, and mean pulmonary pressure. These are shown by the nomogram in Figure 12–3. The solid line drawn across the nomogram illustrates the normal values, showing a mean pulmonary pressure of 5 mm. Hg, a mean circulatory pressure of 7 mm. Hg, and a mean systemic pressure of 7.3 mm. Hg. Note, however, that the 7 mm. Hg and 7.3 mm. Hg levels are near enough to each other to be within the limits of error of measurement. The dashed line drawn across the nomogram illustrates a very high mean pulmonary pressure, such as one might find in an animal or person with severe left heart failure. The values depicted by the intersections of this line on the nomogram are 20 mm. Hg mean pulmonary pressure, 12 mm. Hg mean circulatory pressure, and 10.8 mm. Hg mean systemic pressure. Here again, the mean circulatory pressure and the mean systemic pressure are only about 1 mm. Hg apart.

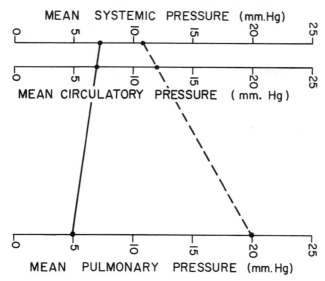

Figure 12–3. Nomogram showing the interrelationships between the mean circulatory pressure, mean systemic pressure, and mean pulmonary pressure. The solid line across the graph shows the normal values. The dashed line shows representative values in serious left heart failure.

Most conditions which elevate the mean systemic pressure, such as increased vasomotor tone or increased blood volume, also increase the mean pulmonary pressure. It is only when a disparity exists between the pumping abilities of the two sides of the heart that mean systemic and mean pulmonary pressures become significantly different from each other (Lindsey, 1957); the dashed curve of Figure 12–3 illustrates about as great a disparity as one would ever expect between mean pulmonary pressure and mean systemic pressure except under very acute conditions.

From this discussion, one can see that the mean circulatory pressure and the mean systemic pressure are almost identical under almost all conditions. The reason is very simply that the mean circulatory pressure is determined 7/8 by the mean systemic pressure and only 1/8 by the mean pulmonary pressure. Furthermore, the mean pulmonary pressure is rarely very much different from the mean systemic pressure. Therefore, for practical purposes one can almost always consider measurements of mean circulatory pressure to be synonymous with measurements of mean circulatory pressure. This explains why we have simply measured the mean circulatory pressure in most of our studies and have not gone to special trouble to measure the mean systemic pressure; that is, the mean circulatory pressure is very easy to measure while the mean systemic pressure is very difficult to measure, and the errors of measurement are such that the difference between the two measurements would be within the limits of error anyway. For this reason, in many places in this text, I use the term "mean systemic pressure" almost synonymously with the term "mean circulatory pressure."

EFFECT ON THE VENOUS RETURN CURVE OF CHANGING THE MEAN SYSTEMIC PRESSURE

Figure 12–4 illustrates four separate venous return curves run in the same animal in which the mean systemic pressure was progressively increased by increasing the blood volume (Guyton, 1955a). The respective mean systemic pressures were 4.7, 6.9, 8.4, and 10.6 mm. Hg. Note that as the mean systemic pressure increased, the venous return curves rose to higher levels. Also the point at which the venous return curve crossed the zero venous return axis shifted progressively to the right. The right atrial pressure at this point of crossing is actually a measure of the mean systemic pressure, because at this point there is no flow in the systemic system, which means that the right atrial pressure is then equal to the mean systemic pressure.

In general, therefore, one can say that an increase in the mean systemic pressure causes an almost parallel shift in the venous return curves upward and to the right. All curves reach a plateau in the negative right atrial pressure range because of venous collapse, as was explained in the previous chapter. However, the greater the mean systemic pressure, the higher the level of the plateau.

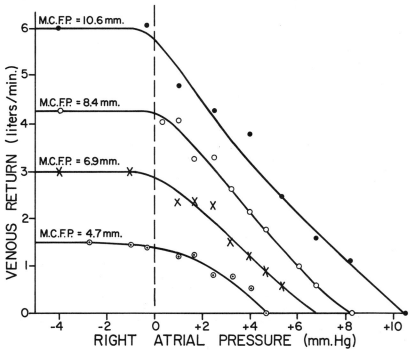

Figure 12–4. Effect on the venous return curve of progressive increase of the mean systemic pressure (measured as the "mean circulatory filling pressure," M.C.F.P.). [Reprinted from Guyton (1955a).]

"Pressure Gradient for Venous Return"

When the resistances in the systemic circulation remain constant, the rate of venous return is proportional to the difference between the mean systemic pressure and the right atrial pressure. We have called this pressure difference the "pressure gradient for venous return" (Guyton, 1955a), the significance of which is demonstrated in Figure 12–5, which shows two separate venous return curves that have been extrapolated from animal experiments to the human being. Curve 1 is a normal venous return curve and curve 2, an elevated curve. In both instances, the resistances in the systemic circulation are equal, but the mean systemic pressure for curve 1 is 7 mm. Hg and for curve 2 is 11 mm. Hg, as illustrated by the fact that these two curves cross the zero flow axis, respectively, at the 7 mm. Hg and 11 mm. Hg right atrial pressure levels.

To demonstrate the significance of the pressure gradient for venous return, two additional scales have been placed at the bottom of the curves. The uppermost of these scales is the pressure gradient for venous return for curve 1, and the lowermost scale is the pressure gradient for venous return for curve 2. In each of the two curves, note that the venous return increases directly in proportion to the pressure gradient for venous return and that, at the same pressure gradients for both curves, the venous returns are also equal. The reason is that the downslope of the venous return curves (we have measured several hundred of them) are all either completely or almost completely straight, demonstrating a linear relationship between the pressure gradient for venous return and venous return itself.

To summarize, when the resistance in the systemic circulation remain

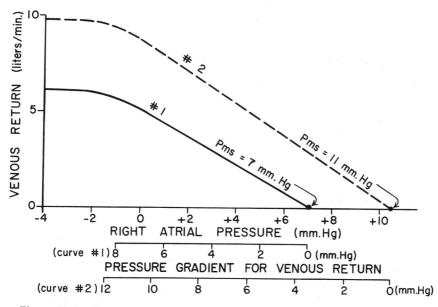

Figure 12–5. Venous return curves extrapolated to the human being: curve 1, normal; curve 2, elevated mean systemic pressure. The lower two scales represent the respective *pressure gradients for venous return* for the two curves.

constant, the venous return is almost directly proportional to the *mean systemic pressure minus the right atrial pressure.*

FACTORS THAT AFFECT THE MEAN SYSTEMIC PRESSURE

It is hoped that by now the reader recognizes the high degree of correlation between mean systemic pressure and venous return. If so, the following sections of this chapter will become especially meaningful, for we now propose to show from a quantitative point of view, as best as we can from the facts known, how different circulatory factors can affect the mean systemic pressure—such factors, for instance, as blood volume, vasomotor tone, and extravascular factors.

Effect of Blood Volume on the Mean Systemic Pressure

Figure 12–6 illustrates the effect on the mean systemic pressure of changing the blood volume in the normal live dog (Richardson, 1961). These experiments were performed in dogs in the following manner: Approximately 10 seconds prior to fibrillating the heart, the blood volume was altered from the normal to any given level by rapid infusion into or removal of blood from the circulation. Then the heart was fibrillated, and the mean circulatory pressure was measured (the mean circulatory pressure considered is essentially equal to the mean systemic pressure, for reasons explained earlier in the chapter). Immediately after making the measurement and after defibrillating the heart, the blood volume was returned to the control value by removal or infusion of blood within the next few seconds. Fifteen minutes later the blood volume was changed to a different value, and the measurement was repeated. The curve illustrated in this figure represents an average curve obtained from ten dogs.

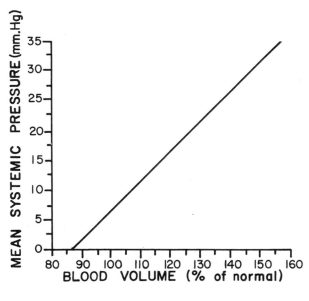

Figure 12–6. Relationship between blood volume and mean circulatory pressure. [Drawn from data in Richardson, Stallings, and Guyton (1961).]

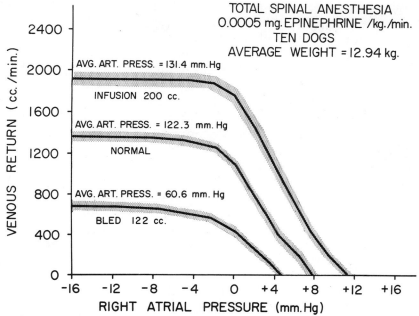

Figure 12–7. Average venous return curves recorded in 10 dogs, showing (a) the average normal curve, (b) the average curve after bleeding the animals an average of 122 ml. of blood, and (c) after returning the removed blood and infusing an additional 200 ml. of blood. These animals were given total spinal anesthesia and a continuous infusion of epinephrine to cause (1) abrogation of all circulatory reflexes and (2) maintenance of the vasomotor tone at a normal level. [Reprinted from Guyton, Lindsey, Kaufmann, and Abernathy (1958d).]

The purpose of making the measurements in this manner was to obtain the true effect on the mean systemic pressure of blood volume changes before reflexes could set in. However, similar measurements were made in five additional dogs in which total spinal anesthesia had been instituted and the vasomotor tone of the animal returned to normal by a continuous infusion of norepinephrine. Such an animal has no reflexes. Nevertheless, the curve obtained in this manner was identical to the one recorded in Figure 12–6.

Several features of the curve in Figure 12–6 should be pointed out. (1) The relationship between blood volume and mean systemic pressure is almost exactly linear. (2) When reflexes do not occur, an instantaneous decrease in blood volume of only 15 per cent decreases the mean circulatory pressure from its normal value of 7 mm. Hg down to zero. (3) An increase in blood volume of 14 per cent doubles the mean circulatory pressure, an increase of 27 per cent triples the mean systemic pressure, and so forth. Thus, only slight variations in the blood volume can alter the mean systemic pressure very markedly.

EFFECT ON THE VENOUS RETURN CURVE OF CHANGING THE BLOOD VOLUME. Figure 12–7 illustrates the alterations in the venous return curve caused by blood volume changes (Guyton, 1957c). These curves are average results obtained in ten separate dogs, each of which had total spinal anesthesia and was given a continuous infusion of epinephrine to maintain its vasomotor tone at a constant level. In other words, all vasomotor reflexes were eliminated to prevent their interference with the results.

The middle curve was obtained at normal blood volume; the bottom curve was obtained after bleeding an average of 122 ml. of blood from the dogs; and the top curve was obtained after returning the blood and infusing an additional 200 ml. of blood. From these curves, as well as those in Figure 12–4, it is readily evident that alteration of the mean systemic pressure caused by changing the blood volume can cause markedly different venous return curves, as was predicted from earlier discussions in the chapter.

EFFECT OF STRESS RELAXATION AND STRESS RELAXATION RECOVERY ON THE MEAN SYSTEMIC PRESSURE. In the course of our studies of the relationship between blood volume and mean systemic pressure, we have noted that, immediately after a large quantity of blood is infused, the mean systemic pressure rises but then falls rapidly during the ensuing few minutes to progressively lower levels. We have interpreted this to mean that a very intense degree of stress relaxtion occurs in the circulation, this allowing the mean systemic pressure to fall even though the blood volume remains greatly elevated. Thus far, however, we have not been able to control all other factors, such as fluid shifts from the circulation, in order to be able to say quantitatively exactly how much stress relaxation does affect the mean systemic pressure over a period of time. Figure 12–8 illustrates approximately the changes in mean systemic pressure that occur following a sudden transfusion (Richardson and Guyton, unpublished observations; Prather, 1969). This figure shows the results of transfusing an animal in less than one minute's time with blood equal to approximately 35 per cent of its own blood volume. The mean circulatory pressure rises instantaneously to 24 mm. Hg, and then, even though the blood volume is presumably maintained at or near this elevated level, the mean systemic pressure falls progressively back toward a lower value. The

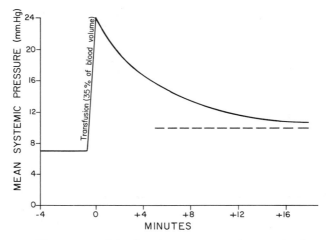

Figure 12–8. Time course of the changing mean systemic pressure after transfusion of a large quantity of blood. We believe this effect to result mainly from stress relaxation.

dashed line is the asymptote which the curve approaches. The approach toward this asymptote has a half-time in the order of 2 to 4 minutes.

After removal of blood from the circulation, a stress-relaxation recovery phenomenon also seems to occur, but here again quantitative results with all other factors completely controlled have not yet been attained. In general, the phenomenon of stress relaxation recovery appears to take place considerably more slowly than that of stress relaxation. However, it must be cautioned that these results are preliminary, and better controlled studies in the future might show considerable differences.

Nevertheless, it is already very obvious that whatever this phenomenon is, and we assume it to be stress relaxation and stress relaxation recovery, it can compensate to a very great extent for the effects of blood volume changes on venous return and cardiac output. Immediately after infusion or removal of large quantities of blood, even when the circulatory reflexes are eliminated, one finds at first extraordinary effects on cardiac output, but then gradually over a period of minutes that cardiac output returns toward normal (Guyton, 1959f). Therefore, this mechanism nullifies much of the effect of changing the blood volume. However, there are limitations to the degree of compensation that can occur, for if the blood volume keeps on changing enough, the mean systemic pressure can still fall to zero or can rise to chronic pressures of more than 20 mm. Hg, as occurs in congestive heart failure (Starr, 1940b).

Effect of Vasomotor Tone on the Mean Systemic Pressure and on Venous Return

Figure 12–9 illustrates the results of an experiment in a dog in which the vasomotor tone was changed through a wide range of values. First, the

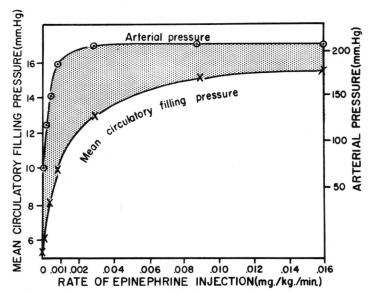

Figure 12–9. Effect on the mean systemic pressure (measured as "mean circulatory filling pressure") and the mean arterial pressure of increasing rates of infusion of epinephrine. [Reprinted from Guyton, Polizo, and Armstrong (1954c).]

dog was given total spinal anesthesia so that all circulatory reflexes were removed. Then epinephrine was infused at progressively greater rates. Note that the mean circulatory pressure rose from the spinal level of 4.5 mm. Hg up to a maximum level of approximately 15 mm. Hg (Guyton, 1954c). Since the vasomotor tone throughout the body was progressively increasing during the course of the experiment, this curve illustrates the relationship between vasomotor tone and mean systemic pressure.

To obtain an idea of how much changing the vasomotor tone can alter the mean systemic pressure, the following quantitative values can be given: (1) At normal vasomotor tone the mean systemic pressure is 7 mm. Hg. (2) Total spinal anesthesia, which removes all vasomotor tone throughout the body, reduces the mean systemic pressure to 5 mm. Hg (Guyton, 1954c). (3) A carotid sinus reflex, which increases vasomotor tone moderately, raises the mean systemic pressure from 7 mm. Hg up to about 10 mm. Hg (unpublished observations). (4) A Cushing reflex (caused by compression of the brain) initiates the most intense physiological increase in vasomotor tone that we have ever observed; this raises the mean systemic pressure to an average of 17 mm. Hg (Guyton, 1952c; Richardson, 1964). (5) Infusion of maximal doses of epinephrine increases the mean systemic pressure to an average value of 19 mm. Hg, and an infusion of norepinephrine increases the pressure to 15 mm. Hg (Guyton, 1954c).

Therefore, between the two extremes of zero vasomotor tone and maximal vasomotor tone, the mean systemic pressure, when the blood volume remains normal, varies between a lower limit of 5 mm. Hg and an upper limit of 15 to 19 mm. Hg. If the blood volume changes simul-

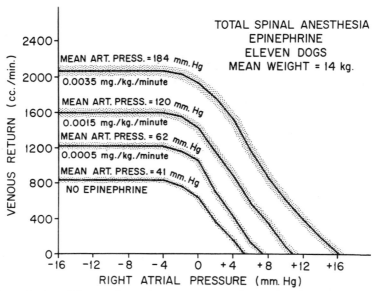

Figure 12–10. Effect on the venous return curve of increasing the vasomotor tone. The animals used in these studies had had total spinal anesthesia to remove all circulatory reflexes, and the curves are mean values from 11 dogs averaging 14 kg. weight. The shaded areas indicate the probable errors of the means. [Reprinted from Guyton, Lindsey, Abernathy, and Langston (1958c).]

taneously, however, this range can be either markedly decreased or increased for obvious reasons.

EFFECT OF CHANGES IN VASOMOTOR TONE ON THE VENOUS RETURN CURVE. Figure 12–10 illustrates the average of four separate venous return curves determined in each of 11 dogs (Guyton, 1958c). The lowest curve was run in dogs with total spinal anesthesia and no epinephrine infusion. The other curves were run in the same dogs but at three different rates of epinephrine infusion, thus obviously increasing the vasomotor tone throughout the animal's circulation. During the measurement of these curves, the blood volume remained normal. Note that the average mean systemic pressure rose from approximately 5 mm. Hg in the spinalized dogs to higher values as the rate of epinephrine infusion increased—to 7 mm. Hg, then to 10.5 mm. Hg, and finally to 16 mm. Hg. Also note that the venous return curves moved upward and to the right as the vasomotor tone increased, thus illustrating that increasing the vasomotor tone alters the venous return curve in the typical manner normally observed when the mean systemic pressure increases.

Effect of Extravascular Factors on Mean Systemic Pressure

The factors discussed thus far that affect the mean systemic pressure, blood volume, and vasomotor tone have been vascular factors. However, compression of the vessels from the outside, which we will call extravascular factors, can also increase the mean systemic pressure. Among these factors are abdominal compression, positive pressure breathing, increased interstitial fluid volume, and muscular contraction.

ABDOMINAL COMPRESSION. Very strong compression with the hands on the abdomen can increase the mean systemic pressure to at least double the normal (Guyton, 1952c). When one remembers that a person often contracts his abdomen during the course of muscular exercise, or even when he becomes startled or excited in any way, one can understand that venous return is markedly affected by many of our normal activities.

POSITIVE PRESSURE BREATHING. In positive pressure breathing, the mean systemic pressure can also increase to at least double the normal (Guyton, 1952c). This effect undoubtedly results partly from translocation of blood from the pulmonary vessels and heart into the systemic circulation and partly from the increased abdominal pressure required for breathing against the positive pressure.

We will recall from the discussions in the previous chapter that positive pressure breathing causes a rise in right atrial pressure, which can markedly impede venous return. Fortunately, this concomitant rise in mean systemic pressure during positive pressure breathing helps to overcome the detrimental effect of positive pressure breathing on venous return. A person can breathe for many minutes against a positive pressure of as much as 20 mm. Hg, which would not be possible without this compensation and the compensations that undoubtedly result from the autonomic reflexes, which further increase the mean systemic pressure. At any rate, the mean systemic pressure must rise to a value greater than the pressure against which a person breathes in order for any blood to return to the heart. Otherwise, there will be no pressure gradient for venous return (Guyton, 1955a).

INCREASED INTERSTITIAL FLUID.   Still another factor that can increase the mean systemic pressure is an increase in interstitial fluid, especially when this is associated with edema and ascites. Edematous fluid sometimes causes a subcutaneous tissue pressure as high as 5 to 10 mm. Hg (Burch, 1937; Wells, 1938; McMaster, 1946), and ascitic fluid can easily increase pressures in the abdomen as high as 10 to 15 mm. Hg (Guyton, 1954a). Obviously, the pressure of this fluid outside the vessels will elevate the mean systemic pressure.

Precise quantitative relationships between increased interstitial fluid and the mean systemic pressure have not yet been determined. However, we have infused animals with Tyrode's solution until serious ascites and edema resulted. In some of these animals, the mean systemic pressure had increased to as much as double the normal (Guyton, 1952c).

When we consider the problems of venous return in relation to cardiac failure in Chapter 26, it will become evident that an increase in mean systemic pressure as a result of increased interstitial fluid can be a very valuable compensatory factor to prevent cessation of venous return, for it is well known that in occasional cases of cardiac failure the right atrial pressure rises as high as 10 to 15 mm. Hg without a very great elevation in blood volume. Under these conditions, were it not for the extravascular compression, the mean systemic pressure probably could not rise high enough to maintain an adequate pressure gradient for venous return to the heart.

MUSCULAR CONTRACTION.   In recent experiments in which we studied the effect of muscular contraction on venous return and cardiac output, we found that strong contraction of the abdominal and hind leg muscles of the dog can increase the mean systemic pressure as much as three to four times, that is, to 20 to 30 mm. Hg (Guyton, 1962b). Furthermore, this increase occurs instantaneously at the beginning of muscular exercise (within the first second), thereby allowing an immediate surge of blood to flow toward the heart and an increase in cardiac output, the increased output actually anticipating the metabolic needs of the muscles. Here one finds once again that an increase in mean systemic pressure is of critical importance in increasing the venous return and consequently in increasing the cardiac output. Since cardiac output regulation during muscular contraction is one of the most important of all the problems to be considered in this book, the effect of muscular exercise on mean systemic pressure will be considered in detail in Chapter 25.

SUMMARY

The thesis of this chapter has been to impress upon the reader that the return of blood to the heart is almost directly proportional to the mean systemic pressure minus the right atrial pressure. Therefore, any factor that increases or decreases the mean systemic pressure will also greatly affect venous return and cardiac output. Among the different factors that have significant effects on the mean systemic pressure, and consequently on the cardiac output, are the blood volume, probably stress relaxation and stress relaxation recovery, vasomotor tone, and such extravascular factors as abdominal compression, positive pressure breathing, interstitial fluid volume, and muscular contraction.

Alterations in blood volume can change the mean systemic pressure from as little as zero up to 40 to 50 mm. Hg when other factors remain constant, and alterations in vasomotor tone can change the mean systemic pressure from 5 to 17 mm. Hg. Also the effects of these different factors can summate. For instance, in cardiac failure an increase both in blood volume and in vasomotor tone can summate together to increase the mean systemic pressure to values far greater than that resulting from either of the two factors alone. Also, all the other factors which affect mean systemic pressure can summate so that the total effect can be far greater than the effect of any one of the factors alone.

Furthermore, if the blood volume falls below normal, the fall in mean systemic pressure can be compensated by an increase in vasomotor tone, and, conversely, if the blood volume rises above normal, compensation can result from a decrease in vasomotor tone.

Chapter 13

EFFECT OF PERIPHERAL RESISTANCE AND CAPACITANCE ON VENOUS RETURN

It is very easy to understand that a change in resistance to blood flow in the systemic circulation can alter the rate at which blood can flow around the circulation. For instance, if the systemic resistance becomes infinite, venous return becomes zero. On the other hand, if the systemic resistance should become zero, blood theoretically would flow instantaneously and in great quantities from the root of the aorta directly to the right atrium.

On the other hand, it is not so easy to understand how alterations in the peripheral capacitances can affect venous return. Yet because an understanding of this, too, is essential to a complete understanding of the problems of venous return, it will be discussed along with the effects of altering the peripheral resistances.

Chapters 15 and 17 will present different types of mathematical analyses of the factors that regulate venous return and cardiac output. An approximate formula for venous return, which is derived in Chapter 15, is the following (Guyton, 1955a):

$$VR = \frac{Pms - Pra}{\dfrac{CvRv + Ca(Rv + Ra)}{Cv + Ca}} \tag{13-1}$$

in which VR equals venous return, Pms is the mean systemic pressure, Pra is the right atrial pressure, Rv is venous resistance from the midpoint of the veins to the right atrium, Ra is arterial resistance from the arterial tree to the midpoint of the veins, Cv is capacitance of the venous tree, and Ca is capacitance of the arterial tree.

Note from the above formula that the numerator is the mean systemic pressure minus the right atrial pressure, which was called in the previous chapter the "pressure gradient for venous return." On the other hand, the denominator is a function of the various resistances and capacitances

222

of the systemic circulation. The discussion, in the present chapter will concern the factors in this denominator and how they affect venous return.

EFFECT OF PERIPHERAL RESISTANCES ON VENOUS RETURN

CALCULATED EFFECT OF PERIPHERAL RESISTANCES ON VENOUS RETURN

Observing the above formula once again, one can see that increasing the resistances in the denominator will decrease the venous return a corresponding amount provided both the venous and arterial resistances are increased proportionately. This effect is demonstrated in Figure 13–1, which shows, first, that when the right atrial pressure is equal to the mean systemic pressure, regardless of the resistance in the systemic circulation, the venous return is zero. Yet when the right atrial pressure is less than the mean systemic pressure, the less the resistance, the greater is the venous return. For instance, at zero right atrial pressure and at some constant positive value for the mean systemic pressure, the venous return increases exactly two fold when the peripheral resistance decreases by one-half. Conversely, the venous return decreases exactly one-half when the resistance is increased two fold.

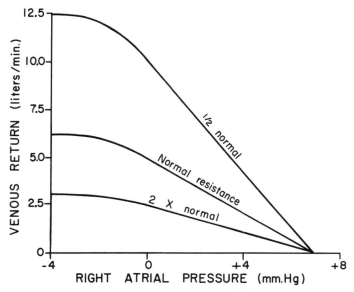

Figure 13–1.   Calculated effects on the venous return curve caused by a two fold increase or a two fold decrease in total peripheral resistance when the resistances throughout the systemic circulation are all altered proportionately.

Downslope of the Venous Return Curve as a Measure of "Resistance to Venous Return"

The denominator of the above formula is actually a resistance, for in a *dimensional* analysis of this denominator one finds that the capacitances cancel out. Therefore, the entire denominator can be called the *resistance to venous return* (Guyton, 1955a). It represents an algebraic average of all the resistances from the different areas of the systemic circulation back to the right atrium when each of these resistances is weighted in proportion to the capacitance of the individual area. When one quantitates the denominator of this equation, he finds that, for any given pressure gradient for venous return, the venous return is inversely proportional to the quantitative value of the "resistance to venous return." He will also find that the slope of the venous return curve is proportional to the quantitative value of the denominator, which means that one can calculate the resistance to venous return from the slope of the venous return curve. If the slope is 5 liters per 7 mm. Hg pressure change (which are approximately the values to be expected in the human being), the resistance to venous return will be 7/5 mm. Hg/liter/min. or 112 dyne sec./cm.^{5} If the slope is 10 liters per 7 mm. Hg, the resistance to venous return will be one-half the above value, and if the slope is 2.5 liters per 7 mm. Hg, the resistance will be two times as great.

To express the above effects another way, a decrease in resistance to venous return rotates the venous return curve in a clockwise direction, the curve approaching the vertical as the resistance approaches zero. An increase in resistance to venous return rotates the curve in the counterclockwise direction, the curve approaching the horizontal as the resistance approaches infinity (Guyton, 1959b).

EXPERIMENTAL EFFECTS OF ALTERING THE PERIPHERAL RESISTANCE

Effect of Opening an A-V Fistula

The systemic resistance can be changed as much as 100 per cent or more, simply by opening or closing an A-V fistula. Figure 13–2 illustrates the effect on the venous return curve of suddenly opening a large A-V fistula, in this instance decreasing the total peripheral resistance suddenly from 3900 dyne sec./cm.^{5} to 1980 dyne sec./cm.^{5} In other words, the total systemic resistance was reduced by 49 per cent. The curves illustrated in this figure represent average curves from ten separate animals (Guyton, 1961b), and the results show that the venous return at each right atrial pressure is increased precisely as it should be in accord with the calculations above. For instance, at a right atrial pressure of −4 mm. Hg, the normal venous return is almost exactly 2000 ml./min. However, when the fistula is opened, the venous return at this same atrial pressure is 3400 ml./min. Note also that when the right atrial pressure was equal to the mean systemic pressure, there was no flow through the circuit either when the fistula was open or closed.

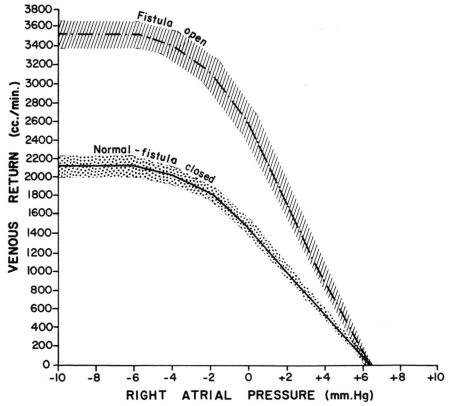

Figure 13–2. Average effect on the venous return curve in 10 areflex dogs of opening a large A-V fistula. Shaded areas indicate probable errors of the means. [Modified from Guyton and Sagawa, (1961b).]

Figure 13–2 illustrates that altering the peripheral resistance does not cause the same change in the venous return curve as altering the mean systemic pressure, for altering the mean systemic pressure shifts the entire curve upward and to the right, whereas altering the systemic resistance simply rotates the curve around an axis at the point where the venous return curve crosses the zero venous return level. The right atrial pressure at this point on the curve, as noted in the previous chapter, is equal to the mean systemic pressure.

Effect of Anemia and Polycythemia on Venous Return and on the Venous Return Curve

It is reasonable to expect that anemia or polycythemia will alter essentially all of the systemic resistances approximately proportionately. Therefore, a decrease in blood viscosity resulting from anemia should, in accordance with the above formula, rotate the venous return curve in a clockwise direction, whereas polycythemia, which markedly increases the blood viscosity and total peripheral resistance, should rotate the venous return curve in a counterclockwise direction.

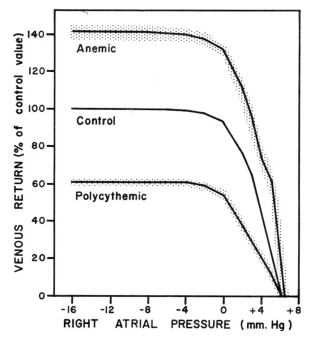

Figure 13-3. Average effects on the venous return curve of altering the total peripheral resistance by creating anemia in 10 dogs and polycythemia in 8 dogs. Shaded areas indicate probable errors of the means. [Reprinted from Guyton and Richardson (1961a).]

Figure 13-3 illustrates the average experimental effect of anemia in ten dogs and polycythemia in eight dogs in which the mean systemic pressure was kept as constant as possible, showing that anemia rotated the curve in a clockwise direction and polycythemia in the counterclockwise direction (Guyton, 1961a).

Once again, one can see from these curves that when the right atrial pressure equaled the mean systemic pressure, in this case averaging approximately 6.5 mm. Hg, there was no venous return, regardless of whether the animal was anemic, normal, or polycythemic. However, at the lower right atrial pressures, the polycythemic animals had an average venous return approximately 61 per cent of the average control value, and the anemic animals had an average venous return approximately 42 per cent greater than the control value. Here again, the experimental results are almost identical to the calculated results as depicted in Figure 13-1.

DIFFERENCE BETWEEN THE EFFECTS OF VENOUS VERSUS ARTERIAL RESISTANCE ON VENOUS RETURN

Calculated Differences

In the above discussion of the effect of resistance on venous return we have considered only proportionate changes in all the resistances in the peripheral circulation. However, if all the resistance change occurs in the venous tree or in the arterial tree alone, one finds that increased arterial resistance hardly affects venous return, while a comparable increase in venous resistance decreases venous return very markedly. This effect can be predicted in the following way from the equation presented earlier in the chapter: The capacitance of the venous tree, Cv, is approximately 18 times as great as the capacitance of the arterial tree, Ca. If we place these values into the above formula, we obtain the following relationship:

$$VR = \frac{Pms - Pra}{\frac{18(Rv) + 1(Ra + Rv)}{19}} = \frac{Pms - Pra}{Rv + \frac{Ra}{19}} \qquad (13-2)$$

Now, if we increase the total peripheral resistance by 20 per cent with all the resistance increase occurring entirely on the arterial side, we can calculate that the venous return will be reduced by only 6 per cent. (In making this calculation we insert the increase in resistance into the formula and utilize the normal ratio of about 7 to 1 for Ra to Rv. Ra is the resistance from the aorta to the midpoint of the veins, while Rv is the resistance from the midpoint of the veins back to the right atrium.) On the other hand, if we increase the total peripheral resistance the same amount but with the increase now occurring entirely on the venous side, we find that the venous return will be reduced by 53 per cent, which means that an increase in resistance occurring entirely in the venous tree should cause approximately nine times as much decrease in venous return as a similar increase occurring entirely in the arterial side of the systemic circulation.

Experimental Results Obtained by Increasing Arterial or Venous Resistances

To study the effect on venous return of altering the arterial resistance, 200-micron microspheres were injected into the aorta to embolize

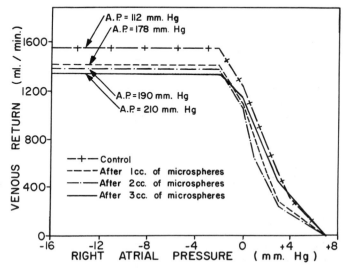

Figure 13–4. The relatively slight effect on the venous return curve of increasing the arterial resistance by injecting microspheres into the aorta to occlude many of the arterioles. Note the several fold increase in total peripheral resistance with only 10 per cent decrease in the plateau of the venous return curve. [Reprinted from Guyton, Abernathy, Langston, Kaufmann, and Fairchild (1959b).]

many of the small arterioles and thereby increase the arterial resistance. To study the effect of altering the venous resistance, the large veins entering the right atrium were gradually compressed (Guyton, 1959b). Figure 13–4 illustrates successive venous return curves determined in the same animal after progressive injection of microspheres. This figure shows that even after the total peripheral resistance had been increased to approximately double the control value, the venous return at the plateau level had decreased from 1530 ml./min. to 1350 ml./min., representing only a 12 per cent decrease in venous return, which accords well with the calculated prediction that increasing the arterial resistance should not reduce the venous return greatly.

Figure 13–5 illustrates average results from ten separate animals of increasing the arterial resistance with microspheres, of increasing the venous resistance by progressive compression of the larger veins entering the right atrium, and of increasing both these resistances simultaneously. Note that when the total peripheral resistance had been increased to about 20 per cent above the control value, the venous return had decreased eight times as much when increasing the venous resistance as when increasing the arterial resistance. This is almost precisely in accord with the above calculations, which gave a predicted nine fold difference between the effects of venous and arterial resistances when the peripheral resistance increased 20 per cent.

These results illustrate that an increase in venous resistance can have quite a different effect on venous return from an increase in arterial resistance. A significant deduction that results from this study is that cardiac

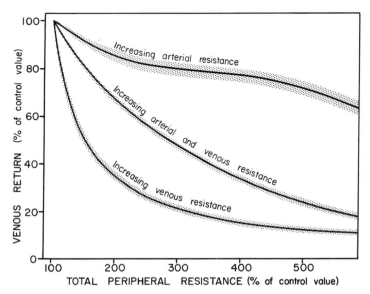

Figure 13–5. Average effects on venous return of (a) increasing arterial resistance versus (b) increasing venous resistance. Fifteen dogs were used in the arterial resistance experiments. The shaded areas represent the probable errors of the mean. [Reprinted from Guyton, Abernathy, Langston, Kaufmann, and Fairchild (1959b).]

output is markedly affected by altering the venous resistance but is little affected by altering the arterial resistance. Yet it is well known that arterial pressure is mainly controlled by altering the arterial resistance. Therefore, it would be theoretically possible to regulate cardiac output almost independently of arterial pressure by altering venous resistance and theoretically possible to regulate arterial pressure almost independently of cardiac output by altering the arterial resistance.

Explanation of the Difference Between the Effects of Venous and Arterial Resistance on Venous Return

Figure 13–6 is a symbolic schema which can help to explain the difference between the effects of arterial and venous resistance on venous return. If the resistance to blood flow from the veins to the heart increases, the pressure in the veins increases. However, since the veins have very large capacitance, about 18 times as much as the arteries, the venous pressure can rise only a few millimeters of mercury before sufficient blood is dammed in the veins to block venous return completely. This pressure rise in the veins, averaging only 7 to 14 mm. Hg, is relatively slight in comparison with the increase in resistance; therefore, the ratio of pressure rise to resistance rise is very low, which causes the systemic flow to decrease drastically. On the other hand, when the arterial resistance increases and

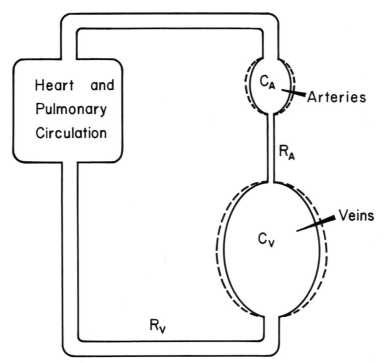

Figure 13–6. Symbolic schema for explaining the difference between the effects of arterial and venous resistance on venous return. See explanation in text. [Reprinted from Guyton, Abernathy, Langston, Kaufmann, and Fairchild (1959b).]

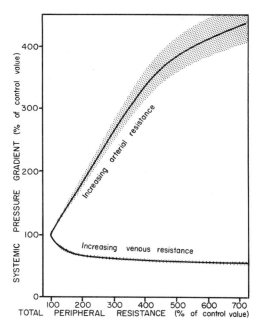

Figure 13–7. Average relationship between total peripheral resistance and systemic pressure gradient from aorta to the right atrium when resistance was increased (a) by injecting microspheres into arteries to increase arterial resistance in 15 dogs, or (b) by inflating pneumatic cuffs around major veins to increase venous resistance in 10 dogs. The dashed line indicates the pressure rise that would have been necessary to compensate completely for the increasing total peripheral resistance. Shaded areas indicate probable errors of the mean. [Reprinted from Guyton, Abernathy, Langston, Kaufmann, and Fairchild (1959b).]

blood begins to dam up in the arteries, only a slight amount of stored blood in the arteries causes the arterial pressure to rise tremendously, the arterial pressure rising almost in proportion to the increase in arterial resistance; therefore, the ratio of pressure rise to resistance rise is almost unity. As a consequence, the flow through the increased arterial resistance hardly changes.

Figure 13–7 explains in another way the difference between the increase in venous resistance and arterial resistance in affecting venous return. Note that when the arterial resistance is increased, the pressure gradient across the systemic circulation increases almost in proportion to the increase in resistance, thereby compensating for the increase in arterial resistance and thereby allowing the flow to remain almost normal. On the other hand, when the venous resistance increases, not only does the systemic pressure gradient fail to increase, but it actually decreases. Hence, with an increased venous resistance there is a reduced systemic pressure gradient for forcing the blood through the system and also an increased total peripheral resistance, each of which reduces the venous return markedly.

EFFECT OF PERIPHERAL CAPACITANCES ON VENOUS RETURN

The capacitance of a segment of the circulation is equal to the quantity of blood that can be stored in that segment for a given rise in pressure; this is usually expressed by the symbol dV/dP.

In the present discussion, it is important that we consider, first, the relative capacitances of the arterial tree versus the venous tree. We determined these relative capacitances by suddenly stopping the heart by electrical fibrillation in nine dogs and pumping blood rapidly from the arterial tree into the venous tree while recording both arterial and venous pressures. By employing a special mathematical procedure, it was possible to calculate both the amount of blood translocated from the arteries to the veins through the pump and that translocated directly through the capillaries from the arteries to the veins during the ensuing few seconds after ventricular fibrillation (Guyton, 1956b). From this study, it was found that for a given change in blood volume, the arterial pressure changed, on the average, 18 times as much as the venous pressure. In other words, the capacitance of the venous tree was 18 times the capacitance of the arterial tree.

Significance of Systemic Vascular Capacitances in Relation to Venous Return

Referring again to Formula 13–1, we see that the denominator includes the capacitances of the arterial and venous vascular trees. These capacitances determine the relative importance of venous and arterial resistances in the regulation of venous return. That is, the reason an increase in venous resistance causes a decrease in venous return eight times greater than does an increase in arterial resistance is that the venous capacitance is far greater than the arterial capacitance. In other words, it is actually the arterial and venous resistances that impede the flow of blood around the circulation, but the capacitances help to determine what happens to the pressures that push the blood through the resistances when one of the resistances changes.

Under steady state conditions, the capacitance of any portion of the systemic circulation can be increased or decreased infinitely without affecting venous return. For instance, if a large blood reservoir is attached to the right atrium and is filled with blood up to a hydrostatic pressure level equal to the pressure level in the right atrium, no effect will be observed on the circulation regardless of how much capacitance the reservoir might have. Yet adding this reservoir to the circuit increases the capacitance of the venous tree, because should the right atrial pressure rise, not only would blood be stored in the venous tree, but it would also be stored in the reservoir. Therefore, even though under steady state conditions the circulation would be normal during changing conditions—that is, as the right atrial pressure rises—the animal would lose a large portion of its blood volume into this extra storage capacitance, and obviously the change would not have the same overall effect on the circulation under these conditions as it would if the reservoir were not attached.

The same analogy can be drawn with the aorta: Under steady state conditions, a reservoir connected to the aorta and filled with blood to a hydrostatic pressure level equal to that in the aorta will have no effect on the circulation as long as the aortic pressure does not change. On the other hand, if changes take place in the circulation which either raise or lower the aortic pressure, blood will, respectively, be stored in the reservoir or removed from the reservoir, which causes the circulatory system to react to the changes in a completely different way from the normal reaction.

Therefore, the present discussion of the relationship between systemic capacitances and venous return will be directed toward analyzing the changes in venous return when the capacitances are abnormal versus when they are normal.

Calculated Effects

Figure 13–8 illustrates four separate curves, three of which were calculated from the formula given earlier in the chapter. Point A represents a normal venous return of 5 liters/minute and a normal right atrial pressure of 0 mm. Hg. The light solid curve is a normal venous return curve. The short dashed curve is the calculated effect on the venous return curve if either the capacitance of the arterial tree should be reduced to one-fourth normal or the capacitance of the venous tree should be increased to four times normal. The long dashed curve illustrates the effect on the venous return curve if the arterial capacitance is increased to four times or the venous capacitance is decreased to one-fourth normal. Though the effects of these changes in capacitance are not tremendous, they can be especially important under certain circumstances.

Experimental Results

The dark solid curve in Figure 13–8 is an average venous return curve determined in ten animals in which the arterial capacitance has been increased to four times normal by connecting an appropriate blood reservoir to the aorta by means of a catheter. This reservoir was a long, linear, vertical tube which had a diameter calculated so that the tube would store three times as much blood for each millimeter of mercury rise in arterial

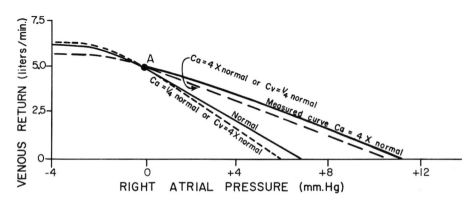

Figure 13–8. Calculated and measured effects on the venous return curve of altering systemic capacitances. The dashed curves represent calculated effects, and the heavy solid curve represents the measured effect of increasing the arterial capacitance to four times normal. (The flow values for the measured curve have been extrapolated from dogs to the human being.)

pressure as would the arterial tree (Guyton, unpublished results). Thus, the total capacitance was increased to equal the capacitance of the arterial tree plus three times more capacitance, or a total of four times normal capacitance.

Note that the measured curve in Figure 13–8 is almost precisely the same as the calculated curve.

Alterations in Capacitance in the Human Being

It is doubtful that the capacitance of the arterial or venous tree ever changes more than two fold even under the most severe pathological conditions. Conditions in which capacitances might change are aortic aneurysm, change in aortic capacitance as a result of age, or increased venous capacitance as a result of varicose veins.

On studying Figure 13–8 and on recognizing that capacitances do not change markedly in the systemic circulation, one can readily see that the effect of capacitance changes on the venous return curve is of more academic importance than practical importance. Perhaps the most important capacitance effect is the greater propensity for a person with severe varicose veins to develop circulatory distress when the venous pressure rises than is true in the normal person (Krug, 1960).

The real value in understanding the effects of capacitance changes on function of the circulation is that once a person has comprehended these effects, he can then understand such problems in circulatory flow as (a) why the mean systemic pressure is exceedingly important in the control of cardiac output, (b) why changes in venous resistance affect cardiac output much more than changes in arterial resistance, and (c) why the cardiac output is limited by venous collapse when the pumping activity of the heart is increased beyond certain critical levels.

IV

GRAPHICAL, ALGEBRAIC, AND COMPUTER ANALYSES OF CARDIAC OUTPUT REGULATION

Chapter 14

GRAPHICAL ANALYSIS OF CARDIAC OUTPUT REGULATION

In Chapters 7 to 13 we have discussed the various factors that affect, first, the ability of the heart to pump blood and, second, the flow of blood through the systemic circulation. The ability of the heart to pump blood can be expressed in terms of "cardiac output curves," and the tendency for blood to flow through the systemic circulation back to the heart can be expressed in terms of "venous return curves." The purpose of the present chapter is to show how these two types of curves can be equated with each other to analyze the effect of many different factors on cardiac output.

EQUATING CARDIAC OUTPUT CURVES WITH VENOUS RETURN CURVES

A cardiac output curve or a venous return curve is a graphical expression of a mathematical equation, each having the same two variables: (1) flow and (2) right atrial pressure. Flow in the circuit is equal to both cardiac output and venous return, except during transient states for only a few seconds at a time. Therefore, if the two mathematical equations are solved by the method of simultaneous equations, one can determine the two unknowns, cardiac output and right atrial pressure (Weber, 1850; Guyton, 1955a, 1962c; Grodins, 1959; Warner, 1959).

The algebraic equations for the cardiac output and venous return curves are often very complicated, as will become evident in Chapter 15. On the other hand, the solution to these equations can be achieved graphically by simply plotting the two curves on the same coordinates as illustrated in Figure 14–1 (Guyton, 1955a, 1958a, 1958b, 1962c). The point at which the two curves cross is the solution to the equation giving the value of the cardiac output and right atrial pressure when the two respective curves are known. The point at which the two curves cross, which is the solution to the equation, is called the *equilibrium point* (Guyton, 1955a).

237

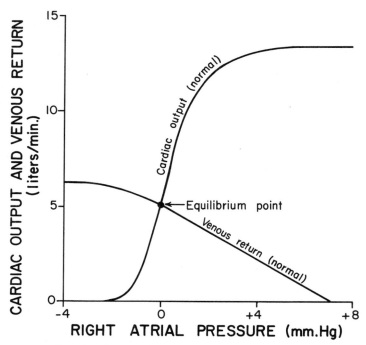

Figure 14–1. Equating the normal cardiac output curve with the normal venous return curve.

Significance of the Equilibrium Point

For a few seconds at a time, the cardiac output can be far greater than the venous return, or conversely the venous return can be far greater than the cardiac output. However, any time the cardiac output becomes greater than the venous return, blood will shift from the pulmonary circulation and heart into the systemic circulation; on the other hand, any time the venous return becomes greater than the cardiac output, blood will shift from the systemic circulation into the heart or pulmonary circulation. Experimental studies have shown that when venous return and cardiac output are temporarily out of equilibrium, the equilibrium is reestablished in approximately six heart beats (Buckley, 1955).

To explain how these principles apply to the equilibrium point, let us assume that 30 ml. of blood is suddenly injected directly into the right atrium, enough to increase the right atrial pressure from its normal value of 0 mm. Hg up to +7 mm. Hg. If one observes Figure 14–1 again, it is immediately evident that at a right atrial pressure of 7 mm. Hg there will be no venous return, but the cardiac output will be over 13 liters/minute. Thus, there is a disparity of 13 liters/minute between cardiac output and venous return. As a result, large quantities of blood shift rapidly from the heart and pulmonary circulation into the systemic circulation, the loss of blood from the heart lowering the right atrial pressure. After 1 second, the right atrial pressure might have fallen to a value of, say, 3 mm. Hg. At this point, as is shown by the figure, the venous return is 3 liters/minute and the cardiac output, 12 liters/minute. Therefore, a disparity of 9 liters/minute still exists between cardiac output and venous return. Consequently, blood continues to be transferred from the pulmonary circulation and heart into the systemic circulation and, as a consequence, the right atrial pressure falls still further. This sequence of events continues during the next few seconds until the right atrial pressure has fallen to the level at which venous return becomes equal to cardiac output. At this point the circulation has reached an equilibrium state. We note in Figure 14–1 that this is also the point at which the cardiac output and venous return curves cross, which explains why this point is called the "equilibrium point."

We can also consider the converse example in which 30 ml. of blood is suddenly removed from the right atrium to lower the right atrial pressure to −4 mm. Hg. In this instance, the cardiac output becomes zero, while the venous return is still 6 liters/minute. As a result, blood now flows rapidly from the systemic circulation into the heart while none is flowing out of the heart and pulmonary circulation. As a result, the volume of the cardiac chambers and pulmonary circulation increases, and the right atrial pressure rises within 1 second from −4 mm. Hg to −2 mm. Hg. At this point the venous return is still 5.75 liters/minute while the cardiac output is only a small fraction of a liter/minute. Therefore, a disparity of over 5 liters/minute still exists between the venous return and cardiac output, with blood continuing to shift from the systemic circulation into the heart and pulmonary circulation. After a few more seconds, the right atrial pressure rises to the point at which cardiac output becomes equal to venous return, which, in the case of Figure 14–1, is zero mm. Hg. Once again, equilibrium has been established.

It should be noted very emphatically that cardiac output and venous return never remain significantly out of equilibrium for longer than a few seconds at a time. Otherwise, either the systemic circulation or the pulmonary circulation would become completely depleted of blood while the opposite circulation would become engorged (Berglund, 1954; Lindsey, 1957, 1959).

Another point which will be emphasized in the remainder of this chapter is that when either the venous return curve or the cardiac output curve becomes altered because of changes in the peripheral circulation or the heart, the equilibrium point immediately shifts to new cardiac output and right atrial pressure values. It is these shifts that are the primary concern of this chapter.

PATTERNS OF CARDIAC OUTPUT AND VENOUS RETURN CURVES

In the previous chapters, it has already been pointed out that there are only a few major patterns of cardiac output and venous return curves. By understanding these patterns and also understanding the conditions which cause them to change in different states of the circulation, one can construct almost exactly the specific type of cardiac output or venous return curve that will exist in almost any circulatory condition and can then plot the curves on the same coordinates to solve for the equilibrium point. This gives the solution to the cardiac output and mean right atrial pressure.

CARDIAC OUTPUT CURVES

In general, only two major patterns of cardiac output curves occur: (1) a pattern of curves that depicts the effects of increased and decreased effectiveness of the heart as a pump, and (2) a pattern that depicts the effects of increased or decreased extracardiac pressure.

Patterns of Cardiac Output Curves in "Hypereffective" and "Hypoeffective" Hearts

It was pointed out in Chapter 9 that almost any factor that increases the effectiveness of the heart as a pump elevates the cardiac output curve and shifts it slightly to the left, whereas almost all factors that decrease the effectiveness of the heart as a pump depress the curve and shift it slightly to the right (Sarnoff, 1955). Figure 14–2 illustrates a "family" of cardiac output curves which depict the ability of the heart to pump blood at all degrees of cardiac effectiveness. The upper solid curve represents approximately the maximum ability of the normal heart to pump blood when it is operating in its most effective state. Obviously, the curve which would depict the minimal ability of the heart to pump blood would be a curve

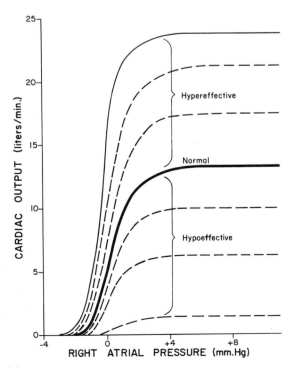

Figure 14–2. Family of cardiac output curves for hypo- and hypereffective hearts.

along the zero cardiac output axis. Between these two extremes are an infinite number of cardiac output curves which can depict the pumping abilities of hearts with any degree of effectiveness of the heart from zero up to an effectiveness approximately two-thirds above normal.

The following is a list of the factors that can cause the heart to become a more effective pump than usual:

1. Sympathetic stimulation, which can increase the cardiac output curve up to approximately 1 2/3 times normal (Sarnoff, 1955).

2. Cardiac hypertrophy, which can increase the cardiac output curve to perhaps as much as two times normal even without sympathetic stimulation. Also, this factor can summate with sympathetic stimulation to produce perhaps a three fold increase in the cardiac output curve; unfortunately precise data on this are not available.

3. Decreased load on the heart. Decreasing the load on the heart to zero systemic resistance can increase the cardiac output perhaps as much as 10 to 20 per cent above normal (Markwalder, 1914), but probably not to a value greater than this because even with zero systemic resistance the right heart still must pump blood against the pulmonary resistance, which becomes a limiting factor in the increase in cardiac output.

4. Inhibition of the parasympathetics to the heart, which can probably increase the cardiac output as much as 20 to 30 per cent, though this depends to a great extent upon the normal degree of vagal inhibition of the heart; unfortunately, precise values for this effect are also yet unknown.

The different factors which can cause a hypoeffective heart are numerous, but we can list some of them as follows:

1. Myocardial infarction
2. Valvular heart disease
3. Vagal stimulation of the heart
4. Inhibition of the sympathetics to the heart
5. Congenital heart disease
6. Myocarditis
7. Cardiac anoxia
8. Diphtheritic or other types of myocardial damage or toxicity.

Though this is but a partial list of the different conditions that can cause a hypoeffective heart, nevertheless it serves to show the types of conditions that can decrease the effectiveness of the heart as a pump. The degree of hypoeffectivity can be either slight or extreme—indeed down to the point of no pumping at all.

Pattern of Cardiac Output Curves Caused by Alteration of Extracardiac Pressure

Figure 14–3 shows the different patterns of curves which occur when the extracardiac pressure is altered. The solid line curves represent the effects of changes in intrapleural pressure. Note that the curve is simply displaced to the right or left by changes in intrapleural pressure. The different types of factors that can alter the cardiac output curve by altering the intrapleural pressure are the following:

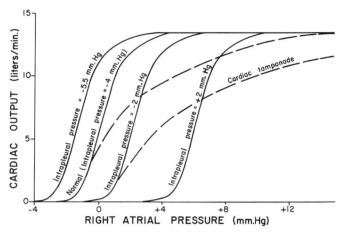

Figure 14–3. Family of cardiac output curves caused by changes in intrapleural pressure and by cardiac tamponade.

1. Cyclic changes during normal respiration (Brecher, 1953a)
2. Negative pressure breathing (Holt, 1943, 1944a)
3. Positive pressure breathing (Holt, 1943, 1944a)
4. Opening the thoracic cage (Fermoso, 1964)
5. Entrapped air or fluid in the intrapleural space.

CARDIAC TAMPONADE. The dashed curves in Figure 14–3 illustrate the effect of cardiac tamponade on the curves. Cardiac tamponade has a different effect from increasing the intrapleural pressure in that it increases the pressure around the heart far more when the heart is distended than when it is not distended (Isaacs, 1954). Therefore, cardiac tamponade shifts the upper portions of the cardiac output curves much more to the right than the lower portions.

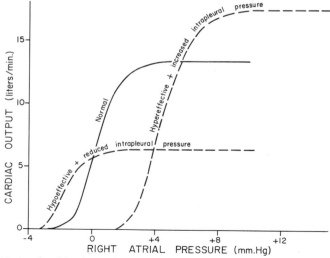

Figure 14–4. Combinations of the two major patterns of cardiac output curves, showing alterations both in extracardiac pressure and in effectiveness of the heart as a pump.

Combinations of Different Patterns of Cardiac Output Curves

Some cardiac output curves show the effects of both a changed degree of effectiveness of the heart and of changed extracardiac pressure. For instance, in Figure 14–4 the short dashed curve shows the effect of intrapleural pressure reduced to approximately 2 mm. Hg below normal, while at the same time the heart is hypoeffective, capable of pumping, at its maximum, only one-half the amount of blood that can be pumped by the normal heart. The long dashed curve of Figure 14–4 illustrates the effects of elevated intrapleural pressure, to approximately 4 mm. Hg above normal, combined with a hypereffective heart capable of pumping at maximal activity approximately 30 per cent more blood than can the normal heart. These are but two of the infinite number of different combinations that can occur between the two major patterns of cardiac output curves.

PATTERNS OF VENOUS RETURN CURVES

There are also two major patterns of venous return curves, (1) a family of curves that results from alterations in the mean systemic pressure (Guyton, 1955) and (2) a family resulting from alterations in "resistance to venous return" (Guyton, 1959b, 1961b). The bases for these were discussed in Chapters 12 and 13.

Patterns of Venous Return Curves Resulting from Altered Mean Systemic Pressure

Figure 14–5 illustrates a family of venous return curves that occurs when the mean systemic pressure is altered. The normal curve is shown when the mean systemic pressure is 7 mm. Hg. The lowest solid curve shows the venous return curve when the mean systemic pressure is one-half normal, or 3.5 mm. Hg, and the solid curve to the far right shows the effect of elevating the mean systemic pressure to 14 mm. Hg. The dashed curves

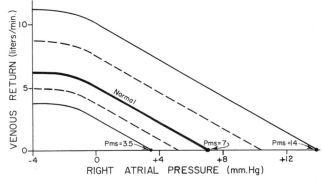

Figure 14–5. Family of venous return curves depicting the effect of altering the mean systemic pressure.

illustrate that there is an infinite number of other curves, all of which parallel each other and each one of which is determined by the level of the mean systemic pressure. Because the mean systemic pressure can fall to as low as zero mm. Hg or rise to as high as 40 mm. Hg, one readily sees that an infinite series of venous return curves exists, which can be applicable to the analysis of cardiac output.

The different factors that can change the mean systemic pressure and that therefore can alter the venous return curve as illustrated in Figure 14–5 are the following:

1. Changes in vasomotor tone (Starling, 1897; Starr, 1940b; Guyton, 1958c)

2. Changes in blood volume (Starling, 1897; Starr, 1940b; Guyton, 1958d)

3. Changes in interstitial fluid volume (Guyton, 1952c)

4. Changes in intra-abdominal pressure (Guyton, 1952c)

5. Changes in muscular compression of the vascular system (Guyton, 1962b).

The methods by which these factors affect the mean systemic pressure, and that therefore affect the venous return curve, were discussed in Chapter 12.

Pattern of Venous Return Curves Resulting from Alterations in "Resistance to Venous Return"

Figure 14–6 illustrates the family of venous return curves resulting from alterations in resistance to venous return. The solid curves represent normal resistance, one-half the normal resistance, and two times the normal resistance. The upper dashed curve represents one-third the normal

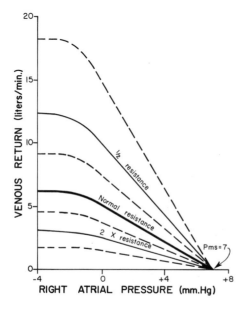

Figure 14–6. Family of venous return curves depicting the effect of altering the "resistance to venous return."

resistance and the lower dashed curve, three times the normal resistance; the other curves indicate that there is an infinite series of such curves. Note that all these curves reach the zero venous return axis at a right atrial pressure of 7 mm. Hg. In other words, the mean systemic pressure is 7 mm. Hg for each of these curves.

The different factors that can affect the resistance to venous return, and that thereby affect the venous return curve, are:

1. Change in the total peripheral resistance resulting from dilatation or constriction of the blood vessels or from increase or decrease in blood viscosity (Guyton, 1961).

2. A-V fistulae or other types of shunts (Guyton, 1961b).

3. Change in the ratio of arterial resistance to venous resistance [discussed in detail in Chapter 13 (Guyton, 1959b)].

4. Alteration in the relative capacitances of the arterial and venous vascular trees (a factor that is usually not to significant but that was discussed in Chapter 13).

Combinations of the Two Patterns of Venous Return

If one knows that the mean systemic pressure has been changed as a result of a blood volume change or some other factor and he knows also that the resistance has been changed, he can determine what the momentary venous return curve of the circulation will be by combining appropriate curves from the two separate patterns. Such combinations of curves are illustrated in Figure 14–7. The short dashed curve represents a decrease in the mean systemic pressure from 7 mm. Hg to 2.3 mm. Hg and a decrease in resistance to venous return to one-third normal. The long dashed curve represents an increase in mean systemic pressure to

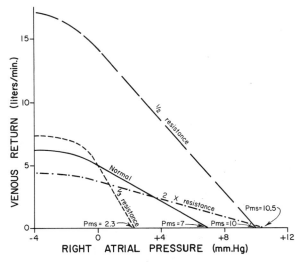

Figure 14–7. Combinations of the two major patterns of venous return curves, illustrating changes both in mean systemic pressure and in "resistance to venous return."

10 mm. Hg and a decrease in resistance to venous return to one-half normal. The dot-dash curve represents an increase in mean systemic pressure to 10.5 mm. Hg and an increase in the resistance to venous return to two times normal.

EXAMPLES OF CARDIAC OUTPUT ANALYSIS BY EQUATING CARDIAC OUTPUT WITH VENOUS RETURN CURVES

Cardiac output and venous return will be analyzed in detail for many different circulatory conditions in the following chapters; however, to indicate briefly the use of this method for cardiac output analysis, three simple examples will be given in Figures 14–8, 14–9, and 14–10.

Effect of an Increase in Mean Systemic Pressure on Cardiac Output

Figure 14–8 illustrates the effect of a single change in the circulatory system, an increase in the mean systemic pressure (Guyton, 1958d). In this example, the heart's pumping ability is not altered at all. Any one of the factors listed earlier in this chapter could be the cause of the increase in mean systemic pressure.

The two solid curves of Figure 14–8 represent the normal venous return and cardiac output curves with an equilibrium point A. However, the mean systemic pressure is then increased to 15 mm. Hg. Once this has occurred, the operating venous return curve immediately changes to the dashed curve. This curve equates with the cardiac output curve at point B, illustrating that the cardiac output has now increased to 10 liters/minute

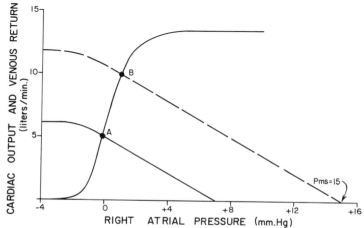

Figure 14–8. Effect on cardiac output and right atrial pressure caused by increasing the mean systemic pressure to +15 mm. Hg without any other simultaneous alteration in the basic factors affecting circulatory function.

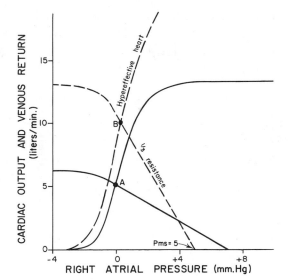

Figure 14–9. Effect on cardiac output and right atrial pressure of making the heart hypereffective, reducing the resistance to venous return to one-third normal, and reducing the mean systemic pressure from 7 to 5 mm. Hg.

and the right atrial pressure has increased to a 1 mm. Hg. In other words, the solution to this problem of cardiac output regulation is the coordinates 10 liters/minute cardiac output and 1 mm. Hg right atrial pressure.

Increased Effectiveness of the Heart as a Pump, Decreased Mean Systemic Pressure, and Decreased Resistance to Venous Return

Figure 14–9 illustrates a more complicated analysis. In this case the heart has become more effective as a pump, which could have resulted from any of the four factors listed earlier in this chapter. The mean sys-

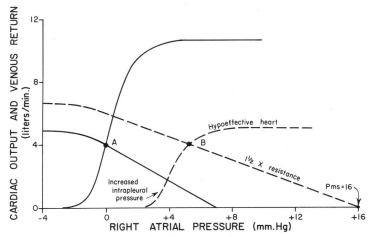

Figure 14–10. Effect on cardiac output and right atrial pressure caused by making the heart hypoeffective, increasing the intrapleural pressure to 4 mm. Hg above normal, increasing the resistance to venous return to 1 1/2 times normal, and increasing the mean systemic pressure to 16 mm. Hg.

temic pressure has been reduced from 7 mm. Hg to 5 mm. Hg, which could have been caused by decreased blood volume, decreased vasomotor tone, or one of the other factors listed earlier in the chapter. Finally, the resistance to venous return has been decreased to one-third normal, which could have resulted from dilatation of all the blood vessels in the systemic circulation, an increased *ratio* of the dilatation of the veins to dilatation of the arteries, an A-V fistula, or several other factors which were listed earlier in the chapter.

Now if we put all these factors together, we find that the cardiac output and venous return curves have become those represented respectively by the dashed curves. The normal cardiac output and venous return curves no longer represent the function either of the heart or of the systemic circulation. The two new curves equilibrate with each other at point B, with a cardiac output of 10 liters/minute and a right atrial pressure of 0.3 mm. Hg. Therefore, if one knows from an analysis of the different segments of the circulation (a) how effective the heart is as a pump, (b) the resistance to venous return, and (c) the mean systemic pressure, he can determine the cardiac output and the right atrial pressure in this manner.

Decreased Effectiveness of the Heart as a Pump, Increased Mean Systemic Pressure, Increased Resistance to Venous Return, and Increased Extracardiac Pressure

Figure 14–10 illustrates the effect on cardiac output and right atrial pressure of changing four different circulatory factors. First, the heart has become much weaker as a pump, as depicted by the lowered cardiac output curve. Second, the intrapleural pressure has been elevated by 4 mm. Hg, as depicted by the shift of the curve to the right. Third, the mean systemic pressure has been increased from 7 to 16 mm. Hg, which is depicted by a shift of the point at which the venous return crosses the venous return axis. Fourth, the resistance to venous return has been increased to 1.5 times normal, which is depicted by a decreased slope of the venous return curve. With these new conditions, one finds that the normal cardiac output and venous return curves no longer depict circulatory function, but that function is now depicted by the dashed curves, which equilibrate with each other at point B, showing a cardiac output of 5 liters/minute and a right atrial pressure of 5.4 mm. Hg. Such a state of the circulation could result easily from an open chest experiment in which the intrapleural pressure is elevated by 4 mm. Hg, in which the heart has become weakened because of surgical procedures around the heart, in which the mean systemic pressure has been increased to $2\frac{1}{3}$ times normal by transfusion, and in which the resistance to venous return has been increased because of pressure on the veins leading to the heart. In other words, if the operating conditions of the circulation are known, one can determine reasonably accurately the applicable cardiac output and venous return curves and from these can then predict the cardiac output and right atrial pressure.

The examples in Figures 14–8, 14–9, and 14–10 are merely representative of large numbers of possible circulatory changes. In Chapters 18 through 27, detailed analysis of the many different types of factors that alter the cardiac output will be presented.

A MORE COMPLEX GRAPHICAL ANALYSIS OF CARDIAC OUTPUT REGULATION

In the First Edition of this book, a much more extensive graphical analysis of cardiac output regulation was presented in detail; it included a combined functional analysis of the two sides of the heart and of both the systemic and the pulmonary circulations, all at the same time. This analysis is particularly useful in understanding the balance of pumping by the two sides of the heart, and especially for understanding shift of blood volume from the systemic circulation into the pulmonary circulation, or vice versa, when unilateral heart failure occurs. However, recent advances in computer technology have facilitated new and very accurate methods for analyzing circulatory function. These are even more accurate in predicting shifts of blood volume from one sector of the circulation to another than are the graphical methods. Therefore, we will not go deeply into the complex graphical method for analysis of cardiac output. Those readers interested in this subject are referred to the First Edition of this book.

However, once one understands the basic principles of the complex graphical analysis, he can "see," all in a single diagram, the complex interrelationships between the two halves of the circulation, especially how the outputs of the two hearts instantaneously adapt to each other. Therefore, a quick description of the basic principles of the complex analysis will be given in the following paragraphs.

The Basic Complex Analysis

Figure 14–11 illustrates on a single graph ventricular output and venous return for each of the two sides of the circulation. Note, however, that the left ventricular output curve and the pulmonary venous return curve utilize a different scale on the abscissa. This scale is labeled "left atrial pressure," and it is in reverse to the scale used for the right side of the circulation, labeled "right atrial pressure." Also, for a given distance along the abscissa, the left atrial pressure changes seven times as much as does the right atrial pressure. The reverse relationship of the two scales and the seven fold difference is calibration factor depict the effect of shifting blood from the systemic circulation into the pulmonary circulation, or in the other direction. Since the capacitance of the systemic circulation is seven times as great as the capacitance of the pulmonary circulation, a shift of blood causes reverse effects in the two circulations, and the effects are seven times as great in the pulmonary circulation as in the systemic circulation.

Note also that the points at which the systemic venous return curve

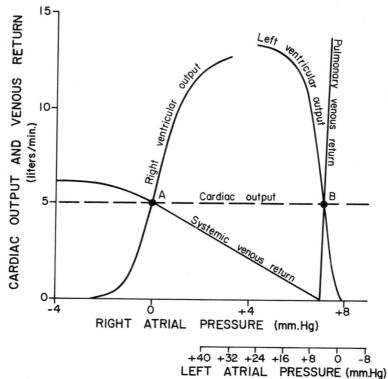

Figure 14–11.   Complex cardiac output analysis for the normal circulatory system.

and the pulmonary venous return curve terminate on the abscissa are always the same point. This is when cardiac output becomes zero—the left atrial pressure equals mean pulmonary pressure and right atrial pressure equals mean systemic pressure. In this figure the systemic pressure is shown to be 7 mm. Hg and the mean pulmonary pressure is 5 mm. Hg. The right ventricular output curve crosses the systemic venous return curve at point A, showing a ventricular output of 5 liters per minute. The left ventricular output curve equates with the pulmonary venous return curve at point B, also with a ventricular output of 5 liters per minute, thus giving an overall cardiac output also of 5 liters per minute.

To understand the functional significance of Figure 14–11, let us assume that a small amount of blood is shifted from the systemic circulation into the lungs. This will decrease the mean systemic pressure in the systemic circulation and drop the systemic venous return curve, causing right ventricular output to fall below the value depicted by point A. However, simultaneously, the shift of blood into the pulmonary system will shift the pulmonary venous return curve to the left in the figure, so that it now equates with the left ventricular output curve at a value much above that depicted by point B. Thus, the outputs of the two ventricles become greatly different, the left ventricle pumping large amounts of blood per minute and the right ventricle pumping small amounts. Consequently, blood will shift from the pulmonary circulation into the systemic circulation, and this shift will continue to occur until the systemic venous return curve shifts to the right and upward and the pulmonary venous return curve shifts to the right and downward enough to bring the two ventricular outputs back to equal levels. In other words, within a few beats of the heart, the outputs of the ventricles become reequilibrated with each other.

Use of the Complex Analysis in Pathological Conditions — Acute Left Ventricular Failure

Figure 14–12 shows the effects that will occur following instantaneous decrease in pumping capability of the left ventricle. The solid curves of this figure are the same as those depicted in Figure 14–11. The initial event is decrease of the left ventricular output curve to the dashed curve labeled "weak left ventricle." This curve equates with the pulmonary venous return curve at point B, giving a left ventricular output of only 1.5 liters per minute. However, the right ventricle is still pumping at a rate of 5 liters per minute. Therefore, several events occur. First, blood begins to shift from the systemic circulation into the pulmonary circulation, elevating the mean pulmonary pressure to approximately 18 mm.

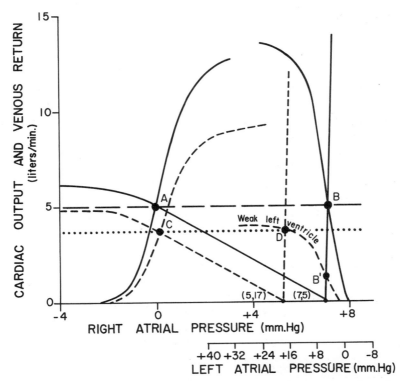

Figure 14–12. Analysis of the circulation, especially cardiac output, when the left ventricle becomes acutely weakened.

Hg, while the mean systemic pressure decreases approximately 5.5 mm. Hg. The shift of these venous return curves caused by transfer of blood from the systemic circulation into the pulmonary circulation is accompanied by the following three effects: (1) the left ventricular output rises to point D, (2) the right ventricular output curve falls to the lower dashed curve because of extra loading of the right ventricle and because weak pumping by the left ventricle results in internal cardiac effects that reduce pumping by the right ventricle, and (3) the right ventricular output falls from point A to point C. Thus, within a few beats of the heart the outputs of the two ventricles have now become adjusted to a new equilibrium level. However, for a transient period of time the left ventricular output had fallen far below that of the right ventricle, and it was the shift of blood into the pulmonary circulation that caused the reequilibration. Note that these effects occur entirely independently of nervous or hormonal controls of the circulation. Indeed, when the nervous system is completely abrogated and the hormonal system is also blocked entirely, readjustment of the outputs of the two ventricles still occurs within a matter of seconds (a few heart beats).

Without further ado one can readily see how this complex type of analysis can be very useful in understanding blood volume shifts between the two major segments of the circulatory system in abnormalities of either side of the heart.

Chapter 15

SIMPLIFIED ALGEBRAIC ANALYSES OF CARDIAC OUTPUT REGULATION

The relationship between cardiac output and other factors in the circulation can be analyzed mathematically in many different ways, each one of the analyses having its own specific meaning. The purpose of the present chapter will be to present some of the simpler of the analyses, and Chapter 17 will present a more complicated analysis, which will take into consideration far more simultaneously acting factors.

RELATIONSHIP OF CARDIAC OUTPUT, STROKE VOLUME OUTPUT, AND HEART RATE

Perhaps the simplest of all the relationships between cardiac output and other parameters of circulatory function is the following:

$$CO = HR \times SVO \qquad (15\text{–}1)$$

in which CO is cardiac output, HR is heart rate, and SVO is stroke volume output.

This relationship, which states simply that the cardiac output is equal to the heart rate times the stroke volume output, has had considerable significance in the past few years because of a controversy over which is the major factor regulating cardiac output—changes in heart rate or changes in stroke volume output. Starling (Patterson, 1914b; Starling, 1918), in expressing his law of the heart, emphasized the importance of an increased stroke volume output for increasing cardiac output when the blood flow from the veins into the heart increases, and subsequent research workers have confirmed that at least under some circumstances marked changes in stroke volume do accompany changes in cardiac output (Sarnoff, 1954a; Chapman, 1960; Wang, 1960). However, Rushmer (1959) has contended that cardiac output is controlled almost entirely by changes in heart rate rather than by changes in stroke volume output.

253

Despite this controversy, Formula 15–1 states simply that changes in either of these two factors can increase the output. Furthermore, there are many instances in which either one of the factors is far more important than the other in determining the output. For instance, in an animal under total spinal anesthesia, the heart rate cannot change significantly; therefore, the cardiac output under these conditions changes almost directly with changes in stroke volume output (Guyton, 1957b). On the other hand, when reflexes are completely active, especially in moderate exercise, the cardiac output seems to be regulated more by changes in heart rate than by changes in stroke volume output (Meek, 1923; Rushmer, 1959). Yet during very severe exercise the output is increased considerably by both these factors at the same time (Wang, 1960; Chapman, 1960).

RELATIONSHIP OF CARDIAC OUTPUT TO THE SYSTEMIC PRESSURE GRADIENT AND SYSTEMIC RESISTANCE

Perhaps the most commonly used expression of the relationship of cardiac output to other circulatory factors is represented by the following formula:

$$CO = \frac{Pa_s}{R_s} \qquad (15\text{--}2)$$

which states that the cardiac output is equal to the mean systemic arterial pressure (Pa_s) divided by the systemic resistance (R_s). However, this formula is based on the assumption that the right atrial pressure is zero, which is not always the case. Therefore, for more accuracy, the following formula should be used:

$$CO = \frac{Pa_s - Pra}{R_s} \qquad (15\text{--}3)$$

which states that cardiac output is equal to the pressure gradient [systemic arterial pressure minus mean right atrial pressure (Pra)] divided by the systemic resistance. In other words, the greater the pressure gradient through the systemic system, the greater the cardiac output. On the other hand, the greater the systemic resistance, the less the cardiac output.

The most usual use of this formula is to determine the systemic resistance when the other factors are known; for this purpose, the formula can be expressed in the following form:

$$R_s = \frac{Pa_s - Pra}{CO} \qquad (15\text{--}3A)$$

Unfortunately, this formula is not very important in understanding the *regulation* of cardiac output, because one cannot predict from the formula what will happen to cardiac output when one of the three factors is changed. The reason for this is that a change in one of the factors usually causes one of the other two to change at the same time. For instance, if the resistance increases, the arterial pressure increases secondarily so that the output is not affected nearly so much as one might expect (Guyton, 1959b). As another example, when the arterial pressure becomes increased, this distends the arterioles (Green, 1944), which thereby reduces the systemic resistance. Therefore, the cardiac output is increased more than would be predicted from the change in pressure alone, and since the interrelationships between the different individual factors in Formula 15–3 are exceedingly variable, it is almost impossible to use this formula accurately for predicting cardiac output.

Relationship of Cardiac Output to the Pulmonary Pressure Gradient and Pulmonary Resistance

We often forget that cardiac output is related to the pressure gradient and the resistance in the lungs in exactly the same way as in the systemic circulation. In other words, the following formula applies:

$$CO = \frac{Pa_p - Pla}{R_p} \qquad (15\text{--}4)$$

in which Pa_p is mean pulmonary arterial pressure, Pla is mean left atrial pressure, and R_p is pulmonary resistance.

Formula 15–4 is also frequently used to determine the pulmonary resistance when the other factors have been measured. But here again it is impossible to analyze what will happen to cardiac output when one of the factors in the formula is changed without knowing also what is happening simultaneously to the other factors. Therefore, this formula, too, is of little use in understanding the regulation of cardiac output.

RELATIONSHIP OF CARDIAC OUTPUT TO RIGHT ATRIAL PRESSURE, MEAN SYSTEMIC PRESSURE, AND "RESISTANCE TO VENOUS RETURN"

In searching for a mathematical expression that would help us understand the *regulation* of cardiac output, it became necessary to derive an expression for cardiac output which is composed of factors that are either entirely or almost entirely independent of each other. The following formula satisfies these requirements (Guyton, 1955b).

$$CO = \frac{Pms - Pra}{\dfrac{Cv_s\,Rv_s + Ca_s\,(Rv_s + Ra_s)}{Cv_s + Ca_s}} \qquad (15\text{--}5)$$

It will be observed that the determinants of cardiac output in this formula are the mean systemic pressure (Pms), the right atrial pressure (Pra), the systemic venous resistance (Rv_s), the systemic arterial resistance (Ra_s), the systemic venous capacitance (Cv_s), and the systemic arterial capacitance (Ca_s). The resistances and capacitances are functions of the dimensions and physical characteristics of the vessels, and the mean systemic pressure is a function of blood volume in the systemic circulation in relation to the capacitances. Furthermore, as pointed out in Chapter 7, relative capacitances of the circulation remains almost constant; therefore, in this formula the different capacitances can be considered to be constants rather than variables. The last determinant of cardiac output in Formula 15–5 is the right atrial pressure, which is determined mainly by the pumping ability of the heart and only slightly by the other factors in this formula. Therefore, all factors in Formula 15–5 that determine cardiac output, with the exception of the right atrial pressure, are mainly independent of the other factors, and even right atrial pressure is almost entirely independent of all the others.

Derivation of Formula 15–5

The real significance of Formula 15–5 cannot be appreciated until one understands the steps by which it is derived. This can be presented best by referring first to Figure 15–1, which illustrates a simplified schema of the circulation that considers the heart and lungs to be a single segment, and the arterial and the venous vascular trees to be two other major segments of the circulation. Resistance Ra_s is the resistance from the mid-point of the arterial vascular tree to the mid-point of the venous tree. The resistance Rv_s is the resistance from the mid-point of the venous tree to the right atrium. The capacitance Ca_s is the capacitance of the arterial tree, and the capacitance Cv_s is the capacitance of the venous tree. The pressure Pa_s is the systemic arterial pressure and the pressure Pv_s is the pressure at the mid-point of the venous tree. The volume EVa is the extra volume in the arterial tree over and above that amount which is required

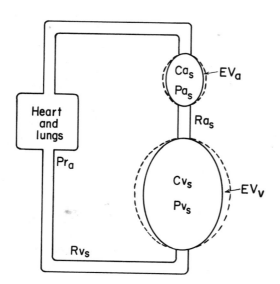

Figure 15–1. Schematized circulatory system used as the basis for deriving Formula 15–5.

to fill the arterial tree without any pressure. The volume EV_V is the extra volume in the venous tree in addition to that amount which barely fills the vessels without any pressure. With this background, we can now derive the equations which will lead to Formula 15–5.

The pressures in the arteries and veins are equal respectively to the right atrial pressure plus the pressure drop from the arteries to the right atrium or from the veins to the right atrium. Thus,

$$Pv_s = CO(Rv_s) + Pra \qquad (15\text{–}5A)$$

$$Pa_s = CO(Rv_s + Ra_s) + Pra \qquad (15\text{–}5B)$$

The extra volume in each of the two major vascular trees is equal to the pressure times the capacitance, the capacitance being defined as dV/dP. Thus, utilizing the pressures from Formulas 15–5A and 15–5B, we derive the following expressions:

$$EVv_s = [CO(Rv_s) + Pra]Cv_s \qquad (15\text{–}5C)$$

$$EVa_s = [CO(Rv_s + Ra_s) + Pra]Ca_s \qquad (15\text{–}5D)$$

The mean systemic pressure is equal to the total extra volume (EV_s) of blood in the systemic circulation above that required to fill the system with no pressure divided by the total capacitance of the systemic circulation (C_s). (At this point it is necessary to explain that the capillaries of the systemic circulation have essentially zero capacitance because they have very little volume and because their very small sizes prevent any significant increase in volume with pressure.) Therefore, for the mean systemic pressure, we can obtain the following expression:

$$Pms = \frac{EV_s}{C_s} \quad \frac{EVv_s + EVa_s}{Cv_s + Ca_s} \qquad (15\text{–}5E)$$

It will be noted from this expression that the total extra volume in the systemic circulation (EV_s) is equal to the sum of the extra volumes in the veins and arteries, and the total capacitance (C_s) of the systemic circulation is equal to the sum of the capacitances of the veins and arteries.

Now by substituting the expressions for the extra volumes in the veins and arteries derived in Formulas 15–5C and 15–5D into the expression 15–5E we can solve for the cardiac output in accordance with the following steps:

$$Pms = \frac{[CO(Rv_s) + Pra]Cv_s + [CO(Rv_s + Ra_s) + Pra]Ca_s}{Cv_s + Ca_s} \qquad (15\text{–}5F)$$

$$Pms = \frac{CO(Rv_s)Cv_s + PraCv_s + CO(Rv_s + Ra_s)Ca_s + PraCa_s}{Cv_s + Ca_s} \qquad (15\text{–}5G)$$

$$Pms = \frac{CO[Rv_sCv_s + (Rv_s + Ra_s)Ca_s] + Pra(Cv_s + Ca_s)}{Cv_s + Ca_s} \qquad (15\text{–}5H)$$

$$Pms = \frac{CO[Rv_s Cv_s + (Rv_s + Ra_s)Ca_s]}{Cv_s + Ca_s} + Pra \tag{15-5I}$$

$$Pms - Pra = \frac{CO[Rv_s Cv_s + (Rv_s + Ra_s)Ca_s]}{Cv_s + Ca_s} \tag{15-5J}$$

$$CO = \frac{Pms - Pra}{\dfrac{Rv_s Cv_s + (Rv_s + Ra_s)Ca_s}{Cv_s + Ca_s}} \tag{15-5}$$

Significance of Formula 15-5

In essence, Formula 15-5 states the following relationships in the circulation:

First, it states that the cardiac output is proportional to the mean systemic pressure minus the right atrial pressure. This effect has also been demonstrated experimentally (Guyton, 1955a).

Second, it states that when the heart fails, which causes the right atrial pressure to rise, the upper limit to which the right atrial pressure can rise is equal to the mean systemic pressure (see Guyton, 1957b).

Third, it states that, however high the right atrial pressure rises, the cardiac output falls proportionately as the right atrial pressure approaches the mean systemic pressure. In other words, these first three relationships emphasize that the difference between the mean systemic pressure and the right pressure is a major determinant of cardiac output.

Fourth, the formula states that if all the resistances in the systemic circulation are increased proportionately, including the venous resistance as well as the arteriolar resistance, the cardiac output will decrease in proportion to the increase in systemic resistances.

Fifth, it states that if all the capacitances of the systemic circulation are altered proportionately without affecting the mean systemic pressure, the cardiac output will be unchanged.

Sixth, the formula states that a given change in venous resistance will cause a far greater effect on cardiac output than a similar change in arterial resistance. This fact becomes even more apparent when we substitute into Formula 15-5 the relative ratios of the venous and arterial capacitances (the venous capacitance being approximately 18 times as great as the arterial capacitance, which was discussed in Chapter 13).

$$CO \propto \frac{Pms - Pra}{\dfrac{18\,Rv_s + 1\,(Rv_s + Ra_s)}{19}} \propto \frac{Pms - Pra}{Rv_s + \dfrac{Ra_s}{19}} \tag{15-5K}$$

This derivation from Formula 15-5 illustrates that a given change in venous resistance under at least some circumstances could cause as much as 19 times as great an effect on cardiac output as the same change in arterial resistance (Guyton, 1959b).

In summary, one can see that Formula 15-5 helps to explain many of the well known phenomena in relation to cardiac output regulation. Most important of these phenomena is the fact that even a very slight acute rise in right atrial pressure as a result of cardiac damage causes a marked decrease in cardiac output (Guyton, 1952c; Fermoso, to be published) and, when the right atrial pressure rises to equal the mean systemic pressure, the cardiac output by that time will have fallen to zero (Guyton, 1957b). Also another important point is the extreme effect of venous resistance on cardiac output, a fact which is demonstrated every day at the operating table when the inferior vena cava is inadvertently compressed even slightly.

Other Derivations from Formula 15–5

The numerator of Formula 15–5 is actually an average pressure gradient—the mean systemic pressure minus the right atrial pressure; this gradient is called the *pressure gradient for venous return* (Guyton, 1955a). On the other hand, the denominator in Formula 15–5 is actually a resistance. Note that the denominator itself is composed of both a numerator and a denominator. Capacitances are present in both the numerator and denominator, and on dimensional analysis they cancel each other out. In other words, the capacitances are only quantitative modifiers of the resistances. Therefore, the entire denominator of Formula 15–5 is a resistance and is called the *resistance to venous return* (Guyton, 1955a). The quantitative value of this "resistance to venous return" is the mean of all the resistances from all the vessels of the systemic circulation to the right atrium when each of these resistances is weighted in proportion to the capacitance of the respective vessel. If we go back to the definition of the mean systemic pressure as presented in Chapter 12, we see that the mean systemic pressure is the mean of all the pressures in all the vessels of the systemic circulation when each of these pressures is weighted in proportion to the capacitance of the respective vessel. Therefore, the analogy of the resistance to venous return to the pressure gradient for venous return is immediately evident. That is, the pressure gradient for venous return is a mean gradient from the systemic vessels to the right atrium, and the resistance to venous return is a mean resistance from the peripheral vessels to the right atrium. The interrelationships of cardiac output with the pressure gradient for venous return and the resistance to venous return can be expressed by the following formula:

$$CO = \frac{\text{Pressure gradient for venous return}}{\text{Resistance to venous return}} \qquad (15\text{–}6)$$

On some occasions it might be important to determine the relative effects on cardiac output of resistance of the large veins near the heart versus resistance of the small veins far away from the heart, or it might be important to determine the relative effects on the cardiac output of the capacitances of the small veins versus those of the large veins. In these cases, the circulatory system would need to be divided into far more segments than the two segments illustrated in Figure 15–1. Should one wish to divide the systemic circulation into n segments, the first segment nearest the right atrium having a pressure of P_1, a capacitance of C_1, and a resistance to the right atrium of R_1, the next segment having a capacitance of C_2, and a resistance from that segment to the preceding segment of R_2, and so forth, Formula 15–5 would become the following (Guyton, 1955b):

$$CO = \frac{Pms - Rra}{\dfrac{R_1C_1 + (R_1 + R_2)C_2 + \ldots + (R_1 + R_2 + \ldots + R_n)C_n}{C_s}} \quad (15\text{–}7)$$

Formula 15–7 represents exactly the same type of formula as Formula 15–5 except that the systemic circulation is divided into any number of segments rather than only two. For almost all practical purposes, such a complicated formula as this is not required, because there are only two major capacitative portions of the systemic circulation, the arteries and the veins. The only important occasion for dividing the systemic circulation into more than two segments is when one wishes to compare the effects of large vein resistance and small vein resistance on cardiac output. The reason for this importance is that there is a reasonable amount of capacitance in both these segments of the venous tree, and there is also a reasonable amount of resistance between the two segments. In the arterial tree, on the other hand, there is essentially no capacitance in the small arteries and arterioles. Therefore, it is almost useless ever to divide the arterial tree into more than one single segment.

Similar Formula for the Pulmonary Circulation

A formula analogous to Formula 15–5 can be derived for the pulmonary circulation:

$$CO = \frac{Pmp - Pla}{\dfrac{Cv_pRv_p + Ca_p(Rv_p + Ra_p)}{Cv_p + Ca_p}} \quad (15\text{–}8)$$

This formula gives one an analysis of the interrelationships between cardiac output, mean pulmonary pressure, left atrial pressure, pulmonary capacitances, and pulmonary resistances. It will be especially valuable in the following chapter for use with other relationships in the circulation to derive a much more complex analysis of circulatory function.

RELATIONSHIP OF CARDIAC OUTPUT TO CAPILLARY PRESSURE, RIGHT ATRIAL PRESSURE, AND VENOUS RESISTANCE

Another extremely important interrelationship between cardiac output and other parameters of circulatory function is the following (Guyton, 1958a, 1959b):

$$CO = \frac{Pc_s - Pra}{Rv_s} \qquad (15\text{-}9)$$

This formula states that cardiac output is equal to a particular pressure gradient divided by a particular resistance. In this case the pressure gradient ($Pc_s - Pra$) is from the mid-point of the capillaries to the right atrium, and the resistance (Rv_s) is from the mid-point of the capillaries to the right atrium. When one realizes that, over the long course of time, capillary pressure is controlled almost entirely independently of all other circulatory functions (it is controlled by the relationship expressed in Starling's law of the capillaries), then Formula 15–9 becomes especially significant.

Starling's law of the capillaries (Starling, 1894) can be expressed by the following relationship:

$$Pc_s = Pt + Pco_p - Pco_t \qquad (15\text{-}10)$$

Formula 15–10 states that in equilibrium conditions the mean capillary pressure (Pc_s) is equal to the tissue pressure surrounding the capillaries (Pt) plus the plasma colloid osmotic pressure (Pco_p) minus the tissue colloid osmotic pressure (Pco_t). If Formula 15–10 is combined with Formula 15–9 to eliminate capillary pressure, we find a new expression:

$$CO = \frac{Pt + Pco_p - Pco_t - Pra}{Rv_s} \qquad (15\text{-}11)$$

Before applying this formula to practical problems we must point out that it can be applied only when capillary pressure is in equilibrium with tissue pressure, plasma colloid osmotic pressure, and tissue colloid osmotic pressure. Sudden changes in circulatory function can throw the capillary pressure far out of equilibrium with these other pressures. Yet over a period of time, usually several hours, fluid will transfer through the capillary membrane, either out of the blood into the tissue spaces or from the tissue spaces into the blood, to readjust capillary pressure in relationship to these other pressures (Starling, 1894). Once the equilibrium has been re-established, the cardiac output can be estimated very exactly from Formula 15–11.

Significance of Formula 15–11

The major significance of Formula 15–11 is that essentially all the factors in this formula besides cardiac output are almost entirely independent of the other factors. That is, tissue pressure is determined by the volume of fluid in the tissue spaces and the physical characteristics of the tissues. Plasma colloid osmotic pressure is determined by the protein concentration of the plasma. Tissue colloid osmotic pressure is determined by the protein concentration of the tissue fluid, and right atrial pressure is determined mainly by the strength of the heart. The venous resistance is determined by the physical dimensions of the venous vasculature and by the viscosity of the blood. Of all these factors affecting cardiac output, the right atrial pressure is the most dependent on the others, and even here the right atrial pressure is dependent almost entirely on the pumping ability of the heart rather than on the other four factors in the right-hand side of this equation. Thus, once again we have a formula similar to Formula 15–5 in which all the factors entering into the determination of cardiac output either are entirely independent or are almost entirely independent of each other. Therefore, this formula can tell us the following significant facts about the regulation of cardiac output.

First, it tells us that an elevated tissue pressure tends to increase the cardiac output.

Second, it tells us that an elevated plasma colloid osmotic pressure tends to elevate the cardiac output.

Third, it tells us that an elevated tissue colloid osmotic pressure tends to decrease the cardiac output.

Fourth, it tells us that an elevated right atrial pressure tends to decrease the cardiac output.

Fifth, it states that, when capillary equilibrium exists, cardiac output is inversely proportional to venous resistance and entirely independent of arterial resistance except insofar as arterial resistance loads the heart and affects right atrial pressure (Pra).

SIGNIFICANCE OF FORMULA 15–11 IN CARDIAC FAILURE. It is well known that patients in cardiac failure often have very severe symptoms of congestive failure and yet have essentially normal cardiac output. This effect can be explained by Formula 15–11, because it is known that patients with severe congestive symptoms not only have a high right atrial pressure, which tends to reduce the cardiac output, but also have a simultaneous elevation of the tissue pressure, which can offset the elevation in right atrial pressure, thus resulting in a nearly normal pressure gradient from the capillaries to the right atrium. In addition, the distention of the veins which occurs in cardiac failure reduces the venous resistance. This would be another factor tending to promote increased return of blood to the heart.

To summarize the importance of Formula 15–11, this is probably the most important of all the formulas in this chapter for predicting the base level of cardiac output, whereas Formula 15–5 is more important for estimating transient changes in cardiac output when different factors are altered in the circulation.

Chapter 16

COMPUTER ANALYSIS OF HEART PUMPING: THE MYOCARDIAL BASIS OF CARDIAC FUNCTION CURVES

This chapter and the following one will give in outline form two separate computer analyses that are helpful in understanding cardiac output and its regulation. This chapter presents an analysis of heart pumping, and the following chapter presents an analysis of total circulatory function.

The analysis of heart pumping shows how one can determine overall pumping performance of the heart from such basic determinants as anatomy of the heart; integrity of the myocardium; the physical laws that govern interactions between tension, pressure, and flow; degree of autonomic stimulation of the heart; pressure load against which the heart must pump; and input pressure to the heart at the right atrium. The major purpose of this chapter is to identify those factors that are most important in determining the overall pumping capability of the heart. Another goal is to show how cardiac function curves, as described in previous chapters, can be derived mathematically from the basic determinants of cardiac function.

Quantitative Factors That Affect Heart Pumping

While a multitude of factors have been proposed to influence cardiac function, it can be reasoned that some factors are much more important than others, with a few ultimately having a dominant role in the final determination of the cardiac function curve. Distinction between factors of primary importance and those of lesser importance is made difficult by the complex interactions that occur. For instance, the dimensions of the heart affect the amount of tension that the myocardium can develop, and they also influence the effectiveness of this tension in generating intraventricular pressure. Ventricular pressure, on the other hand, affects ventricular dimensions by influencing the patterns of inflow and outflow of blood. This situation is further complicated by the fact that the rate of change of ventricular dimensions affects the tension developed in the myocardium, since this tension is a function of the velocities of shortening of the individual sarcomeres. Such interaction suggests that a rigorous analysis, similar to that which will be applied to the whole circulation in the following chapter, can also be appropriately applied to basic heart pumping mechanics. For this reason the following presentation is mathematical, with the various physiological relationships being expressed as algebraic and differential equations. The equations in turn have been combined into a composite block diagram, a mode of communication that presents complex mathematical interrelationships in a straightforward fashion. The basic rules for block diagram notation will be outlined in a later paragraph.

The ultimate utility of a detailed mathematical analysis is to predict the performance of the intact system and to determine the interaction of the various components within the system. Correlation between the mathematical predictions and experimental observations helps determine whether proper concepts have been selected from the multitude of concepts available. Agreement between the performance of the model and the experimental data is evidence (though not proof) that the concepts contained in the model are important ones.

In this case, a mathematical model of the intact ventricle will be connected to a simple mathematical description of the circulatory system. The sarcomeres in the ventricular muscle of the model will be stimulated rhythmically, and the events of the cardiac cycle will be observed. Subsequently, the model's cardiac sensitivities to extrinsic stimuli will be evaluated.

Examples will be developed to demonstrate how extrinsic stimuli, such as changes in sympathetic stimulation or heart rate, can affect specific intracardiac mechanisms and alter the cardiac function curve. A variety of intracardiac factors can participate in this phenomenon; for instance:

1. Cardiac function is affected by the basic anatomy of the heart, and function is altered by hypertrophy, congenital anomaly, or infarction.

2. Cardiac function is affected by the ability of the individual sarcomeres to develop adequate tension. This tension is a function of both inotropic and chronotropic factors, which include the effects on the heart of sympathetic and parasympathetic activity, cardiac drugs, and electrolytes.

3. Cardiac function is affected by the circulatory system immediately adjacent to the ventricle, particularly the valves. Loss of valve patency or improper valve opening or closing can dramatically alter the cardiac function curve.

Although space permits the development of only a few examples, it is important to remember that all of the vast variety of changes in cardiac function have an intracardiac basis and can be analyzed within this framework.

Only function of the left ventricle will be analyzed, but this is appropriate since the left ventricle does the major work in propelling blood into the periphery and because the left heart is most prone to catastrophic failure. All of the general concepts and physical principles that apply to the left ventricle also apply qualitatively to the right ventricle. These same concepts can be made to apply quantitatively to the right ventricle by tailoring them to the right ventricle's unique features, such as a different basic shape and decreased wall thickness.

Events of the Cardiac Cycle

This chapter relates cardiac function to the pulsatile, second by second filling and emptying of the heart, in contrast to the usual considerations of cardiac output, which describe average outflow from the heart over a relatively long period of time. The cardiac function curve, of course, is directly related to pulsatile events in that the blood flow values presented on the ordinate of the function graph are the arithmetic mean of a series of pulsatile outflow cycles. Pulsatile outflow in turn is a function of proper filling of the heart and the ability of the heart to empty into the aorta.

In a normal cardiac cycle, the left ventricle reaches its minimum volume at the end of systole. Diastole begins as left atrial pressure exceeds ventricular pressure, the mitral valve opens, and the ventricle begins to fill. The increasing ventricular volume is associated with increasing ventricular dimensions and decreasing wall thickness. Filling slows as atrial pressure decreases and ventricular pressure increases, the latter being a function of the increased ventricular volume and the compliance of the myocardium. Diastole is completed at the termination of atrial contraction, and end-diastolic volume is defined as this final volume.

Systole begins with a brief period of isometric contraction. During this time ventricular pressure is greater than atrial pressure but less than aortic pressure and, consequently, both the mitral and aortic valves remain closed. Although the volume of the ventricle is constant during this period, ventricular shape changes, the ventricle assuming a slightly more spherical shape and the ventricular wall increasing in thickness at its equator (Feigl, 1964; Bove, 1971b). Ventricular pressure rises very rapidly during this period, concomitant with little decrease in sarcomere length. The maximum rate of increase of ventricular pressure with time, dp/dt, is often used as an index of the integrity of the myocardium (Mason, 1969), but the precise significance of this determination is not yet clear (Noble, 1972).

Ejection of blood from the ventricle starts when ventricular pressure exceeds aortic pressure and the aortic valve opens. Outflow quickly rises to a peak flow that is three to four times the mean outflow. As systole continues, outflow decreases and finally ceases as aortic pressure increases to impede flow, the momentum of the blood decreases, the myocardium begins to relax, and the aortic valve closes. A brief period of isometric relaxation follows, during which ventricular volume is constant but ventricular pressure is rapidly decreasing. When ventricular pressure falls below left atrial pressure, the mitral valve opens and the next diastole begins.

The entire cardiac cycle requires about 8/10 of a second at normal heart rate, with diastole occurring during 60 per cent and systole occurring during 40 per cent of the cycle. This ratio holds for only normal heart rates, however; systole occupies a greater fraction of the cycle as heart rate increases (Bazett, 1920).

Diastole and systole appear superficially to be two unrelated events in that they occupy two separate and distinct time periods and in one instance the myocardium is contracting and in the other instance it is not. Both diastole and systole contribute to the final determination of the cardiac function curve, but not separately. Most importantly, the ventricular filling during diastole determines the ventricular pressure generated during the subsequent systole.

COMPUTER ANALYSIS OF LEFT VENTRICULAR FUNCTION

This analysis consists of three steps: (1) identifying important determinants of ventricular function and expressing these factors in mathematical form, (2) combining the various components in the form of a systems analysis for an intact ventricle, and (3) running the analysis on a computer to observe how it responds both normally and following changes in extrinsic influence.

A block diagram of the left ventricle is shown in Figure 16–1. This diagram is no more than a compact expression of a family of equations. Each line in the diagram represents a variable. The relationship between any two variables (lines) is given by the intervening block, with each block, according to shape and notation, representing a fundamental mathematical operation. Addition and subtraction are denoted by a circle containing a capital sigma, such as block 1, where proper polarities are shown using peripheral pluses and minuses. Multiplication by a constant or by a variable is represented by blocks having the format of block 6. Division is demonstrated by block 16, where the line ending on the long axis of the block, in this case the line originating at block 5, is the divisor. Integration is denoted by block 2, where the entering arrow represents the derivative of a given variable and the exiting line represents instantaneous value of the variable itself. Finally, when the relationship between two variables is best expressed as a graphical function, this function is incorporated directly into the block diagram as shown in block 7. (A desirable feature of the block diagram approach, besides compactness, is that the relationship between any two variables is immediately evident, which is not the case when equations are tabulated in the classic form. In addition, the block diagram approach presents the mathematical expressions in a format that facilitates computer programming, which is part of the eventual solution of the equations.)

It is often convenient to include an immense amount of detail in mathematical analysis of this type; however, this detail often makes communication very difficult when relationships of little importance obscure the most important relationships. In this instance we have limited the analysis to a minimum of detail, divided into four general sections. They are:

1. *Anatomy of the ventricle.* Blocks 1 to 6 describe a basic geometric figure and relate sarcomere length and minor axis radius to ventricular volume.

2. *Myocardial muscle mechanics.* Blocks 7 to 15 express the complex relationship between total tension in the myocardium and the length and velocity of shortening of the sarcomere, and include rhythmic depolarization of the sarcomeres, and chronotropic and inotropic influences.

3. *Conversion of wall tension to intraventricular pressure.* Blocks 16 to 18 contain the physical principles used to calculate ventricular pressure. These blocks give the relationship between ventricular pressure, wall tension, and ventricular volume.

4. *The circulatory system immediately adjacent to the left ventricle.* This section interfaces the left ventricle to the inflow (left atrium) and outflow (ascending aorta) regions of the circulation and provides an environment for proper evaluation of the ventricle. Blocks 19 to 27 describe the outflow

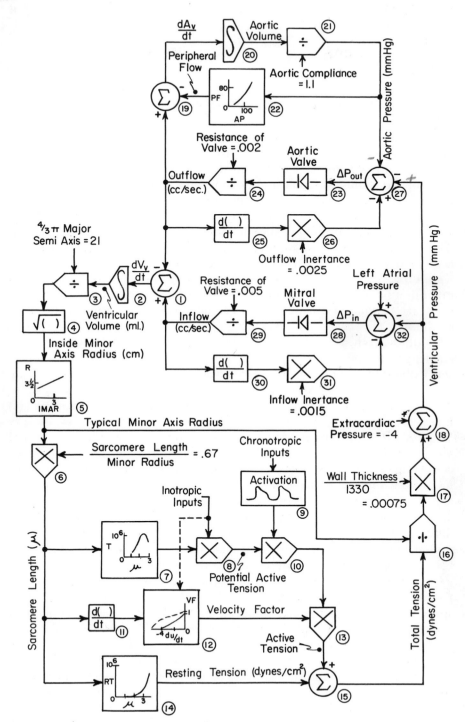

Figure 16-1. A systems analysis in block-diagram form, depicting function of the left ventricle and of the immediately adjacent circulation.

area, including the aortic valve, while blocks 28 to 32 describe the inflow area. Provision is made at this point in the model for changing left atrial pressure and, consequently, end-diastolic volume of the ventricle.

The rationale behind these four major subdivisions of the model is detailed in the following sections.

THE ANATOMY OF THE LEFT VENTRICLE

The gross anatomy of the left ventricle has been thoroughly investigated (Brecker, 1963). Briefly, the ventricle resembles a thick-walled, irregular ellipsoid with both valves, the aortic and mitral, at the upper aspect (or base) of the chamber. Upon blunt dissection the myocardium shows three distinct muscle layers running at angles to each other such that the inner layer is nearly perpendicular to the outer layer (Robb, 1942) and with the majority of fibers running perpendicular to the major axis (Streeter, 1969). The transition from one layer to another may be less abrupt than classically thought, though, with fiber orientation undergoing continuous change within the ventricular wall (Streeter, 1966). Each muscle layer consists of a great number of muscle fibers, which are composed of myofibrils; these, in turn, are composed of sarcomeres, the basic contractile unit of the myocardium.

Although the shape of the ventricle has been accurately described, the challenge has been to find a *simple* geometric shape that adequately represents this shape. The use of a geometric figure is essential (1) to relate changes in ventricular volume to changes in sarcomere length and, (2) to convert wall tension to intraventricular pressure at various ventricular volumes. In general, consideration (2) above has promoted the use of very simple shapes. The geometric figures commonly used include the cylinder, an ellipsoid of revolution, the sphere, and a nonspecific geometric figure consisting of a series of stacked rings resembling donuts. Criteria for selection of a geometric figure include ease of mathematical manipulation and accurate representation over the normal range of volumes.

Use of the cylinder as an approximation is desirable because the cylinder is easy to describe mathematically and because it approximates the minimal amount of shortening that occurs along the major axis of the ventricle during systole. The sphere, on the other hand, has the desirable property of having uniform wall tension throughout when considered a uniformly thick, isotropic elastic body. The ellipse of revolution (elliptical spheroid or prolate spheroid) comes closest to modeling the actual shape of the ventricle as determined by casts made after rapid fixation (Ross, 1967a) and cineangiograms made during life (Dodge, 1960, 1966; Arvidsson, 1961). These observations show that the ventricle is markedly prolate along the major axis that joins the base to apex, with the major axis being approximately twice the length of the minor axes. A variety of mathematical techniques are used to extract the dimensions of the ventricle from cineangiograms (Davila, 1966b), allowing ventricular volume to be calculated from the volume formula for an elliptical spheroid:

$$V = \frac{4}{3}\pi R^2 L \qquad (16-1)$$

where R is the minor radius and L is the major semiaxis. The ventricle, in actuality, has a very irregular geometric shape, but fortunately the ellipsoid has been shown to be a suitable geometric representation over the normal range of volumes (Davila, 1966b).

The mass of the left ventricular wall has been determined by weighing at autopsy, qualified by subjective decisions of exactly which tissue to include (Reiner, 1959), and by using cineangiography to visualize the inner and outer aspects of the ventricle (Rackley, 1964; Kennedy, 1966). In this latter technique, the volume of ventricular muscle is first estimated, and muscle mass is then calculated by multiplying the volume by the specific density of cardiac muscle. A reasonable estimate of normal left ventricular mass in man is 190 grams (Kennedy, 1966).

Block 1 of Figure 16–1 shows that the rate of change of ventricular volume (ml./sec.) is equal to the inflow minus the outflow. Block 2 states that ventricular volume is equal to the integral of the rate of change of ventricular volume. Blocks 3 and 4 calculate the minor radius of the ventricular cavity from ventricular volume, using an ellipsoidal shape with a constant major axis (Rushmer, 1955; Bove, 1971b). The major axis is assumed to be 10 centimeters long (Falsetti, 1970), making the divisor of block 3 equal to 21.

The elongation and contraction of sarcomeres ringing the inner radius are not typical of sarcomeres throughout the ventricular wall (Ross, 1967a). The more external sarcomeres are less sensitive to change in cavity volume in terms of both magnitude of length change and velocity of length change. For this reason, the minor radius at the endocardium is used to estimate the length of a minor radius part way through the ventricular wall. The approximation uses the elliptical shape, a constant wall thickness at the apex, and a constant ventricular muscle mass of 190 grams. This relationship is shown in block 5, with the output of the block defined as a typical minor axis radius. Block 6 calculates sarcomere length in microns from the typical minor axis radius. Microscopic examination of the myocardium has shown that sarcomere length is slightly greater than 2 microns at normal end-diastolic volumes (Spotnit, 1966; Sonnenblick, 1967a). Using a normal end-diastolic volume of 140 cc. (Folse, 1962; Kennedy, 1966), the multiplier at block 6 becomes 0.67.

The combined function of blocks 1 to 6 is to calculate the minor radius and the sarcomere length in the circumscribed muscle fibers around this radius for a given ventricular volume in the human left ventricle.

MUSCLE MECHANICS

Contraction of cardiac muscle plays a central role in determining the cardiac function curve, in that sarcomeres supply the force necessary to raise intraventricular pressure to the aortic pressure level during systole.

When the myocardium fails to generate this force in an organized and forceful way, the cardiac function curve is severely compromised. Notable examples of this are seen following myocardial infarction or in the presence of specific myopathies. When the myocardium is healthy, on the other hand, the sarcomeres are capable of producing forces that can elevate intraventricular pressure to levels of 250 mm. Hg or more.

Development of force by the sarcomeres is a complex function of sarcomere length, velocity of shortening, and time (i.e., state of excitation). When extrinsic chronotropic and inotropic influences are considered, the situation becomes even more complex. Considerable research effort has been spent quantitating the development of force in cardiac muscle as a function of these variables, and a variety of experimental procedures have been employed. Development of analogies between heart muscle and skeletal muscle has for the most part proved to be of only qualitative use because of some major differences between the two tissues (Huxley, 1961; Spiro, 1964). Most information available today has come from (1) studying papillary muscles excised from experimental animals and (2) observing the performance of the intact ventricle and developing inferences about the myocardium.

Isometric Tension

Some doubt still remains as to whether the papillary muscle is quantitatively representative of the entire myocardium, but there is no doubt that it is qualitatively representative. The muscle has proved to be a very suitable cardiac tissue to study because it can be removed easily from the ventricle and because its cylindrical shape makes it convenient to mount for testing. The preparation usually used is to suspend a papillary muscle in a special holding apparatus and then to suffuse the muscle with an oxygenated physiological solution (Abbott, 1957; Sonnenblick, 1962a). Various combinations of forces, lengths, and velocities can be generated and measured. Developed tension can be determined by dividing developed force by the cross sectional area of the muscle. The proper units for tension in the centimeter-gram-second system of measurement are dynes/centimeter squared. Frequently, though, investigators express this tension in terms of the mass that the muscle preparation will lift; that is, in terms of grams/centimeter squared. The two quantities are related by an acceleration term due to gravity; at the earth's surface a mass of 1 gram generates a force of approximately 980 dynes, allowing easy conversion between the commonly used system and the more rigorous system.

When a papillary muscle is made to contract isometrically, the tension developed is a function of the sarcomere length, as shown in Figure 16–2. Active tension is negligible below sarcomere lengths of 1.5 microns, but above this length active tension increases sharply and reaches a maximum at around 2.2 microns; then it decreases back toward zero at lengths greater than 3 microns (Sonnenblick, 1963). Presumably this dependence of active tension on length is a function of the degree of intermeshing of actin and myosin filaments within the sarcomere, with too little or too great intermeshing allowing less development of force than at optimum intermeshing.

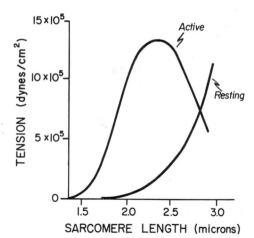

Figure 16-2. Estimated active and resting tensions in the myocardium as a function of sarcomere length.

The maximum amount of isometric tension that a sarcomere can develop varies, depending on the experimental methods used and the inotropic state of the muscle. Papillary muscle preparations typically develop between 4×10^5 and 7×10^5 dynes/centimeter squared (Sonnenblick, 1962a, 1962b, 1964; Spann, 1967; Noble, 1969; Brutsaert, 1970), but greater tensions have frequently been observed (Sonnenblick, 1962b; Downing, 1964; Parmley, 1969). It is not clearly understood, though, whether these tensions are typical of the intact myocardium. It may well be that some feature of the experimental preparation, such as surface suffusion with a bloodless solution, prevents development of normal tensions. It may also be that papillary muscle, due to its unique function, develops a lesser maximum tension than the myocardium as a whole, although there is no morphological basis for this idea.

Data from studies of the intact ventricle suggest that tensions considerably greater than those typically shown by papillary muscle can be developed in the intact myocardium. Wall tensions have been estimated in the intact ventricle using intraventricular pressures, dimensions obtained by cineangiography, and an assumed geometric shape. These tensions, observed following *normal* filling and during a period in systole when *marked outflow* is occurring, range typically between 3×10^5 and 6×10^5 dynes/centimeter squared (Sandler, 1963; Goult, 1968; Hood, 1969; Falsetti, 1970, 1971). It can be reasoned that both the normal filling pressure and the velocity of shortening of the sarcomeres (2 microns/second or greater) cause these tensions to be less than the maximum possible isometric tension. Normal filling means that the sarcomeres are shorter than the length at which maximum tensions can develop, while the marked velocities of shortening mean that a tension less than isometric is being produced. There is a good possibility that maximum isometric tension in these instances could be greater than 1.5×10^6 dynes/centimeter squared. Indirect estimation is subject to the criticism that these tensions are derived, whereas in the papillary muscle preparation the tension is measured directly. Though this is a partially valid objection, in that the selection of the mathematical technique used in the analysis biases the final estimate of developed tension, it is unlikely that this is a source of major error.

An estimate of maximum isometric tension that is consistent with evidence obtained directly from papillary muscle and indirectly from the intact ventricle is a maximum active tension for a sarcomere of 1.4×10^6 dynes/centimeter squared (acknowledging that this value is sensitive to a variety of inotropic influences). These relationships are shown in blocks 7 and 8 of Figure 16–1.

Activation

The instantaneous tension of a sarcomere is a function of whether the sarcomere is activated, deactivated, or in transition between the two states. Analysis of the function of the intact ventricle is further complicated by the fact that the sarcomeres in the myocardium do not all depolarize and repolarize in complete synchrony. This lack of homogeneity during depolarization and repolarization can be correlated with the normal electrocardiogram. The depolarization process starts regionally at the beginning of the QRS complex and lasts throughout the duration of the QRS complex, a period of a few hundredths of a second, as depolarization spreads throughout the ventricle (Harris, 1941). Depolarization is uniform throughout the ventricle during the ST segment but becomes regional again during the T wave, with repolarization processes taking somewhat longer than depolarization.

The development of maximum active tension does not occur simultaneously with depolarization. There is an additional delay while electrical and mechanical events are coupled (Wiggers, 1917; Sonnenblick, 1967b).

Activation of the sarcomeres as a function of time is shown in blocks 9 and 10. The duration of a complete cardiac cycle is proportional to the reciprocal of heart rate, with activation occurring over approximately 40 per cent of the cycle at normal heart rate. The leading and trailing edges of the activation wave form have been "blurred" to represent (1) regional depolarization and repolarization, and (2) a smooth transition to and from active tension as a function of activation-contraction coupling. The trailing edge of the wave form is less abrupt than the leading edge, because ventricular repolarization is less synchronous than ventricular depolarization, and because the period of transition from the active state is longer than the period of transition into the active state (Sonnenblick, 1967b).

The Effect of Velocity of Sarcomere Shortening on Developed Tension

A reciprocal relationship between developed tension and velocity of shortening was initially observed in skeletal muscle by Hill (1938), who characterized the relationship as a displaced hyperbola. This same reciprocity occurs in papillary muscle (Sonnenblick, 1962b), as demonstrated by the fact that contraction at increasing isotonic loads causes decreasing velocity of contraction. The situation in cardiac muscle is not a simple one, though, because the length and inotropic state of the muscle affect the relationship of force to velocity. Typically, in papillary muscle a velocity of sarcomere shortening of one micron per second decreases developed tension to 50 to 60 per cent of maximum (Sonnenblick, 1965a), and this tension falls to zero at a velocity of shortening of 3 to 4 microns per second (Sonnenblick, 1962b, 1965a). This same phenomenon has been observed in the intact ventricle, in which tension is calculated from intraventricular pressure and anatomy of the ventricle, while velocity of fiber shortening is calculated from changes in ventricular volume (Fry, 1964; Ross, 1966). It appears from this data that developed tension falls to about 50 per cent of maximum at 2 microns shortening per second. Blocks 11 through 13 in Figure 16–1 present a composite of these concepts, decreasing the potential active tension in response to fiber shortening.

Resting Tension

When not depolarized, cardiac muscle develops a tension that is predominantly a function of the length of the sarcomeres. This tension is negligible at sarcomere lengths less than 1.6 microns but rises very quickly in an exponential fashion at lengths greater than this as shown in Figure 16–2 (Sonnenblick, 1963; Spotnitz, 1966). Resting tension is considerable at the sarcomere lengths at which maximum active tension is developed, in contrast to the resting tension of skeletal muscle, which is negligible at the muscle lengths where maximum active tension occurs (Spiro, 1964).

The myocardial resting length-tension relationship is important to overall cardiac function because this relationship helps to determine the amount of ventricular filling that will occur for any given filling pressure. Specifically, as filling proceeds, the ventricular volume increases, the average sarcomere length increases, the resting tension in the wall increases, and eventually a pressure is generated that equals left atrial pressure, terminating the filling process.

Block 14 describes resting tension as a function of sarcomere length, and block 15 adds resting tension to active tension to get the total tension in dynes/centimeter squared in the ventricle wall. This tension is tangential to the ventricle wall at the equator and at a point within the wall as determined by the length of the typical minor axis radius. Because of the shape of the ventricle, the tension developed in this region is very important in determining overall ventricular function and can be considered typical of tensions occurring elsewhere in the ventricle.

CONVERSION OF WALL TENSION TO VENTRICULAR PRESSURE

Expulsion of blood from the ventricle ultimately depends on developing an intraventricular pressure greater than the existing aortic pressure. The intraventricular pressure is not only a function of the tension in the ventricular wall but also a function of the anatomy of the ventricle, and this must be considered in any analysis. Basically, the ventricle is assumed to be an elastic body of simple geometric shape such as a sphere or an ellipse, and tension in the wall is converted to pressure according to the laws that are appropriate to this geometric body. A variety of schemes have been used, ranging from very simple to very complex, using geometric shapes of all types, approximating the walls of the ventricle as thin or thick, and assuming even or uneven distribution of tension within the wall (Sandler, 1963; Wong, 1968; Hood, 1969; Mirsky, 1969; Falsetti, 1970).

The most direct approach to converting tension to pressure uses Laplace's law for thin-walled, elastic surfaces. This law states that the pressure within a thin-walled, elastic shell is a function of wall tension and the radii of curvature of the shell, as shown in Equation 16–2:

$$P = T \cdot t \cdot (1/R_1 + 1/R_2)$$

where P = pressure in dynes/cm.^{2}
T = wall tension in dynes/cm.^{2} (16–2)
t = wall thickness in cm.
$R_1 R_2$ = radii of curvature in cm.

Although this formula can be applied directly to elliptical spheroids, it reduces to very simple forms when applied to either cylindrical or spherical shells. One of the radii of curvature of a cylinder is infinite and, therefore, Equation 16–2 reduces to:

$$P = \frac{T \cdot t}{R} \qquad (16\text{--}3)$$

where R is the radius of the cylinder. When a spherical shell is assumed, both radii of curvature are equal and Equation 16–2 reduces to:

$$P = \frac{T \cdot t \cdot 2}{R} \qquad (16\text{--}4)$$

While both of these simple expressions can be used to relate ventricular pressure to wall tension, the assumptions of both a thin wall and a simple geometric shape are potential sources of inaccuracy.

The following rationale was used to generate the relationship depicted in blocks 16 to 18 of Figure 16–1. The ventricle was assumed to be an elliptical spheroid, with one radius of curvature being the typical minor axis calculated in blocks 2 to 5. The other radius of curvature (the longitudinal) is equal, at the equator, to the major semiaxis squared, divided by the minor radius of curvature. This longitudinal radius of curvature is typically seven or more times the minor axis radius (Bove, 1970b) and, therefore, the $1/R_2$ term in Equation 16–2 was considered to be negligible in comparison to $1/R_1$. While it is not actually negligible, the error introduced partially offsets errors resulting from the assumption that the ventricular wall is an isotropic, elastic medium during contraction. The ratio of tension to the dominant radius of curvature is calculated at block 16.

Wall thickness, t, was assumed to be constant at one centimeter (Falsetti, 1970). This requires some explanation in light of the fact that the wall thickness of the ventricle increases considerably during systole. The isometric length-tension diagram presented in Figure 16–2 and block 7 gives tension per square centimeter produced by the sarcomeres. The data that determine the shape of this function are customarily computed using the force developed at any instant and the cross sectional area of the papillary muscle at resting length. During contraction, muscle volume is conserved (Abbott, 1962; Baskin, 1967) and the fiber assumes an increased cross sectional area as the muscle shortens. If tension were calculated in terms of the dynamic cross sectional area at every muscle length, the curve in block 7 would be depressed at shorter muscle length (because the developed forces are now spread over a greater cross sectional area), but this depression is completely compensated for by assuming a constant wall thickness at block 17. Pressure, in dynes/centimeter squared, is converted to pressure in mm. Hg by multiplying by 1/1330. The result is added to mean extracardiac pressure, normally equal to −4mm. Hg (Coleridge, 1954) at block 18 to complete the translation of wall tension into ventricular pressure.

If the wall thickness is a considerable fraction of inner radius, the assumption of a thin-walled shape is not warranted. Formulas have been developed for thick-walled shapes to include tension gradients within the ventricular wall. These formulas represent the concept that wall tension is greater along the inner aspect of the ventricular wall because the inner layers more directly support the intraventricular pressure than do the outer layers. This creates a tension profile which is highest at the endocardium, decreasing in a nonlinear fashion as the pericardium is approached (Hood, 1969). The average tension in the wall is determined by integrating along the tension profile, and is a function of inner and outer radii and wall thickness. Although these formulas are quite elaborate, they can be easily manipulated using modern digital computing techniques.

It has been difficult to ascertain which of the great variety of available formulas is the most accurate and most applicable to ventricular dynamics. The difficulty arises primarily because direct measurements of tension in the ventricular wall are very difficult to obtain, causing a paucity of experimental data. In the final analysis most of these formulas, whether simple or complex, agree with each other within 10 to 20 per cent or less (Hood, 1969; Mirsky, 1969; Falsetti, 1970), and until proved otherwise, the relationships of blocks 16 to 18 can be considered acceptably accurate.

Potential errors arise in both thin-walled and thick-walled approximations when the myocardium is assumed to be isotropic. The implication is that homogeneous elastic properties allow active tension to develop in a fiber in mutually perpendicular directions. This, in fact, is not the case. The muscle fibers have a very specific orientation and develop tension only along one axis, behaving as an anisotropic material. The assumption of isotropicity can be compensated for by: (1) assuming a more cylindrical shape (as was done in this model), in which case pressure is generated mainly by tension developed in the radial direction, with tension developed in the axial direction making little contribution; or (2) assuming a decreased wall thickness. This is equivalent to compressing two mutually perpendicular muscle layers into a single layer with complete superposition of the fibers, transforming a thick anisotropic myocardium into the thinner isotropic myocardium. Such a compression can be handled mathematically by using a wall thickness in computations that is less than the actual wall thickness. It is interesting to note that if Laplace's law for a thin-walled sphere is used to calculate pressure, and if wall thickness of one-half the actual wall thickness is used in the calculation, the expression reduces to Laplace's law for thin-walled cylinder (see Equations 16–3 and 16–4). Items (1) and (2), therefore, represent two different initial viewpoints but have the same ultimate effect on the pressure-tension relationship.

THE PERIPHERAL CIRCULATION NEAR THE LEFT VENTRICLE

The ventricle must be interfaced to the proper inflow and outflow conduits in order to evaluate ventricular performance, both in actuality and in this analysis. The peripheral circulation immediately adjacent to the left ventricle can alter cardiac function, for instance, when incompetent valves or unusually high aortic blood pressures occur. This influence has necessitated extending the analysis to include descriptions of the mitral and aortic valves, and the inflow and outflow regions near the ventricle.

Outflow

Blocks 19 to 21 describe a segment of aorta as a single compartment, while a single block (#22) represents the remainder of the peripheral circulation. Block 19 states that the net rate of change of volume of the aorta is equal to flow from the ventricle into the compartment minus peripheral flow leaving the compartment, while block 20 shows that the volume of the compartment is the integral of this net rate of change. A compliance of 1.1 ml./mm. Hg is used in block 21 to calculate aortic pressure from aortic volume. While the compliance of the aorta is curvilinear (Roy, 1881), in this instance we have assumed linearity without introducing appreciable error.

Peripheral flow as a function of aortic pressure is calculated in block 22. The function shows that this relationship is not linear, with no flow occurring at pressures below 20 mm. Hg. Total resistance decreases (i.e., increased slope of the curve) as aortic pressure increases (Read, 1957; Green, 1964). The function in block 22 is an approximation in that the pressure-flow relationship of the peripheral circulation has been shown to be sensitive to the pulsatile part of the flow through the system; that is, it has been shown to be frequency-sensitive. This approximation probably does not seriously alter the performance of the model, though, because the dominant component of the impedance to flow occurs at constant flow (Patel, 1963; O'Rourke, 1966).

The hemodynamics of the aortic valve are described by blocks 23 and 24. Resistance to blood flow in this region is a function of both (1) the viscosity of the blood and the dimensions of the region in accordance with Poiseuille's law, and (2) the diminution of cross sectional area in the region of the aortic valve in accordance with Bernoulli's equation (Gorlin, 1951; Rodrigo, 1953). The net effect is normally a pressure drop of several mm. Hg., and this can be modeled most conveniently using simple proportionality as shown in block 24.

The momentum of the outflowing bolus of blood can make an important contribution to the transfer of blood from the ventricle to the major arteries. Early in systole, energy is transferred from the myocardium to the blood as it is accelerated, and then later in systole this energy is given up as the blood is decelerated. Accelerating blood requires an additional pressure gradient along a vessel to maintain flow, while decelerating blood permits a decreased pressure gradient along the vessel in the same circumstances (Spencer, 1956). Spencer (1962) measured the pressure gradient across the aortic valve during the cardiac cycle and found this gradient to be *negative* during the latter part of systole. That is, while positive outflow is occurring during this period, the aortic pressure is greater than the ventricular pressure, owing to inertial effects. The pressure gradient in a given region is altered in proportion to the rate of change of velocity of the blood and the inertance of the blood, which in turn is a function of the mass of the blood divided by the square of the cross sectional area of the conduit (Spencer, 1962). Inertance is a distributed phenomenon, and unfortunately its effect can only be approximated when studied in a compartmentalized model, represented here by blocks 25 and 26.

Block 27 summates the pressure effects to get the pressure gradient in the region of the aortic valve, completing the description of the circulation near the outflow side of the left ventricle.

Ventricular Filling

The same physical principles which apply to the outflow side of the ventricle also apply to the inflow side of the ventricle, as represented by blocks 28 to 32. Blocks 28 and 29 describe the mitral valve, while blocks 30 and 31 describe the inertance in this region.

Block 32, the final block in the model, sums pressures on the filling side of the ventricle and introduces left atrial pressure to the model. This pressure ultimately determines how much blood the ventricle will pump during a cardiac cycle and is the primary point of "communication" between the ventricle and the immediately preceeding portions of the circulation.

A note of apology: This description of the circulation could be criticized as being a gross oversimplification. And indeed it is. A considerable amount of additional detail could be added; in fact, nearly every block is itself the basis for a separate, detailed mathematical analysis. Our purpose in this chapter, though, is to analyze the function of the intact ventricle in terms of the most important individual components that help to determine this function. For this purpose, only a skeletal description of the remainder of the circulation is necessary.

PERFORMANCE OF THE INTACT VENTRICLE

Complex interactions occur when the individual components of ventricular function are combined into an intact ventricle. While the number of possible mathematical investigations (simulations) is large, several specific phenomena are of greatest interest. (1) How do ventricular anatomy, resting muscle mechanics, and the conversion of tension to pressure interact to form the diastolic pressure-volume curve? (2) What are the pulsatile events of the normal cardiac cycle? (3) How does the average outflow from the ventricle change in response to changing left atrial pressure in normal and abnormal instances?

The Diastolic Pressure-Volume Curve

During diastole, filling continues until intraventricular pressure rises to equal the filling pressure from the left atrium. The volume at which filling terminates increases as filling pressure increases. At low filling pressures (that is, less than 10 mm. Hg) the ventricle is very compliant, with large increments in volume being obtained for small increments in filling pressure. As filling pressure increases to values that are greater than normal, compliance decreases in a continuous fashion, and eventually only very small increases in volume can be obtained from further increases in filling pressure.

The diastolic pressure-volume curve of the intact left ventricle is determined by the relationship of ventricular volume to sarcomere length, the relationship of sarcomere length to tension, and the relationship of tension to intraventricular pressure. Increased ventricular volume leads to increased sarcomere length as a function of the anatomy of the ventricle. Volume increases much more rapidly than sarcomere length; for instance, Sonnenblick (1967a) observed an increase in sarcomere length from 1.8 to 2.25 microns as intraventricular volume increased three and one-half fold. At each sarcomere length, there is a corresponding resting tension, increasing in exponential fashion as sarcomere length increases, as shown in Figure 16–2. Finally, diastolic pressure is a function of resting muscle tension, as operated on by the tension-pressure relationships of the ventricle. The exact relationships have been diagrammed in Figure 16–1.

The pressure-volume relationship of the intact ventricle predicted by the mathematical analysis is shown in Figure 16–3. The ventricle has negligible volumes at negative pressures, is very compliant within the normal end-diastolic pressure range, and is much less compliant at higher diastolic pressures and volumes. The features of this curve are identical to those observed in experimental animals (Griggs, 1960; Spotnitz, 1966; Kelley, 1971) when the difference in ventricle size is taken into account. There is a limited amount of information available about human diastolic pressure-volume relationships, but some data have been obtained from angiography (Folse, 1962; Kennedy, 1966), indicator-dilution studies, and transseptal catheterization (Braunwald, 1961a). The angiographic observations have characterized the normal end-diastolic operating region of the ventricle as the shaded area shown in Figure 16–3; estimations of end-diastolic volume from indicator-dilution procedures are consistently greater than this, and are thought to be in error (Hallerman, 1963; Bartle, 1966).

In summary, Figure 16–3 shows the normal diastolic pressure-volume relationship in the left ventricle. This relationship is consistent with the theoretical analysis, data from animal experimentation, and human obser-

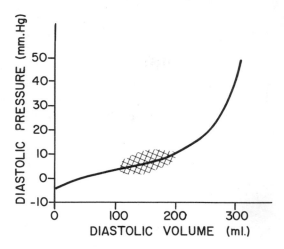

Figure 16–3. Human left ventricular diastolic pressure-volume curve from the mathematical analysis. Pressure is referred to atmospheric pressure. Cross-hatched area shows region of normal values at end-diastolic in adult human beings. [From Kennedy (1966) and Folse (1962).]

vations. The great sensitivity of diastolic volume to changes in pressure over the normal pressure operating range allows significant changes in stroke volume to be obtained from small changes in filling pressure, while the decreased sensitivity at increased volumes protects the ventricle from overdistention.

Computer Prediction of Pulsatile Events

The pulsatile events of two cardiac cycles, as obtained from the mathematical analysis, are shown in Figure 16–4. A summary of the other important concomitant data is presented in the legend.

In each cardiac cycle there is complex interaction between the various determinants of left ventricular function. At the onset of systole the ventricular pressure rises very rapidly, exceeding aortic pressure in a few hundredths of a second, and the aortic valve opens. However, marked outflow does not occur immediately because of the inertia of the blood; sarcomere contraction continues in a predominantly isometric fashion. Then ventricular pressure falls as outflow increases because the outflowing blood shows decreasing acceleration while the sarcomeres shorten at increasing velocity. This temporary trough in ventricular pressure reaches a minimum when acceleration of outflowing blood reaches zero (the peak of the outflow profile) and velocity of sarcomere shortening is at a maximum. After this, ventricular pressure increases toward a second maximum, augmented by deceleration of outflowing blood and decreased velocity of sarcomere shortening. During this phase of systole, decreased ventricular volume causes two partially offsetting events. One is decreased potential tension due to sarcomere shortening, while the other is increased effectiveness of conversion of developed tension to intraventricular pressure because of a shortened minor axis. The pressure gradient across the aortic valve is directed opposite to outflow during the latter part of systole, owing to the momentum of the outflowing (decelerating) blood. A smooth transition to diastole is followed by (1) a continued fall in aortic pressure due to blood

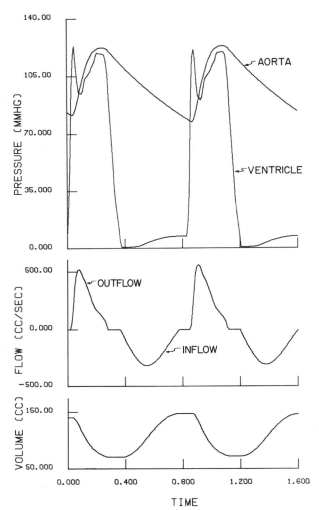

Figure 16–4. Pressure, flow, and volume relationships predicted by the computer analysis of pumping by the human left ventricle. Mean aortic pressure = 101 mm. Hg; left atrial pressure = 5 mm. Hg; cardiac output = 5.12 l/min.; heart rate = 72 beats/min.; end-diastolic sarcomere length = 2.08μ; end-systolic sarcomere length = 1.73μ; ejection fraction = 52 per cent; maximum tension, early systole = 540 $\times$ 10^3 dynes/cm.^{2}; maximum tension, late systole = 435 $\times$ 10^3 dynes/cm.^{2}

run-off from the aorta into the periphery and (2) a rise in ventricular pressure as inflow fills the ventricle.

These events are shown again in Figure 16–5, which displays high fidelity pressure and flow curves obtained from anesthetized dogs (Spencer, 1962). The reasonable correlation between the experimentally observed events and predicted events adds credibility to the mathematical analysis, suggesting that the concepts included in this analysis are important ones. Describing a complex, distributed system such as the ventricle and surrounding circulation in terms of simple compartments inevitably leads to some unavoidable differences between the performances of the real and

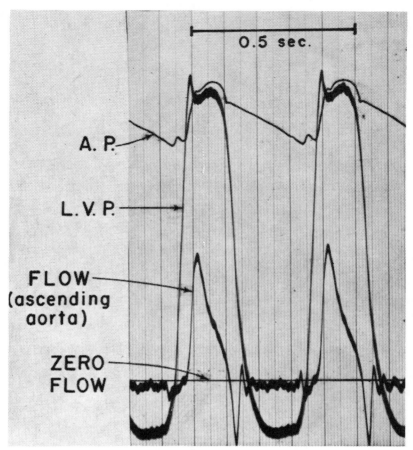

Figure 16–5. High fidelity pressure and flow curves recorded from aorta and left ventricle of an anesthetized dog. [Reproduced from Spencer (1962) by permission of the American Heart Association, Inc.]

the mathematical systems. In this instance there appear to be few major differences.

The Normal Left Ventricular Function Curve

An increase in left atrial pressure causes both increased ventricular filling and increased ejection. This phenomenon has been observed and averaged over many heart cycles at different left atrial pressures to obtain the cardiac function curve shown in Figure 16–6. The curve is typical of those observed in both experimental animals and human subjects (Patterson, 1914a, 1914b; Sarnoff, 1955; Bishop, 1964; Sagawa, 1967a) when the animal data are properly extrapolated to human size. In particular, the response of normal human subjects to blood volume expansion has been determined by Braunwald (1961b) as depicted by the shaded areas in the figure. Ventricular output is very sensitive to left atrial pressure changes below about 12 mm. Hg, but becomes less sensitive at pressures greater

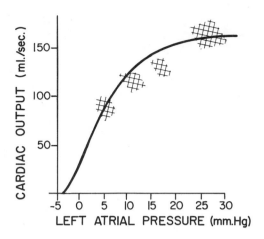

Figure 16–6. Normal left ventricular function curve from the mathematical analysis. Shaded areas summarize the response of five normal subjects to autotransfusion. [From Braunwald (1961b).]

than this, reaching a maximum (plateau) at left atrial pressures above 20 mm. Hg. The plateau in this instance occurs at approximately twice normal output.

Patterns of Cardiac Function Curves

Subsequent chapters describe changes in cardiac function due to a variety of physiological and pathological stimuli. The ultimate effect of these stimuli depends on how they alter the cardiac function curve; yet in every instance these changes in overall function have a basis in one or both ventricles, and more specifically a basis in a particular intraventricular mechanism. Several examples are illustrated in Figure 16–7.

1. *Increased contractility.* Sympathetic stimulation was simulated by changing the inotropic input to block 8 in Figure 16–1 to 75 per cent above normal and by stretching the velocity function in block 12 to the left, representing an increase in the maximum velocity of contraction of the sarcomeres (Sonnenblick, 1962b). Cardiac function in this case is markedly elevated, with the plateau of the function curve being approximately 70 per cent above normal, an elevation that has been frequently observed experimentally (Sarnoff, 1954).

2. *Chronotropic influence.* Tachycardia was simulated by increasing heart rate from 72 beats per minute to 130 beats per minute. The activation wave form in block 9 of Figure 16–1 was altered to include this increase in heart rate and an increase in systolic-diastolic ratio from 0.67 to 1.5 in proportion to the normal chronotropic adjustment during tachycardia (Bazett, 1920). The resulting augmentation in cardiac function is shown in Figure 16–7 (for experimental correlation, see Sugimoto, 1966).

3. *Increased intrathoracic pressure.* Extracardiac pressure was increased from −4 to +6 mm. Hg at block 18, simulating the increased intrapleural pressures that can occur during positive pressure ventilation. The alteration in the cardiac function curve is characterized by a shift to the right, with no alteration in the height of the plateau (Fermoso, 1964).

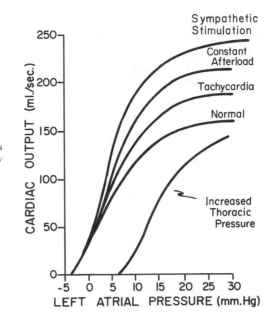

Figure 16–7. Predicted alterations of the cardiac function curve caused by several extrinsic influences.

4. *Aortic pressure afterload.* The cardiac function of the left ventricle is dependent on the aortic pressure against which the ventricle must pump. In the intact circulation, aortic pressure increases as outflow from the left ventricle increases in a manner that is dependent on the characteristics of the total peripheral resistance. Experimentally, two different preparations are commonly used when left ventricular function is determined. They are:

a. To pump into an intact circulation and allow aortic pressure to increase without constraint. This increase is not linearly related to the increase in flow, as discussed before, because the increasing aortic pressure distends the vasculature and lowers total peripheral resistance. The utility of this preparation is that it mimics the restrictions placed on the *in situ* ventricle, and for this reason the results are considered in this text to be normal ventricular function.

b. To hold aortic pressure constant. This preparation (Patterson, 1914b; Sagawa, 1967a) uses a Starling resistor adjusted to produce an afterload equal to a predetermined pressure, usually normal arterial pressure. Markedly elevated cardiac function curves are produced because aortic pressure (afterload) does not increase as outflow increases. The condition of constant afterload has been simulated by setting the output of block 21 of Figure 16–1 equal to 100 mm. Hg, resulting in the function curve shown in Figure 16–7. The difference between the normal and constant afterload function curves demonstrates that marked variations in ventricular function can occur according to afterload conditions (Sagawa, 1967a); the protocol used in generating these curves must be identified in each instance.

Cardiac function curves for the entire heart-lung compartment are similar to those of the left ventricle, but must be thought of as a mathematical composite of function of the right and left ventricles and the pulmonary circulation. The composite is special in that the pumping abilities of the right and left hearts are cascaded within the heart-lung compartment. Cascading causes the heart-lung compartment to have both greatly increased sensitivity to input pressure changes and greatly decreased sensitivity to output pressure changes in comparison with those of either ventricle taken separately.

SUMMARY

This chapter has shown how one can use a mathematical analysis, followed by solution of the analysis by a computer, to predict cardiac pumping capability under various conditions. It has also demonstrated how all the basic determinants of heart pumping, such as myocardial strength, proper function of the heart valves, dimensions of the heart, mass of cardiac muscle, and so forth, can affect the heart's pumping ability. The analysis has been used to compute cardiac function curves for different heart conditions, showing that function curves derived in this analytical manner are almost identical to those presented in previous chapters based on actual measurement in animal and human experiments. A graphical method using these function curves to predict cardiac output in various circulatory conditions was presented in Chapter 14. In the next chapter these same function curves will be employed in a computer analysis of the entire circulatory system, an analysis that can be run on a computer to predict most aspects of cardiac output regulation. Finally, most of the succeeding chapters of this text will demonstrate how abnormalities of cardiac function affect both the cardiac function curve and the regulation of cardiac output.

Chapter 17

COMPUTER ANALYSIS OF TOTAL CIRCULATORY FUNCTION AND OF CARDIAC OUTPUT REGULATION

In this chapter we will use the same basic mathematical techniques as those explained in the previous chapter, but this time they will be used to analyze function of the total circulation rather than function of the heart alone. In the analyses of this chapter, we will use cardiac function curves to depict the heart's ability to pump blood instead of using the computer analysis of the previous chapter. The reader should recognize, however, that at each point where we do utilize cardiac function curves, the computer analysis, or one very similar to it, could be substituted. Such a substitution would allow one to demonstrate how individual factors, such as cardiac mass, strength of the heart muscle, valve function, and so forth, affect the overall circulation. However, it is also possible to see how these factors affect overall circulatory function by simply inserting the appropriate cardiac function curves that have already been derived from the computer analysis of heart pumping or that have been measured experimentally. For instance, if the cardiac mass is changed, the cardiac function curve changes. We can insert the appropriately changed cardiac function curve into the analysis of this chapter without again going through the complexities of the heart pumping analysis of the previous chapter.

Three separate analyses will be presented in this chapter: first, a very simple one presented primarily for conceptual reasons; second, an analysis of intermediate complexity that allows one to determine the effects of the more important control factors on cardiac output; and third, a very complex analysis that allows one to predict the effect of almost any circulatory change on cardiac output and its regulation.

285

SIMPLIFIED ANALYSIS OF THE TOTAL CIRCULATION AND OF CARDIAC OUTPUT REGULATION

Figure 17–1 illustrates a simplified analysis of total circulatory function, depicting especially the interrelationships between cardiac output, arterial pressure, total peripheral resistance, blood volume, and extracellular fluid volume (Guyton, 1967). It is based on the following highly simplified concept: the heart pumps whatever amount of blood flows into the right atrium. In other words, this analysis assumes that the heart is an automaton that is capable of pumping either zero amount of blood or infinite amount of blood, depending on how much blood flows from the veins into the heart. It also assumes that increased inflow of blood into the heart does not increase the right atrial pressure. These principles are very much the same as those stated by the Frank-Starling law of the heart: within physiological limits, the heart pumps whatever amount of blood enters it, and does so without a significant rise in right atrial pressure (Starling, 1918).

Individual Blocks of the Simplified Analysis

Block 1 of the simplified analysis shows the effect of arterial pressure on urinary output by the kidneys (Selkurt, 1946). The output is expressed as output of extracellular fluid, which means output of both water and extracellular electrolytes. Note that as the arterial pressure increases, loss of

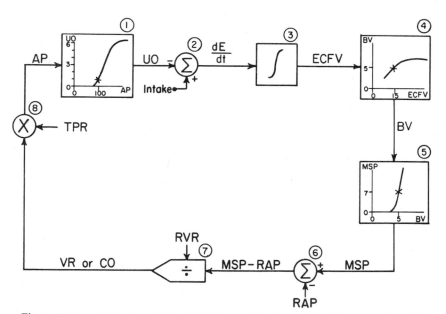

Figure 17–1. A simple analysis of circulatory function and cardiac output regulation, showing interrelationships between cardiac output, arterial pressure, total peripheral resistance, extracellular fluid volume, and blood volume. [From Guyton and Coleman (1967).]

extracellular fluid through the kidneys increases markedly, increasing about six fold for an arterial pressure rise from its normal value of 100 mm. Hg. up to 200 mm. Hg.

Block 2 subtracts the output of extracellular fluid from the intake of extracellular fluid. The intake is the intake of water and salt by mouth minus losses of both of these substances through other routes besides the kidneys. The output of block 2 is the rate of change of extracellular fluid volume (dE/dt).

Block 3 integrates the rate of change of extracellular fluid volume, and its output (E) is the instantaneous quantity of extracellular fluid in the body. This will be increasing if dE/dt is positive, and it will be decreasing if dE/dt is negative. Or it will be constant if dE/dt is zero, which represents the steady state condition of the circulation.

Block 4 depicts the relationship between extracellular fluid volume and blood volume in the normal person. It shows that as the extracellular fluid volume increases, the blood volume also increases. However, when the extracellular fluid volume rises above a critical level of approximately 22 liters, the blood volume, which by that time has risen to about 7 liters, will not increase significantly more because by that time the interstitial fluid pressure will have risen from its normal subatmospheric value to a supra-atmospheric level at which edema fluid collects very rapidly in the interstitial spaces instead of remaining in the circulation.

Block 5 illustrates the relationship between blood volume and the mean systemic pressure (Richardson, 1961), showing that as the blood volume increases the mean systemic pressure also rises.

Block 6 subtracts the right atrial pressure from the mean systemic pressure to determine the difference between these two values. It was pointed out in Chapter 15 that this difference is called the "pressure gradient for venous return" because venous return is, within limits, proportional to this difference (Guyton, 1957b).

Block 7 divides the pressure gradient for venous return by the "resistance to venous return." The output of this block is equal to the venous return itself, which in turn is equal to cardiac output because the output of the heart must equal the input to the heart over any significant period of time. The term "resistance to venous return" includes resistance in all the peripheral vessels of the body that impede flow of blood toward the right atrium. It is mainly determined by venous resistance but to a lesser extent by capillary and arteriolar resistances, as explained in Chapter 13 (Guyton, 1959b).

Block 8 multiplies cardiac output times total peripheral resistance to give arterial pressure, which is the output from this block.

Function of the Simplified System for Circulatory Control

The total analysis in Figure 17–1 represents a typical negative feedback control system, which can be explained as follows: Beginning at block 1, if the arterial pressure becomes higher than normal, the output of the kidneys also becomes too great. As a result, the extracellular fluid volume begins to decrease, the blood volume decreases, the mean systemic pressure decreases, the pressure gradient for venous return (MSP–RAP) decreases, venous return and cardiac output decrease, arterial pressure decreases, and renal output from the kidneys decreases back to that level which becomes equal to the intake of extracellular fluid. Thus, the entire system approaches a steady state level of function at which the intake and output of extracellular fluid become equal — that is, dE/dt becomes zero. Once the system has approached this point, all of the individual functional elements of the system will have reached a steady state and will not change further until some change is introduced into the system.

Some of the changes that might be introduced into the control system of Figure 17–1 are changes in (1) total peripheral resistance, (2) resistance to venous return, (3) right atrial pressure, (4) intake of water and electrolytes, (5) function of the kidney as depicted by the curve in block 1, (6) the relationship between extracellular fluid volume and blood volume (changes caused by altered capillary dynamics, plasma proteins, or so forth) as depicted in block 4, and (7) the relationship between blood volume and mean systemic pressure as depicted by the curve in block 5 (changes caused by such effects as sympathetic stimulation, stress relaxation of the circulation, or so forth).

A special feature of circulatory control as depicted by the analysis of Figure 17–1 is its slowness to come to equilibrium. For instance, if the extracellular fluid volume becomes abnormally elevated, which in turn increases blood volume, cardiac output, and arterial pressure, the entire system returns to a steady state only after many hours or days. That is, it takes a long time to rid the body of the extra extracellular fluid volume and thereby to bring the urinary output into equilibrium with the fluid intake.

Some of the important principles of cardiac output regulation that can be discerned from this simplified analysis of circulatory dynamics are the following.

Effect on Cardiac Output of Increasing the Right Atrial Pressure

Block 6 of the analysis shows that as the right atrial pressure rises to approach the mean systemic pressure, the pressure gradient for venous return approaches zero. Therefore, venous return and cardiac output also approach zero. The usual cause of the rising right atrial pressure is failure of the heart. Therefore, this analysis predicts the effect that one would expect in progressive failure of the heart to the point that it cannot pump blood at all; namely, a rise of right atrial pressure to equal the mean systemic pressure and a decrease in cardiac output to zero.

Effect of Increased Total Peripheral Resistance

Block 8 shows that an increase in total peripheral resistance will immediately increase the arterial pressure and will have essentially no immediate effect on cardiac output. However, the increase in arterial pressure will cause the kidneys to increase their output of water and salt from the body and, therefore, will decrease the extracellular fluid volume, blood volume, and mean systemic pressure. As a result, both venous return and cardiac output slowly decrease over a period of hours or days. The decrease in cardiac output continues until the arterial pressure falls all the way back to its normal value, because it is only at the normal value of arterial pressure that the kidneys will excrete the normal amount of extracellular fluid per day. Since the arterial pressure has returned to normal, but the total peripheral resistance is still elevated, one can see that the final net result of increasing the total peripheral resistance is to decrease the cardiac output by a proportionate amount. This is the effect that occurs when an A–V fistula is closed (Warren, 1951b). Conversely, decreasing the total peripheral resistance by opening an A–V fistula automatically increases the cardiac output by a reciprocal amount.

Effect of Increasing the Blood Volume

If the blood volume is suddenly increased by transfusion, the immediate effect is to increase the mean systemic pressure, which in turn increases cardiac output markedly. If the reflexes were intact and if the phenomenon of local tissue vascular control were also functioning normally, these would very rapidly return the cardiac output back to normal. However, these two elements of circulatory control are not depicted in Figure 17–1, and in the absence of their functioning, the cardiac output would become elevated and would also cause elevated arterial pressure. As a result, the kidneys would excrete excess amounts of fluid, thereby decreasing the extracellular fluid volume to a progressively lower level. Finally, the decrease in extracellular fluid volume would cause the blood volume to decrease back toward normal. These, indeed, are the effects that occur following massive transfusion of blood, though the timing of the events is altered considerably by other circulatory factors that are not depicted in Figure 17–1 but that will be presented in the other two analyses to be discussed in this chapter.

AN INTERMEDIATE ANALYSIS OF CIRCULATORY FUNCTION AND OF CARDIAC OUTPUT REGULATION

Figure 17–2 illustrates a circulatory function analysis of intermediate complexity (Guyton, 1967, 1969b). Blocks 1 through 8 are exactly the same as those depicted in the analysis of Figure 17–1. However, several important additional functions and controls of the circulatory system have been added, including especially the following: (1) control of the circulation by the autonomic nervous system, (2) the role of local tissue vascular control in circulatory function, and (3) the role of heart function in determining total circulatory function.

It will not be possible to explain in detail all the features of this analysis, but it and the very complex analysis to follow are presented not for their details but to illustrate the manner in which and the extent to which overall

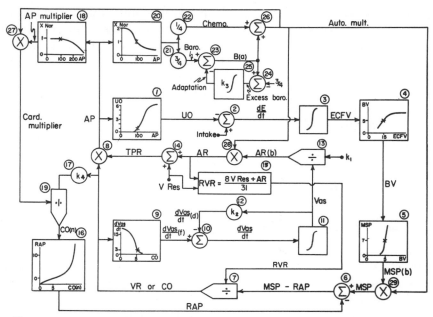

Figure 17–2. A more complex analysis of circulatory function and cardiac output regulation. This analysis includes all the factors illustrated in Figure 17–1, plus the role of the heart itself, the mechanism of local vascular control, and the function of the circulatory reflexes. [From Guyton and Coleman (1967).]

circulatory function and cardiac output regulation can be related to function of the basic circulatory components. However, we will describe in summary fashion the general principles of these more complex analyses.

Effect of Local Vascular Control on Circulatory Function

Blocks 9 through 14 illustrate the manner in which local blood vessels and their local controls help to regulate overall function of the circulation. Blocks 9 through 12 show that when the blood flow through the tissues increases (that is, when the cardiac output increases), an intrinsic effect occurs in the tissues themselves to cause decreased vascularity of the tissues (Johnson, 1960, 1964; Jones, 1964; Granger, 1969). Conversely, a decrease in blood flow through the tissues will increase the vascular dimensions and thereby promote increased flow through the tissues. This is an automatic, local protective mechanism present in all or almost all tissues, and it helps to gear the blood flow through the tissues to the metabolic needs of the tissues. Blocks 13 and 14 calculate the effect of changes in tissue metabolism on arterial resistance. When the metabolism increases, k_1 decreases, the arterial resistance decreases, total peripheral resistance decreases, resistance to venous return decreases, and cardiac output increases. All these effects can be discerned by following the appropriate lines through the different blocks of the analysis.

The effect of the local tissue mechanism for vascular control on overall circulatory function and on cardiac output regulation is to adjust cardiac output to the blood flow needs of the tissues.

This mechanism can often act extremely rapidly, such as within seconds after the onset of muscle activity, and it can be the cause of changes in cardiac output as great as several hundred per cent. In addition, there is also a much more slowly acting component of this mechanism resulting from increase or decrease in numbers of vessels or in physical sizes of the vessels (Korner, 1959). This slower component is called a change in "vascularity," and it requires days, weeks, or months to develop completely.

Role of the Heart in Circulatory Control

Blocks 16 through 19 and block 27 depict the role of the heart in circulatory control. The curve in block 16 is a function curve of the heart-lung portion of the circulation, except that its coordinates have been reversed from the usual way of depicting these curves, showing cardiac output on the abscissa and right atrial pressure on the ordinate. That is, as the venous return (and cardiac output) increases, the right atrial pressure increases in accord with the curve function of this block.

Block 17 represents the strength of the heart, which can be changed by changing the value of k_4.

Block 18 shows the effect of arterial pressure load on heart function, this effect being mediated through blocks 27 and 19.

The output of the heart function block (block 16) feeds into the remainder of this circulatory analysis by way of its effect on right atrial pressure. That is, as the venous return increases, the right atrial pressure also increases, and this acts at block 6 to decrease the venous return back toward a lower value. Likewise, if the strength of the heart is decreased by changing k_4 in block 17, right atrial pressure will rise and venous return will change accordingly.

Effect of the Nervous System on Circulatory Function and on Cardiac Output Regulation

Blocks 20 through 30 illustrate various effects of the autonomic nervous system on circulatory control. Block 20 shows the effect of changing arterial pressure in activating or depressing various components of the autonomic nervous system, while block 21 illustrates the effect on the baroreceptors and block 22 the effect on the chemoreceptors. Blocks 23 through 25 represent adaptation of the baroreceptors (also called "resetting" of the baroreceptors (McCubbin, 1956; Kezdi 1967). That is, when arterial pressure is increased to a new level and remains at that level, the baroreceptors are stimulated strongly at first but then adapt to a new level of pressure, losing their excess stimulation in the process.

Block 26 summates the effects of both the baroreceptors and the chemoreceptors; this summation is called the "autonomic multiplier." Block 27 shows the effect of the autonomic multiplier on cardiac function; block 28 shows the effect on arterial resistance; block 29, the effect on the mean systemic pressure (Richardson, 1964); block 30, the effect on the kidneys to alter urinary output (Langston, 1959).

Some Predictions From the Intermediate Analysis of Circulatory Function

Though the simplified analysis of circulatory function presented earlier in this chapter is a very important one conceptually, it lacks so many of the important circulatory controls that it cannot predict circulatory function with a high degree of quantitative validity. On the other hand, the intermediate analysis of Figure 17–2 is a very useful one even quantitatively despite the fact that it, too, still lacks many of the details of circulatory regulation. To give an example of the validity of this analysis, the effect of reduced cardiac strength will be discussed in the following section.

Prediction by the Intermediate Analysis of the Effects of Reduced Cardiac Strength

Figure 17–3 shows the computed effects of reducing the pumping ability of the heart first to 0.5 normal (as depicted by change in constant k_4 in block 17 of the analysis), and later to 0.33 times normal. Note that reduction in cardiac pumping ability to 0.5 normal reduced the predicted arterial

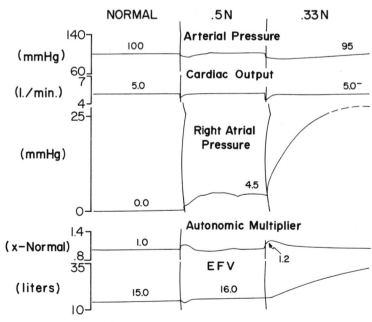

Figure 17–3. Computed effects, using the systems analysis of Figure 17–2, of reducing the pumping ability of the heart to 0.5 normal, and to 0.33 normal. Note that the effects of reducing the heart pumping ability to 0.5 normal are not significant enough to be measurable in a human being. However, reducing the pumping ability of the heart to 0.33 normal causes drastic effects, particularly a markedly increased extracellular fluid volume and right atrial pressure. [From Guyton and Coleman (1967).]

pressure and cardiac output very slight amounts at first. However, the autonomic system helped to compensate for these effects; and the extracellular fluid volume increased a small amount, which in turn increased the tendency for venous return. As a result, the right atrial pressure rose from zero to 4.5 mm. Hg while the cardiac output and arterial pressure both returned essentially to normal within a few hours.

When the cardiac pumping ability was decreased to 0.33 normal, the circulatory changes were much more drastic, because at this level of cardiac pumping the heart approaches that level of failure that compromises blood flow to the tissues. The immediate effect is further reduction in arterial pressure and cardiac output. However, the autonomic system prevents severe decrease in these, and very soon the kidneys cause retention of enough fluid in the body to elevate both cardiac output and arterial pressure back toward normal. However, because the heart is not quite strong enough ever to return cardiac output and arterial pressure all the way to normal, the kidneys continue to retain fluid indefinitely, causing progressive, generalized edema and very marked elevation in right atrial pressure. In other words, somewhere between 0.5 and 0.33 normal cardiac pumping ability, the heart of this simulated person reaches a critical level which elicits extreme peripheral circulatory adaptations in an attempt to overcome the deficiency of the heart. This is the well-known stage of severe peripheral congestion and edema in decompensated congestive heart failure.

One can see from this analysis that the computer predictions are essentially what one actually sees in a human patient when the pumping ability of his heart is progressively reduced: first, a stage of compensatory heart failure with nothing more than mild retention of fluid and moderate elevation of right atrial pressure, but second, a much more drastic stage of decompensated heart disease in which both cardiac output and arterial pressure may be near to normal, but the circulation develops severe evidences of both congestion and edema.

A COMPLEX ANALYSIS OF CIRCULATORY FUNCTION AND CARDIAC OUTPUT REGULATION

Figure 17–4 illustrates a very complex analysis of circulatory function, an analysis that can be used to analyze the effects of most circulatory changes on cardiac output and its regulation. Obviously, so many factors are considered in this analysis that it will not be possible to explain the details here. However, some of its details were explained in the original publication (Guyton, 1972). The larger labels of the diagram, such as "Circulatory Dynamics," "Autonomic Control," "Capillary Membrane Dynamics," and "Kidney Dynamics and Excretion," are self-descriptive. These depict eighteen different functional components that play major roles in overall circulatory regulation and control. We will give here only a general outline of this systems analysis and its theory of operation.

The section on circulatory dynamics includes in blocks 1 through 33

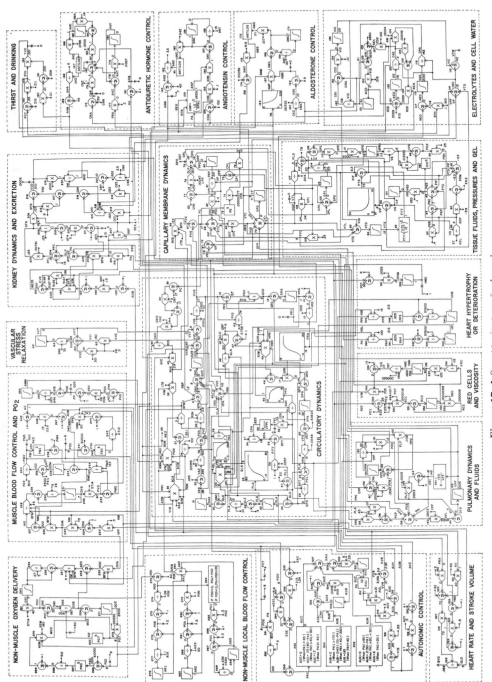

Figure 17-4 *See opposite page for legend.*

Figure 17–4. Systems analysis diagram for regulation of the circulation. Units are the following: volume in liters; mass in grams; time in minutes; chemical units in milliequivalents; pressure in millimeters of mercury; control factors in arbitrary units but in most instances expressed as the ratio to normal—for instance, a value of 1 represents normal. Normal values are given on the lines that represent the respective variables.

The following is a list of the important dependent and independent variables in the analysis (additional variables are present for purposes of calculation but generally have no physiological significance). [From Guyton, Coleman, and Granger (1972).]

AAR – afferent arteriolar resistance

AHM – antidiuretic hormone multiplier, ratio of normal effect

AM – aldosterone multiplier, ratio of normal effect

AMC – aldosterone concentration

AMM – muscle vascular constriction caused by local tissue control, ratio to resting state

AMP – effect of arterial pressure on rate of aldosterone secretion

AMR – effect of sodium to potassium ratio on aldosterone secretion rate

AMT – time constant of aldosterone accumulation and destruction

ANC – angiotensin concentration

ANM – angiotensin multiplier effect on vascular resistance, ratio to normal

ANN – effect of sodium concentration on rate of angiotensin formation

ANP – effect of renal blood flow on angiotensin formation

ANT – time constant of angiotensin accumulation and destruction

ANU – nonrenal effect of angiotensin

AOM – autonomic effect on tissue oxygen utilization

APD – afferent arteriolar pressure drop

ARF – intensity of sympathetic effects on renal function

ARM – vasoconstrictor effect of all types of autoregulation

$AR1$ – vasoconstrictor effect of rapid autoregulation

$AR2$ – vasoconstrictor effects of intermediate autoregulation

$AR3$ – vasoconstrictor effect of long-term autoregulation

AU – overall activity of autonomic system, ratio to normal

AUB – effect of baroreceptors on autoregulation

AUC – effect of chemoreceptors on autonomic stimulation

AUH – autonomic stimulation of heart, ratio to normal

AUK – time constant of baroreceptor adaptation

AUL – sensitivity of sympathetic control of vascular capacitance

AUM – sympathetic vasoconstrictor effect on arteries

AUN – effect of CNS ischemic reflex on autoregulation

AUV – sensitivity control of autonomics on heart function

AUY – sensitivity of sympathetic control of veins

AUZ – overall sensitivity of autonomic control

AVE – sympathetic vasoconstrictor effect on veins

$A1K$ – time constant of rapid autoregulation

$A2K$ – time constant of intermediate autoregulation

$A3K$ – time constant of long-term autoregulation

$A4K$ – time constant for muscle local vascular response to metabolic activity

BFM – muscle blood flow

BFN – blood flow in non-muscle, non-renal tissues

CA – capacitance of systemic arteries

CCD – concentration gradient across cell membrane

CHY – concentration of hyaluronic acid in tissue fluids

CKE – extracellular potassium concentration

CKI – intracellular potassium concentration

CNA – extracellular sodium concentration

CNE – sodium concentration abnormality causing third factor effect

CPG – concentration of protein in tissue gel

CPI – concentration of protein in free interstitial fluid

CPN – concentration of protein in pulmonary fluids

CPP – plasma protein concentration

CV – venous capacitance

DAS – rate of volume increase of systemic arteries

DFP – rate of increase in pulmonary free fluid

DHM – rate of cardiac deterioration caused by hypoxia

DLA – rate of volume increase in pulmonary veins and left atrium

DLP – rate of formation of plasma protein by liver

DOB – rate of oxygen delivery to non-muscle cells

DPA – rate of increase in pulmonary volume

DPC – rate of loss of plasma proteins through systemic capillaries

DPI – rate of change of protein in free interstitial fluid

DPL – rate of systemic lymphatic return of protein

DPO – rate of loss of plasma protein

DRA – rate of increase in right atrial volume

DVS – rate of increase in venous vascular volume

EVR – postglomerular resistance

EXC – exercise activity, ratio to activity at rest

EXE – exercise effect on autonomic stimulation

GFN – glomerular filtration rate of undamaged kidney

GFR – glomerular filtration rate

GLP – glomerular pressure

Legend continued on following page.

GPD—rate of increase of protein in gel
GPR—total protein in gel
HM—hematocrit
HMD—cardiac depressant effect of hypoxia
HPL—hypertrophy effect on left ventricle
HPR—hypertrophy effect on heart, ratio to normal
HR—heart rate
HSL—basic left ventricular strength
HSR—basic strength of right ventricle
HYL—quanity of hyaluronic acid in tissues
IFP—interstitial fluid pressure
KCD—rate of change of potassium concentration
KE—total extracellular fluid potassium
KED—rate of change of extracellular fluid concentration
KI—total intracellular potassium concentration
KID—rate of potassium intake
KOD—rate of renal loss of potassium
LVM—effect of aortic pressure on left ventricular output
MMO—rate of oxygen utilization by muscle cells
MO2—rate of oxygen utilization by non-muscle cells
NAE—total extracellular sodium
NED—rate of change of sodium in intracellular fluids
NID—rate of sodium intake
NOD—rate of renal excretion of sodium
OMM—muscle oxygen utilization at rest
OSA—aortic oxygen saturation
OSV—non-muscle venous oxygen saturation
OVA—oxygen volume in aortic blood
OVS—muscle venous oxygen saturation
O2M—basic oxygen utilization in non-muscle body tissues
PA—aortic pressure
PAM—effect of arterial pressure in distending arteries, ratio to normal
PC—capillary pressure
PCD—net pressure gradient across capillary membrane

PCP—pulmonary capillary pressure
PDO—difference between muscle venous oxygen Po2 and normal venous oxygen Po2
PFI—rate of transfer of fluid across pulmonary capillaries
PFL—renal filtration pressure
PGC—colloid osmotic pressure of tissue gel
PGH—absorbency effect of gel caused by recoil of gel reticulum
PGL—pressure gradient in lungs
PGP—colloid osmotic pressure of tissue gel caused by entrapped protein
PGR—colloid osmotic pressure of interstitial gel caused by Donnan equilibrium
PIF—interstitial fluid pressure
PLA—left atrial pressure
PLD—pressure gradient to cause lymphatic flow
PLF—pulmonary lymphatic flow
PMO—muscle cell Po2
POD—non-muscle venous Po2 minus normal value
POK—sensitivity of rapid system of autoregulation
PON—sensitivity of intermediate autoregulation
POS—pulmonary interstitial fluid colloid osmotic pressure
POT—non-muscle cell Po2
POV—non-muscle venous Po2
POY—sensitivity of red cell production
POZ—sensitivity of long-term autoregulation
PO2—oxygen deficit factor causing red cell production
PPA—pulmonary arterial pressure
PPC—plasma colloid osmotic pressure
PPD—rate of change of protein in pulmonary fluids
PPI—pulmonary interstitial fluid pressure
PPN—rate of pulmonary capillary protein loss
PPO—pulmonary lymph protein flow
PPR—total protein in pulmonary fluids
PRA—right atrial pressure
PRM—pressure caused by compression of interstitial fluid gel reticulum

PRP—total plasma protein
PTC—interstitial fluid colloid osmotic pressure
PTS—solid tissue pressure
PTT—total tissue pressure
PGV—pressure from veins to right atrium
PVG—venous pressure gradient
PVO—muscle venous Po2
PVS—average venous pressure
QAO—blood flow in the systemic arterial system
QLN—basic left ventricular output
QLO—output of left ventricle
QOM—total volume of oxygen in muscle cells
QO2—non-muscle total cellular oxygen
QPO—rate of blood flow into pulmonary veins and left atrium
QRF—feedback effect of left ventricular function on right ventricular function
QRN—basic right ventricular output
QRO—actual right ventricular output
QVO—rate of blood flow from veins into right atrium
RAM—basic vascular resistance of muscles
RAR—basic resistance of non-muscular and non-renal arteries
RBF—renal blood flow
RC1—red cell production rate
RC2—red cell destruction rate
RCD—rate of change of red cell mass
REK—percent of normal renal function
RFN—renal blood flow if kidney is not damaged
RKC—rate factor for red cell destruction
RMO—rate of oxygen transport to muscle cells
RPA—pulmonary arterial resistance
RPT—pulmonary vascular resistance
RPV—pulmonary venous resistance
RR—renal resistance
RSM—vascular resistance in muscles
RSN—vascular resistance in non-muscle, non-renal tissues
RVG—resistance from veins to right atrium
RVM—depressing effect on right ventricle of pulmonary arterial pressure
RVS—venous resistance

SR—intensity factor for stress relaxation
SRK—time constant for stress relaxation
STH—effect of tissue hypoxia on salt and water intake
SVO—stroke volume output
TRR—tubular reabsorption rate
TVD—rate of drinking
VAS—volume in systemic arteries
VB—blood volume
VEC—extracellular fluid volume
VG—volume of interstitial fluid gel
VGD—rate of change of tissue gel volumes
VIB—blood viscosity, ratio to that of water
VIC—cell volume
VID—rate of fluid transfer between interstitial fluid and cells
VIE—portion of blood viscosity caused by red blood cells
VIF—volume of free interstitial fluid
VIM—blood viscosity (ratio to normal blood)
VLA—volume in left atrium
VP—plasma volume
VPA—volume in pulmonary arteries
VPD—rate of change of plasma volume
VPF—pulmonary free fluid volume
VRA—right atrial volume
VRC—volume of red blood cells
VTC—rate of fluid transfer across systemic capillary membranes
VTD—rate of volume change in total interstitial fluid
VTL—rate of systemic lymph flow
VTS—total interstitial fluid volume
VTW—total body water
VUD—rate of urinary output
VV7—increased vascular volume caused by stress relaxation
VVR—diminished vascular volume caused by sympathetic stimulation
VVS—venous vascular volume
Z8—time constant of autonomic response

Figure 17–4. Continued

296

the basic flow of blood around the circulation. Blocks 16 and 28 represent, respectively, the function curves for the right ventricle and the left ventricles. Block 50 represents the loading effect of pulmonary arterial pressure on the right ventricle, and block 59 represents the loading effect of aortic pressure on the left ventricle.

Block 1 subtracts systemic venous pressure (PVS) from aortic pressure (PA) to give the pressure gradient for the systemic circulation (PGS). Block 2 calculates the blood flow through the nonrenal, nonmuscle portion of the circulation by dividing the pressure gradient of the systemic circulation by the resistance to blood flow through this portion of the circulation (RNS). Block 3 calculates blood flow through the muscles in a similar manner, and block 207 (in the "Kidney Dynamics" section) calculates renal blood flow. The blood flows through these separate sectors are summated at block 4 to give the rate of blood flow through the systemic circulation (QAO). Block 5 calculates the rate of change of blood volume in the systemic veins by adding the systemic blood flow, subtracting the flow of blood from the veins into the right atrium, and adding any rate of increase in blood volume caused by absorption of fluid into the systemic capillaries. Block 6 integrates the rate of change of blood volume in the veins to give the actual volume in the veins (VVS). Block 7 calculates the excess venous volume above that volume that barely fills the veins without any increase in pressure. Block 8 calculates the effect of stress relaxation on the veins, and block 9 calculates the venous pressure. Blocks 10 through 15 calculate flow of blood from the veins into the right atrium and the resultant right atrial pressure. Blocks 16 through 21 calculate the pumping of blood through the right heart into the pulmonary artery and also calculate the pulmonary arterial pressure. Blocks 22 through 27 calculate blood flow through the pulmonary system and determine the left atrial pressure. Blocks 28 through 33 calculate the pumping of blood through the left heart and the development of pressure in the aorta. Thus, beginning with block 1 and returning to block 33, a circuit has been completed representing flow of blood around the systemic circulation.

The other seventeen sections of the systems analysis calculate different accessory functions that help to control the blood flow around the basic circuit in blocks 1 through 33. For instance, Blocks 66 through 82 calculate capillary dynamics and transfer of fluid and proteins through the capillary membrane. Blocks 83 through 113 calculate various factors relating to interstitial fluid dynamics. And blocks 114 through 142 calculate the dynamics of fluid and electrolyte exchanges between interstitial fluids and intracellular fluid. Similarly, there are sections for calculating the effects of aldosterone, angiotensin, and antidiuretic hormone on the control of the circulation; a section for determining the interactions between kidney dynamics with circulatory function; another for autonomic nervous control of the circulation; three sections for calculating blood flow and tissue P_{O_2} respectively in the nonmuscle and muscle tissues; one section to calculate the effect of pulmonary dynamics and pulmonary interstitial fluids on overall function of the circulation; another for calculating red cell volume, hematocrit, and viscosity and their effects on circulatory function; another section for calculating heart rate and stroke volume; and a final section for calculating the effect of either heart hypertrophy or heart deterioration on circulatory function.

PREDICTIONS OF CIRCULATORY FUNCTION USING THE COMPLEX ANALYSIS

Later in this text different predictions of circulatory function, as derived from this complex analysis, will be discussed in relation to specific aspects of cardiac output control, especially control of cardiac output during (1) muscle exercise, (2) when an A–V shunt is opened or closed, and (3) in congestive heart failure. However, to illustrate the more universal applicability of this complex analysis of circulatory function, we will present here two brief experiments performed with the complex analysis to predict, first, the changes in cardiac output, arterial pressure, and other circulatory parameters during the onset of salt loading hypertension and, second, the changes in cardiac output, extracellular fluids, and other factors in hypoproteinemia.

Changes in Circulatory Function During Onset of Salt Loading Hypertension

Figure 17–5 gives computer predictions, as recorded directly from the screen of an oscilloscope output from the computer, of important circulatory changes during the development of salt loading hypertension. At the beginning of this simulated experiment, control values for seven different parameters of circulatory function were recorded: (1) extracellular fluid volume, (2) blood volume, (3) degree of autonomic stimulation (in terms of the degree of excitation of the sympathetic nervous system), (4) cardiac output, (5) total peripheral resistance, (6) arterial pressure, and (7) urinary output.

After one and one-half days of recording control values, 70 per cent of the kidney mass was removed, and the salt intake was increased to four times normal. The immediate effect of removing the kidney mass was to reduce urinary output to one-third normal, but this lasted for only a few hours. The increase in salt intake caused increased thirst and, therefore, greatly increased drinking of water. As a result of this the extracellular fluid volume and the blood volume both began to rise, but the rising arterial pressure elicited baroreceptor reflexes which reduced the degree of sympathetic stimulation to a lower level. This decrease in sympathetic stimulation (plus the direct effect of a rising arterial pressure to stretch the arteries) decreased the total peripheral resistance and kept the arterial pressure from rising as much as the cardiac output rose. Finally, the rising arterial pressure caused the kidney to begin to excrete greater amounts of water and electrolytes, and after a few days the extracellular fluid volume and blood volume, though remaining elevated, returned slightly toward normal.

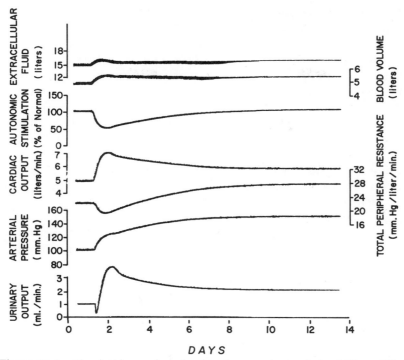

Figure 17–5. Simulated experiment, using the complex analysis of Figure 17–4, to show changes in seven different parameters of circulatory function during the onset of salt loading hypertension. This figure illustrates an initial increase in cardiac output but a decrease in total peripheral resistance during the initial onset of salt loading hypertension. The total peripheral resistance rises later, and the cardiac output returns almost to normal once the hypertension has become established. [From Guyton, Coleman, and Granger (1972).]

After the initial decrease in total peripheral resistance, this began to rise for two reasons: first, the baroreceptor reflexes which had been depressing the total peripheral resistance were beginning to adapt and, second, the local tissue blood flow control mechanism reacted to the excess blood flow through the tissues, causing progressive closure of some of the peripheral vessels. At the end of about three days, the total peripheral resistance had risen to its initial control value and thereafter it continued to rise to levels far above normal. As this occurred, the cardiac output returned toward normal and the arterial pressure rose to still higher values. Simultaneously, the baroreceptors continued to adapt so that the level of autonomic stimulation was also returning toward normal. And the increased resistance in the arterioles decreased systemic capillary pressure; this returned the interstitial fluid volume (and, therefore, also the extracellular fluid volume) back toward normal. Thus, in the end-state of the simulated experiment, the extracellular fluid volume, blood volume, cardiac output, and degree of autonomic stimulation were all so near to their control values that one could not call them abnormal, even though all of them had been abnormal during the onset of the hypertension. The only two factors that were abnormal at the end of the experiment were the increased arterial pressure and the increased total peripheral resistance.

If one did not know the sequence of changes during the onset of this type of hypertension, he would naturally assume the increase in arterial pressure was caused by the increased total peripheral resistance. However, if one studies all the transient events carefully, he will come to an entirely different conclusion. The initial event in causing the elevated arterial pressure was increased cardiac output and not increased total peripheral resistance. Indeed the total peripheral resistance actually fell at first, while the arterial pressure was rising. Furthermore, the arterial pressure had already risen more than two-thirds of the total rise before the total peripheral resistance rose even the slightest bit above normal. Thus, the simulation shows the increase in total peripheral resistance to follow the rise in arterial pressure rather than to precede it. And the final conclusion is that the basic cause of the increase in arterial pressure in salt loading hypertension is increased cardiac output and that the increase in total peripheral resistance is a secondary rather than a primary event.

Thus, one can see that use of a systems analysis such as this for analyzing circulation regulation can demonstrate many features of circulatory function that are not self-evident from simple logic.

One might suspect at first that the curves in Figure 17–5 are nothing more than an abstract exercise in computer technology. However, curves obtained experimentally in both animals (Langston, 1963; Douglas, 1964; Coleman, 1969) and human beings during development of salt loading hypertension (Coleman, 1970b) are almost exact duplicates of those obtained from the computer. The fact that the computer curves have been derived from a circulatory system which itself is built from very simple discrete, experimentally demonstrated circulatory components makes one realize that such a computer analysis is in reality an expression in mathematical form of the physical and engineering principles of circulatory function.

Effect of Hypoproteinemia on Circulatory Function

Figure 17–6 illustrates the computer-predicted effects that would occur if the plasma protein were progressively depleted. This figure shows curves representing: (1) cardiac output, (2) arterial pressure, (3) total plasma protein, including that in the interstitial spaces, (4) interstitial fluid pressure, (5) plasma volume, (6) interstitial total fluid volume, (7) interstitial gel fluid volume, and (8) urinary output.

At the end of two days of control measurements, the circulatory system was made to lose plasma protein at a rapid rate, as depicted by the third curve in the figure. The major effect of this was to decrease the plasma colloid osmotic pressure. Therefore, fluid transuded through the capillary membrane into the interstitial spaces and increased the interstitial fluid volume while at the same time slightly decreasing the plasma volume. The decrease in plasma volume caused a decrease in cardiac output and a slight decrease in arterial pressure, both of which effects are well known to occur when a person loses plasma protein rapidly. However, the effects

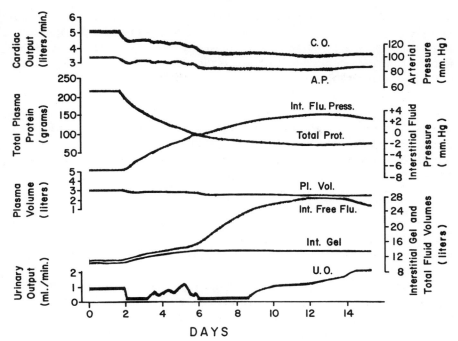

Figure 17-6. Simulated experiment, using the complex analysis of Figure 17-4, to show the effects on eight different parameters of circulatory function caused by progressive hypoproteinemia. This figure illustrates the lability of the circulatory system (especially cardiac output and arterial pressure) and the development of pitting edema. [From Guyton, Coleman, and Granger (1972).]

were not too severe until the total protein fell below a critical level of about two-fifths the normal amount. At this point, the interstitial fluid pressure had risen from its normally negative value of about -6 mm. Hg to a pressure level equal approximately to atmospheric pressure, and the total interstitial fluid volume began to increase markedly; the additional increase in fluid volume was free fluid rather than interstitial gel fluid. Consequently, the tissues at this point began to develop pitting edema, in contrast to the nonpitting consistency of normal tissues.

Note also in the analysis that during the development phase of the edema, urinary output remained very low, usually at a level approximately equal to the obligatory urinary daily output. However, once the edema had reached a stable state, urinary output became essentially normal. Then, toward the extreme right of the figure the total protein was allowed to rise very slightly, and this very minute increase in protein caused (1) almost immediate absorption of much of the free fluid from the tissue spaces, (2) greatly increased urinary output, (3) a decrease in interstitial fluid pressure, (4) increased cardiac output, and (5) increased arterial pressure.

This simulated experiment illustrates many of the known features of hypoproteinemia, such as the following: (1) extreme lability of urinary output, with greatly decreased urinary output during the onset of edema and greatly increased urinary output during resorption of edema; (2) typically decreased cardiac output and slightly decreased arterial pressure that occur because of diminished plasma volume; (3) only slight increase in interstitial fluid volume as the first half of the plasma protein is lost and still no evidence of pitting edema, because essentially all of the fluid in the interstitial fluid spaces up to a critical point is contained in the interstitial fluid gel and is not free interstitial fluid; however, when the total protein falls below a critical value of about two-fifths normal, severe pitting edema begins to occur; (4) failure of pitting edema to occur as long as the interstitial fluid pressure remains less than zero mm. Hg (less than atmospheric pressure) and development of very severe pitting edema when the interstitial fluid pressure rises greater than zero mm. Hg (Guyton, 1963b).

SUMMARY

In this chapter three different analyses of total circulatory function have been presented. Each of these has its importance in demonstrating the concepts or details of cardiac output regulation. Study of the components that make up the analyses can be extremely useful in helping one understand the basic determinants of circulatory function and cardiac output regulation. In support of the validity of the analytical results, computer solutions of several different types of simulated experiments have been presented, demonstrating that the computer results are almost exactly the same as those measured in actual animal or human experiments. Additional simulations of this type will be discussed in relation to muscle exercise, arteriovenous fistulas, and congestive heart failure.

Fortunately, it is not necessary to understand the details of the complex analyses in this chapter to understand most of the important aspects of cardiac output regulation. Most of the remainder of this text is devoted to relatively simple logical or graphical procedures for analyzing most of the important events in cardiac output regulation. Unfortunately, however, these procedures fail to show how all the other aspects of circulatory function change at the same time that the cardiac output is being regulated. This is one of the prime values of these much more complex computer analyses of circulatory function.

V

REGULATION OF CARDIAC OUTPUT IN SPECIFIC PHYSIOLOGICAL AND PATHOLOGICAL STATES

Chapter 18

AUTONOMIC REGULATION OF CARDIAC OUTPUT

IMPORTANCE OF AUTONOMIC REGULATION

Several physiologists have proposed that cardiac output is regulated mainly by the autonomic nervous system (Warren, 1945, 1948b; Stead, 1947a, 1947b; Rushmer, 1959). Yet when we recognize that the cardiac output of animals with total sympathetic block (Guyton, 1962b), with blocked pressoreceptor reflexes (Leusen, 1956a), or with total destruction of the central nervous system (Dobbs, 1971) increases during muscular exercise in the same way as in normal animals, it becomes evident that the circulatory system can get along without autonomic regulation and that at least a large share, if not the major share, of cardiac output regulation occurs by means other than autonomic regulation.

Yet it is also true that stimulation of either the sympathetic nervous system or the parasympathetic nervous system can effect major alterations in cardiac output, under some conditions increasing output to as great as double the normal and under other conditions actually decreasing cardiac output to zero. Therefore, before attempting to describe the effect of special circulatory states, such as exercise, arteriovenous fistulas, or cardiac failure, on cardiac output, it is necessary to consider the effect of autonomic stimulation on cardiac output, and especially the effect of reflexes that operate through the autonomic nervous system.

MECHANISMS BY WHICH THE AUTONOMIC NERVOUS SYSTEM CAN AFFECT CARDIAC OUTPUT

In the preceding chapters, it has been emphasized that cardiac output can be affected by both cardiac and peripheral circulatory factors. Furthermore, the effects of autonomic stimulation on both these factors were discussed in Chapters 9, 12, and 13. In the present chapter we need, therefore,

305

only to review these effects on the heart and peripheral circulation and then to see how they can operate together to affect cardiac output.

AUTONOMIC EFFECTS ON THE HEART

Autonomic stimulation of the heart can affect cardiac output in three important ways: by affecting the heart rate, by affecting the strength of contraction of the heart, and by affecting the level of the mean circulatory pressure.

Heart Rate

Even the normal heart is constantly affected by parasympathetic and sympathetic tone; that is, impulses at very low frequencies are constantly being transmitted from the nervous system by both parasympathetic and sympathetic nerves to the heart. In the normal animal, parasympathetic tone, which reduces the heart rate, is probably several times as great as sympathetic tone (Rushmer, 1958; Carsten, 1958; Folkow, 1956; Mc-Michael, 1944; Robinson, 1966; Stone and Bishop, 1968; Levy and Zieske, 1969a; Warner and Russell, 1969), which means that the parasympathetic impulses transmitted through the vagus nerves actually hold the heart rate in check. Cutting the two vagus nerves or administering atropine to block the parasympathetic endings will allow the heart rate to increase about 35 per cent. On the other hand, section of the cardiac sympathetic nerves causes the heart rate to decrease a few per cent (Beck, 1958; Bronk, 1936; Robinson, 1966; Stone, 1967). And when the sympathetic nerves are subjected to strong stimulation while the parasympathetic nerves are simultaneously inhibited, the heart rate can increase to at least double the normal, and occasionally to as high as two and one-half to three times the normal (Rushmer, 1959).

Recent evidence suggests that the interrelationship between the parasympathetic and the sympathetic nerves in controlling heart rate is complex, the influence of either one on heart rate being largely determined by the level of activity of the other (Robinson, 1966; Warner and Russell, 1969; Levy and Zieske, 1969a). An example of this interrelationship can be seen in Figure 18-1, which shows results from the study of Levy and Zieske. To obtain these results, the cardiac sympathetic nerves and the vagal nerves to the heart were stimulated separately at various frequencies. Two important features can be derived from this figure. First, it is evident that the depressing effect of increased parasympathetic activity on heart rate is greater when the level of sympathetic activity is high than when the level of sympathetic activity is low. Second, the influence of sympathetic activity on heart rate is greater when the parasympathetic activity is low than when the parasympathetic activity is high. Indeed, when the vagus nerve was stimulated at a frequency of 8 pulses per second, the effect on heart rate of increasing sympathetic activity from zero to 4 pulses per second was almost negligible. Thus, although the precise nature of the interrelation-

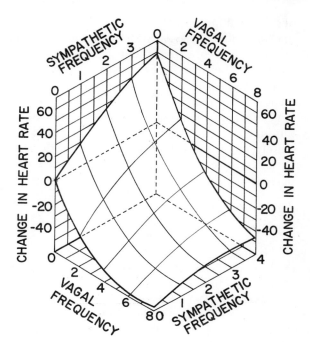

Figure 18–1. A three dimensional plot showing the relationship between sympathetic stimulation frequency, parasympathetic stimulation frequency, and heart rate. [Redrawn from Levy and Zieske (1969a).]

ship is still uncertain, it is evident that the influence of either set of nerves on heart rate is highly dependent upon the other set of nerves.

When the parasympathetic nerves to the heart are stimulated maximally by direct stimulation of the vagus nerves, the heart rate often decreases temporarily to zero. Ordinarily the atria remain stopped as long as the stimulation continues, but the ventricles "escape" from atrial control within 5 to 10 seconds and begin to beat at their own intrinsic rate of 20 to 35 beats per minute. During the short interval before the ventricles escape, a period of 5 to 10 seconds, the cardiac output falls to zero as a result of the complete cessation of heart beat. When the ventricles escape, however, the cardiac output returns to as much as 75 to 90 per cent of normal (unpublished observations), the precise degree of return depending on other circulatory conditions besides heart rate.

If all other factors remain constant, the cardiac output is affected by heart rate in approximately the following manner (Landowne, 1950; Miller, 1962; Ross, 1965; Sugimoto, 1966; Braunwald, 1967; Cowley and Guyton, 1971): As the heart rate increases from normal to higher rates, maximal cardiac output is reached at a heart rate of approximately 120 to 140 beats per minute, and as the rate rises above this level the cardiac output progressively decreases because of decreased diastolic filling of the ventricles resulting from the greatly shortened diastolic filling time.

On the other hand, if the heart rate decreases to less than 120 to 144 beats per minute, the cardiac output also decreases. However, the decreased cardiac output is not proportional to the decrease in heart rate because the degree of filling of the ventricles becomes enhanced during the prolonged diastolic filling periods, which increases the stroke volume and in this way offsets to a great extent the decrease in output that one might predict. For instance, when the heart rate falls from the normal of 70 to 80 beats per minute to as low as 20 beats per minute, the cardiac output does not decrease 70 per cent as one might suspect, but instead decreases only 20 to 30 per cent. Further decrease in heart rate to less than about 20 beats per minute, however, does cause the output to fall drastically, now approximately in proportion to the additional decrease in rate because the ventricles have reached their maximal stroke volume output and cannot compensate further (see Miller, 1962, for studies in dogs).

Strength of Heart Beat

It has long been known that both the parasympathetic and sympathetic nerves can affect the strength of the atrial beat and that sympathetic stimulation has a substantial influence on the strength of the ventricular beat (Sarnoff, 1954a; Anzola 1956b; Folkow, 1956; Carsten, 1958; Randall and McNally, 1960; Zimmerman, 1960; Braunwald, 1963a; Kot, 1963; Randall, 1967). Maximal sympathetic stimulation ordinarily increases the strength of the ventricular beat to approximately 60 to 70 per cent above normal. On the other hand, complete abrogation of sympathetic impulses to the heart decreases the strength of ventricular contraction perhaps 10 to 20 per cent.

Only recently has the study of DeGeest (1956a) demonstrated that parasympathetic stimulation can also affect the force of ventricular contraction, although to a much lesser degree than can sympathetic stimulation. The original results of DeGeest have been confirmed by numerous other studies (Buccino, 1966; Levy, 1966a, 1966b; Daggett, 1967; Randall, 1968, 1971; Levy and Zieske, 1969b; Priola, 1969; Wildenthal, 1969a, 1969b; Pace, 1970a; Pace and Keefe, 1970b). On the basis of these studies, it appears that parasympathetic stimulation can depress the strength of ventricular contraction by approximately 5 to 10 per cent if the heart is also under the influence of a normal level of sympathetic stimulation. However, at maximal levels of sympathetic stimulation, the influence of parasympathetic stimulation on ventricular contractile force is increased. Under this condition, parasympathetic stimulation can depress the strength of ventricular contraction by as much as 15 to 20 per cent (Levy, 1966a, 1969b).

That parasympathetic nerves can affect ventricular muscle as well as atrial muscle is also suggested by histochemical studies, which have demonstrated a preponderance of cholinergic nerve fibers in atrial muscle and a small to moderate number in ventricular muscle (Jacobowitz, 1967). Sympathetic, or adrenergic, fibers are abundant in both atrial and ventricular muscle. Thus, these histochemical findings are in agreement with the results of functional studies which indicate that both parasympathetic and sympathetic nerves have an influence on the strength of atrial as well as ventricular contraction, although the sympathetic influence predominates in the ventricle.

Effect of Cardiac Stimulation on the Mean Circulatory Pressure

Another interesting means by which the heart can affect cardiac output is by changing the mean circulatory pressure, which can be explained as follows: The average volume of the cardiac chambers, which often hold as much as 500 ml. of blood at one time, can change from time to time, depending upon the degree of autonomic stimulation (Gauer, 1955; Rushmer, 1959; Kjellberg, 1952). Sympathetic stimulation decreases the cardiac volume, particularly that of the ventricles, whereas parasympathetic stimulation increases the cardiac volume. The autonomic effect on heart size comes about because of changes in heart rate as well as changes in cardiac strength. That is, a decreased heart rate allows more filling time and consequently an increased cardiac volume, while an increased rate decreases the volume for opposite reasons. Also, a decreased strength of contraction prevents the heart from expelling as much blood as usual, resulting in increased heart volume, while an increased strength of contraction decreases the heart volume.

Thus, sympathetic stimulation causes large volumes of blood to be displaced from the heart into the remainder of the circulation, and parasympathetic stimulation causes large volumes to be stored in the heart. The displacement of blood into the peripheral vessels increases the mean circulatory pressure, which in turn increases both the mean systemic pressure and the mean pulmonary pressure, thereby benefiting blood flow through the peripheral vasculature. One can estimate from the quantity of blood displaced in this manner that this effect can increase the mean circulatory pressure by as much as 20 to 30 per cent [estimations based on Richardson's data (1961) for the relationship between blood volume and mean circulatory pressure], which can then increase the cardiac output by almost the same amount for reasons to be discussed below.

AUTONOMIC REGULATION OF FACTORS IN THE PERIPHERAL CIRCULATION, AND THEIR EFFECTS ON CARDIAC OUTPUT

It is a major mistake to consider that autonomic regulation of cardiac output is mediated only through the heart, because the autonomic nervous system affects cardiac output at least as much if not more through its effects on the peripheral circulation as through its effects on the heart. The two effects on the peripheral circulation that are of major importance for cardiac output regulation are changes in mean circulatory pressure and in resistance to venous return.

Effect of Autonomic Stimulation on the Mean Circulatory Pressure

Total abrogation of sympathetic impulses to the circulation reduces the mean circulatory pressure from the normal value of 7 mm. Hg down to an average of about 5 mm. Hg (Guyton, 1954c). On the other hand, maximal sympathetic stimulation, such as that caused by eliciting a maximal central nervous system ischemic reflex or by infusing a maximal amount of a sympathomimetic amine, increases the mean circulatory pressure to an upper maximal level of 17 to 20 mm. Hg (Guyton, 1954c; Richardson, 1964). Since mean circulatory pressure is one of the principal determinants of the amount of blood that will flow from the peripheral vasculature into the heart (Guyton, 1955b; also see Chapters 11 through 13), this variation under the influence of autonomic impulses is one of the major contributors to the regulation of cardiac output.

The effect on venous return of autonomic stimulation of the peripheral circulation has also been studied by many other investigators in other ways. Several workers have demonstrated that sympathetic stimulation results in constriction of the veins (Kelly, 1956; Shadle, 1958; Davis, 1963; Zingher and Grodins, 1964; Baum and Hosko, 1965; Browse, 1966; Zimmerman, 1966; Guntheroth, 1971). In addition, Alexander (1954, 1955, 1956), Merritt (1959), and Mellander (1960) have shown that venous constriction produced by sympathetic stimulation increases the venous return. Eckstein (1957) has shown the same effect following epinephrine and norepinephrine infusion. Also, Adriani (1940), Doud (1940), and Trapold (1957) have shown that spinal anesthesia or ganglionic blocking agents can cause peripheral vascular paralysis with consequently decreased venous return. Finally, Page (1955) and Weissler (1957b) have shown, respectively, a depressed venous return in postural hypotension and in vasodepressor syncope.

Resistance to Venous Return

The effect of autonomic stimulation on the "resistance to venous return" is usually slight in comparison with its effect on total peripheral resistance for the following reasons: First, the resistive factors affecting the "resistance to venous return" are located mainly in the veins (to a greater extent in the large veins than in the small veins), as was discussed in Chapter 13, whereas essentially all the increase in peripheral resistance following sympathetic stimulation occurs in the arterioles. Therefore, sympathetic stimulation has little effect on the resistance to venous return from the peripheral vasculature (Guyton, 1958c), as is evident from the discussion in Chapter 13.

A second factor that keeps autonomic stimulation from significantly affecting the resistance to venous return results from the incompressibility of blood, as follows: When the sympathetic nervous system stimulates all the blood vessels of the circulatory system at once, constriction of any one segment of these vessels must be accompanied by dilatation of another segment. Studies on sympathetic stimulation, and particularly on infusion of sympathomimetic drugs, have shown that when the arterioles constrict, the venous tree dilates very slightly (Guyton, 1958c). In slight to moderate sympathetic stimulation, this dilatation of the venous tree is sufficient to overcome the slight detrimental effect of arteriolar constriction on venous return, but when the degree of sympathetic stimulation is extremely powerful, sympathetic stimulation then increases the resistance to venous return as much as 10 to 20 per cent.

RELATIVE SIGNIFICANCE OF CARDIAC AND PERIPHERAL FACTORS IN AUTONOMIC REGULATION OF CARDIAC OUTPUT

Cardiac Effects

Figure 18-2 illustrates the normal venous return curve and four separate cardiac output curves: a normal cardiac output curve, a cardiac output curve during sympathetic stimulation of the heart, a normal cardiac output curve when the chest is open, and a cardiac output curve during sympathetic stimulation of the heart when the chest is open. The equating point of the normal venous return curve and the normal cardiac output curve is point A, with a cardiac output of 5 liters/minute and a right atrial pressure of zero. Now if the heart is maximally stimulated by the sympathetics, we change from the normal cardiac output curve to the dashed curve shown to the left, which equates with the venous return curve at point D. This represents an increase in cardiac output of approximately 5 per cent. In other words, maximal sympathetic stimulation of the heart can increase the cardiac output only very slightly (Carrier, unpublished observations). The reason for this is the following: Even the normal heart can pump essentially all the blood that will return to it from the systemic circulation, and making the heart a far stronger pump cannot make it pump any more because the veins collapse and thereby prevent more blood from flowing into the heart (Holt, 1941, 1959; Duomarco, 1946, 1950d; Guyton, 1954a, 1962a). In other words, cardiac output in this normal state of the circulation is limited more by the peripheral circulation than by the heart itself.

Since many studies of the effect of sympathetic stimulation on cardiac output have been performed in opened chest animals, we also need to analyze the benefits that sympathetic stimulation can have under this condition. The two curves to the right represent, respectively, the normal curve and the curve following sympathetic stimulation in the opened chest dog. The equating point of the normal curve with the venous return curve is point B, whereas that for the stimulated heart is point C. Note that sympathetic stimulation in this instance increases the cardiac output from 2.6 liters to approximately 3.1 liters, which represents an increase of about 25 per cent. This analysis gives almost exactly the same results as those recorded in actual experiments by Fermoso (1964) and agrees also with results obtained by Shipley and Gregg (1945) in opened chest dogs in which they found an increase in cardiac output of 27 to 30 per cent on maximal stimulation of the stellate ganglion.

To summarize, the degree of increase in cardiac output that can result from cardiac stimulation depends to a great extent on other factors besides the degree of cardiac stimulation. In the normal animal, the increase in cardiac output that results from cardiac stimulation alone is usually insignificant. However, it is emphasized that the permissive level of cardiac

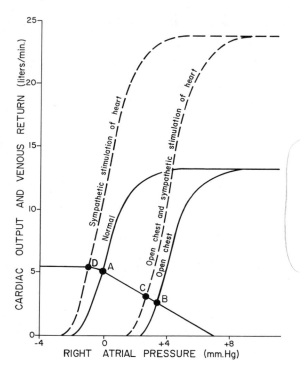

Figure 18–2. Effect on cardiac output of sympathetic stimulation of the heart in the closed chest animal (as depicted by the left two cardiac output curves) and in the opened chest animal (as depicted by the right two cardiac output curves).

pumping is greatly influenced by the degree of autonomic stimulation; parasympathetic stimulation or sympathetic inhibition lowers the permissive level of pumping, and parasympathetic inhibition or sympathetic stimulation greatly increases the permissive level of pumping. The increase in the permissive level of cardiac pumping which occurs with cardiac stimulation is especially important under certain circulatory conditions, such as cardiac failure, extreme exercise, arteriovenous fistulas, an opened chest, and others, as will be pointed out in later chapters. Under these conditions, autonomic stimulation of the heart is one of the truly important means for increasing cardiac output.

Peripheral Effects

Figure 18–3 illustrates the effect of peripheral stimulation alone on cardiac output. The data for this analysis were determined in dogs in which the pumping action of the heart was controlled by passing the blood first from the right atrium through an external controlled perfusion system and then back into the pulmonary artery (Guyton, 1958c; also see Chapter 12). In this way, it was possible to keep cardiac function from changing during the course of the experiments even though the degree of peripheral stimulation was changed. The second curve from the top represents approximately the venous return curve that one records during moderate sympathetic stimulation, and the uppermost curve represents a venous return curve that one records during maximal sympathetic stimu-

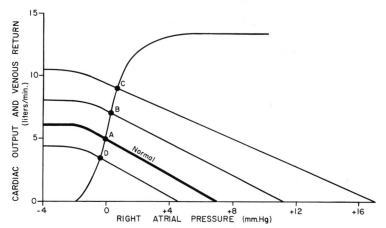

Figure 18–3. Effect on cardiac output of sympathetic stimulation of the peripheral circulation without stimulation of the heart, illustrating a very significant change in cardiac output even when the pumping ability of the heart was controlled very precisely.

lation, such as occurs during a maximal central nervous system ischemic response. We find the normal equilibrium point of the circulation to be point A where the normal venous return curve and the normal cardiac output curve cross. Should all sympathetic tone be lost, the cardiac output, even without any change in cardiac function, should fall from 5 liters per minute to approximately 3.4 liters, or a reduction of 32 per cent. On the other hand, maximal sympathetic stimulation of the peripheral circulation should increase the cardiac output to point C at a value of 9 liters per minute, or an 80 per cent increase.

Thus, we see that alterations in the peripheral circulation from zero sympathetic tone to maximal sympathetic tone can change the cardiac output from approximately 30 per cent below normal up to approximately 80 per cent above normal. It is evident, therefore, that under normal operating conditions, sympathetic control of cardiac output through the peripheral factors is considerably greater than through the cardiac factors. However, again we must caution that this applies only to conditions in which other factors besides alterations in vasomotor tone are not at work, for in exercise, cardiac failure, and other conditions one finds that cardiac stimulation sometimes plays as great a role as peripheral stimulation.

Effect of Sympathetic Stimulation on Cardiac Output When Considering Both Cardiac and Peripheral Factors

Figure 18–4 illustrates an analysis for the combined effects of both cardiac and peripheral factors on cardiac output. The very heavy solid curves represent the normal effects. The short-dashed curves represent total loss of sympathetic tone. The long-dashed curves represent moderate sympathetic stimulation, and the dot-dashed curves represent maximal

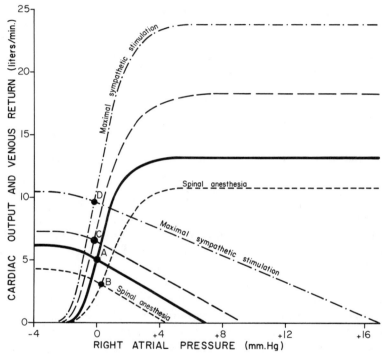

Figure 18–4. Effect on cardiac output of combined stimulation of the heart and of the peripheral vasculature, showing an increase in cardiac output of 25 per cent during moderate sympathetic stimulation, an increase of 92 per cent during maximal sympathetic stimulation, and a decrease of 40 per cent when all sympathetic tone in the body is abrogated by total spinal anesthesia.

sympathetic stimulation. These results fit with measurements of the effects of sympathetic stimulation or of sympathomimetic drugs on cardiac output (Isschutz, 1948; Delaunois, 1954; Gilmore, 1954; Levy, 1957; Richardson, 1965).

From this combined analysis one can see that complete loss of sympathetic tone reduces the cardiac output from 5 liters to slightly more than 3 liters, a reduction of as much as 40 per cent. However, one must qualify this by stating that this depends to a very great extent on the patient's or the animal's position. If the subject is lying in a slightly headdown position, the marked reduction in mean circulatory pressure will be offset by the low hydrostatic level of the heart so that the cardiac output may be normal or even greater than normal (Smith, 1949). This effect will be discussed in much more detail in Chapter 20 in relation to the effect of orthostatic factors in the regulation of cardiac output.

Moderate sympathetic stimulation increases the cardiac output from point A to point C, with an increase in output of about 25 per cent, and strong sympathetic stimulation increases the cardiac output up to point D, which represents 9.6 liters per minute or an increase to 92 per cent above normal.

It should be noted especially in Figure 18-4 that the greater the degree of sympathetic stimulation, the lower the right atrial pressure becomes, even though the cardiac output rises. This observation has been used by Rushmer (1959) to state that Starling's curves of the heart (cardiac function curves) have little to do with the regulation of cardiac output. However, one can see from this figure that one can actually predict from the curves the decrease in right atrial pressure.

EFFECT OF PARASYMPATHETIC STIMULATION ON CARDIAC OUTPUT

Because of the sparsity of parasympathetic nerve fibers to the peripheral vasculature, parasympathetic stimulation has no measurable effect on the peripheral vascular system, and it is generally agreed that it affects cardiac output only through its effects on the heart. As pointed out earlier, the parasympathetic nerves affect the heart primarily through their influence on heart rate. A reduction in heart rate to approximately 20 beats per minute reduces the cardiac output to about 30 per cent below normal, whereas a further reduction in rate below 20 beats per minute ordinarily reduces the cardiac output in proportion to the additional decrease in rate. Very powerful parasympathetic stimulation can actually stop the heart completely for a short period of time, in which case the cardiac output becomes zero. Then the ventricles escape and beat at a rate of 20 to 40 beats per minute; the cardiac output at this time returns to approximately 85 per cent of normal. Thus, for sustained periods of time very strong parasympathetic stimulation can reduce the cardiac output to about 15 per cent below the normal control level. However, the cardiac reserve becomes almost nonexistent, since the permissive level of cardiac output is greatly reduced, so that factors that normally increase the output would be unable to do so.

It will be recalled from the discussion earlier in this chapter that parasympathetic stimulation also affects the pumping ability of the heart by depressing cardiac contractility. However, under normal circumstances this effect is so small that it may be considered negligible, and only under conditions of very intense sympathetic stimulation does this depressing effect of the parasympathetic nerves become substantial.

It was also pointed out earlier in the chapter that the heart is normally under a considerable degree of parasympathetic tone. Removal of this tone by administering atropine to an animal or by cutting the vagus nerves has essentially the same effect on cardiac output as moderate sympathetic stimulation of the heart without simultaneous sympathetic stimulation of the peripheral vasculature. Therefore, we can refer back to Figure 18–2 to see the approximate effect one observes on abrogating parasympathetic tone to the heart—that is, only a very slight effect on cardiac output, in the order of 5 to 15 per cent. Indeed, we have cut the vagi a number of times while recording the cardiac output, and ordinarily this has hardly caused a measurable effect on the cardiac output except under unusual circulatory conditions.

EFFECT OF CENTRAL NERVOUS SYSTEM STIMULATION ON CARDIAC OUTPUT

Literally hundreds of research studies have reported the effects of central nervous system stimulation on arterial pressure, pulse rate, cardiac diameters, and other facets of circulatory function besides cardiac output (Kabat, 1935; Hoff, 1936; Pitts, 1941; Kaada, 1951; Wall, 1951; Uvnas, 1954, 1967; Hoff, 1963; Manning, 1965; Hilton, 1966; Smith, 1966a; Hockman, 1969; Gebber, 1969; Forsyth, 1970a,b; Chalmers and Wurtman, 1971; and many others), but few reports can be found regarding the effects of central nervous system stimulation on cardiac output. However, we know that stimulation of the cerebral cortex, the hypothalamus, or the diencephalic and medullary centers can mimic almost any type of sympathetic or parasympathetic stimulation, even to the extent of sometimes stopping the heart beat or at other times producing heart rates and arterial pressures equal to the maximum that can be achieved by maximal sympathetic stimulation. Therefore, it is reasonable to believe that different types of central nervous system stimulation can also cause both minimal and maximal autonomic effects on cardiac output, ranging from a decrease in cardiac output to as low as zero for short periods of time up to as high as 100 per cent above normal.

Rushmer and Smith (1959) found that stimulation in the fields of Forel in the diencephalic portion of the central nervous system can cause both cardiac and peripheral vascular changes that contribute significantly to an increase in cardiac output. Manning (1958) and Brucke (1951) have also localized a number of hypothalamic areas in which stimulation can cause essentially the same effects. More recently, Folkow and coworkers (1966, 1968) demonstrated that stimulation of the defense area of the hypothalamus caused an increase in cardiac output of approximately 100 per cent, this increase in output being due to an increase both in stroke volume and in heart rate. Furthermore, following stimulation of this hypothalamic region, there was a significant increase in central venous pressure, implying an increase in mean systemic pressure. These investigators also localized and stimulated the depressor area of the medulla, which resulted in a decrease of cardiac output to approximately 50 per cent of normal. Concomitant with the decrease in cardiac output there occurred a diminution in stroke volume, heart rate, and central venous pressure. The results of these studies show clearly that stimulation of certain areas of the central nervous system can produce cardiac and peripheral vascular effects identical to those obtained by direct stimulation of the autonomic nerves.

EFFECT OF AUTONOMIC REFLEXES ON CARDIAC OUTPUT

Thus far, we have considered the effects on cardiac output of direct stimulation of the sympathetic or the parasympathetic nervous system. However, these effects are of importance only insofar as the sympathetic and parasympathetic nervous systems can be activated during the normal course of bodily operation. Many discrete circulatory reflexes, activated during exercise and during other conditions that are stressful to the circulation, are especially important in increasing the cardiac output. The effects of a few of these will be discussed.

EFFECT OF THE PRESSORECEPTOR REFLEX ON CARDIAC OUTPUT

When one thinks of circulatory reflexes, he almost immediately thinks of the pressoreceptor reflex (also called the baroreceptor reflex) simply because this reflex has been studied far more than all the other cardiovascular reflexes put together. The primary pressoreceptors are the carotid sinus pressoreceptors, located in the walls of the internal carotid arteries slightly above the carotid bifurcation, and the aortic arch baroreceptors, located within the walls of the aortic arch. Stimulation of the pressoreceptors occurs by the stretching of the arterial wall consequent to the pressure within the arteries, and the pressoreceptor impulses are transmitted to the medulla of the brain by appropriate nerves; carotid pressoreceptor impulses are transmitted by the Hering nerve, a branch of the glossopharyngeal nerve, and aortic pressoreceptor impulses are transmitted through the vagus nerves. In general, the pressoreceptor impulses inhibit sympathetic stimulation of the entire circulatory system and enhance parasympathetic stimulation of the circulatory system.

It is universally recognized that the pressoreceptor reflex is primarily concerned with the regulation of arterial pressure and has relatively little effect on cardiac output. For instance, the results of many studies show that the average increase in cardiac output resulting from elicitation of a maximal carotid sinus reflex by a large reduction in arterial blood pressure is perhaps approximately 10 to 15 per cent, although the individual results are highly variable (Charlier, 1947a,b, 1948a,b; Vleeschhouwer, 1950; Kenney, 1951; Leusen, 1954, 1956a,b; Brind, 1956; Polosa, 1961; Groom, 1962; Corcondilas, 1964; Iriuchijima, 1968). We too have studied the effect of the carotid sinus reflex on cardiac output using a continuous cardiac output recorder and have found the same type of variability as that described in the literature. Our results have shown the reflex to increase cardiac output 10 to 35 per cent in some animals, as illustrated in Figure 18–5, and to reduce the output as much as 20 per cent in other animals. Also, we found that the response could be altered from a positive to a negative response in the same animal, a positive response usually occurring when the blood volume is normal or reduced as a result of hemorrhage, and a negative response occurring following a large infusion of fluid. The average results of our studies were approximately the same as that shown in the literature, cardiac output increasing approximately 10 to 15 per cent as a result of a maximal carotid sinus reflex.

The carotid sinus reflex, however, causes only about one-half the effect of the total pressoreceptor reflex, for it is elicited only by the carotid pressoreceptors and does not involve the aortic pressoreceptors. The results of a recent study by Allison (1969) demonstrate that maximal elicitation of the aortic pressoreceptor reflex by a reduction of blood pressure within the isolated aortic arch from approximately 100 to zero mm. Hg can cause an increase in cardiac output of approximately 5 per cent. Therefore, we can

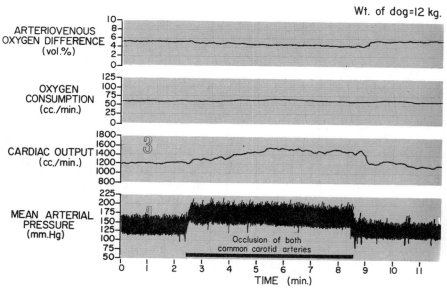

Figure 18–5. Continuous recording of cardiac output, arterial pressure, A-V oxygen difference, and rate of oxygen consumption during the elicitation of a maximal carotid sinus reflex by compression of both common carotid arteries. This was the greatest increase in cardiac output recorded in these studies. Note the slow and relatively slight rise in cardiac output. (Courtesy of Drs. T. Q. Richardson and J. Fermoso.)

estimate that the total pressoreceptor reflex could, on the average, increase the cardiac output about 20 per cent. This amounts to almost a negligible effect in comparison with the several hundred per cent increase that can result from a large transfusion of blood. Therefore, we can conclude that the pressoreceptor reflex has a very weak effect on cardiac output and it is too variable to be of significant value in cardiac output regulation.

If we refer back to Figure 18-4 and observe the long dashed curves of the analysis, we will see that the analysis predicts that the cardiac output should be increased by about 20 per cent by a maximal pressoreceptor reflex, which causes only moderate sympathetic stimulation.

EFFECT OF THE CENTRAL NERVOUS SYSTEM ISCHEMIC REFLEX AND ASPHYXIA ON CARDIAC OUTPUT

Studies in our laboratory on the central nervous system ischemic reflex caused by increasing the intracranial pressure (also called the Cushing reflex) have shown this reflex to cause four to six times as great a degree of sympathetic stimulation as does the carotid sinus reflex (Guyton, 1952b; Sagawa, 1961a). These differences have been estimated by determining the amount of epinephrine or norepinephrine required to mimic the response of each reflex. Invariably, the amount of epinephrine or norepinephrine required to mimic the effect of the central nervous system ischemic reflex has been four to six times as great as the amount needed to mimic a carotid sinus reflex. Another interesting observation is that the central nervous system ischemic reflex, when maximally elicited, will cause as great a sympathetic effect as will maximal infusion of norepinephrine (Richardson, 1964, 1965). For this reason, we have come to consider the central nervous system ischemic reflex to be either the, or one of the, most powerful physiological stimulators of the sympathetic nervous system in the body. Also, studies on the effects of asphyxia have indicated this to cause a degree of sympathetic stimulation similar to that caused by the ischemic reflex. For these reasons, it is important to know the effect of these extremely powerful autonomic reflexes on cardiac output.

Figure 18-6A illustrates the effect on cardiac output caused by an almost maximal central nervous system ischemic reflex, showing records of arteriovenous oxygen difference, rate of oxygen consumption, right atrial pressure, mean arterial pressure, and cerebrospinal fluid pressure. Note that the ischemic reflex does not cause the cardiac output to rise instantaneously but only after a delay of several minutes. This delay is caused at least partly by an initial but transient extreme slowing of the heart initiated by strong vagal impulses from the medulla. Yet once the steady state has been reached, the cardiac output uniformly reaches a level averaging 80 to 100 per cent above the control. Note especially that the change in cardiac output predicted by the analysis of Figure 18-4 was also to about 80 to 100 per cent above the control level. This increase in cardiac output caused by the central nervous system ischemic reflex has also been observed by Rodbard (1954) and especially by Richardson (1965) in a very complete study.

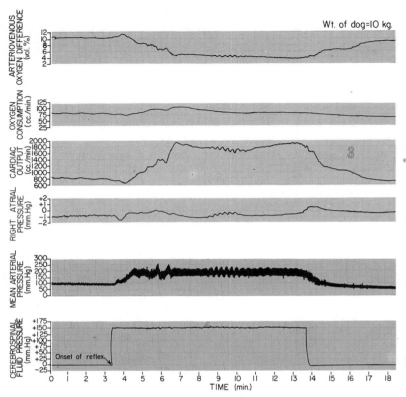

Figure 18–6A. Continuous recording of cardiac output and other parameters in a dog during almost maximal elicitation of the central nervous system ischemic reflex. [Richardson and Fermoso (1965).]

THE "ABDOMINAL COMPRESSION REACTION"

Another factor discovered by Youmans and his colleagues (Gilfoil, 1959) that is closely allied with the autonomic control of the circulation is the "abdominal compression reaction." Though this reaction has not yet been studied fully, it seems to affect the mean circulatory pressure in the following way: When the pressures in the thoracic vessels tend to fall too low, a reflex similar to the autonomic reflexes automatically causes the abdominal muscles to tighten. Since abdominal contraction can increase the mean circulatory pressure by as much as 100 per cent (Guyton, 1962b), this "abdominal compression reaction" might well prove to be one of the most important of all reflex controllers of cardiac output.

EFFECT OF NEGATIVE REFLEXES

The pressoreceptor reflex can act in a negative manner as well as in a positive manner. That is, a rise in systemic arterial pressure can cause loss

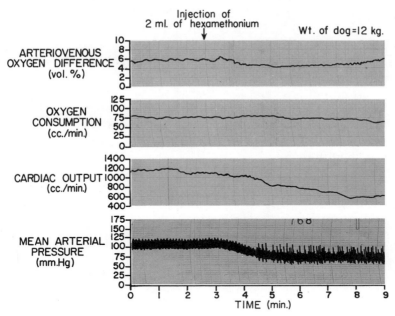

Figure 18–6B. Effect on cardiac output and other parameters of administering an autonomic paralyzing dose of hexamethonium to a dog. (Courtesy of Drs. T. Q. Richardson and J. Fermoso.)

of vasomotor tone and a decrease in cardiac output. It is possible too that other reflexes exist—such as those initiated by receptors in the heart, pulmonary circulation, and great veins—that can cause negative reflexes. Still another type of negative reflex at times possibly results from pain, causing a loss of vasomotor tone and perhaps a decrease in cardiac output.

The actual extent to which a negative pressoreceptor response can decrease cardiac output is uncertain. However, it has been shown in dogs that a negative aortic pressoreceptor response caused by increasing the pressure in the isolated aortic arch to approximately 300 mm. Hg causes a reduction in cardiac output of approximately 10 to 15 per cent (Allison, 1969). An in humans, it has been shown that direct electrical stimulation of the sinus pressoreceptors causes a reduction in cardiac output of about 10 per cent (Epstein, 1969). If we consider the effects of aortic arch and carotid sinus pressoreceptors to be additive, we see that the simultaneous stimulation of both pressoreceptor mechanisms would perhaps cause a reduction in cardiac output of approximately 20 per cent.

The negative pressoreceptor reflex is not a very strong negative reflex, but we can assume that there are at least some reflexes that can completely abrogate all sympathetic tone to the circulatory system. We must then attempt to assess the extent to which cardiac output would be reduced under these conditions. According to the analysis presented in Figure 18–4, the cardiac output should decrease to an average of 50 to 60 per cent of normal. Figure 18–6B shows an actual record in a dog of abrogating all autonomic activity by infusing a dose of hexamethonium, a dose far greater than that normally given to patients. It can be seen that the cardiac output does indeed decrease to approximately the level predicted by the analysis given earlier in the chapter. We have also observed such a reduction in cardiac output when total spinal anesthesia is instituted.

To round out our numbers, we can say that complete loss of sympathetic activity probably reduces the cardiac output to about one-half normal, while maximal sympathetic activity increases the output to about two times normal. Thus, the total range of sympathetic control of cardiac output is about four fold.

Chapter 19

EFFECT OF TISSUE OXYGEN NEED ON CARDIAC OUTPUT

One of the most important features of cardiac output regulation is that the output almost exactly parallels the level of metabolism in the animal. For instance, if the metabolic level is low, the cardiac output will also be low, and if the metabolic level is high, the cardiac output likewise will be high.

In the past several years, a host of investigations have been performed in an attempt to explain this intimate relationship between metabolism and cardiac output and, more specifically, to determine the precise nature of the controlling mechanism which regulates cardiac output at a level that almost exactly meets the metabolic requirements of the body. On the basis of these studies, it has now become widely recognized that the single factor most responsible for the significant linkage between metabolic rate and cardiac output is the tissue need for oxygen (Douglas, 1922; Grollman, 1930b; Chiodi, 1941; Keys, 1943; Ershler, 1943; Whitehorn, 1946; Feldman, 1948; Nahas, 1952; Hurlimann, 1953; Gorlin, 1954; Cross, 1958, 1959; Huckabee, 1960; Chidsey, 1961; Jones and Berne, 1964b, 1965; Bergofsky, 1966; Whalen, 1967; Duling, 1970; Bachofen, 1971b; Costin, 1970; and many others).

In our laboratories we have also studied the relationship between tissue oxygen demand and cardiac output. Our studies have dealt both with the effect of oxygen lack on local tissue vasodilatation (Crawford, 1959; Ross, 1962; Carrier, 1964, 1966; Guyton, 1964; Fairchild, 1966; Walker and Guyton, 1967) and with the effect of whole body oxygen need on the cardiac output (Öberg, 1961; Granger and Guyton, 1969; Banet and Guyton, 1971; Guyton, 1971). The purpose of this chapter, therefore, will be to discuss the effect of oxygen need on both local blood flow and total cardiac output. A final purpose of this chapter will be to discuss some of the possible mechanisms by which the oxygen need of the tissues can regulate the rate of blood flow to these tissues.

323

EFFECT OF METABOLISM AND TISSUE OXYGEN INSUFFICIENCY ON LOCAL BLOOD FLOW

LOCAL EFFECT OF METABOLISM ON BLOOD FLOW

Almost from the earliest measurements of blood flow, it has been known that the rate of flow through any tissue of the body, with very few exceptions, increases in proportion to the metabolism of the tissue. For instance, blood flow through a single skeletal muscle is increased when the muscle is stimulated either electrically (Stainsby, 1962, 1964a, 1964b) or during normal muscular exercise (Barcroft, 1953), the flow often rising as high as 15 times the normal rate during the intervals between contraction. Simultaneously, large quantities of nutrients, especially oxygen, are removed from the blood.

Figure 19-1 illustrates the effect of increased muscle activity on local blood flow (Barcroft, 1953), showing the high degree of dependence of blood flow on the degree of tissue activity. Furthermore, experiments in which the sympathetic nerves to the muscles have been blocked completely still show this increase in blood flow during muscular activity. Note especially that the blood flow rises to 15 times the control value during the periods of relaxation between contractions.

Results similar to those shown in Figure 19-1 have been observed in all

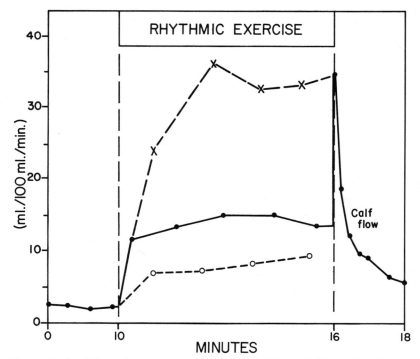

Figure 19-1. Effect of exercise on blood flow in the calf, illustrating the extreme dependence of blood flow on the degree of tissue activity. Dots = mean rate of flow; crosses = flow during a few seconds relaxation; circles = flow during sustained contraction. [Redrawn from Barcroft and Swann (1953).]

the following different conditions: (1) Blood flow through essentially all tissues of the body increases when the overall metabolic rate is increased in thyrotoxicosis (Lequime, 1940; Charlier, 1946; Stead, 1950), or following dinitrophenol poisoning (Stainsby, 1962). (2) Blood flow is increased in any local tissue that is heated (Kunkel, 1939; Barcroft, 1943). (3) Blood flow increases markedly in glands that are actively secreting. (4) Blood flow increases in areas of the brain that are highly activated (Schmidt, 1950). (5) Coronary blood flow decreases when the metabolic activity of the heart is reduced by fibrillation (Berne, 1964a, 1964b).

In addition to *changes* in blood flow induced by altering the rate of metabolism, one also finds even during normal metabolism that blood flow in the more active tissues of the body is far greater than that in the less active tissues. For instance, there is little blood flow in fibrous tissue, while that in the brain, the thyroid gland, the adrenal gland, and the liver is always very great. In other words, blood flow is proportional among the tissues approximately in accord with their metabolic needs. In this way, an adequate supply of nutrients is assured to each of the tissues for the job that it is to perform. (The skin and kidneys are two major exceptions to this general rule. These two tissues perform special functions that require excessive flow, the first a temperature controlling function and the second a blood clearing function.)

LOCAL EFFECT OF OXYGEN AND OXYGEN INSUFFICIENCY ON BLOOD FLOW

In an attempt to explain the high degree of correlation between local metabolism and local blood flow, the effects of many different metabolic factors on local blood flow have been studied. Some of these metabolic factors are changes in blood oxygen concentration (Gregg, 1940; Bing, 1949; Foltz, 1950; Katz, 1955, 1958; Berglund, 1957; Braunwald, 1958; Feinberg, 1958; Crawford, 1959; Yonce, 1959; Ross, 1962; Bergofsky, 1966; Daugherty, 1967a, 1967b; Walker, 1967; Costin, 1970), changes in carbon dioxide concentration (Crawford, 1959; Kontos, 1967, 1968, 1971; Whelan, 1967; Haddy, 1968), many types of protein derivatives (Anrep, 1935, 1944; Barsoum, 1936; Patterson, 1955; Webster, 1967), changes in potassium concentration (Driscol, 1957; Kjellmer, 1961; Bevan, 1963; Skinner, 1967a, 1970; Scott, 1970), changes in osmolality (Skinner, 1970; Overbeck, 1970; Gazitua, 1971), and breakdown products of adenine nucleotides (Berne, 1963; Imai, 1964; Richman, 1964; Katori, 1966; Rubio, 1969a, 1969b; Forrester, 1969; Olsson, 1970; Dobson, 1971). On the basis of these and many other studies, it has become widely accepted that the high degree of correlation between local metabolism and local blood flow in some way involves the balance between oxygen delivery to the tissues by the blood and the local tissue need for oxygen.

At present, there is much disagreement regarding the precise mechanism by which the tissue need for oxygen regulates the blood flow to the tissues, although almost everyone agrees that the tissue demand for oxygen is indeed involved in this regulation [an exception to this occurs in the brain, where carbon dioxide is just as potent a regulator of flow (Schmidt, 1950; Yoshida, 1966; Severinghaus, 1967; Shapiro, 1966a, 1966b; Raper, 1971; Sundt, 1971)]. Therefore, in the following few paragraphs the circulatory response to various conditions that disrupt the normal balance between oxygen delivery and tissue oxygen demand will be discussed. These conditions include changes in arterial oxygen saturation, brief periods of complete occlusion of blood flow to a local tissue, and variations of perfusion pressure to local tissues.

Response of Local Blood Flow to Changes in Arterial Oxygen Saturation

Figure 19–2 illustrates the response of local blood flow in the hindleg of a dog to changes in arterial oxygen saturation (Crawford, 1959). At the beginning of this experiment, the oxygen saturation of the arterial blood entering the leg was 97 per cent; the concentration then was suddenly changed to 30 per cent. Within the next minute or two, the blood flow rose from 80 ml./min. to 163 ml./min. Furthermore, the response began immediately upon entry of the desaturated blood into the vascular tree, thus demonstrating an immediate vasodilator response caused by oxygen deficiency. The half-time of the response was approximately 20 to 30 seconds, and the response was almost complete within 2 minutes.

Figure 19–2 also demonstrates an immediate return of blood flow to the control level when the arterial blood saturation was suddenly changed back to 97 per cent. Again, the half-time of the response was 20 to 30 seconds.

Figure 19–3 illustrates the progressive effect on blood flow in the dog's

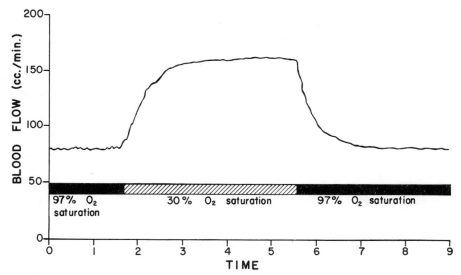

Figure 19–2. Effect of acute changes in arterial oxygen saturation on arterial blood flow to the hind limb of a dog. Note especially the rapidity of the reaction.

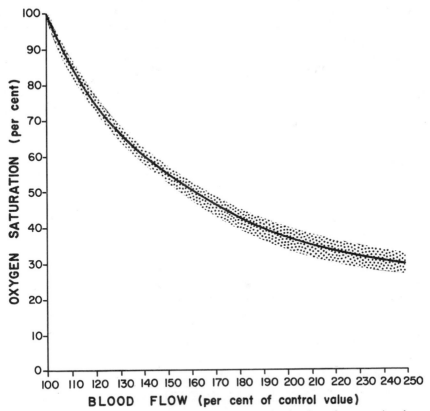

Figure 19-3. Effect on blood flow in the hind limb of a dog of progressive decrease in arterial oxygen saturation (average results from 10 dogs; the shaded area represents probable errors of the means). [Reprinted from Crawford, Fairchild, and Guyton (1959).]

hindleg of gradually decreasing the arterial oxygen saturation (Crawford, 1959), showing that as the oxygen saturation fell from 100 per cent down to 30 per cent the blood flow progressively increased to 250 per cent of normal, thus illustrating that the greater the degree of oxygen insufficiency, the greater the blood flow becomes.

Importance of Oxygen Regulation of Local Blood Flow

Obviously, when the arterial oxygen saturation falls, the increase in blood flow helps to compensate for the decreased transport of oxygen to the tissues. As a result, the total amount of oxygen transported to the tissues falls much less than the oxygen saturation. To determine the total inflow of oxygen to the tissues, one can simply multiply the oxygen saturation of the arterial blood times the blood flow to the tissues.

Figure 19-4 presents findings from ten experiments, showing the effect on rate of oxygen inflow to the hindleg of the dog caused by decreas-

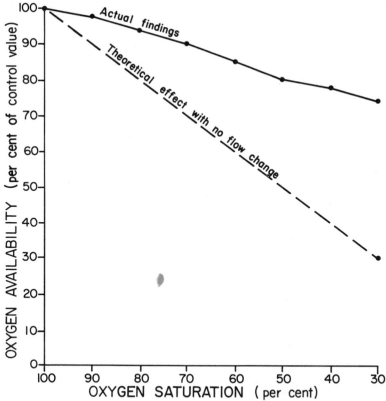

Figure 19-4. Effect of progressive decrease in arterial oxygen saturation on oxygen transport to the hind limb of a dog. The dashed curve shows the theoretical effect if no increase in flow had occurred. The solid curve shows the actual findings, illustrating approximately 65 per cent compensation (average results from 10 dogs). [Reprinted from Crawford, Fairchild, and Guyton (1959).]

ing the arterial oxygen saturation. The dashed curve shows the theoretical effect on oxygen inflow had there been no increase in flow with decreasing oxygen saturation. The solid curve, on the other hand, shows the actual findings, illustrating that the percentage decrease in oxygen inflow, on the average, was approximately one-third the percentage decrease in oxygen saturation. This experiment illustrates that the immediate increase in blood flow in response to oxygen lack helps the tissues to maintain an adequate oxygen supply even in the face of decreased arterial oxygen saturation.

"LOOP GAIN" OF THE OXYGEN REGULATORY SYSTEM. The "loop gain" of a feedback regulatory system is a measure of its effectiveness as a regulator; gain is equal to the ratio of the compensatory effect resulting from the feedback system to the remaining displacement of the controlled factor from the desired control level. To describe this in relation to Figure 19-4, we see that, when the oxygen saturation was 30 per cent, the oxygen inflow to the hindlimb would also have been 30 per cent of normal *had there been no blood flow change*. However, after the blood flow increase, the oxygen inflow to the hindlimb was 75 per cent of normal. The degree of compensation, therefore, was 75 minus 30, or 45 per cent. On the other hand, the displacement of the oxygen inflow even after compensation was still 22 per cent below normal (97–75), and the ratio of 45 to 22 is 2.0.

A more recent study by Walker and Guyton (1967) provided results very similar to those seen in the study of Crawford (1959). In this latter study, the gain of the oxygen regulatory system was approximately 2.5 when the arterial oxygen saturation was reduced to 30 to 35 per cent. However, when the arterial oxygen saturation was reduced only to approximately 45 per cent, the gain of the regulatory system was approximately 3.5, and at arterial oxygen saturations between 45 per cent and the normal arterial oxygen saturation, the gain of this regulatory system was even higher, the compensatory effect being nearly 100 per cent in some cases. Thus, we can see that the gain of the oxygen regulatory system is actually very high for one of the control systems of the body. For instance, the well-known carotid sinus control system usually has a gain of less than 2 (Scher, 1962). The analysis of loop gain provided above emphasizes the significance of the local oxygen need mechanism for regulating local blood flow.

Response of Local Blood Flow Following Brief Periods of Occlusion

When the blood flow to a local tissue such as the hindlimb is occluded for 30 seconds to 10 minutes and the occlusion is suddenly removed, the blood flow increases immediately to exceedingly high levels and then gradually returns to normal. This response is termed *reactive hyperemia* and has been observed in most tissues, especially in skeletal muscle (Wood, 1955; Patterson, 1955, 1956; Blair, 1959; Crawford, 1959; Hyman, 1963; Coffman, 1963; Fairchild, 1966), cardiac muscle (Coffman, 1960; Gregg, 1963; Rubio, 1969a, 1969b; Jones, 1970), and skin (Lewis, 1924; Di Palma, 1942; Jepson, 1954). When the occlusion lasts for more than approximately one minute, the blood flow often rises to approximately 4 to 5 times normal before it begins to return to normal. Therefore, it is obvious that during the period of occlusion, something takes place in the peripheral vasculature to cause a marked vasodilatation. It is not difficult to see that the vasodilatation which occurs during a hyperemic response could result from the same mechanism that causes vasodilatation during increased metabolic activity. That is, during the period of occlusion the balance between oxygen delivery and oxygen demand by the local tissues is obviously disrupted. In some manner, this causes vasodilatation in the tissues in an effort to increase the local blood flow and, consequently, the oxygen delivery to the tissues.

The results of several studies suggest an involvement of oxygen in the reactive hyperemic response. For instance, in a study by Fairchild, Ross, and Guyton (1966), reactive hyperemia was caused in the hindlimb of dogs by occluding arterial inflow for three to ten minutes. In some experiments, a normal reactive hyperemic response was obtained. In others, on release of the occlusion the limbs were perfused with blood that had had all of its oxygen removed. Figure 19–5 shows the results of this procedure. Graph A shows a normal hyperemic response following a ten minute occlusion; in

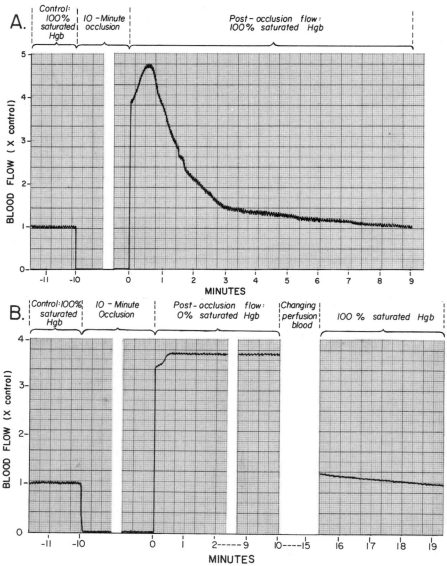

Figure 19-5. A, Typical reactive hyperemia response in a perfused hindlimb of a dog when the limb was perfused with 100 per cent oxygen-saturated blood, both before and after the period of occlusion. B, Record of blood flow showing (a) a control period—perfusion with 100 per cent oxygen-saturated blood, (b) a 10 minute period of occlusion, (c) a period of hyperemia following release of the occlusion—perfusion with 0 per cent oxygen-saturated blood, and (d) a period of recovery from the hyperemia—perfused again with 100 per cent oxygen-saturated blood. (From Fairchild, 1966.)

this experiment, the hindlimb was perfused with 100 per cent saturated blood following the release of the occlusion. Note particularly that following release of the occlusion, blood flow rises abruptly to approximately five times normal but begins to return toward normal in approximately one minute. Graph B shows a hyperemic response obtained when the limb was perfused with deoxygenated blood following release of the occlusion. Note that following the initial rise in blood flow, blood flow does not begin to fall back toward normal as long as the limb is perfused with deoxygenated blood. However, when the limb is once again perfused with 100 per cent saturated blood, the blood flow begins to return to its normal level. Thus, these experiments illustrate that oxygen is necessary for the blood vessels of the hindlimb to constrict back toward normal during the hyperemic response, and that oxygen lack causes the vessels to remain dilated.

The effectiveness of the oxygen system for regulating local blood flow may be estimated from the reactive hyperemic response. To do this, the excess quantity of blood delivered to the local tissue immediately following release of the occlusion is compared to the flow debt produced during the period of the occlusion. To illustrate this point, the normal hyperemic response shown in Figure 19–5 has been redrawn in Figure 19–6. The area marked D indicates the actual flow debt produced during the ten minute occlusion, and the area marked R indicates the hyperemic flow above the normal level following release of the occlusion. Thus, the area R is the repayment flow. It may be calculated that area R is approximately 70 per cent of area D, which means that the flow debt produced during the period of occlusion is approximately 70 per cent repaid immediately following the release of the occlusion.

The ten minute period of occlusion used in the study of Fairchild is a relatively long period of occlusion, and much higher gains may be observed when shorter periods of occlusion are used. For instance, Coffman (1963) reported that reactive hyperemia in skeletal muscle completely repaid the flow debt produced by a 30 second occlusion. This was true whether the muscle was resting or was contracting very strongly.

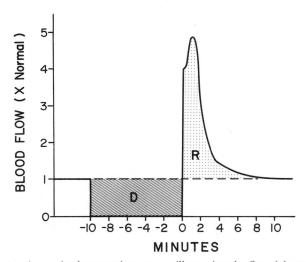

Figure 19–6. A reactive hyperemic response illustrating the flow debt produced during occlusion of hindlimb blood flow (area D) and the repayment flow following release of the occlusion (area R). In this example, R is 70 per cent of D, indicating a 70 per cent repayment of the flow debt.

Response of Local Blood Flow to Variations in Perfusion Pressure

Nearly all tissues display an intrinsic ability to maintain a constant blood flow despite changes in the pressure tending to force blood through that tissue. Such an ability to maintain a constant blood flow is termed *autoregulation.* The earliest experiments that suggested an autoregulatory type of behavior were probably those of Bayliss (1902), who observed this phenomenon in the hindlimbs of cats and dogs when the arterial pressure was either increased or decreased. Since the earlier experiments of Bayliss, autoregulation has been observed in the kidney (Rein, 1931; Selkurt, 1946; Haynes, 1953; Navar, 1970a, 1970b), skeletal muscle (Folkow, 1949, 1964; Jones and Berne, 1964b, 1965; Stainsby, 1964a, 1964b), brain (Fog, 1937; Lassen, 1959; Sokoloff, 1960; Rapela, 1964; Yoshida, 1966), intestine (Johnson, 1960, 1964; Hinshaw, 1962), myocardium (Eckel, 1949; Osher, 1951; Berne, 1959, 1964a, 1964b), and liver (Torrance, 1958; Brauer, 1964).

Figure 19–7 shows the phenomenon of autoregulation in the isolated hindlimb of a dog as recorded in our laboratories. This figure shows autoregulation in the hindlimb both when the perfusion pressure is increased abruptly and when the perfusion pressure is reduced abruptly. The perfusion pressure, the difference between arterial and venous pressure, is denoted by the long dashed line marked P, and the hindlimb blood flow is denoted by the solid curve marked F. Note that when the perfusion pressure is suddenly increased from 100 to 140 mm. Hg, the blood flow rises rapidly to approximately three times normal but returns within approximately 40 seconds to a steady state flow only slightly above normal. The tremendous increase in flow is due both to the increase in perfusion pressure and to a decrease in vascular resistance caused by passive distention of the vessels. Note that the flow returns to a level only approximately 10 per cent above normal despite the fact that perfusion pressure is sustained at a level 40 per cent above normal. Just the opposite occurs when perfusion pressure is abruptly reduced, as can be seen on the right hand side of Figure 19–7. When the perfusion pressure is reduced from 100 to 60 mm. Hg, blood flow almost completely ceases initially, but then rises to a steady state level only slightly below normal despite the fact that perfusion pressure remains greatly reduced.

Again, it is not difficult to understand that the phenomenon of autoregulation could be due to the same mechanism that regulates flow during either increased or decreased metabolic activity. Thus, a decrease in perfusion pressure would tend to cause a proportional decrease in local blood flow and, consequently, in oxygen delivery to the tissues. In some way, this causes vasodilatation, which returns blood flow toward its normal level. Inversely, when perfusion pressure is suddenly increased, there is a tendency toward a proportional increase in oxygen delivery to the local tissues. However, the vessels rapidly constrict, which reduces blood flow and oxygen delivery back toward the normal level.

The effectiveness of autoregulation in maintaining a normal blood flow despite variations in perfusion pressure is illustrated in Figure 19–8. This

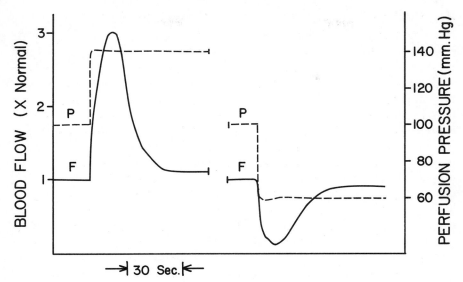

Figure 19–7. Autoregulation in the hindlimb when the perfusion pressure is increased and decreased. Hindlimb blood flow is represented by the solid curve marked F, and perfusion pressure is indicated by the dashed curve marked P. Note the rapidity of autoregulation when the perfusion pressure is either increased or decreased.

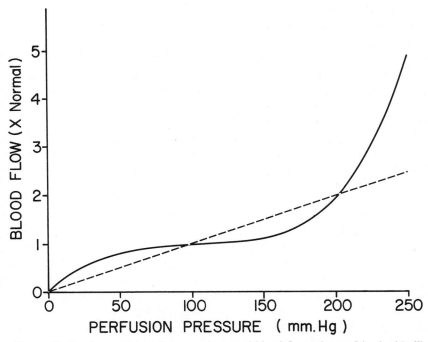

Figure 19–8. A comparison between the actual blood flows observed in the hindlimb at various perfusion pressures (solid curve) with the theoretical flows predicted if the hindlimb vasculature were a system of passive nondistensible tubes (dashed line). Note that within the physiological range of perfusion pressure, autoregulation largely compensates for changes in perfusion pressure. [Redrawn from Walker and Guyton (1967).]

figure shows the steady state flows observed in the hindlimb of the dog when perfusion pressure was varied over a wide range. The actual steady state flows observed are denoted by the solid curve, while the dashed line represents the theoretical flows that would have been observed in a passive, nondistensible tube. Thus, the effectiveness of the hindlimb vasculature as a regulator of blood flow when the perfusion pressure is changed may be derived from the difference between the theoretical blood flows represented by the dashed line and the actual flows represented by the solid curve. Note that within the perfusion pressure range of approximately 60 to 150 mm. Hg, the autoregulation mechanism maintains blood flow within approximately 10 per cent of normal, even though theoretical change in flow is as much as 50 per cent. Thus, within the normal physiological range of perfusion pressures, the gain of the autoregulation mechanism was approximately 3 to 4, which is actually a very high gain for a physiological control system. However, at perfusion pressures either below approximately 60 mm. Hg or above approximately 150 mm. Hg, the gain of the autoregulation mechanism becomes reduced. This is caused by the fact that at either very low or very high perfusion pressures, the vasculature of the hindlimb becomes either maximally dilated or maximally constricted. Thus, at extremely low and extremely high perfusion pressures, the vasculature behaves as a system of passive, distensible tubes.

POSSIBLE MECHANISMS BY WHICH TISSUE OXYGEN DEMAND REGULATES LOCAL BLOOD FLOW

It has been pointed out in the preceding paragraphs that nearly all tissues have an intrinsic ability to regulate the local blood flow and that this local regulation of flow is intimately related to the local tissue demand for oxygen. In recent years, many investigators have carried out an intense search for the precise mechanism by which the local oxygen need regulates local blood flow. From this search, a number of opinions have emerged, but nearly all of these belong to one of two more general concepts. The first of these general concepts is that tissue oxygen insufficiency causes the release of a metabolic vasodilator substance from the tissues. This vasodilator substance then supposedly causes local vasodilatation and a consequent increase in local blood flow. The second concept states that there is no necessity for predicting the release of an intermediate vasodilator substance, since oxygen, or oxygen insufficiency, has a direct effect on the vascular smooth muscle of the local tissues. Thus, according to this theory, any time local blood flow is insufficient to meet the requirements of the local tissue, the oxygen tension within the tissue begins to fall, and the reduced oxygen tension within the vascular smooth muscle causes relaxation of the muscle and, consequently, vasodilatation.

Because of the extreme difficulty in distinguishing between the direct effect of oxygen on vascular smooth muscle and the indirect effect of oxygen lack in causing the release of local metabolic vasodilators, it cannot be stated with any degree of certainty which of these two concepts is the correct one. On the basis of numerous studies, it is even feasible to predict that both mechanisms are effective in controlling local blood flow. Some of the more important studies supporting these concepts will be reviewed below.

The Vasodilator Concept

As was pointed out earlier, the possible involvement of a number of metabolic vasodilators in the regulation of local blood flow has been investigated, but in recent years only three of these have received much attention. These are potassium, local osmolality, and adenosine, a breakdown product of tissue adenosine triphosphate.

POTASSIUM. A number of studies have shown that the potassium ion causes relaxation of the vascular smooth muscle and vasodilatation (Dawes, 1941; Emanuel, 1959; Kjellmer, 1960, 1961, 1965; Overbeck, 1961; Lowe and Thompson, 1962; Glover, 1963; Scott, 1965, 1970; Skinner and Costin, 1970, 1971). Furthermore, an almost equal number of investigations have demonstrated that potassium is released from skeletal muscles during exercise (Kjellmer, 1960, 1961, 1964; Kilburn, 1966; Laurell and Pernow, 1966; Skinner and Powell, 1967a,b). The results of these studies have prompted the idea that potassium released from the local tissues, especially skeletal muscle, may be a factor responsible for the regulation of local blood flow during conditions of increased metabolic activity, or during other conditions which disrupt the balance between oxygen delivery and tissue oxygen demand.

Upon examination of these results, one sees that it is highly improbable that the potassium mechanism is the sole mechanism regulating local blood flow. For instance, Skinner and Powell (1967a) demonstrated that a 300 to 400 per cent increase in the potassium concentration of the blood perfusing an isolated skeletal muscle produced, at most, a 30 per cent reduction in vascular resistance. This potassium-induced reduction in vascular resistance is comparatively small in view of the tremendous decrease in vascular resistance which occurs during maximal exercise. Indeed, during maximal muscular exercise, the vascular resistance of skeletal muscle is reduced to approximately 10 to 20 per cent of normal.

Another factor which leads one to question the importance of potassium in local blood flow regulation is that during moderate muscular exercise, the concentration of potassium in the venous blood draining the muscles rises only moderately when compared to the tremendous concentrations of potassium used by Skinner and Powell, as well as others, to elicit vasodilatation in skeletal muscle. For instance, increases in venous blood potassium concentrations of as little as 10 to 15 per cent and, at most, 75 to 100 per cent have been measured during moderate to severe muscular exercise. In this regard, Scott (1970) infused potassium into isolated skeletal muscles of dogs at a rate which raised the venous potassium concentration by 1.2 mEq. per liter. This caused a reduction in vascular resistance of the skeletal muscle to 91 per cent of the control level. In the same animals, exercise raised the potassium concentration 1.6 mEq. per liter but caused a five times greater reduction in vascular resistance. It is also significant that the same investigators failed to find any significant rise in the potassium concentration of venous blood draining the isolated muscle during reactive hyperemia.

In summary, it may be stated that no definite conclusions regarding the potassium vasodilator mechanism may be reached. Such a mechanism almost certainly exists, but its significance is still highly questionable.

OSMOLALITY. The belief that increased osmolality may play a role in the regulation of blood flow in contracting skeletal muscle stems from the finding that the venous blood draining skeletal muscles is increased during muscular contraction, and that an increase in local osmolality causes dilatation of the local vascular bed (Marshall and Shepherd, 1959; Mellander, 1967; Gray, 1968; Lundvall, 1969; Overbeck, 1970; Skinner and Costin, 1970; Gazitua, 1971). The increase in regional osmolality observed during skeletal muscle contraction is caused by the release of hydrogen, potassium, and magnesium ions as well as certain organic compounds from the muscles, and release of these substances is most likely due to the relative oxygen insufficiency in the active tissues.

Mellander (1967) observed that moderate stimulation of an isolated skeletal muscle resulted in an increase in venous osmolality of approximately 1 to 10 per cent and that the magnitude of this increase in osmolality was directly related to the magnitude of the reduction in skeletal muscle vascular resistance. He also observed that when similar increases in venous osmolality were produced by infusion of hypertonic solutions into the skeletal muscle, the resultant decrease in vascular resistance was approximately 60 to 80 per cent as great as that observed during stimulation of the muscle. These results indicate that an increase in regional osmolality could account for a large portion of the vasodilatation which occurs during exercise. However, the concept of an osmolality mechanism for regulating local blood flow has been largely discredited by the recent study by Scott (1970), who demonstrated that the increase in venous osmolality during skeletal muscle contraction is only transient. That is, when an isolated skeletal muscle was stimulated for several minutes, venous osmolality initially increased but gradually returned to the control level, even though the stimulation of the skeletal muscle and a tremendous increase in skeletal muscle blood flow were sustained.

ADENOSINE. The adenosine vasodilator theory, which has been promoted primarily by Berne and coworkers (Berne, 1963, 1964a, 1964b; Katori and Berne, 1966; Imai, 1964; Rubio, 1969a, 1969b; Dobson, 1971), is the following: Any condition which disturbs the balance between oxygen delivery to the tissues and the tissue oxygen demand causes the tissue to become hypoxic, and the oxygen insufficiency of the tissues retards the intracellular process of oxidative phosphorylation. A normal rate of oxidative phosphorylation is necessary for the reutilization of adenosine triphosphate breakdown products by the cell, and when the process is retarded, these breakdown products begin to accumulate within the cell. One of these breakdown products, adenosine, can pass very easily through the cell membrane, so that during periods of hypoxia, relatively large quantities of adenosine pass into the interstitial spaces. Adenosine is a very potent vasodilator, and when the concentration of adenosine increases in the interstitial fluid, this causes an intense vasodilatation of the local vasculature. Oxygen delivery to the local tissue then increases until the rate of oxidative phosphorlyation within the tissue is increased to the level required by the metabolic activity of the tissue.

Adenosine has been proposed primarily as the physiological regulator of coronary blood flow, although recent evidence suggests that it may also be effective in regulating skeletal muscle blood flow. Evidence which supports the belief that adenosine is a regulator of coronary blood flow includes the following: (1) The myocardial concentration of adenosine triphosphate decreases during hypoxia (LePage, 1946; Danforth, 1960; Benson, 1961; Berne, 1963; Gerlach and Deuticke, 1963; Imai, 1964; Richman and Wyborny, 1964; Braasch, 1968; Olsson, 1970). These findings demonstrate that the process of oxidative phosphorylation is, indeed, retarded by hypoxia. (2) Concomitant with a decrease in the concentration of myocardial adenosine triphosphate during hypoxia, the concentrations of adenosine within the myocardial tissue and in the coronary venous effluent increases (Richman and Wyborny, 1964; Katori, 1966; Rubio, 1969a). In addition, the quantities of adenosine released from the heart are roughly proportional to the degree of cardiac hypoxia (Katori and Berne, 1966). (3) The concentration of adenosine in the myocardial tissue after 30 to 60 seconds of coronary occlusion is sufficient to account for the increase in coronary blood flow observed during the ensuing period of reactive hyperemia (Rubio, 1969a). (4) Even in the normal fully oxygenated myocardium, adenosine is continually released into the interstitial spaces at a relatively slow rate (Rubio, 1969b). This means that the adenosine vasodilator mechanism would be capable of decreasing coronary blood flow as well as increasing it. That is, during conditions of myocardial overoxygenation, the release of adenosine by the myocardial cells could be reduced to subnormal levels, which would result in an increase in myocardial vascular resistance and a decrease in coronary blood flow.

It is apparent that the adenosine vasodilator theory can explain the regulation of coronary blood flow. There is, however, one factor which makes its importance questionable. This is that during prolonged periods of myocardial hypoxia, the myocardial concentration of adenosine triphosphate may be reduced to extremely low levels, which implies that the potential source for adenosine is not unlimited. Thus, it is possible, though not proved, that during such prolonged periods of hypoxia, other mechanisms must operate to maintain increased myocardial blood flow.

The role of adenosine in the regulation of skeletal muscle blood flow is far more uncertain. It is known that the process of oxidative phosphorylation is also retarded in skeletal muscle during hypoxia and that the skeletal muscle levels of adenosine triphosphate are, consequently, reduced. However, because cardiac muscle and skeletal muscle possess somewhat different metabolic pathways, it is not certain that large quantities of adenosine are released from skeletal muscle as a result of the adenosine triphosphate degradation. Nevertheless, Dobson (1971) was recently successful in detecting significantly increased quantities of adenosine in the venous effluent of the isolated dog hindlimb following a moderate period of ischemia. This finding indicates that adenosine may play a greater role than previously believed in the regulation of skeletal muscle blood flow. However, much more work needs to be done to elucidate further its importance here as well as in cardiac muscle.

The Direct Oxygen Theory

In the past ten years, several investigators, from our own as well as other laboratories, have proposed that oxygen and oxygen lack have a direct effect on vascular smooth muscle and that this action of oxygen is an important factor in the regulation of local blood flow. The experimental evidence which supports this proposal is the following:

It has been shown in several investigations that the contractile strength of vascular smooth muscle decreases when its oxygen tension is reduced and increases when its oxygen tension is raised (Kovalcik, 1963; Carrier, 1964, 1966; Lundholm and Mohme-Lundholm, 1965; Smith and Vane, 1966; Detar and Bohr, 1968). Figure 19–9 shows results from the study of Carrier (1964), who perfused isolated arterial segments, one-half to one millimeter in diameter, with blood having various oxygen tensions. Note that when the oxygen tension was reduced to less than 100 mm. Hg, the isolated vessel segment began to dilate, and the vascular conductance consequently increased. Indeed, when the oxygen tension was reduced to 30 mm. Hg, the vascular conductance increased to approximately two and one-half times normal. Carrier also observed that the vasodilatory response to hypoxia was greater in small vessels than in larger vessels, and it may, therefore, be predicted that in vessels smaller than one-half millimeter in diameter, the conductance may be increased to an even greater degree during hypoxia.

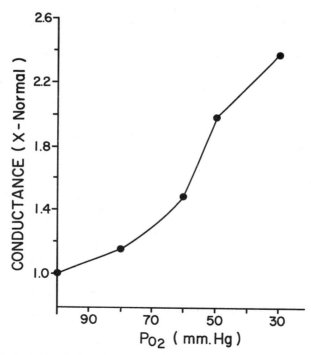

Figure 19–9. The relationship between vascular conductance and oxygen tension in small isolated arterial segments. [Redrawn from Carrier, Walker, and Guyton (1964).]

Results similar to those of Carrier have been observed in the smooth muscle of isolated aortic strips (Smith and Vane, 1966b; Detar and Bohr, 1968). Detar studied the contractile response of isolated aortic strips to epinephrine when the oxygen tension of the bathing medium was varied between 100 and zero mm. Hg. He observed that the contractile strength of the muscle was directly proportional to the oxygen tension, falling to nearly zero when the oxygen tension of the bathing fluid was zero.

Observations on the microcirculation are consistent with the results of the above studies on the vascular muscle of large and small arteries. Duling (1970) has microscopically observed changes in the diameter of arterioles in the hamster cheek pouch when the Po_2 of the arteriolar wall, as determined with an oxygen electrode, was either increased or decreased. Thus, the diameter of the arterioles increased when the Po_2 was reduced and decreased when the Po_2 was increased. Dollery (1968) made similar observations on the arterioles of the human retina. Since these studies were not performed in the isolated vasculature, the results cannot exclude the possibility that vasodilators released by the surrounding tissues during the hypoxia were responsible for the arteriolar vasodilatation. However, the results are consistent with the concept that oxygen directly affects the smooth muscle of the vascular wall.

On the basis of studies such as the ones cited above, it is almost certain that the contractile force of arteriolar smooth muscle is directly related to its oxygen tension. However, it has been difficult to understand the means by which arteriolar oxygen tension is changed during conditions which are known to increase local blood flow. Thus, since the arterioles are in close proximity to arterial blood, it would be expected that the oxygen tension of the arteriolar wall is always very close to that of arterial blood. If this is true, it is easy to understand the arteriolar dilatation which occurs when arterial blood oxygen tension is reduced, but it is much more difficult to understand arteriolar vasodilatation during increased tissue metabolism or following a reduction in perfusion pressure, conditions under which arterial blood oxygen tension is not reduced. This dilemma can perhaps be resolved by the recent findings of Duling and Berne (1970), who demonstrated that oxygen begins to diffuse from the blood into the tissues long before the blood reaches the capillaries; that is, the oxygen tension of the blood first begins to be reduced in the small arteries and arterioles. Since the rate at which oxygen diffuses from these vessels is proportional to the ratio of metabolic rate to blood flow, it can be shown that either an increase in metabolic activity of the tissues or a reduction in blood flow through the local tissues would cause a consequent reduction in arteriolar oxygen pressure. This can be clarified by referring to Figure 19–10, which shows a simplified diagram of a vessel segment in the microcirculation and the oxygen tensions of the blood and vascular wall at various distances along this vessel segment. For simplification, point A on this vessel represents the point at which oxygen first begins to diffuse out of the vessel into the tissues, and point B represents the point on the vessel where oxygen ceases to diffuse into the tissues. The upper curve in the figure represents the oxygen tensions of the blood and vascular wall at various distances between

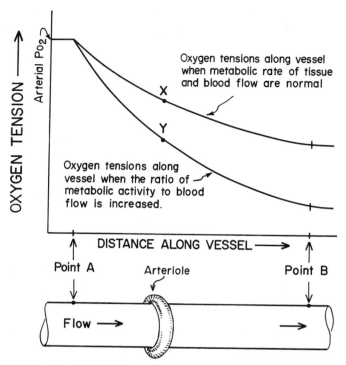

Figure 19–10. A simplified diagram showing the oxygen tension of the blood and vascular wall at various distances along a vascular segment of the microcirculation. Point A on the vessel represents the point at which oxygen first begins to diffuse from the vessel into the surrounding tissues, and point B represents the point at which oxygen ceases to diffuse from the vessel. The upper curve of the graph represents the oxygen tensions of the blood and vascular wall at various distances along the isolated vascular segment when the metabolic rate of the surrounding tissues and the blood flow are normal. Point X on the upper curve represents the normal oxygen tension of the arteriole. The lower curve represents the oxygen tensions when the ratio of metabolic activity to blood flow is increased; that is, when either metabolic activity is increased or blood flow is decreased. Point Y on the lower curve represents the arteriolar oxygen tension under these conditions.

points A and B when the rate of tissue metabolism and the blood flow to the tissue are normal. Under these conditions, the P_{O_2} of the vessel wall at point A is equal to the normal arterial blood P_{O_2}; the P_{O_2} of the vessel wall at point B is equal to the normal venous P_{O_2}; and the P_{O_2} represented by point X is the normal oxygen tension of the arteriolar smooth muscle. The lower curve represents the oxygen tensions at various distances along the vessel when either metabolic rate is increased or blood flow to the tissue is decreased. Either of these conditions causes an increased extraction of oxygen from each volume of blood passing through the vessel, such that the blood and vessel wall oxygen tensions at all points between points A and B are lower than normal. Thus, the oxygen tension of the arteriolar wall is now reduced to point Y, which would result in dilatation of the arteriole. One can readily see that if the arteriole were located at point A on the vessel, or if no oxygen diffused from the vessel prior to point A, the oxygen tension of the arteriolar wall would not have been affected by either an increase in metabolic activity or a reduction in blood flow.

Another factor which indicates that oxygen may directly be responsible for local blood flow regulation and which seems to discredit an indirect vasodilator mechanism is that venous blood removed from the right heart causes vascular dilatation, while the same blood removed from the arteries immediately after it passes through the lungs causes vascular constriction (Crawford, 1959). Therefore, if a vasodilator material were present in the venous blood, it either would have to be removed by the lungs or would have to be destroyed within the blood before it is recirculated to the local tissues. None of the metabolic vasodilators discussed above is removed by the lung, and only the vasodilator adenosine is known to be destroyed rapidly in the blood. In fact, adenosine is destroyed so rapidly in the blood, it is doubtful that it could be the factor responsible for vasodilatation when venous blood removed from the right heart is reinfused into a local tissue.

To summarize the possible mechanisms for regulation of local blood flow, we can only say that the tissue oxygen need is involved, but that it is uncertain whether the involvement of oxygen is through its direct action on the vascular smooth muscle, or through the action of oxygen lack, in causing the release of a vasodilator substance from the tissues. It is quite possible that the two mechanisms act in concert to produce a more precise control of local blood flow. Evidence for such a dual mechanism may be seen in the results of the study by Skinner and Powell (1967a), who showed that when an isolated skeletal muscle was perfused with blood that was both hyperkalemic and hypoxic, the fall in vascular resistance of the muscle was greater than that observed when it was perfused with blood that was either hyperkalemic or hypoxic. It is possible that the direct vasodilator action of oxygen lack is also enhanced by increased concentrations of some of the other proposed vasodilator substances released from the tissues, although much more research needs to be performed in this area.

LONG-TERM EFFECT OF OXYGEN LACK ON TISSUE BLOOD FLOW

The acute increase in blood flow resulting from decreased oxygen concentration in the arterial blood, as discussed above, can compensate for up to 70 per cent of the expected deficiency of oxygen transport to the tissues. Yet if the arterial oxygen saturation is decreased to very low values, there finally comes a point beyond which the acute vasodilation can dilate the blood vessels no further. Thereafter, further decreases in arterial oxygen saturation will result in serious deficiency of oxygen transport to the tissues.

Fortunately, when the acute oxygen lack regulatory mechanism cannot ensure adequate quantities of oxygen to the tissues, a long-term effect gradually occurs over a period of several days to several months to cause further increase in blood flow to the local tissues. This effect consists of an opening of previously closed vessels, an anatomical enlargement of existing vessels, and possibly even a growth of new vessels into the oxygen-deficient tissues, which is called "increased vascularization." This long-term phenomenon has been demonstrated both when an animal is subjected to low ambient oxygen (Huerkamp, 1950; Opitz, 1950; Clark, 1953; Becker, 1955; Valdiver, 1956, 1958, 1960; Korner, 1959; Smith and Crowell, 1967a; Diemer, 1968; Cassin, 1971) and in local hypoxia of tissues resulting from an occlusion of the arterial supply; the effect has been shown especially in the heart in response to occlusion of the coronary arteries or in response to anemia (Zoll, 1951; Eckstein, 1955, 1957). A particularly interesting study was that of Dollery (1968), who demonstrated that when the small vessels of the retina were occluded by embolization, two stages of autoregulation occurred to correct for the low blood flow beyond the embolus. The first stage consisted of dilatation of the small vessels, which is the intrinsic type of acute regulation described above. The second stage of compensation did not become apparent until several days following the occlusion, when the blood vessel seemed to stretch anatomically rather than simply to dilate. This second stage is a long-term type of regulation which occurs upon chronic exposure to tissue oxygen deficiency.

It is probable that the tissue demand for oxygen plays a very important role in the long-term regulation of blood flow as well as in the acute regulation of flow. The reason for believing this is that hypoxia causes increased vascularity, and hyperoxia causes decreased vascularity. This effect is emphasized by the study of Patz (1965), who observed that when newborn infants were put into an oxygen tent for therapeutic purposes, the excess oxygen was associated with an almost immediate cessation of new vascular growth in the retina of the eye and even degeneration of some of the capillaries that had already been formed. Furthermore, when the infants were removed from the oxygen tent, there was a very rapid proliferation of the retinal vessels to make up for the sudden decrease in the available oxygen. Thus, although the precise mechanism by which increased tissue vascularization occurs is almost completely unknown, it is almost certain that the tissue demand for oxygen is involved in this type of local blood flow regulation.

Overall Loop Gain of the Combined Acute and Long-term Vasodilator Effects

Unfortunately, quantitative studies have not yet been carried out to determine how effective the long-term vascularization mechanism is in providing continued oxygen supply to the tissues. Since we do not know the gain of the long-term blood flow regulatory mechanism, we can only state that the overall loop gain of the combined, acute and long-term mechanisms must be greater than the gain of the acute mechanism alone. Thus, since the acute mechanism regulating local blood flow has a gain which averages approximately 3, the overall gain must be greater than this, perhaps as high as 10 to 15. This means that a decrease in oxygen saturation of the arterial blood from 100 per cent to 30 per cent would result in an almost immediate increase in local blood flow to approximately 2.7 times normal, but after the second or long-term compensation occurs, the local blood flow would increase to over three times normal, thus delivering almost normal amounts of oxygen to the tissues despite the low arterial oxygen saturation. Obviously, this is a very high theoretical gain, but it demonstrates that in the long run, the degree of oxygenation of tissues perhaps has the most profound effect of any single factor on the regulation of local blood flow.

COMPARISON OF OXYGEN CONTROL OF BLOOD FLOW WITH NERVOUS CONTROL OF FLOW

Blood flow to almost all local areas of the body is determined both by local regulatory factors and by nervous regulation. In large portions of the body's tissues, the local control of flow is far more important than the nervous factors. For instance, in skeletal muscles, which comprise almost one-half of the entire body weight, the autonomic nerves to the muscle vessels can be completely removed or pharmacologically blocked and, still, insofar as can be measured, the same vasodilating effect of exercise occurs as is true when the nerves are intact (Barcroft, 1952). Furthermore, our own studies have shown equally as great a correlation between local blood flow and arterial oxygen saturation in animals under total spinal anesthesia as in normal animals (Ross, 1962). In addition, the results of many investigations demonstrate that the local tissues still show reactive hyperemia and autoregulation after denervation (Hyman, 1963; Jones and Berne, 1964b, 1965; Bache and Ederstrom, 1965; Walker and Guyton, 1967).

In certain specialized tissues, however, the local factors are not pre-potent over the nervous factors. For instance, in the skin, the nervous factor predominates, and the local metabolism factor enters into the control of skin blood flow only when the flow to the skin falls to drastically low levels. For instance, when the flow is completely cut off for 20 to 30 minutes, typical reactive hyperemia occurs in the skin vessels, thus illustrating an important metabolically activated blood flow control system under these circumstances. However, under normal circumstances, the blood flow to the skin is controlled almost entirely by the nervous system for the purpose of regulating body temperature; the flow required for this purpose is usually far greater than that required to supply adequate nutrition to the skin (Green, 1959; Hertzman, 1959). The kidneys are another tissue whose blood flow is controlled to a considerable extent by the nerves, the nerves in this way helping to regulate urine formation.

REGULATION OF TOTAL CARDIAC OUTPUT AND ITS RELATIONSHIP TO THE REGULATION OF LOCAL BLOOD FLOW

The discussion to this point has concerned the effects of oxygen and oxygen insufficiency on local blood flow. Now we would like to see how these local effects relate to the control of total cardiac output. Since cardiac output is the sum of the blood flows to all local tissues, we would expect that the same mechanism which controls local blood flow is also important in the regulation of cardiac output.

EFFECT OF OVERALL BODY METABOLISM ON CARDIAC OUTPUT

The best example of the effect of metabolism on cardiac output is in severe muscular exercise. Cardiac outputs in human beings as high as five to six times normal have been reported during extremely strenuous exercise in well trained athletes (Christensen, 1931; Ekblom and Hermansen, 1968) and even in normal persons, cardiac outputs during heavy exercise as high as four times normal are regularly reported (Chapman, 1960; Wang, 1960; Widimsky, 1963; Astrand, 1964; Khouri, 1965; Damato, 1966; Gilbert, 1971). Furthermore, the cardiac output increases almost in direct proportion to the increase in level of body metabolism during the exercise, which, can be seen very precisely by referring back to Figure 1–1 in Chapter 1.

Other significant studies have shown a high degree of correlation between thyrotoxicosis and cardiac output, the cardiac output increasing approximately in proportion to the increase in basal metabolism. Also, in hypothyroidism, the cardiac output decreases, likewise approximately in proportion to the decrease in basal metabolism (Lequime, 1940; Charlier, 1946; Kattus, 1955; Stead, 1950). Finally, chemical factors that increase the metabolism, such as epinephrine or dinitrophenol (Stainsby, 1962; Banet and Guyton, 1971), all increase the cardiac output. Thus, the correlation between metabolism and cardiac output can probably be accepted without question.

AUTOREGULATION OF THE TOTAL SYSTEMIC CIRCULATION AND ITS RELATION TO CONTROL OF CARDIAC OUTPUT

It was pointed out earlier in this chapter that most tissues of the body show the phenomenon of autoregulation, local blood flow being maintained at a nearly constant level despite large changes in perfusion pressure. Since cardiac output is the sum of the local blood flows to all tissues, it may be expected that cardiac output is also autoregulated to a large degree despite great changes in arterial pressure. Recent studies from our laboratories have demonstrated that this is, indeed, the case (Granger and Guyton, 1969; Coleman, 1971; Guyton, 1971; Shepherd, to be published).

Granger (1969) studied the phenomenon of autoregulation in the total systemic circulation in dogs in which sympathetic influences were completely removed by decapitation and destruction of the spinal cord by alcohol. In his procedure, epinephrine and norepinephrine were infused at a constant rate to produce a normal level of sympathetic tone in the systemic vasculature, arterial pressure was controlled by adjusting the height of a blood reservoir connected to a systemic artery, and cardiac output was measured continually using the cardiac output recorder developed in our laboratories and described in Chapter 2. The changes in cardiac output, oxygen consumption, A–V oxygen difference, and right atrial pressure in one animal when arterial pressure was abruptly reduced are shown in Figure 19–11. Note that when arterial pressure was reduced rapidly from over 100 mm. Hg to approximately 50 mm. Hg, cardiac output fell rapidly to approximately 50 per cent of control. Following the abrupt reduction in cardiac output, autoregulation began to occur, and cardiac output gradually rose over the ensuing several minutes almost to its control level. Granger calculated that the average open loop gain of the autoregulation control system for the entire systemic circulation was 3.32, indicating more than 75 per cent compensation. It should be noted that this very closely approximates the open loop gain of autoregulation in most local tissues.

The study of Granger especially suggests that the factors responsible for regulation of local blood flow are also important in the regulation of cardiac output, and reemphasizes that this factor is the tissue need for oxygen. It may be seen in Figure 19–11 that when arterial pressure was abruptly reduced, the quantity of oxygen extracted from the blood as it passes through the tissues, the A–V oxygen difference, was rapidly increased, so that oxygen consumption was not reduced nearly as much as cardiac output. Furthermore, as cardiac output returned toward its control level, oxygen consumption and the A–V oxygen difference also returned toward normal. It was observed in this study that the average compensation for oxygen consumption was about 50 per cent better than the compensation for cardiac output; that is, as long as oxygen consumption was

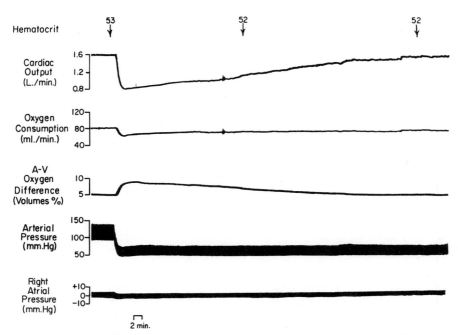

Figure 19–11. Effects of a single step decrease in arterial pressure on cardiac output, oxygen consumption, A-V oxygen difference, and right atrial pressure. [From Granger (1969), by permission of The American Heart Association, Inc.]

markedly different from normal, the cardiac output continued to return toward the control level, but when oxygen consumption had returned almost to the control level, the cardiac output thereafter failed to change further. This implies that the factor most precisely controlled is the oxygen delivery to the tissue and that changes in both the rate of blood flow to the tissues and the quantity of oxygen extracted from the blood are important mechanisms in regulating the oxygen delivery to the tissues.

Shepherd (to be published) has further studied the relationship between blood flow and oxygen extraction in maintaining a constant whole body oxygen consumption following changes both in arterial pressure and in the concentration of oxygen in the inspired air. Using the same animal preparation as Granger, the control A-V oxygen difference was altered by infusing epinephrine at various rates. It was found that within a wide range of initial A-V oxygen differences, oxygen consumption was maintained almost completely constant despite changes in arterial pressure or inspired oxygen. However, when the initial A-V oxygen difference was low, oxygen consumption was maintained primarily by an increase in oxygen extraction, and when the initial A-V oxygen difference was very high, increased blood flow played the major role in maintaining oxygen consumption. Indeed, when the initial A-V oxygen difference was as high as 10 ml. per 100 ml. of blood, cardiac output increased to 500 per cent normal when the concentration of oxygen in the inspired air was reduced to 8 per cent. Thus, this study also emphasizes that the oxygen delivery to the tissues is one of the most rigidly regulated systems in the body.

EFFECT OF OXYGEN INSUFFICIENCY ON CARDIAC OUTPUT

In the same way that an increase in metabolism increases cardiac output, so does oxygen insufficiency. Increases in cardiac output to as much as two or more times normal have been observed in simple anoxia resulting from reduced ambient oxygen concentration (Gorlin, 1954; Grollman, 1930b; Cross, 1958, 1959; Murray and Young, 1963a; Vogel and Harris, 1967; Richardson, 1967; Bing, 1969; Carrell and Milhorn, 1971), cyanide poisoning (Huckabee, 1960; Öberg, 1961; Krasney, 1971), and carbon monoxide poisoning (Chiodi, 1941; Öberg, 1961). Identical effects occur in all three types of anoxia, the cardiac output rising on the average to almost 100 per cent above normal at optimal levels of anoxia. When the degree of anoxia increases above this critical level, however, the heart begins to fail, and the cardiac output then falls instead of rising as the degree of anoxia increases still further.

Öberg, in our laboratory, has made very precise studies of the changes in cardiac output at various levels of cyanide and carbon monoxide poisoning, both of which gave almost identical results. Figure 19–12 illustrates the average effect of continuous cyanide infusion on the cardiac output in ten dogs when the average infusion rate was just sufficient to cause death in about 60 minutes. Note that immediately after the cyanide begins to take effect, the cardiac output begins to rise, this resulting from a decreasing peripheral resistance. After reaching a peak almost double

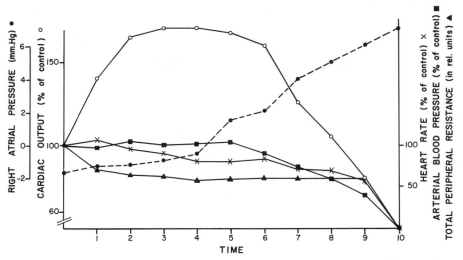

Figure 19-12. Effect of cyanide infusion on the cardiac output. Coincident with the fall in cardiac output toward the end of the infusion, multiple signs of cardiac failure were observed as discussed in the text. (Öberg and Guyton, unpublished observations.)

the normal, the cardiac output begins to decline, and the right atrial pressure begins to rise, illustrating beginning failure of the heart. From these studies we see the two different effects of anoxia on cardiac output; first, an increase in output in the early stages caused primarily by decreased peripheral resistance [which decreases to about one-fifth normal in maximal cyanide anoxia (Öberg, unpublished observations] and, second, a decrease in cardiac output at a later stage when the heart begins to fail because of cardiac anoxia. Jose and Stitt (1969) have also observed this failure of the heart during severe hypoxia. These experiments demonstrate that the peripheral effect begins long before the cardiac reserve is used up. As a result, blood flows through the systemic circulation into the heart more easily than usual, and the heart, in accordance with Starling's law of the heart, simply pumps this blood back around the circuit again and again at a more rapid rate than usual.

It was pointed out earlier in this chapter that the effects of hypoxia on local blood flow are almost as great in the absence of nervous control of the vascular system as in its presence. However, it has recently become obvious that nervous reflexes do play a significant role on the effects of hypoxia on total cardiac output; this is especially true of nervous reflexes involving the capacitance vessels or the veins. For example, Smith and Crowell (1967b) observed that when intact animals were respired with 8 per cent oxygen, cardiac output was increased by approximately 50 per cent, and this increase in output was associated with a dilatation of the peripheral resistance vessels and a 25 per cent increase in the mean systemic pressure and pressure gradient for venous return, indicating reflex constriction of the veins. On the other hand, when the animals were given total spinal anesthesia, this same degree of hypoxia caused no significant increase in cardiac output, even though there was still a tremendous dilatation of the peripheral resistance vasculature. The failure of cardiac output to rise significantly was caused by an absence of venous constriction. Indeed, there was actually a drop in the mean systemic pressure and the pressure gradient for venous return during hypoxia in the animals given spinal anesthesia. Similar findings have been made by others (Korner, 1969, 1970; Uther, 1970; Banet and Guyton, 1971). Banet and Guyton studied the effects of dinitrophenol on cardiac output in decapitated dogs with the spinal cord destroyed. They observed that in intact animals, dinitrophenol resulted in an increase in cardiac output of approximately 200 per cent, but in the totally denervated dogs, the same dosage of dinitrophenol increased cardiac output only 50 per cent. This relatively small increase in cardiac output resulted despite the fact that the degree of vascular dilatation was approximately the same as that observed in the intact dogs. The results of Banet also demonstrated that if the vasculature of the totally denervated dogs was expanded with blood or dextran, thus increasing the mean systemic pressure, dinitrophenol caused an increase in cardiac output almost identical to that seen in the intact animals. And in the cyanide studies of Öberg cited above, it was noted that the increase in cardiac output caused by the anoxia was somewhat greater in intact animals than in animals with total autonomic block. Thus, all of these studies demonstrate that nervous reflexes are important in maintaining or even increasing the mean systemic pressure and the pressure gradient for venous return during hypoxia, thereby permitting the full effect of local hypoxic vasodilatation on cardiac output to occur.

Severe hypoxia ultimately results in a reduction in cardiac contractility, but there is substantial evidence that during moderate hypoxia or during the initial stages of severe hypoxia, the cardiac contractility is actually increased (Kahler, 1962a; Downing, 1963, 1966; DeGeest, 1965b, 1965c; Penna, 1965; Levy and Zieske, 1968). This increase in cardiac contractility amounts to approximately 30 to 40 per cent and is due to an increase in the sympathetic stimulation of the heart. The exact mechanism by which sympathetic activity is increased during hypoxia is somewhat uncertain, but it appears to be caused by oxygen insufficiency in the central nervous system. Thus, this reflex is probably very similar to the central nervous system ischemic reflex described in the preceding chapter and is another example of the means by which nervous reflexes affect cardiac output during hypoxia.

ANALYSIS OF THE EFFECT OF OXYGEN LACK ON CARDIAC OUTPUT

Figure 19–13 shows an analysis of the effects of anoxia on cardiac output. The solid curves represent the normal venous return and cardiac output curves, with the equilibrium point at point A, with a cardiac output of 5 liters per minute and a right atrial pressure of zero. However, after hypoxia has begun to take effect, as in the cyanide poisoning studies illustrated in Figure 19–12, the resistance to venous return decreases moderately. As explained in Chapter 13, under these conditions the venous

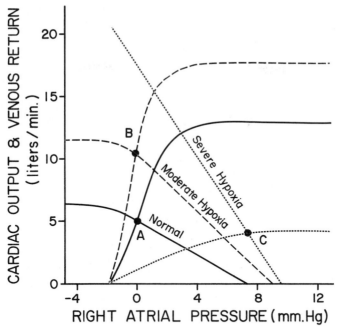

Figure 19–13. Analysis of the effect of hypoxia on cardic output. Point A represents the normal condition, point B represents moderate hypoxia, and point C represents severe hypoxia. See explanation in text.

return curve rotates upward. The dashed curve illustrates the venous return curve under these conditions and shows a reduction in the resistance to venous return of approximately 50 per cent. Note also that the venous return curve under these conditions has been shifted slightly to the right, indicating a slight increase in the mean systemic pressure. Furthermore, as a result of increased sympathetic stimulation of the heart, the cardiac output curve (dashed curve) is shifted upward during moderate hypoxia such that the new equilibrium point is now point B. Note that under these conditions the cardiac output is increased approximately 100 per cent, which is the result shown by many animal and human experiments. This increase in cardiac output occurs even though right atrial pressure is not changed or is even slightly reduced, which is the result shown by Smith and Crowell (1967b).

As the hypoxia becomes progressively more severe, the heart begins to weaken, causing the cardiac output curve to fall drastically. Indeed, it can fall all the way to zero if the hypoxia is severe enough. Thus, the dash-dot curves of Figure 19–13 illustrate the effect of very severe, but not quite yet lethal, hypoxia, showing a greatly depressed cardiac output curve and a further rotated venous return curve which is also shifted slightly further to the right. These two curves now equate with each other at point C, showing a cardiac output of 3.8 liters per minute, which is considerably depressed below the normal, and a right atrial pressure of approximately 7 mm. Hg. Any additional increase in the severity of the hypoxia further reduces the cardiac output because of the progressively deteriorating heart.

Computer Simulation of Circulatory Dynamics During Hypoxia

Figure 19–14 shows simulated changes in the oxygen tension of the muscle venous effluent, cardiac output, arterial pressure, total peripheral resistance, heart rate, and urinary output when the arterial oxygen saturation was abruptly reduced to 60 per cent for a period of five minutes and then suddenly returned to 100 per cent. Following the onset of hypoxemia, the venous oxygen tension decreased during the ensuing one to two minutes to approximately one-half its normal value, indicating that the muscles of the body had become severely hypoxic. Following the onset of the reduction in venous oxygen tension, cardiac output began to rise and, after three minutes of hypoxemia, plateaued at a value of approximately 180 per cent its control value. Associated with the increase in cardiac output, total peripheral resistance was reduced to slightly less than one-half its normal value, and systemic arterial pressure decreased from 100 mm. Hg to approximately 84 mm. Hg. The reduction in total

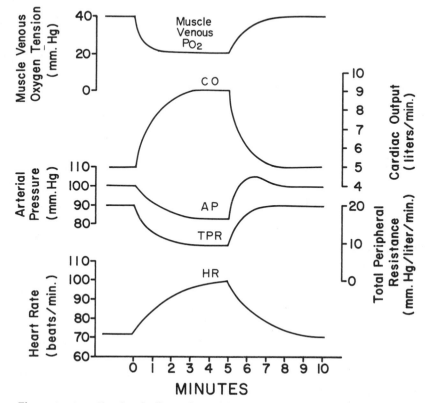

Figure 19–14.   Simulated effects of arterial hypoxemia on circulatory dynamics.

peripheral resistance and the consequent increase in cardiac output were due to the intrinsic mechanism which is present in nearly every tissue of the body and which regulates the local blood flow to meet the demand of the local tissues for oxygen. Note particularly that the simulated increase in cardiac output is precisely that predicted for moderate hypoxia by the graphical analysis of Figure 19–13.

During the period of hypoxemia the heart rate increased from its normal value of 72 beats per minute to approximately 100 beats per minute, indicating an increased sympathetic stimulation of the heart, resulting primarily from activation of the chemoreceptors.

Following the return of arterial oxygen saturation to its normal value of 100 per cent, cardiac output and muscle venous Po_2 returned to their control values over the ensuing two to three minutes. The failure of oxygen tension and cardiac output to return to their control values immediately after the cessation of the hypoxemic period is evidence of an oxygen debt acquired during the hypoxic period. As this debt was repaid, venous Po_2 and cardiac output reapproached their prehypoxemic values.

TISSUE NEED FOR OXYGEN AS A COMMON DENOMINATOR IN CARDIAC OUTPUT REGULATION

In this chapter the correlation between metabolism and cardiac output has been emphasized, and attempts have been made to establish a probable link between tissue oxygen need and the increased cardiac output that is observed during increased tissue activity. The different studies on hypoxia have all demonstrated that hypoxia in itself can increase the cardiac output to about two times normal. On the other hand, it is also known that when the overall rate of metabolism of the body is greatly increased, such as during exercise, the cardiac output can increase from four to five times normal. This appears to be a discrepancy that would rule out tissue oxygen insufficiency as the major cause of the increased cardiac output in exercise. However, it should be recalled that the failure of cardiac output to increase above two times normal in hypoxia is caused by cardiac debility resulting from the hypoxia. Such debility of the heart does not occur when the metabolic rate of the body increases, because then plenty of oxygen is available to the heart. For instance, in severe exercise, the increased metabolism of the muscle is not associated in any way with a decrease in oxygen availability to the heart. Consequently, it is reasonable to expect that under these conditions, the heart would pump far more than two times the normal cardiac output. This fits with the concept that (1) increased tissue metabolism increases the local need of the tissues for oxygen, (2) the local need of the tissues for oxygen in turn increases local tissue blood flow, and (3) the increased local blood flow throughout the body then causes a summated increase in flow back to the heart with a consequently increased cardiac output. The primary value of nervous reflexes in this scheme is that they maintain or enhance the arterial pressure, thereby allowing the local oxygen insufficiency mechanism to increase cardiac output to its fullest extent.

In summary, the thesis that has been developed in the chapter is the following: The tissues themselves regulate their own blood flow in proportion to their need for oxygen, and this intrinsic regulation of local blood flow is the one most important factor governing the tendency for blood to return from the systemic circulation to the heart and thereby to regulate the cardiac output.

Chapter 20

EFFECT OF BLOOD VOLUME CHANGES AND ORTHOSTATIC FACTORS ON CARDIAC OUTPUT

Often it is stated that changes in blood volume have no significant effect on cardiac output. However, any time one records cardiac output continuously and infuses even a small quantity of blood, plasma, gelatin solution, or dextran solution into an animal, he will see an instantaneous rise in output such as that illustrated in Figure 20–1 (Guyton, 1958d, 1959f; Fleming, 1957; Haynes, 1945; Ferguson, 1953, 1954; Schnabel, 1959; Sunahara, 1955; Holt, 1944b; Fletcher, 1945; Frye, 1960; Balent, 1961; Conway, 1966; Robinson, 1966; Prather, 1969). This effect is even more marked in the sympathectomized animal (Guyton, 1958d; Chien, 1961). After the initial rise, the output then falls gradually back toward normal during the ensuing 10 to 60 minutes. Bleeding causes exactly the opposite results, as shown in Figure 20–2, except that recovery of normal cardiac output is not likely to be so rapid (Guyton, 1958d; Fleisch, 1936; Warren, 1945; Root, 1947; Eckstein, 1947a; Remington, 1950a, b; Conway, 1966). Likewise, diminishing "effective" blood volume by using tourniquets to pool blood in the limbs causes the cardiac output to fall (Fitzhugh, 1953; Judson, 1955). Finally, a particularly interesting study was that performed by de Burgh Daly in 1925 in which he showed that changing the blood volume of a closed circuit heart-lung preparation causes instantaneous changes in cardiac output in exactly the same way as in the intact animal, the output rising with increased volume and falling with decreased volume.

From these simple experiments it is evident that blood volume does have much to do with cardiac output, but from many other studies it is equally as evident that very powerful compensatory mechanisms are available in the body to compensate for this effect so that it often cannot be seen in clinical or experimental studies (Warren, 1945, 1948; Reeve, 1960; Frye, 1960; Chien, 1961). Therefore, two of the purposes of this chapter are to discuss the instantaneous effects of blood volume changes on cardiac output and to discuss the compensatory mechanisms that can nullify the effects of volume changes on cardiac output.

353

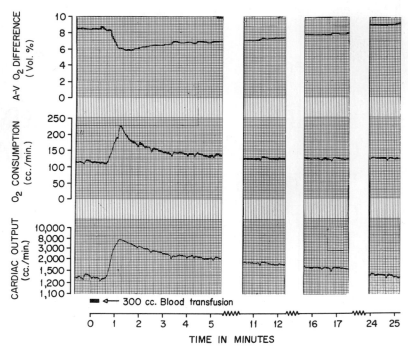

Figure 20–1. Effect of transfusion on the cardiac output, O_2 consumption, and A-V O_2 difference in a 11 kg. anesthetized dog, as recorded by the continuous Fick recorder. [Reprinted from Guyton, Farish, and Abernathy (1959f).]

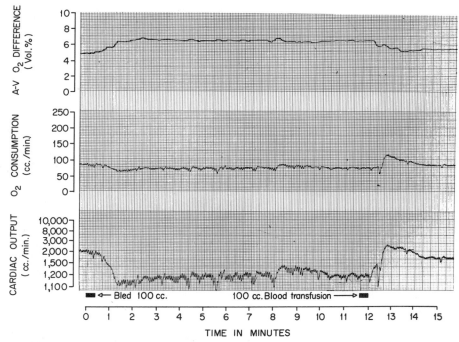

Figure 20–2. Effect of hemorrhage on cardiac output, O_2 consumption, and A-V O_2 difference in a 14 kg. anesthetized dog, as recorded by the continuous Fick recorder. [Reprinted from Guyton, Farish, and Abernathy (1959f).]

A third purpose of this chapter is to discuss the changes in cardiac output that occur with changes in bodily position, that is, to discuss the effects of orthostatic factors on cardiac output.

BASIC MECHANISMS BY WHICH BLOOD VOLUME CHANGES CAN AFFECT CARDIAC OUTPUT

An increase in blood volume alters the cardiac output mainly by increasing the degree of filling of the systemic circulation, which causes rapid flow of blood into the heart, increased filling of the heart, and consequently increased cardiac pumping. Increased filling of the systemic circulation affects the flow of blood into the heart in two different ways: by increasing the *mean systemic pressure* (Guyton, 1955b; Richardson, 1961; Harlan, 1967; Prather, 1969) and by decreasing the *resistance to venous return* (Guyton, 1958d).

Effect of Blood Volume Changes on Mean Circulatory and Mean Systemic Pressures

The effect of blood volume changes on mean circulatory pressure was discussed in Chapter 12 where it was pointed out that an instantaneous increase in blood volume of approximately 14 per cent will raise the mean circulatory pressure from the normal value of 7 mm. Hg up to approximately 14 mm. Hg; that is, to double the normal (Richardson, 1961; Harlan, 1967). Furthermore, Figure 12–6 in Chapter 12 illustrates that this relationship between blood volume and mean circulatory pressure is approximately linear. However, the immediate rise in mean circulatory pressure following an acute increase in blood volume lasts for less than a minute, the mean circulatory pressure then returning toward a value only slightly above normal with a half-time of approximately 2 to 4 minutes. The significance of this return of the mean circulatory pressure toward normal as a compensatory mechanism will be discussed more fully later in the chapter.

When blood is removed from the circulation, the mean circulatory pressure falls; this is exactly opposite to the effect of increasing the blood volume. An acute decrease in blood volume of approximately 15 per cent will reduce the mean circulatory pressure from 7 mm. Hg to zero, but here again the mean circulatory pressure rises slowly back upward over the next few minutes.

It is important at this point to recall the relationship between mean circulatory pressure, mean systemic pressure, and mean pulmonary pressure. Mathematically, the approximate relationship between these different pressures is the following (see Chapter 12):

$$\text{Pmc} = \frac{7\,\text{Pms} + \text{Pmp}}{8} \qquad\qquad \textbf{(20–1)}$$

This formula shows that the mean systemic pressure and mean circulatory pressure are very closely related, because seven-eighths of the mean circulatory pressure is determined by the mean systemic pressure and only one-eighth by the mean pulmonary pressure. Therefore, in general, one can state that when the mean circulatory pressure is altered in response to blood volume changes, there is an almost corresponding alteration in mean systemic pressure.

If the mean systemic pressure is changed in response to blood volume changes, the *pressure gradient for venous return* in the systemic circulation is also altered (see Chapter 12), and therefore the tendency for blood to return to the heart is correspondingly changed, thus affecting the cardiac output. In short, an increase in blood volume tends to increase the cardiac output, and a decrease in blood volume tends to decrease the cardiac output.

Effect of Blood Volume Changes on Resistance to Venous Return

Though the major means by which alterations in blood volume alter cardiac output is through changes in mean circulatory pressure, alterations in volume also change the *resistance to venous return* to some extent (Guyton, 1958d). It will be recalled from the discussion in Chapter 13 that when the resistance to venous return changes, the tendency for blood to return to the heart changes oppositely. If we now refer to Figure 12–7 (Chapter 12), which illustrates the effect of changing blood volume on venous return, it is evident that as the blood volume increases, the resistance to venous return (which is proportional to the reciprocal of the slope of the venous return curve) decreases, allowing the blood to flow back to the heart more rapidly, with a consequent further increase in cardiac output.

One can explain the decrease in resistance to venous return with increasing blood volume simply on the basis of enlargement of the peripheral vasculature, for it will be recalled from Chapter 13 that the resistance to venous return is an algebraic average of all the resistances to blood flow from the different parts of the systemic circulation back to the right atrium. When the vessels in the periphery become dilated as a result of an increase in blood volume, one would obviously expect a decrease in the resistance to venous return. This is precisely what is observed when the blood volume is increased (Guyton, 1958d).

SIMPLIFIED GRAPHICAL ANALYSIS OF THE EFFECT OF BLOOD VOLUME CHANGES ON CARDIAC OUTPUT

Utilizing the information presented above, and also referring back to Chapter 12 in which the effects of changes in blood volume on the venous return curve were presented in detail, we can now analyze graphically the effect of blood volume changes on cardiac output. Figure 20–3

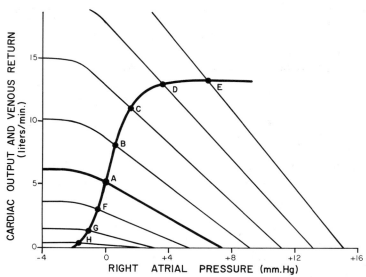

Figure 20–3. Graphical analysis of the instantaneous effects on cardiac output of instantaneous changes in blood volume.

illustrates by the two dark curves an analysis for the normal circulation, showing that the normal venous return curve and the normal cardiac output curve equilibrate at point A, with a cardiac output of 5 liters per minute and a right atrial pressure of 0 mm. Hg. The venous return curves lying to the right of the normal curve illustrates the effects of progressively greater blood volumes on the venous return curve, and the equilibrium points of these curves with the cardiac output curve represent the *immediate* effects on cardiac output after *sudden* increases in blood volume. For instance, an increase in blood volume sufficient to increase the mean systemic pressure by 2 mm. Hg will increase the cardiac output from 5 liters per minute to approximately 8 liters per minute (point B), and an increase in blood volume sufficient to increase the mean systemic pressure 4 mm. Hg will increase the cardiac output up to approximately 11 liters per minute (point C), and so forth.

On the other hand, the venous return curves to the left of the normal curve show the effect on cardiac output of *suddenly* decreasing the blood volume. For instance, a decrease in mean circulatory pressure from 7 mm. Hg to 5 mm. Hg will immediately reduce the cardiac output from 5 liters to approximately 3 liters per minute (point F). Likewise, point G illustrates the effect on cardiac output of reducing the mean systemic pressure to 3 mm. Hg, while point H illustrates the effect of reducing this pressure to 1 mm. Hg.

Thus, Figure 20–3 illustrates that an increase in blood volume shifts the venous return curve to the right (which results from increased mean systemic pressure) and also rotates the curve very slightly clockwise (which results from decreased resistance to venous return). Both these effects tend to increase the cardiac output, because either shifting of the whole curve to the right or rotating the upper part of the curve to the right will have a similar effect in increasing the level of the equilibrium point with the cardiac output curve.

It should be noted, however, that this analysis in Figure 20–3 shows only the *instantaneous* effect on cardiac output caused by increasing or decreasing the blood volume, because, within a matter of seconds, various compensatory effects begin to occur which tend to return the cardiac output toward normal, as will be discussed.

COMPENSATORY MECHANISMS THAT OFFSET THE EFFECTS OF BLOOD VOLUME CHANGES

We know at least three very important compensatory mechanisms that can offset to a very great extent the effects of blood volume changes on cardiac output: (1) nervous reflex compensations, (2) stress relaxation or stress relaxation recovery of the vascular system, and (3) readjustment of the blood volume itself back toward normal.

Compensatory Effects of Nervous Reflexes

Unfortunately, we cannot truly assess the value of the nervous reflexes in compensating for cardiac output changes caused by altered blood volume. Many investigators believe that the autonomic reflexes do have significant compensating effect (Warren, 1945, 1948; Frye, 1960; Chien, 1961; Werko, 1962). However, it is also true that the autonomic reflexes have relatively little effect on cardiac output in contrast to their rather marked effect on arterial pressure. In the case of blood removal, this is particularly well illustrated by the study of Chalmers and coworkers (1967), who compared the circulatory responses to a 26 per cent reduction in blood volume in animals both with and without a functional sympathetic nervous system. In animals without a functional sympathetic nervous system, the reduction in blood volume resulted in an immediate fall of about 40 per cent in both cardiac output and arterial pressure. In animals with intact sympathetics, cardiac output was reduced by approximately 30 per cent, only slightly less than that observed in animals without sympathetics. However, in these animals with intact sympathetics, the compensation in arterial pressure was significantly greater, since pressure suffered a reduction of only 15 per cent following hemorrhage. The relatively small effect of sympathetic stimulation upon cardiac output may also be seen in Figure 18–6 of Chapter 18, which shows a continuous recording of cardiac output when a maximal carotid sinus reflex was elicited. Here, the increase in cardiac output was only approximately 15 per cent, which is not a large alteration when we consider that blood volume changes can affect cardiac output as much as several hundred per cent.

If autonomic reflexes do play a role in compensating for the cardiac output changes, these reflexes are probably mediated by the pressoreceptors. For instance, Kumada and Sagawa (1970) have recently demonstrated that aortic pressoreceptor activity is diminished by 21 per cent in response to a 10 per cent reduction in blood volume, and is increased by 31 per cent following a 20 per cent expansion of the blood volume. In each instance, the resultant change in arterial pressure was only approximately 6 per cent. It is likely that similar changes occur in carotid pressoreceptor activity following reductions or increases in blood volume. Thus, following a change in blood volume, the entire reflex would be expected to function in the following manner: Within a few seconds after a rapid infusion of blood equal to 25 per cent of the subject's own blood volume, the cardiac output might rise as high as 300 per cent above normal (see Fig. 20–1), while the arterial pressure might rise simultaneously to about one and two-thirds times normal. This rise in arterial pressure would cause an increase in the activity of the aortic and carotid sinus pressoreceptors, resulting in parasympathetic stimulation of the heart and inhibition of the sympathetics to the entire circulatory system. These effects would be expected to decrease the heart rate and the peripheral vascular tone. The decreased vascular tone (Alexander, 1954, 1955, 1956) should decrease the mean systemic pressure, which should help to return the cardiac output toward normal. Thus, on two accounts, this inverse pressoreceptor reflex should tend to reduce the cardiac output toward normal, first, by reducing the effectiveness of the heart as a pump and, second, by reducing the pressure gradient for venous return (mean systemic pressure minus right atrial pressure).

Precisely the opposite compensatory effects would be expected to occur following a decrease in blood volume (Page, 1955; Chalmers, 1967; Kumada, 1970), because a decreased arterial pressure causes the aortic pressoreceptor and carotid sinus pressoreceptor nerve activity to diminish (Kumada, 1970), which results in a diminution of parasympathetic stimulation to the heart and an increase in sympathetic stimulation of the entire circulatory system.

Even though the pressoreceptor reflex does not seem to be very powerful as a compensatory mechanism for cardiac output changes, it is still possible that other less well known reflexes originating in the pulmonary circulation, in the heart, or in the veins might play a more significant role in such compensations (Frye, 1960; Gupta, 1966). A particular study which indicates that this might be true is one by Frye and his colleagues, in which they showed that in the normal human being moderate changes in blood volume caused by transfusion and bleeding are often not accompanied by significant changes in cardiac output, whereas in the same individual treated with a ganglionic blocking agent to block the reflexes a very marked change occurs in cardiac output when the blood volume is altered. Yet, unfortunately, not enough is known about the effect on cardiac output of the different extrapressoreceptor reflexes to say which one, if any, might be causing these compensatory effects. Heymans (1958) has discussed many different possible reflexes arising in the veins, heart, and pulmonary circulation, any one or all of which might be responsible for the effects.

In very severe hemorrhage, still another powerful reflex, the central nervous system ischemic reflex, may enter into the compensatory mechanism for helping to maintain the cardiac output. Sagawa (1961a, b, 1962) has shown that a fall in arterial pressure below 50 mm. Hg elicits this reflex extremely powerfully, causing 4 to 6 times as much sympathetic stimulation as does the pressoreceptor reflex. Furthermore, Richardson and Fermoso (1964) showed that a maximal central nervous system ischemic reflex can increase the mean circulatory pressure to two and one-half times its normal value. This tremendous increase in mean circulatory pressure together with the effects of sympathetic stimulation on the heart may result in an increase in cardiac output of between 50 and 100 per cent above its normal level (Richardson, 1965). This increase in cardiac output occurs despite an increase in afterload, the arterial pressure, to as high as 200 mm. Hg. Thus, the central nervous system ischemic response can affect cardiac output far more than the pressoreceptor reflex, and it may well be an extremely important "last ditch stand" mechanism to prevent decreased cardiac output in the terminal stages of severe hemorrhage, after the arterial pressure has fallen very low.

Readjustment of Blood Volume

After a massive transfusion, all the pressures in the circulation, including the capillaries, rise immediately, causing fluid to begin transuding outward through the capillary walls into the interstitial spaces (Guyton, 1950, 1951a; Pappenheimer, 1953) and through the glomeruli into the urine (Smith, 1956; Guyton, 1969a). Within one to 24 hours, the blood volume ordinarily readjusts either to normal or almost to normal (Gregersen, 1959; Prather, 1969). And, as the blood volume returns to normal, the mean systemic pressure, the peripheral resistance, and the cardiac output also return to normal so that again normal cardiovascular dynamics will ensue.

Conversely, after hemorrhage, essentially opposite effects occur. First, large quantities of protein pass by way of the lymphatics from the interstitial fluid to the blood to replenish the plasma protein, and additional protein is formed in the next few days by the liver, thereby increasing the quantity of plasma protein back toward normal (Wasserman, 1956). Simultaneously, the plasma volume returns to normal, or even above normal, usually to a level sufficient to make up for the defect in blood volume caused by the loss of the red blood cells as well as by the loss of plasma. This increase in plasma volume is caused by two events: First, following hemorrhage, all the pressures within the circulatory system, including the capillaries, are reduced. The reduction in capillary pressure causes fluid to move from the interstitial spaces into the vascular system, thus increasing plasma volume (Gregersen, 1959; Öberg, 1964; Haddy, 1965; Chalmers, 1967). Second, the decrease in arterial pressure causes a reduction in the filtration of fluid into the glomeruli and, thus, a reduction in fluid loss through the kidneys (Baer, 1970; Fourcade, 1971; Navar, 1971). The rise of blood volume back toward normal following hemorrhage is ordinarily a slower process than the decrease in blood volume following transfusion. Nevertheless, within 24 to 48 hours the blood volume is usually back to normal, or almost to normal, unless the animal or human being is in a dehydrated state. As a result, the cardiovascular dynamics also return toward normal.

From the above discussion it may be seen that the readjustment of blood volume is one of the most important mechanisms for offsetting the effects of blood volume changes on cardiac output. Although this mechanism acts much more slowly than others, it has the unique ability to correct completely for any changes in blood volume.

Compensatory Effects of Stress Relaxation and Stress Relaxation Recovery

A phenomenon called "stress relaxation" and "stress relaxation recovery" has been known for a long time to occur in the vascular system, especially in the veins (Alexander, 1953). This effect, which was discussed in Chapter 12, results from an intrinsic ability of the vascular walls to stretch slowly when the pressure rises and to contract slowly when the pressure falls.

Unfortunately, quantitative studies on the compensatory effects of stress relaxation and stress relaxation recovery following blood volume changes are meager. Yet, it is evident that the compensation in cardiac output that occurs following transfusion or hemorrhage is far too great to be explained by nervous reflexes and often occurs too rapidly to be explained by adjustments in blood volume. Preliminary results, from studies in our laboratory, on the effects of stress relaxation on the mean circulatory pressure were illustrated in Figure 12–8 of Chapter 12. These studies suggested that over a period of 10 to 20 minutes, the mean circulatory pressure might return as much as three-fourths of the way back toward normal simply as a result of stress relaxation after a large transfusion. More recent results from our laboratories (Prather, 1969) have confirmed our earlier observations and have even further elucidated the importance of stress relaxation in correcting for the effects of changes in blood volume on cardiac output. Results of this more recent study are shown in Figure 20–4, which shows the effects of rapidly expanding the blood volume of dogs with 500 ml. of either Tyrode's solution, whole blood, or dextran. Note that following the infusion of Tyrode's solution, the blood volume returned to near its normal level in approximately 80 minutes, this rapid reduction in blood volume being due to the fluid shift mechanisms discussed previously. Due to their greater colloid osmotic pressure, the whole blood and the dextran solutions remained within the vascular system for a much longer period of time. Following the infusion of whole blood, the blood volume was still approximately 17 per cent above control after 2 hours, and following the infusion of dextran, the blood volume was approximately 35 per cent above normal after 2 hours. Note, however, that the mean circulatory pressure and the cardiac output had returned to their normal levels 2 hours following the infusion, regardless of what type of solution was used to expand the blood volume. The substantial increase in blood volume with no increase in mean circulatory pressure shows that 2 hours after the infusion of whole blood, there was an expansion of the vasculature amounting to approximately 17 per cent of

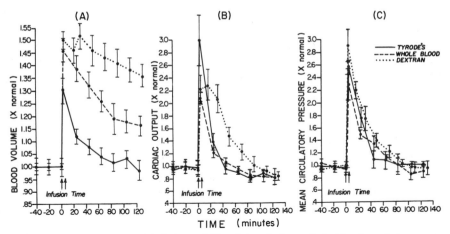

Figure 20–4. Effects of infusion of Tyrode's solution, whole blood, and dextran on (A) blood volume, (B) cardiac output, and (C) mean circulatory pressure. Vertical bars represent standard error of the mean. [From Prather (1969).]

its original volume, and 2 hours following the infusion of dextran solution, there was a 35 per cent expansion of the vascular system. Since at this time both the cardiac output and the arterial pressure (not shown) had returned to approximately their original level, and since reflex vascular dilatation is initiated by an increase in either arterial pressure or cardiac output, it is probable that no portion of this vascular expansion was due to nervous reflex dilatation. Rather, these results illustrate that the phenomenon of stress relaxation is a very powerful mechanism for returning cardiac output to its normal level following expansion of the blood volume. In fact, these results indicate that the stress relaxation compensatory mechanism is actually more powerful in compensating for the effects of blood volume changes on cardiac output than are the circulatory reflexes. However, a major difference in the function of the two mechanisms lies in the fact that the reflexes begin to act in approximately 4 to 5 seconds and reach their maximum activity in some 30 to 40 seconds, while the stress relaxation mechanism is only beginning within this period of time, and becomes maximally effective only over a period of 30 minutes to several hours. Therefore, the reflexes would be expected to cause almost immediate, partial compensation, while the stress relaxation mechanism would cause a more delayed, though more powerful, compensation.

When the blood volume is decreased, opposite effects occur. The mean systemic pressure at first falls very low because of the decreased blood volume, but over a period of a few minutes the vascular system seems to tighten down around the smaller quantity of blood, a phenomenon known as stress relaxation recovery. This increases the mean circulatory pressure back toward normal and partially compensates for the decreased cardiac output in the same way that stress relaxation compensates for the excess cardiac output following a blood volume increase.

Unfortunately, we need to know much more about the effects of stress relaxation and stress relaxation recovery as a compensatory mechanism in circulatory dynamics. We especially need to know *where* in the circulation stress relaxation occurs, because its degree seems to be much greater than can be accounted for by the veins alone (Porciuncula, 1964). Perhaps the liver, the spleen, or even the tissue capillary circulation all enter into the effect. A reason for believing that these other structures, rather than the veins, might play the major role in the stress relaxation mechanism is that the half-time of the effect in the whole body is perhaps 2 to 10 minutes (see Chapter 12), while that in the larger veins is less than one minute (Alexander, 1953).

Graphical Analysis of the Compensations That Occur Following a Massive Transfusion

The solid curves in Figure 20–5 illustrate normal cardiovascular dynamics, with normal equilibrium at point A. Then a sudden massive transfusion is given to the animal (about 20 per cent of its blood volume infused over a few seconds), causing the mean systemic pressure to rise from 7 mm. Hg to 16 mm. Hg. Simultaneously, the increased volume dilates the peripheral vessels and causes the resistance to venous return to decrease. Therefore, the venous return curve becomes changed to the one represented in the figure by the long dashes. During the first few seconds after this transfusion, the efficacy of the heart still has not changed. Therefore, the normal cardiac output curve still depicts the ability of the heart to pump blood. The new venous return curve equates with the normal cardiac output curve at point B, with a cardiac output of 13

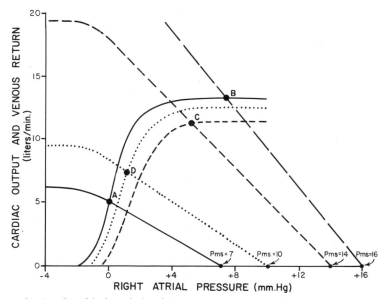

Figure 20–5. Graphical analysis of the acute effects on cardiac output of infusion of blood equal to 20 per cent of the blood volume (point B), followed by reflex compensation (point C), and followed after another 10 minutes by stress relaxation compensation (point D).

liters/minute and a right atrial pressure of 7.4 mm. Hg, which illustrates the immediate effect of cardiac output and right atrial pressure.

Within the next 4 to 5 seconds, however, the reflexes discussed above begin to take effect, reducing the effectiveness of the heart as a pump, as indicated by the short dashed cardiac output curve, and reducing the mean systemic pressure from 16 to 14 mm. Hg, thus resulting in another venous return curve as illustrated by the short dashed curve. These two short dashed curves equate with each other at point C, which represents the approximate effect one observes about 30 seconds after the massive transfusion, with a cardiac output of 11 liters per minute and a right atrial pressure of 5.3 mm. Hg.

During the ensuing 10 minutes, stress relaxation presumably occurs throughout the circulation, which further reduces the mean systemic pressure from approximately 14 to 10 mm. Hg. This causes the venous return curve to take the shape of the one illustrated by the dots. The cardiac output, as a result, falls, thus reducing the arterial pressure, which in turn reduces the reflex inhibition of the heart and allows the heart to become more powerful, as illustrated by the dotted cardiac output curve. These two dotted curves equilibrate with each other at point D, which shows a cardiac output of approximately 7 liters per minute and a right atrial pressure of 1.2 mm. Hg 10 minutes after the massive infusion.

Gradually, over a period of several hours, fluid loss from the circulation causes the mean systemic pressure to fall essentially back to normal, also returning the venous return curve to normal. As this occurs, the arterial pressure falls, and the inhibition of the heart ceases entirely, until finally the cardiac output curve is also back to normal. Thus, once again, the circulatory system is equilibrated at point A, with a normal cardiac output and a normal right atrial pressure.

Following hemorrhage, essentially the reverse effects occur; these will be discussed in more detail in the following chapter, which deals specifically with cardiac output in hemorrhagic and other types of shock.

EFFECT OF ORTHOSTATIC FACTORS ON CARDIAC OUTPUT

BASIC EFFECT OF THE ERECT POSTURE ON THE CIRCULATION

All investigators in the field of circulatory physiology recognize that when the body is in the erect position the weight of the blood in the circulation can cause very high hydrostatic pressures in the lower part of the body and research in "pooling" of the blood and reduced cardiac output (Lawrence, 1927; Sweeney, 1937; Mayerson, 1943; Hellerbrandt, 1943; Donald, 1953; Wang, 1960; Bevegard, 1960; Reeves, 1961b; Pentecost, 1963; Ward, 1966; Frohlich, 1967; Abel, 1968; Tarazi, 1970). In the present section we wish to evaluate the manner in which these hydrostatic pressures can affect cardiac output.

Figure 20–6 will be used to help explain mathematically the basic factors involved in orthostatic changes in cardiac output. Figure 20–6A shows a heart that at the moment is not pumping any blood at all and shows the circulatory system in a lying position. For the sake of this analysis, the circulatory system is represented by a cylinder 160 cm. in length (approximately the length of the human being), having a diameter of 5.75 cm. and holding 5000 ml. of blood. In the supine position, the mean pressure in the circulatory system, when the heart is not pumping any blood, is approximately 7 mm. Hg (which is equal to the mean systemic pressure) or 10 cm. of water. Thus, the pressure in the circulation in Figure 20–6A tending to push blood into the heart is shown to be 10 cm. of water.

Now let us turn the person to an upright position as shown in Figure 20–6B. Approximately 40 cm. of the circulatory system is now above the level of the heart, and approximately 120 cm. is below the heart. Furthermore, the vasculature of the circulation is highly distensible. If we apply the known average factor for the overall distensibility of the circulation, a value that has been determined by Richardson (1961), we can analyze

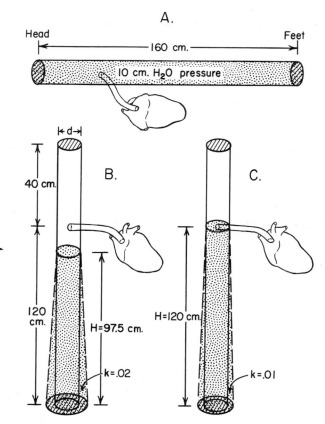

Figure 20–6. Schematic representation of the effect of orthostatic factors on cardiac output. Explanation in the text.

the effect of the shift from the supine to the standing position on translocation of the blood in the circulation. This normal distensibility factor for the entire circulation is 0.02 ml./ml./cm. of water pressure, which can readily be calculated from the relationship between blood volume and mean circulatory pressure as shown in Figure 12–6 of Chapter 12. Now we can calculate how much of the blood will shift from the upper part to the lower part of the circulation as illustrated in Figure 20–6B.

The volume of blood in each unit segment of the circulation is shown by the following expression (if we consider the density of blood to be 1):

$$\Delta V = \left(\frac{\pi d^2}{4} + \frac{k\pi d^2}{4} H \right) \Delta H \qquad (20\text{–}2)$$

in which V is volume, d is diameter of the cylinder representing the circulation in Figure 20–6, k is the distensibility factor in ml./ml./cm. of water pressure, and H is the height of the column of blood in cm. from the respective segment (ΔH) to the top surface of the blood. Now, if we integrate this, we find the relationship between the volume and total height of the column of blood in the upright position to be the following:

$$V = \frac{\pi d^2}{4} H + \frac{k\pi d^2}{8} H^2 \qquad (20\text{–}3)$$

and now solving for the total height of the column, we find the following relationship:

$$H = \frac{\sqrt{1 + \dfrac{8kV}{\pi d^2}} - 1}{k} \qquad (20\text{–}4)$$

If we study the significance of Formula 20–4, we can see the effect of different factors on the height of the blood column in the circulatory system in the upright position as follows:

Effect of Blood Volume

Formula 20–4 shows that the greater the blood volume, the greater will be the height of blood in the circulation, and, conversely, the less the blood volume, the lower will be the height of the column of blood.

Effect of Vascular Distensibility on the Height of the Column of Blood

The extent to which blood will settle to the lower part of the circulation is proportional to the degree of vascular distensibility. Thus, the greater the degree of distensibility, the lower becomes the height of the blood column.

Applying Formula 20–4 to the schematic circulation of Figure 20–6, we find in Figure 20–6B that when k is equal to the normal value of 0.02

ml./ml./cm. of water pressure, when the blood volume is 5000 ml., and when the basic undistended diameter of the system is 5.75 cm., the height of the blood column in the upright position would be 97.5 cm. One can readily see that this height of the blood column would not be sufficient for any of the blood to reach the level of the heart; consequently, no blood could flow into the heart under these conditions. However, one will also recognize two differences between this model and the normal circulatory system. First, the circulatory system is not a cylindrical column, and most of the blood of the body is actually located in blood vessels very near the heart. For this reason the degree of settling of blood to the lower part of the body is far less than that actually illustrated in Figure 20–6B. Second, there are compensatory mechanisms in the circulatory system that prevent this excessive settling of blood. Yet this analysis does show how the different factors interrelate with each other to cause decreased cardiac output when the body is in the erect position.

If we change the degree of distensibility of the circulation from the normal value of 0.02 ml./ml./cm. water pressure to a value of 0.01, we find now that the height of the blood column in the upright position will be 120 cm., as illustrated in Figure 20–6C. Since the heart is located 120 cm. above the lowest end of the column, blood now will barely enter the heart. If the degree of distensibility of the circulatory system decreases to a still lower factor, the height of the blood column will rise progressively above the level of the heart and will, therefore, allow progressively more and more blood to flow into the heart and consequently a greater and greater cardiac output.

To summarize, the greater the distensibility of the circulation, the greater will be the depressant effect of the erect position on cardiac output.

FACTORS THAT HELP TO COMPENSATE FOR POOLING OF BLOOD IN THE LOWER PART OF THE CIRCULATION. At least two different factors are known to help compensate for the tendency of blood to pool in the dependent areas of the body on standing: skeletal muscle contraction and autonomic reflexes.

When one stands, he immediately contracts essentially all the musculature of his body, and especially important in relation to the prevention of orthostatic depression of cardiac output is probably one's tendency to tighten the muscles of his legs and abdomen (Guyton, 1962b; Gilfoil, 1959). An increase in abdominal muscular contraction causes a direct increase in the pressure in the intra-abdominal vessels, and contraction of the leg muscles compresses the leg vessels sometimes to a pressure of 100 mm. Hg or more. Furthermore, intermittent muscular movements cause blood to flow upward along the veins as a result of the venous pump mechanism, which was described in Chapter 10 (Beecher, 1936a; 1936b; Bowers, 1945; Desliens, 1946; Pollack, 1949a, 1949b; Hickam, 1949; Walker, 1950; Hojensgard, 1952; Wang, 1962; Daly, 1965; Stegall, 1966). This keeps the hydrostatic pressures of the leg from rising nearly as high as would otherwise be the case. Indeed, Stegall (1966) has shown that movement of the leg in a standing man reduces the pressure in the veins of the ankles from over 90 mm. Hg to less than 10 mm. Hg. This same investigator estimated that during running, the contraction of the leg muscles contributed over 30 per cent of the energy required to circulate the blood.

The importance of muscular contraction in preventing orthostatic depression of cardiac output has been illustrated in many tilt-table studies in which the subjects have been kept in a state of complete relaxation during tilting to the erect position so that they will not contract their skeletal muscles. If one succeeds in preventing contraction of the skeletal muscles, sufficient blood will flow into the dependent areas of the body, as predicted by the analysis in Figure 20–6B, to cause fainting (Mateeff, 1932; Mayerson, 1939; Brogdon, 1940; Allen, 1945; Eichna, 1947; Hickam, 1951; Ward, 1966; Newberry, 1967). In other words, the upper level of the column of blood under these conditions is not high enough to allow blood to flow into the heart.

The second factor that helps to compensate for orthostatic depression of cardiac output is autonomic reflexes. Even normally, there is a tendency for the cardiac output to decrease about 20 to 40 per cent when one rises to the standing position (Lawrence, 1927; Sweeney, 1937; Mayerson, 1943; Hellerbrandt, 1943; Donald, 1954; Wang, 1960; Ward, 1966; Abel, 1968), and this effect undoubtedly would be much more severe if the reflexes (the same ones as those discussed above that compensate for decreased blood volume) should not become excited. The reflexes, however, increase the vascular tone throughout the body, which in effect decreases the basic undistended "diameter" of the circulation and perhaps also decreases the distensibility factor k in Equation 20–4 and thereby makes the height of the column of blood in the circulation higher than would otherwise be the case.

The autonomic and skeletal muscle compensatory mechanisms are both undoubtedly very important in normal compensations for orthostatic depression of cardiac output, though the exact quantitative value of each is as yet unknown. One of the particular reasons for believing both mechanisms to have major importance is that a person who has recently been completely sympathectomized has a tendency to faint upon first standing. This is analogous to the tilt-table experiments in normal persons under completely relaxed conditions, and it illustrates the value of the reflex increase in sympathetic tone to help prevent the orthostatic decrease in cardiac output. However, within a few months after the total sympathectomy, the person usually will not faint upon standing, illustrating that some development has taken place during the period of time to compensate automatically for the orthostatic tendency to depress the cardiac output. One could easily postulate that the skeletal muscle factor has simply become considerably more potent to take the place of the lost autonomic factor.

Studies on the autonomic factor in dogs indicate that the time required for it to develop fully is about 20 to 40 seconds. Obviously, if the skeletal muscle factor did not operate during the first few seconds after standing, almost everyone would faint before the autonomic factor could achieve its results. Therefore, even though the autonomic compensatory mechanism has received far more emphasis in the past than has the skeletal muscle mechanism, it is now apparent that the skeletal muscle mechanism is at least equally important (Gilfoil, 1959; Guyton, 1962b; Stegall, 1966).

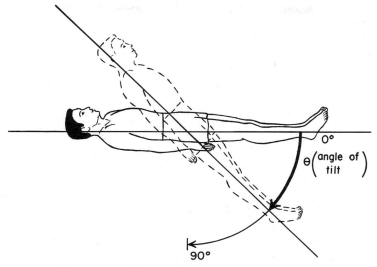

Figure 20–7. Schema showing the angle of body tilt.

Orthostatic Factors at Different Angles of Body Tilt

One can readily understand that the effects of hydrostatic pressure on the circulation vary at different angles of body tilt. Figure 20–7 illustrates the supine position as the 0 angle of tilt and the erect position as the 90 degree angle of tilt. The hydrostatic forces operating along the linear direction of the body change in proportion to the sine of angle theta. To calculate the effects of angulated position of the body on the hydrostatic pressures, Formula 20–4 can be altered to the following expression:

$$H' = \frac{\sqrt{1 + \dfrac{8k \sin \theta \ V}{\pi d^2}} - 1}{k \sin \theta} \tag{20–5}$$

in which H′ is the *length* of the column of blood from the feet to the level to which the blood vessels are filled. In other words, the hydrostatic pressure and the degree of distention of the vessels in the lower part of the body are directly proportional into the sine of the angle of tilt from the horizontal position.

Effect of Angular Acceleration on Orthostatic Depression of Cardiac Output

Angular acceleration intensifies the hydrostatic pressures at the different levels in the circulation (Newberry, 1967). For instance, a force of 2 g causes twice as much hydrostatic pressure as does the normal acceleration of gravity (1 g). Therefore, to utilize Formula 20–4 in predicting the effect of angular acceleration on orthostatic translocation of blood in the body, we can alter it as follows:

$$H = \frac{\sqrt{1 + \frac{8kgV}{\pi d^2}} - 1}{gk} \qquad (20\text{-}6)$$

in which g equals the normal acceleratory force of gravity.

GRAPHICAL ANALYSIS OF THE EFFECT OF ORTHOSTATIC FACTORS ON CARDIAC OUTPUT

A graphical analysis of the different orthostatic effects on cardiac output is essentially the same as that for any other factor which would decrease the mean systemic pressure. If we refer back to Figure 20-6, we will note that a basic condition for this figure was that the heart was not pumping blood. The mean force in the circulation pushing the blood back toward the heart when the heart is not pumping blood is equal to the mean systemic pressure. In the erect position, the mean force pushing the blood back toward the heart is equal to the difference between the level of the top of the column of blood in the circulation and the level of the heart itself. Therefore, this difference is equal to the "effective" mean systemic pressure. Thus, in Figure 20–6B, there is actually no force pushing blood into the heart, because the top of the blood column is beneath the level of the heart. In Figure 20–6C, the blood level is at the level of the heart, which would be an effective mean systemic pressure of zero. This still would cause no blood to flow into the heart. Compensatory factors, such as (1) compression of the vasculature by the abdominal muscles, (2) decrease in the distensibility factor k, or (3) increased blood volume—any one of these—will raise the height of the blood column above the level of the heart and cause a significant cardiac output. Thus, Figures 20–6B and 20–6C are comparable to low mean systemic pressures, and any condition in which the top of the blood column in the circulation is more than 10 cm. above the level of the heart would be comparable to an elevated mean systemic pressure.

Figure 20–8 illustrates by the solid curves a cardiac output analysis for the normal circulation with the equilibrium at point A. Tilting the relaxed person on a tilt-table to the upright or nearly upright position is likely to cause systemic circulatory conditions similar to those depicted by the dashed venous return curve, resulting from a reduced "effective" mean systemic pressure. The reduced cardiac output would then elicit circulatory reflexes, as described earlier in the chapter, and cause the cardiac output curve to rise to the dashed curve, thus establishing a new equilibrium at point B. Note that the cardiac output is at this point 1 liter per minute below normal, and the right atrial pressure has been reduced by approximately 1 mm. Hg.

The dotted curves of Figure 20–8 illustrate the approximate effect one would have with both a mild loss of blood plus a tilt to the upright position, showing a greatly reduced "effective" mean systemic pressure, a reflex in-

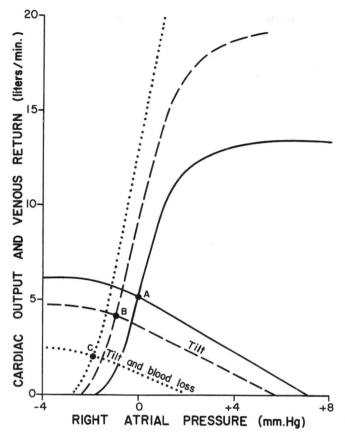

Figure 20–8. Graphical analysis of the effect of tilt (point B) and of tilt plus blood loss (point C) on cardiac output and right atrial pressure.

crease in pumping efficacy of the heart, and a cardiac output reduction to 2 liters/minute with a right atrial pressure reduction to minus 2 mm. Hg.

Obviously, the precise graphical analysis will depend upon (1) the degree of tilt, (2) the amount of blood loss, and (3) the extent of the compensatory factors. However, Figure 20–8 does illustrate the general pattern of changes one would expect from orthostatic factors affecting the cardiac output.

Chapter 21

CARDIAC OUTPUT IN CIRCULATORY SHOCK

A Definition of Circulatory Shock

Many physiologists believe there to be no single definition for circulatory shock because it has many different causes (Davis, 1949; Wiggers, 1950). However, circulatory shock always has one common denominator: The cardiac output is insufficient to supply the tissues of the body with their normal nutritive needs. Therefore, for the purpose of the discussion in the present chapter we can use the following definition of circulatory shock: *Circulatory shock is a state of the circulation in which tissues in widespread areas of the body are being damaged by nutritive insufficiency resulting from inadequate cardiac output.*

In the past several years, probably no other subject has been investigated more thoroughly than circulatory shock, and it has become apparent that nearly every system of the body is impaired to some degree by the inadequate cardiac output. Consequently, it is impossible to cover this subject thoroughly with the space of a single chapter, and emphasis will be placed only on those hemodynamic events which directly affect the cardiac output.

BASIC FACTORS THAT CAN INITIATE SHOCK

One can readily see that any condition which reduces the cardiac output can cause shock and that these conditions can be divided into two different categories, those which affect the peripheral circulation to reduce the cardiac output and those which affect the heart to reduce the cardiac output.

Peripheral Circulatory Factors That Can Result in Shock

The discussions in Chapters 12 and 13 pointed out that two particular circulatory factors, besides the functional state of the heart, are extremely

372

important in helping to determine the level of cardiac output. These are the *mean circulatory pressure* (Guyton, 1955b) and the *resistance to venous return* (Guyton, 1959b, 1961a, b). The lower the mean circulatory pressure or the greater the resistance to venous return, the less becomes the cardiac output. Therefore, a peripheral circulatory type of shock can result from either of these two factors.

TYPES OF SHOCK CAUSED BY LOW MEAN CIRCULATORY PRESSURE. The mean circulatory pressure, as was explained in Chapter 12, is actually a measure of the ratio of blood volume to capacitance of the circulation. If the blood volume is small in relation to the capacitance of the circulation, the mean circulatory pressure will be low. And if the blood volume is normal but the capacitance of the circulatory system is greater than normal, the mean circulatory pressure will also be low. Therefore, remembering these two possible means by which the mean circulatory pressure can be reduced, we can summarize some of the different possible causes of shock resulting from diminished mean circulatory pressure.

1. *Decreased blood volume,* such as occurs in hemorrhagic hypertension (Blalock, 1927; Werle, 1942; Wiggers, 1944b; Walcott, 1945; Ingraham, 1945; Opdyke, 1946; Remington, 1950a, b; Sapirstein, 1960; Handley, 1950; Crowell, 1955, 1958, 1959, 1961, 1962; Weale, 1958; Fine, 1963; Simeone, 1965; Shubin, 1969; and many others) or following loss of plasma in burns or trauma (Johnson, 1931; Blalock, 1933a; Ross, 1957; Clemedson, 1958; Wise, 1959; Clowes, 1960; Hershey, 1964; Shubin, 1969) obviously can decrease the mean circulatory pressure and thereby cause shock.

2. *Dehydration of the body,* with decreased extracellular fluid volume and diminished plasma volume, can also reduce the mean circulatory pressure and thereby contribute to the development of shock (Hardy, 1944; Shubin, 1969).

3. *Decreased vasomotor tone resulting from inhibition of the vasoconstrictor nerves or excitation of the vasodilator nerves* can cause the capacitance of the circulatory system to increase and, since the blood volume still remains normal, the mean circulatory pressure becomes greatly reduced, thus leading to shock (Barcroft, 1944, 1945; Weissler, 1957b).

4. *Vasodilatation resulting from anaphylactic shock, bacterial toxicity, nitrites, or other vascular paralytic agents* can also lead to a reduced mean circulatory pressure and thereby cause shock (Weiss, 1937; Wilkins, 1937, 1938; Chien, 1966a; Hinshaw, 1966; Solis, 1966; Spink, 1966; Tsagaris, 1967; Elsberry, 1969; and many others).

5. *Sudden enlargement of the vascular system* caused by removal of ascites, decreased skeletal muscular tone, removal of a large abdominal tumor, or any other condition that suddenly removes pressure from around the vascular tree can also reduce the mean circulatory pressure and result in shock. Indeed, simply tilting a relaxed person to the upright position often causes fainting, particularly after a bout of heavy exercise, this resulting from pooling of blood in the lower part of the body; if the experiment is continued long enough, serious shock can result (Mateeff, 1932, 1934; Mayerson, 1939; Brogdon, 1940; Allen, 1945; Eichna, 1947; Hickam, 1951). This is called "orthostatic" shock.

GRAPHICAL ANALYSIS OF THE DECREASED CARDIAC OUTPUT RESULTING FROM DECREASED MEAN CIRCULATORY PRESSURE. Figure 21-1 illustrates a graphical analysis of the changes in the circulatory system following severe acute hemorrhage. The very dark curves depict the function of the normal circulation, with equilibrium at point A, at a cardiac output of 5 liters per minute and right atrial pressure of 0 mm. Hg. If a large amount of blood is suddenly removed from the circulation, the mean circulatory pressure might be reduced immediately to only 1 mm. Hg. The venous return curve, therefore, would change to that illustrated by the very light solid curve at the bottom of the graph (Guyton, 1958d). If we assume that this occurred before any compensatory factors could result, the cardiac output curve would still remain normal. The new venous return curve and the normal cardiac output curve would equate at point B, which shows a cardiac output of approximately 0.6 liters per minute and a right atrial pressure of -1.3 mm. Hg.

Within 20 to 40 seconds after the acute bleeding, however, circulatory reflexes will have taken place, which will change both the venous return curve and the cardiac output curve. For instance, the sympathetic reflexes will cause the mean circulatory pressure to rise back toward normal;

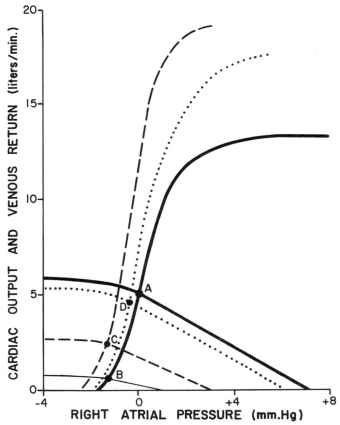

Figure 21-1. Shock caused by decreased mean systemic pressure; some of the compensatory effects that can help to overcome the shock are also shown.

therefore, the mean systemic pressure is shown to rise back to 3 mm. Hg, which is precisely the results found by Smith (unpublished observations), and the new venous return curve is now represented by the dashes. Simultaneously, reflexes to the heart make it a stronger pump so that the cardiac output curve now becomes that represented also by dashes (Regan, 1954; Sarnoff, 1954a). These two curves equate at point C, which shows that 20 to 40 seconds after removal of this large amount of blood, the cardiac output has returned to 2.5 liters per minute, and the right atrial pressure has now become −1.4 mm. Hg.

During the next 20 minutes to an hour, the stress relaxation recovery mechanism, which was discussed in the previous chapter, seems to compensate some for the reduced blood volume, and a reasonable amount of fluid may also be absorbed into the circulatory system through the capillaries to return the blood volume back part way toward normal. Therefore, a new pair of venous return and cardiac output curves becomes applicable, as shown by the dotted curves of Figure 21–1. The mean systemic pressure is shown to have risen back to 6 mm. Hg, and the heart is now shown to be only slightly stimulated by sympathetic reflexes because the cardiac output is almost back to normal. The new point of equilibrium is point D, with a cardiac output of 4.5 liters per minute and a right atrial pressure of −0.4 mm. Hg. Later in the chapter we will see that the animal does not always recover from the hemorrhagic hypotension, for sometimes a state of severe shock develops and the circulation deteriorates rather than recovers, as shown in Figure 21–1.

SHOCK CAUSED BY INCREASED RESISTANCE TO VENOUS RETURN. A classic example of shock caused by increased resistance to venous return is that which results from compression of the large veins entering the heart. For instance, positive intrathoracic pressure can compress the veins entering the chest, thereby increasing the resistance to venous return, and, if continued long enough, can result in shock. Likewise, compression of the inferior vena cava in the region of the liver, either during operative procedures or as a result of a tumor, can lead to shock simply because of increased resistance to venous return, which prevents adequate flow of blood from the peripheral vessels into the heart (Smith, 1952; Farber, 1954; Ohara, 1957). Finally, it has also been shown that a marked increase in blood viscosity can increase the resistance to venous return enough either to cause shock or at least to predispose to shock (Seligman, 1946; Crowell, 1959).

GRAPHICAL ANALYSIS OF THE EFFECT ON CARDIAC OUTPUT OF INCREASED RESISTANCE TO VENOUS RETURN. Figure 21–2 illustrates the manner in which an increase in resistance to venous return reduces cardiac output. The very dark curves represent the normal state of the circulation. Then, suddenly, the resistance to venous return is increased three fold. For the first few seconds after this has occurred, the cardiac output curve remains normal while the venous return curve is reduced to the lowest solid curve of the figure (Guyton, 1959b, 1961a). This curve equates with the normal cardiac output curve at point B, giving a cardiac output of 1.5 liters per minute and a right atrial pressure of −1 mm. Hg. However, within 20 to 40 seconds this very low cardiac output causes

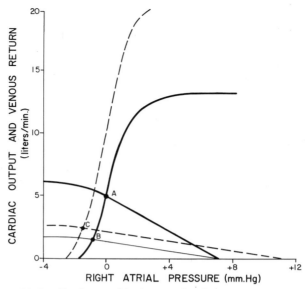

Figure 21–2. Shock caused by increased resistance to venous return.

circulatory reflexes which change both the venous return and the cardiac output curves, giving the two dashed curves. These curves illustrate an increase in the mean systemic pressure up to 11 mm. Hg and also a considerable increase in the ability of the heart to pump blood. These two curves equate at point C, with a cardiac output of 2.5 liters per minute and a right atrial pressure of -1.5 mm. Hg. Obviously, if a state such as this should continue for a long period of time, serious damage to the tissues of the body could result. Thus, a very great increase in resistance to venous return, such as can occur when the major veins entering the heart are compressed, can easily cause serious circulatory shock.

Cardiac Causes of Shock

Since cardiac output is determined by both peripheral and cardiac factors, any cardiac condition that reduces the ability of the heart to pump can result in shock equally as much as can factors that reduce the tendency of the blood to return to the heart. Among the different cardiac conditions that can cause shock are: acute myocardial damage resulting from coronary thrombosis, serious valvular heart disease, myocardial failure, cardiac tamponade, myocarditis, decompensated congenital heart disease, or any other factor that reduces the ability of the heart to pump blood. The effects of these conditions will be discussed in detail in Chapters 26 and 27, but for the time being we will give a simple analysis in Figure 21–3 to show how any one of them can cause shock.

In Chapter 9 it was pointed out that, regardless of what cardiac factor reduces the heart's ability to pump blood, the usual effect on the cardiac

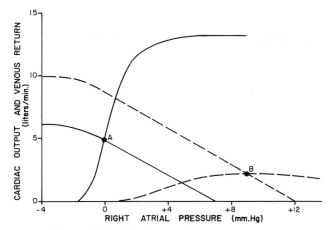

Figure 21-3. Shock caused by cardiac damage.

output curve is to shift it downward and to the right. The solid curves in Figure 21-3 represent the normal state and the dashed curves, the effect of serious cardiac debility. Let us assume, for instance, that the ability of the heart to pump blood becomes so poor and the cardiac output is reduced so low that circulatory reflexes become highly activated. And let us assume that even after activation of these reflexes, the ability of the heart to pump blood is still no greater than that represented by the dashed cardiac output curve. However, the circulatory reflexes elevate the mean systemic pressure to a level of 12 mm. Hg which causes the new venous return curve to become that represented also by a dashed curve. The two dashed curves equate with each other at point B, which shows the cardiac output to be 2 liters per minute and the right atrial pressure 9 mm. Hg. Thus, once again, we have a state of shock, this time not caused by a peripheral abnormality but simply by reduction in the ability of the heart to pump blood.

THE PROGRESSIVE STAGE OF SHOCK

Most physiologists divide shock into two separate stages representing different degrees of severity called *compensated shock* and *progressive shock*. Compensated shock can also be called "recovering shock" and progressive shock can be called "degenerating shock." That is, if the shock is not too severe, the animal or human being will recover automatically. On the other hand, if the shock becomes more severe than a certain critical degree, the shock itself breeds more shock, resulting in progressively more severe shock until death ensues. We will discuss in this section the factors that determine whether the shock will be of the recovering type (compensated shock) or of the degenerating type (progressive shock).

The Critical Point Between Recovering Shock and Progressive Shock

Figure 21–4 illustrates results obtained from a series of experiments in 36 dogs divided into six separate groups, with six animals in each group (Guyton, 1961c). The animals in the first group were bled until their control arterial pressures fell to an average of 80 mm. Hg; the average course of the arterial pressure during the ensuing 4 to 6 hours is illustrated by curve number 1 of the figure. The next 6 animals were bled until the arterial pressure fell to an average of 63 mm. Hg; the next six to an average of 49 mm. Hg; the next six to an average of 44 mm. Hg; the next six to 35 mm. Hg; and the final six to 17 mm. Hg. The respective arterial pressure curves for these animals during the ensuing few hours are shown in the figure. In general, all the animals lived if they were bled to arterial pressures above 47 mm. Hg, whereas those bled to pressures below 47 mm. Hg died. These experiments illustrate that an animal can be bled to a rather critical arterial pressure level and still recover, but beyond this he will die. On studying Figure 21–4, one sees that death, when it occurs, is not instantaneous but instead that the arterial pressure falls gradually over a period of several hours. In other words, the animals represented by the lower three curves were all in *progressive shock*, while the animals represented by the top three curves were all in *recovering shock*. Though the cardiac outputs were not measured in the particular animals studied in these experiments, more recently we have shown, using a continuous cardiac output recorder, that this same general pattern occurs also for cardiac output (Stone and Guyton, unpublished observations). That is, if the animals are bled below a critical cardiac output level, they go into progressive shock, and the circulation eventually deteriorates to the stage of death, whereas, if the cardiac output is above the critical level by even a few milliliters per minute, recovery will eventually take place.

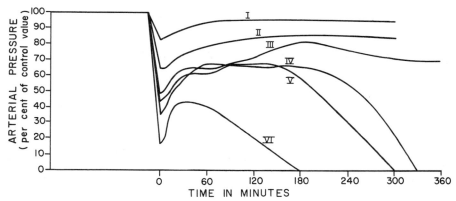

Figure 21–4. Effect of different degrees of bleeding on the subsequent course of the systemic arterial pressure. Each curve represents average effects from six different animals. All animals represented by the first three curves recovered, while all animals represented by the last three curves died. [Reprinted from Guyton and Crowell (1961c).]

The point of this discussion, therefore, is that a cardiac output difference of only a few milliliters or an arterial pressure difference of only a few millimeters of mercury can determine whether an animal in shock will proceed in a progressive downhill direction or in an uphill direction. Furthermore, an animal very near the critical balance point may go for many hours, with arterial pressure or cardiac output changes so slight that one cannot determine whether recovery will take place or whether the shock will progress to death. Even the slightest alteration in the circulation during this period can make the animal go either way; a few milliliters of bleeding will cause progression of the shock or a few milliliters of blood given by transfusion or other therapy will make the animal enter the recovery cycle, which usually leads to complete recovery within a few hours once it starts.

In the following few sections, we will attempt to give the reasons for this critical balance between the recovering type of shock and the progressive type of shock.

Positive Feedback as the Cause of Progression in Shock

It was pointed out above that severe shock breeds more shock; this type of effect is called positive feedback (Guyton, 1961c). That is, severe shock affects the circulation itself in such a way to make the shock still more severe. Then the more severe shock causes more effect on the circulation to make the shock still more severe. Thus, each increase in the degree of shock causes another increase, and after many cycles of such feedback the shock becomes so intense that death ensues.

CIRCULATORY DETERIORATION RESULTING FROM POSITIVE FEEDBACK DURING SHOCK. At least five different types of positive feedback can occur in shock to breed more shock. These are the following:

1. As shock becomes more severe, nutrition to the brain becomes reduced, and eventually the vasomotor and respiratory centers begin to fail (Beck and Dontas, 1955; Rothe, 1963). Failure of the vasomotor center reduces vascular tone, which allows the mean systemic pressure to fall; this in turn causes the cardiac output to fall to a still lower level. Respiratory failure results in decreased oxygenation of the tissues throughout the body, and this too can cause increased circulatory deterioration, leading to increased degrees of shock. Respiratory failure occurs only very late in shock and therefore contributes only to the terminal phases of progressive shock.

2. In severe shock, even the blood vessels themselves will not receive adequate nutrition. Thus, in addition to the failure of the vasomotor center itself, this inadequate nutrition of the blood vessels can result in a reduced vascular tone, a reduced mean circulatory pressure, and a further reduction in the cardiac output. It is not certain which of these two factors, vasomotor center failure or vascular deterioration, is more important in causing peripheral vascular failure in severe shock, although it is certain that such failure occurs (Alexander, 1955; Chien 1958; Mellander, 1963; Hershey, 1964; Rothe and Selkurt, 1964; Rothe, 1966; Longnecker and Abel, 1969; Smith, unpublished observations). The im-

portance of this peripheral vascular failure in reducing cardiac output during severe shock may be seen in the results of the study by Smith (unpublished observations), who showed that dogs in very severe shock had mean circulatory pressures of less than 50 per cent of normal, even though their blood volumes were completely normal.

3. In addition to its effect on vascular tone, the diminished cardiac output causes the peripheral vasculature to fail in such a manner that substantial quantities of fluid are actually lost from the blood into the extravascular spaces. Possible explanations for this loss of blood volume during shock are the following: (a) The diminished vascular nutrition may lead to an increased capillary permeability, thus causing an increased capillary filtration of fluid (Landis, 1934; Fell, 1966). (b) A decreased precapillary resistance with a concomitant increase in postcapillary resistance may occur in shock. This would result in an increase in capillary pressure and an increase in the capillary filtration of fluid, even with no increase in capillary permeability (Mellander and Lewis, 1963; Lundgren, 1964; Hollenberg, 1970a, 1970b). (c) A unique mechanism of fluid loss is seen in the small intestine during shock (Porciuncula and Crowell, 1963; Bounous, 1966; Glenert and Pedersen, 1967; Smith, 1967c; Sutherland 1968; Cook, 1971). Loss of whole blood into the intestinal lumen often occurs, and this is believed to be due to both an enzymatic destruction of the gut mucosa and a rise in intestinal capillary pressure caused by portal congestion.

Regardless of the precise mechanisms involved, it is obvious that loss of blood volume would cause reduction in the mean systemic pressure and further decrease in the cardiac output.

4. Blood flow through some of the vascular beds becomes so sluggish during shock that blood begins to clot in the small vessels (Crowell, 1955). Obviously, this can lead to still further sluggishness of blood flow and consequently to still more severe shock. How important this factor is in the progression of shock is yet to be determined, but Crowell's studies indicate that anticoagulants can protect at least to some extent against progression of shock.

5. Another very important factor that causes shock to progress is cardiac deterioration resulting from positive feedback (Wiggers, 1942, 1945, 1947a; Wegria, 1943; Meneely, 1946; Rodes, 1949; Burdette, 1950; Edwards, 1954; Regan, 1954; Hackel, 1955; Hift, 1958; Caliava, 1959; Crowell, 1961b, 1962, 1965, 1969; Gomez, 1964; Glaviano, 1965; Lefer, 1966; Siegel, 1970; Bethea, 1972). The positive feedback which results in progressive cardiac deterioration operates in the following manner: Many different studies have shown that the ability of the heart to pump blood is highly dependent on the transport of oxygen, and perhaps other nutrients, to the heart by the coronary vessels (Case, 1954, 1955; Sugimoto, 1968, Beneken, 1969, Abel and Reis, 1970). Thus, if the coronary blood flow decreases, the pumping ability of the heart also decreases. Furthermore, if the degree of shock becomes severe enough, the shock itself can decrease the blood flow through the coronary system sufficiently to cause the heart to begin to fail. As the heart fails, the cardiac output falls still more, resulting in further nutritive deficiency in the myocardium. Conse-

quently, the heart fails still more, the cardiac output falls more, and the cycle continues again and again, resulting in positive feedback that eventuates in death of the animal.

Figure 21–5 illustrates the probable basic steps in this positive feedback cycle that cause deterioration of the heart in shock. The figures shows that after hemorrhage the cardiac output falls to a low level and oxygen transport to the tissues becomes reduced. The tissues then begin developing an oxygen debt (Crowell, 1964; Jones, 1968a), which probably leads to additional, as yet unknown, intermediate effects that in turn cause cardiac failure. This leads to further decrease in oxygen transport, and the cycle repeats itself again and again, causing the cardiac failure to become progressively more severe.

Although the cardiac deterioration observed in shock is believed by most investigators to be due to a reduced coronary blood flow, some persons feel that the cardiac depression is caused by a toxic substance released from the hypoxic tissues of the body (Brand and Lefer, 1966; Lefer, 1967, 1970, 1971; Glenn, 1970, 1971; Lovett, 1971; Wangensteen, 1971). This toxic substance has been termed the myocardial depressant factor (MDF), and a positive feedback mechanism involving MDF would operate as follows: Any factor initiating a severe reduction in cardiac output would cause the various tissues of the body to become hypoxic. This tissue hypoxia would result in MDF being released from the tissues. MDF is then transported by the blood to the heart, where it in some way depresses cardiac contractility, which results in an even more reduced cardiac output, a greater degree of tissue hypoxia, and the release of more MDF from the tissues. Thus, according to this scheme, cardiac contractile strength would be progressively diminished until the heart fails completely.

Later in the chapter, in the discussion of "irreversibility of shock," we will present experimental data showing that the pumping ability of the heart decreases markedly during the progressive stage of shock and

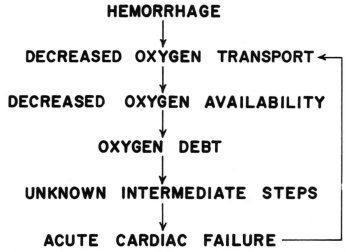

Figure 21–5. Sequence of the positive feedback mechanism that causes cardiac deterioration in shock. [Reprinted from Guyton and Crowell (1961c).]

that this is one very important contributing factor to the progression of shock.

Negative Feedback as a Deterrent to the Progression of Shock

In many chapters of this book we have discussed the compensatory mechanisms that tend to return the cardiac output toward normal when it becomes abnormal. All these compensatory mechanisms are negative feedback processes (Guyton, 1961c). For instance, the pressoreceptor reflex, one of the most important of all the compensatory mechanisms, operates in the following manner: If the arterial pressure falls too low, the number of impulses transmitted by the pressoreceptors becomes reduced; this in turn reduces the inhibitory effect of these impulses on the sympathetic centers of the brain and thereby allows massive discharge of sympathetic impulses throughout the body. At the same time, the parasympathetic fibers to the heart are inhibited. As a result of both the sympathetic and parasympathetic effects, the heart becomes a much stronger pump. Also, the sympathetic impulses to the peripheral circulation increase the mean systemic pressure and the total peripheral resistance. As a consequence, the cardiac output and arterial pressure rise back toward normal. In other words, the initiating effect, a decrease in pressure, results in an increase in pressure. That is, the response is *negative* to the initiating factor.

Two other negative feedback compensatory mechanisms which help to prevent the progression of shock are: (1) the stress-relaxation recovery mechanism in which a decrease in mean circulatory pressure causes the blood vessel tone to increase. The increased tone, in turn, causes the mean circulatory pressure to rise back toward normal. Thus, a fall in mean circulatory pressure is followed by a rise in mean circulatory pressure back toward normal, the response being *negative* to the original effect. (2) the capillary fluid shift mechanism also provides a negative feedback compensatory mechanism. That is, if the blood volume falls very low, the capillary pressure eventually falls very low, and fluid is pulled osmotically into the blood through the capillaries, resulting in an increase in blood volume. Here again, a fall is followed by an increase, a response that is *negative* to the initiating effect.

These negative feedback mechanisms all operate in opposition to the different positive feedbacks discussed above that tend to cause circulatory deterioration. If the negative feedback is greater than the positive feedback, one would expect recovery rather than deterioration of the circulation. However, to be more precise in determining whether the animal will recover or deteriorate, we need to analyze mathematically the relationship of positive feedback to negative feedback.

Mathematical Analysis to Determine Whether Recovery or Progression Will Occur in Shock

MATHEMATICAL ANALYSIS OF POSITIVE FEEDBACK. Before attempting to analyze whether an animal in shock will progress to more serious

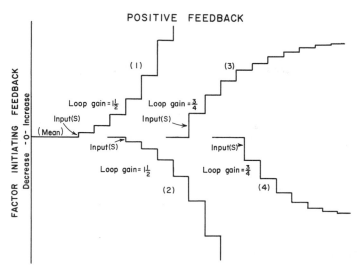

Figure 21-6. Graphical representation of positive feedback. In curves 1 and 2 the loop gain is greater than 1, and in curves 3 and 4 the loop gain is less than 1, illustrating that the total accumulative effect is infinite when the gain is greater than 1 but is finite when the gain is less than 1. [Reprinted from Guyton and Crowell (1961).]

shock or will recover, we need first to reduce the concepts of positive and negative feedback to mathematical terms. Figure 21–6 illustrates different types of positive feedback. Curve 1 shows positive feedback in a positive direction. Let us assume that we have some factor that is normally controlled to a mean value of 0. However, a sudden change from the mean occurs, which is called in Figure 21–6 the "input" and is designated by the symbol "S," which stands for the input stimulus. In Curve 1 we assume that the positive feedback has a "loop gain" of $1\frac{1}{2}$. In other words, the input causes a feedback $1\frac{1}{2}$ times as great as the input and in the same direction as the input. Thus, after one cycle of feedback, a second effect occurs another $1\frac{1}{2}$ times as great as the initial input effect. The second effect then causes another cycle of positive feedback, and the cycles continue on indefinitely. Thus, after each cycle of feedback, the total cumulative effect becomes progressively greater and greater, as illustrated by Curve 1 until finally, if the loop gain remains $1\frac{1}{2}$, the total effect will be infinite.

Curve 2 shows exactly the same effect but in a negative direction. Here the input is negative, and the positive feedback causes a further negative effect $1\frac{1}{2}$ times the input. The second cycle of feedback causes an effect $1\frac{1}{2}$ times the previous effect, and after many cycles of such feedback the total effect in the negative direction eventually becomes infinite in that direction.

There is a very marked difference between having a loop gain of greater than 1 and having a loop gain of less than 1, which is borne out by Curves 3 and 4 in Figure 21–6. In these two curves the inputs are relatively great but the loop gain is only $\frac{3}{4}$. Therefore, the effect of the first cycle of positive feedback is considerably less than the input, and the effect of the next cycle is still less. Consequently, the effect of the feedback will eventually die out. In other words, when the loop gain is less than 1, the effect is not infinite but instead is some finite value.

Mathematically, one can express positive feedback by the algebraic series as follows:

$$\text{Total response} = S + SG_p + SG_p^2 + \cdots \cdots + SG_p^\infty \qquad (21\text{--}1)$$

This is an infinite series which is divergent for values of positive loop gain (G_p) greater than 1 and convergent for values less than 1. In other words, if the gain is greater than 1, the total response becomes infinite, whereas if the gain is less than 1, the total response is some finite value, illustrating a very critical difference that occurs in the total response when the gain changes very minutely from slightly below 1 to slightly above 1.

Formula 21–1 can be algebraically reduced to the following formula:

$$\text{Total response} = \frac{S\,(G_p^\infty - 1)}{G_p - 1} \qquad (21\text{--}2)$$

If we substitute in this formula a value for G greater than 1, it becomes

$$\text{Total response} = \frac{S\,(\infty - 1)}{G_p - 1} = \infty \qquad (21\text{--}3)$$

From this, one can see that positive feedback with a loop gain greater than 1 will lead to a vicious cycle that eventuates in an infinite response.

Yet if we substitute in Formula 21–2 a gain of less than 1, the formula becomes

$$\text{Total response} = \frac{S\,(0 - 1)}{G_p - 1} = \frac{S}{1 - G_p} \qquad (21\text{--}4)$$

which shows that the effect does not continue on to an infinite response when the positive feedback gain is less than 1.

MATHEMATICAL ANALYSIS OF NEGATIVE FEEDBACK. Negative feedback causes a reduction in the input stimulus rather than an exacerbation. This effect is illustrated in Figure 21–7, which shows, first, a factor being controlled to a mean value and then a sudden input stimulus that changes the factor to some value away from the mean value. The negative feedback then causes this to return toward the mean level.

The mathematical analysis of negative feedback is precisely the same as that for positive feedback except that a negative gain is substituted in Formula 21–1 above, giving the following series:

$$\text{Total response} = S + S\,(- G_n) + S\,(- G_n)^2 + \cdots \cdots + S\,(- G_n)^\infty \quad (21\text{--}5)$$

which is the same as the following:

$$\text{Total response} = S - SG_n + SG_n^2 - SG_n^3 + SG_n^4 + \cdots \cdots + S\,(- G_n)^\infty \qquad (21\text{--}6)$$

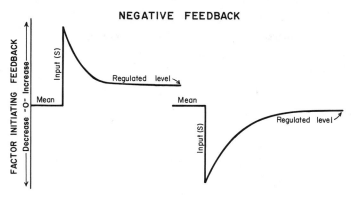

Figure 21–7. Compensatory nature of negative feedback. [Reprinted from Guyton and Crowell (1961c).]

This formula in turn can be reduced to the following simple expression:

$$\text{Total response} = \frac{S}{1 + G_n} \tag{21-7}$$

INTERACTION OF POSITIVE AND NEGATIVE FEEDBACK MECHANISMS IN DETERMINING WHETHER SHOCK WILL PROGRESS OR PROCEED TO RECOVERY. From the above analysis we see that positive feedback will cause a vicious cycle only when the loop gain of the feedback system is greater than plus 1. In the case of cardiac deterioration, for instance, a gain greater than 1 could be explained as follows: If an initial fall in arterial pressure causes sufficient damage to the heart that the subsequent fall in arterial pressure is greater than the initial fall, then the gain will be greater than 1. However, if the subsequent fall in pressure is less than the initial fall, the gain of the loop will be less than 1. Only when the gain is greater than 1 will an infinite positive feedback effect ensue.

Negative feedback is opposite to positive feedback in that it tends to reduce abnormalities in the controlled factor rather than to enhance them. Thus, when the arterial pressure and cardiac output fall below normal, all the negative feedback compensatory mechanisms, including the reflexes, the stress-relaxation recovery mechanism, and fluid shifts, will oppose the positive feedback. Therefore, we need now to combine our mathematical analyses of positive and negative feedbacks to determine the net, simultaneous effect of both these feedbacks on the circulation during shock. The following formula gives this analysis:

$$\text{Total response} = S + S\,(G_p - G_n) + S\,(G_p - G_n)^2 + \cdots + S\,(G_p - G_n)^\infty \tag{21--8}$$

in which G_p is positive gain and G_n is negative gain. This formula reduces to

$$\text{Total response} = \frac{S\,[(G_p - G_n)^\infty - 1]}{(G_p - G_n) - 1} \tag{21-9}$$

And when $G_p - G_n$ is greater than 1, Formula 21–9 reduces to

$$\text{Total response} = \frac{S(\infty - 1)}{(G_p - G_n) - 1} = \infty \qquad (21\text{–}10)$$

But when $G_p - G_n$ is less than 1, Formula 21–9 reduces to

$$\text{Total response} = \frac{S}{1 - (G_p - G_n)} \qquad (21\text{–}11)$$

APPLICATION OF THE ABOVE ANALYSIS TO SHOCK. To understand the significance of this mathematical analysis we need to know some of the precise values of the different positive and negative feedback gains. In the early phases of progressive shock, a positive feedback that is of particular significance is the one affecting the heart itself (see the discussion earlier in the chapter). At arterial pressure levels of around 100 mm. Hg, the gain of this positive feedback is very slight, probably in the order of 0.02 to 0.1, because a moderate *change* in coronary perfusion pressure at this pressure level hardly affects cardiac function (Case, 1954, 1955; Sugimoto, 1968). However, on the basis of a series of hemorrhage experiments, we have estimated that the gain rises to about 1 when the arterial pressure falls to approximately 50 mm. Hg (Guyton, 1961c; Sugimoto, 1968), and, when the arterial pressure falls below 50 mm. Hg, the gain rises to progressively greater than 1, probably reaching 2 to 3 by the time the arterial pressure has fallen to 40 mm. Hg and reaching even considerably higher values at pressures of 30 and 20 mm. Hg. The reason that the very high gains occur at these low pressures is that the pumping force of the heart becomes highly dependent, at low perfusion pressures, on the exact level of the perfusion pressure (Case, 1954). Therefore, a very slight fall in coronary perfusion pressure can set off a marked positive feedback.

Another positive feedback mechanism which occurs in shock is the one by which fluid is lost from the blood and the blood volume is consequently reduced. Thus, in severe shock, the pooling of blood in the systemic vasculature, the increase in capillary permeability, and possibly other factors cause an increase in the capillary filtration of fluid. This obviously reduces the blood volume, decreases the mean systemic pressure, and increases the severity of the shock. However, this positive feedback mechanism probably plays a minor role, since even in very severe shock, the blood volume is reduced by only approximately 10 per cent. Furthermore, fluid is lost from the blood only during the very late stages of shock; indeed, in the earlier stages of shock, fluid is actually absorbed by the capillaries, and this mechanism, therefore, has a negative gain rather than a positive gain early in shock.

In the case of the negative feedback mechanisms, the pressoreceptor reflex has a gain at 100 mm. Hg mean pressure of approximately 2 (Scher, 1962; Hatakeyama, 1961). However, the gain of this reflex becomes almost 0 once the arterial pressure has fallen below 50 mm. Hg (Heymans, 1958).

The negative feedback gain of the stress relaxation recovery mechanism might be as great as 3 to 4 even at pressure levels of 50 mm. Hg, though this response has not been studied adequately enough to talk intelligently about it. However, if the blood volume continues to diminish, or if other factors causing shock continue to progress, the stress relaxation recovery mechanism reaches its limit and thereafter loses all its gain.

The fluid shift mechanism has a very high negative gain during the early stages of shock, but, as pointed out earlier, this mechanism actually fails during the later stages of shock.

Another very important negative feedback mechanism which becomes activated when arterial pressure is reduced to very low levels is the central nervous system ischemic response. The average gain of this mechanism in dogs is approximately 7.7 (Sagawa, 1961a, 1967b). However, it is believed that the gain of this powerful mechanism is reduced to approximately zero in very severe shock. One reason for believing this is the following: The central nervous system ischemic response normally has a very powerful effect on the mean systemic pressure. Elicitation of the reflex can increase the mean systemic pressure to as high as two and one-half times normal (Richardson and Fermoso, 1964). Smith (unpublished observations) has recently demonstrated that the gain of the system regulating the mean systemic pressure is substantially reduced in severe shock. Thus, under normal conditions the gain of this system was approximately 3, but in very severe shock the gain had fallen to approximately zero.

Therefore, in severe shock the gains that need to be considered most seriously are the negative gains of the pressoreceptor reflex and the central nervous system ischemic reflex, and the positive gain of cardiac deterioration. When the arterial pressure is reduced to very low levels, the negative gains of the pressoreceptor system and the central nervous system ischemic reflex are reduced to essentially zero, while the positive gain of the cardiac deterioration has now risen to 1 or higher. Thus, we see that the positive feedback has now become greater than the negative feedback by a factor of 1. Therefore, at arterial pressures below 50 mm. Hg, a vicious cycle of deterioration takes place, whereas at pressure levels above 50 mm. Hg, the vicious cycle of deterioration should not take place, but, indeed, recovery should ensue. Referring back to Figure 21–4, we see that these are essentially the result one finds in shock.

CARDIAC OUTPUT IN THE IRREVERSIBLE STAGE OF SHOCK

Definition of Irreversible Shock

After shock has progressed long enough, transfusion or any other type of therapy becomes incapable of saving the life of the patient or animal. Therefore, the subject is then to be in the *irreversible stage of shock.* Figure 21–8 shows the initial effect of acute hemorrhage on cardiac output and the typical changes in cardiac output during the progressive stage

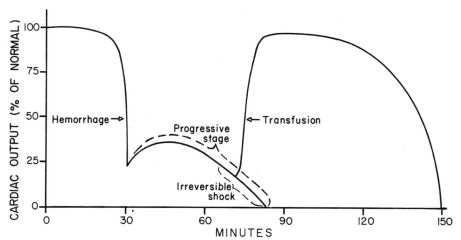

Figure 21–8. Progressive deterioration of cardiac output during the progressive stage of shock following severe hemorrhage, and failure of transfusion to effect permanent recovery once the irreversible stage of shock has been reached.

of shock down to death. If a transfusion is given to an animal in the early phases of the progressive stage of shock, the arterial pressure rises very rapidly back toward normal, and the animal eventually recovers. However, once the circulatory system has deteriorated beyond a certain critical point, transfusion or any other type of therapy will not save the life of the animal even though for temporary periods of time transfusion can often return the cardiac output and arterial pressure all the way to normal, as illustrated in Figure 21–8 by the curve labeled "transfusion" (Wiggers, 1945; Crowell, 1962). That is, the heart is often still capable of pumping large quantities of blood if sufficient blood is made available to the input side of the heart. However, some of the intrinsic factors of the heart have already become so damaged that the heart continues to deteriorate until complete failure ensues. Thus, one is often completely fooled by the return of normal cardiac output or normal arterial pressure following transfusion, for this may be of only temporary benefit to the animal.

Association of the Irreversible Stage of Shock with Oxygen Debt

Crowell and Smith (1964) have recently demonstrated that there is a high degree of correlation between the amount of oxygen debt that an animal builds up during shock and the onset of the irreversible stage of shock. That is, because of poor circulation of blood, the tissues of the body begin immediately in shock to suffer an oxygen deficit. If the shock is very severe, this oxygen debt builds up very rapidly, whereas if the shock is not so severe, the oxygen debt builds up very slowly. Regardless of how rapidly the oxygen debt builds up, when it reaches an average value of approximately 120 ml. of oxygen per kilogram of body weight, the animal will have reached the irreversible stage of shock (the value

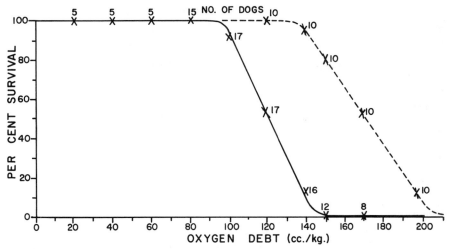

Figure 21-9. Survival rates of dogs following various degrees of oxygen debt in hemorrhagic shock without digitalization (solid curve), and after digitalization with strophanthin (dashed curve). The numbers represent the number of dogs in each group. (Courtesy of Dr. J. W. Crowell.)

is higher than this when the heart is digitalized, as will be discussed later). Figure 21-9 shows Crowell's results, illustrating by the solid curve that essentially all nondigitalized dogs in shock with oxygen debts less than 100 ml./kg. will survive following adequate transfusion, and essentially all with oxygen debts above 150 ml/kg. will die, with an average LD-50 of approximately 120 ml./kg. oxygen debt.

The results of Crowell and Smith (1964) were confirmed by Jones (1968a), who demonstrated that when dogs were hemorrhaged, the time required by the animals to reach the irreversible stage of shock was directly related to the time required for an oxygen deficit of 120 ml. per kg. to build up. Thus, animals in which the LD-50 oxygen debt built up slowly required greater lengths of time to reach the irreverisble stage of shock, while animals in which the LD-50 oxygen debt built up rapidly reached the irreversible stage of shock much more rapidly.

When an animal has incurred a lethal amount of oxygen debt, treatment by transfusion may cause the heart to pump a normal output for as long as 30 minutes to an hour, and even part of the oxygen debt may be repaid, but, unfortunately, by this time so much damage has resulted that the oxygen debt cannot be repaid rapidly enough to prevent the downhill trend toward death.

Cardiac Failure as the Cause of the Irreversible Stage of Shock

Other studies by Crowell have demonstrated that proper use of transfusion can correct any problem of venous return even in the irreversible stage of shock (Crowell, 1961b, 1962). Despite this, all possible therapeutic measures cannot make the heart continue to pump adequate

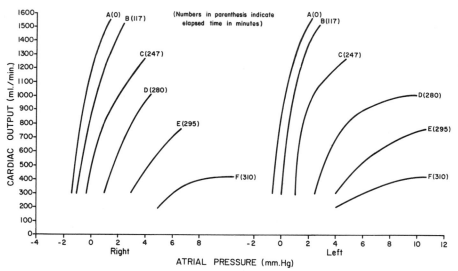

Figure 21–10. Progressive deterioration of the output curves in the progressive stage of shock. The shock was caused by bleeding the animal until the arterial pressure fell to 30 mm. Hg, at which level the pressure was held for the duration of the experiment. The numbers on the curve represent the time in minutes from the initial hemorrhage. [Reprinted from Crowell and Guyton (1962).]

quantities of blood, once irreversible changes have begun, to cause recovery of the animal.

The deterioration of the heart in the irreversible stage of shock was demonstrated in several different ways: First, at the point at which irreversibility began, the atrial pressures also showed a concomitant rise, and, even when sufficient blood was infused into the animal to raise both the right and left atrial pressures as high as 30 to 50 mm. Hg, the heart still could not pump an adequate blood flow. This finding showed that the venous return under these conditions was many times more satisfactory than normally so that the cause of the circulatory deterioration was definitely cardiac failure rather than depressed venous return. In other words, regardless of the original initiating cause of the shock, which might well have been blood loss, trauma, dehydration, or another cause, the final deterioration of the heart that occurs in the irreversible stage of shock seems to be the principal factor that prevents the recovery.

Another method by which Crowell demonstrated cardiac failure in the irreversible stage of shock was to record, using a continuous cardiac output recording apparatus, the actual ventricular output curves during the different stages of shock (Crowell, 1962). Figure 21–10 illustrates these recordings, showing, first, normal ventricular output curves (curves A) and then two other sets of curves later in the progressive stage of shock (curves B and C). The last three curves for each ventricle were recorded after the irreversible period of shock had been reached. Note that these curves keep shifting to the right and downward, illustrating serious deterioration of the heart as the shock progresses, and particularly after the irreversible stage has set in. Similar depression of the cardiac output curve in shock has been recently observed by Bethea and coworkers (1972).

Delay of the Irreversible Stage of Shock by Digitalization

In the preceding few paragraphs, we have discussed the fact that cardiac failure is one of the essential causes of the irreversible stage of shock. If this is true, then digitalization, which usually increases the strength of a seriously failing heart, should be beneficial in delaying the stage of irreversibility in shock. This effect has been definitely demonstrated by Crowell (1961a).

Figure 21–9 illustrates by the dashed curve at the right the survival of dogs at different levels of oxygen debt during shock after strophanthin had been given. From this, one can see that, if the heart is digitalized, the animal can withstand a considerably higher degree of oxygen debt and still survive than is the case without digitalization. These results substantiate the fact that cardiac failure is one of the most important occurrences in the irreversible stage that prevents recovery from shock.

GRAPHICAL ANALYSIS OF PROGRESSIVE AND IRREVERSIBLE SHOCK

Figure 21–11 illustrates a sequential graphical analysis of the different stages of shock following severe hemorrhage. The very dark curves repre-

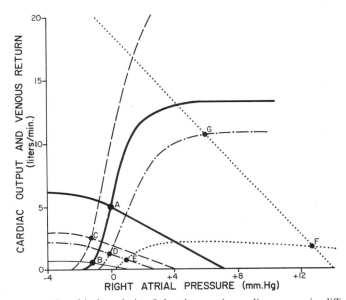

Figure 21–11. Graphical analysis of the changes in cardiac output in different stages of shock, showing also the failure of transfusion to revive the animal once the irreversible stage of shock has been reached.

sent an analysis for the normal circulatory conditions. Then, suddenly, the animal is bled very severely so that its mean systemic pressure falls to 1 mm. Hg and its venous return curve falls to the very light solid curve at the bottom of the graph. During the first few seconds after this bleeding, the heart is still capable of pumping blood in a relatively normal fashion. Therefore, the new curve equates with the cardiac output curve at point B, showing a cardiac output of about 0.6 liters per minute.

After reflexes and stress relaxation recovery have caused compensation for 10 to 15 minutes, the mean systemic pressure might well have risen back to 4 mm. Hg, causing the venous return to rise up to the dashed curve of the figure. Also, circulatory reflexes have made the heart a stronger pump, and the new cardiac output curve is illustrated also by a dashed curve. These new cardiac output and venous return curves equate with each other at point C, giving a cardiac output of 2.4 liters per minute and a right atrial pressure of -1.5 mm. Hg.

A cardiac output of 2.4 liters per minute is approximately at the critical value between progression of shock and recovery from shock. Let us assume that the animal, after a period of several hours, takes a turn for the worse—that is, that the positive feedback factors of deterioration become sufficiently greater than the negative feedback factors to cause the animal to enter a vicious cycle of circulatory deterioration. After another hour or so, the cardiac output curve has fallen from the dashed curve to the dashed-dot curve. Furthermore, two separate factors now might be causing the venous return curve to fall back toward a lower value. First, poor blood supply to the vasomotor center might by this time be causing decreased vasomotor impulses to the peripheral vasculature, thereby resulting in a reduced mean systemic pressure, and, second, the local lack of nutrition to the blood vessels might cause weakening of the musculature or loss of fluid because of increased capillary permeability, both of which would also reduce the mean systemic pressure. Therefore, the venous return curve falls from the dashed curve to the dot-dashed curve. The dot-dashed venous return and cardiac output curves equate at point D, which depicts a cardiac output of 1.25 liters per minute and a right atrial pressure of -0.2 mm. Hg. This cardiac output, obviously, is far below that required to sustain the tissues of the body, and the shock now would progress very much more rapidly until death occurs.

The very rapid progression of the shock leads to further deterioration in the cardiac output curve, and after 20 to 30 minutes one finds a curve such as that illustrated by the dotted cardiac output curve. This equates with the dot-dashed venous return curve at point E, showing that the cardiac output has now fallen to 0.7 liter per minute, and the right atrial pressure has risen to $+1$ mm. Hg. However, to show that the heart is truly in the irreversible state, we now give a massive transfusion, which elevates the mean systemic pressure to 14 mm. Hg. If the heart has any significant pumping ability at all, the cardiac output should rise immediately to normal or perhaps even far above normal. However, since the cardiac output curve has fallen to the level of the dotted curve, the equilibrium point is at point F, with a cardiac output of about 1.7 liters per minute and a right atrial pressure of almost 13 mm. Hg. In other words, after this therapeutic procedure the tendency for venous return is far greater than normal, but the ability of the heart to pump the blood is so greatly depressed that the animal cannot recover. Thus, in the irreversible stage of shock, the simple therapeutic measure of transfusion can overcome any of the presently known peripheral factors that cause shock, but transfusion cannot cause the heart itself to recover. If, however, the transfusion had been given somewhat earlier in the progressive stage of shock, when the heart was only beginning to deteriorate, as represented by the dot-dashed cardiac output curve, the equilibrium point would have been at point G, which represents a cardiac output of slightly over twice normal. This obviously would have resulted in excellent transport of oxygen to the tissues, and one suspects that the heart probably would have been able to repay its oxygen debt and recovered. Therefore, the dot-dashed curve represents the cardiac situation in the progressive stage of shock before irreversibility, while the dotted curve represents the cardiac situation in the progressive stage of shock after irreversibility has taken place.

Chapter 22

EFFECTS ON CARDIAC OUTPUT OF ALTERATIONS IN PERIPHERAL RESISTANCE—ESPECIALLY THE EFFECTS OF ANEMIA AND POLYCYTHEMIA

BASIC EFFECTS OF RESISTANCE ALTERATIONS ON CARDIAC FUNCTION

Changing the resistance either in the systemic circulation or pulmonary circulation can affect cardiac output in two basic ways: by changing the load on one or both of the ventricles and by changing the ease with which blood flows through either the systemic circulation or the pulmonary circulation.

The effect on ventricular output of changing the load is considerable, even in the normal physiological range. Indeed, when the resistive load on either ventricle is doubled *while keeping the atrial pressure constant*, the ventricular output usually falls to about 70 per cent of its previous value (Sarnoff, 1955; Herndon, 1969). In other words, at each atrial pressure, the ventricular output is approximately reciprocally related to the square root of the resistive load. Therefore, it is evident that a changing load on either ventricle can have an exceedingly important effect on the cardiac output.

Yet marked changes in systemic resistance normally have very little effect on the *total* cardiac output curve in the normal operating physiological range of the heart. The reason for this was discussed in Chapter 9 but may be repeated briefly as follows: When the systemic resistance increases very greatly, the back-loading effect on the left ventricle causes a small amount of blood to dam up in the pulmonary circulation. As a consequence, the left atrial pressure automatically rises a millimeter or so of mercury, which in turn causes the left ventricle to pump the necessary

394

amount of blood to keep the cardiac output at almost what it was prior to the rise in systemic resistance. The slight rise in left atrial pressure is hardly enough to affect right ventricular function so that the right atrial pressure does not change a perceptible amount. Thus, the resistive load in the systemic circulation can change very greatly with relatively negligible alteration in the total function curve of the heart. This important fact was first demonstrated by Markwalder and Starling in 1914. Therefore, most of the effect on cardiac output caused by systemic resistance changes results from the effect of these changes on venous return, which will be discussed below.

EFFECT OF RESISTIVE ALTERATIONS ON VENOUS RETURN

In general, when the resistance to blood flow changes *proportionately* in all portions of the systemic circulation, the venous return varies almost exactly inversely with the change in resistance (see Chapter 13 for a detailed discussion). However, if the alterations in resistance *are not proportional* in all parts of the circulation, an alteration in venous resistance will affect venous return about 8 to 10 times as much as a similar alteration in arterial resistance (Guyton, 1959b).

Indeed, many different investigators have pointed out the extreme depressing effect that increased venous resistance has on cardiac output (Smith, 1952; Farber, 1954; Ohara, 1957; Guyton, 1959b; Holt, 1943, 1944a), while others have pointed out the very slight effect on cardiac output caused by considerable compression of the aorta (Markwalder, 1914; Horvath, 1958) or of occluding the arterioles with microspheres (Guyton, 1959b). For detailed discussions of this difference, the reader is referred to Chapter 13, and for a mathematical analysis explaining the difference, he is referred to Chapter 14.

RELATIONSHIP OF VISCOSITY AND RESISTANCE TO HEMATOCRIT

One of the most common causes of resistance changes is a change in the hematocrit, which changes the blood viscosity (Fahraeus, 1931; Whittaker, 1933; Levy, 1953; Olson, 1964; Chien, 1966b; Skovborg, 1968; Merrill, 1969; Benis, 1970; Snyder, 1971). Therefore, before attempting to discuss the effects of anemia and polycythemia on cardiac output, we need to describe the effect of hematocrit changes on blood viscosity.

Figure 22–1 illustrates two different relationships between hematocrit and viscosity determined in different ways (Whittaker, 1933). The upper curve represents typical viscosity measurements made in a high speed glass viscometer, and the lower curve illustrates the typical relationship between hematocrit and viscosity as determined from blood flow measurements in the hindlimb of a dog. Note especially that the viscosity determined in the viscometer is far greater than that determined in the hindlimb of the dog. Our problem in the discussion of the present chapter is to decide which of these relationships should be used. In many physiological circles it has be-

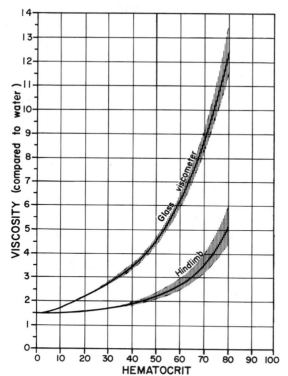

Figure 22-1. Effect of hematocrit on blood viscosity. The upper curve illustrates the effect as measured in a high speed glass viscometer, and the lower curve illustrates the effect as measured in the hindlimb of a dog. [Modified from Whittaker and Winton (1933).]

come customary to use the viscosity measurements in the hindlimb of the dog as the standard, but in the present studies we will use both these measurements and will see how each fits the experimental results.

EFFECT OF ANEMIA ON CARDIAC OUTPUT

MECHANISMS BY WHICH ANEMIA CAN AFFECT CARDIAC OUTPUT

We know at least five different alterations in the circulation during anemia that could affect cardiac output:

Decrease in "Resistance to Venous Return"

Referring again to Figure 22-1, we see that a decrease in hematocrit from a normal value of 45 down to a severely anemic value of 10 to 15 will decrease the viscosity, as determined in the glass viscometer, from approximately four times that of water down to about two times that of water, or about a 50 per cent decrease. However, if we use the values for viscosity obtained in the hindlimb of the dog, the change in viscosity would be from 2 down to 1.5, or a 25 per cent decrease. Therefore, we can say that the "resistance to venous return" in severe anemia probably decreases between 25 and 50 per cent, and that for lesser degrees of anemia it decreases some intermediate amount (Guyton, 1961).

Vasodilation Resulting from Anemia

In Chapter 19 it was pointed out that decreased oxygen transport to the tissues causes a local effect to result in vasodilation. Therefore, it is reasonable to expect that anemia would cause at least some vasodilatation.

If we consider both the decrease in viscosity and vasodilatation, we could calculate that the "resistance to venous return" could easily be decreased by 50 per cent or more in very *severe* anemia. The actual reduction in the resistance to venous return which occurs in moderate anemia is illustrated in Figure 22–2, which shows a control venous return curve and the average venous return curve measured in ten dogs with a mean hematocrit

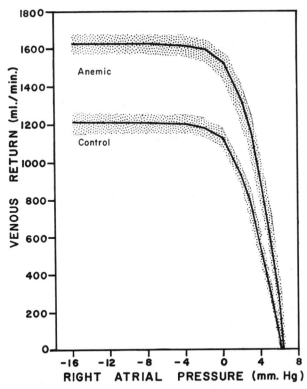

Figure 22–2. Effect on the venous return curve of changing the hematocrit from the control value of 39 down to an anemic value of 21. The results are from 10 dogs, and the shaded areas represent the probable errors of the mean. [Modified from Guyton and Richardson (1961a).]

of 21. In this particular figure, the resistance to venous return decreased 35 per cent as a result of the moderate anemia.

From the results illustrated in Figure 22–2, it is impossible to quantitate the relative roles of decreased viscosity and vasodilatation in reducing the decreased resistance to venous return. However, an attempt will be made to do this later in the chapter.

Decreased Resistive Load on the Heart

Decreasing the resistance to flow through both the systemic and pulmonary circulations will decrease the resistive load on *both ventricles* of the heart. It can be calculated from the studies of Sarnoff (1955) and Herndon (1969) on the effects of load on ventricular function, and from the viscosity measurements discussed above, that this effect can increase the output of the heart at constant atrial pressures as much as 10 to 20 per cent.

Reflex Stimulation of the Circulation

It is reasonable to expect that lack of adequate oxygen transport to the tissues could cause reflex stimulation of the circulation through the chemoreceptor mechanism. However, the results of actual studies on the importance of the autonomic nervous system in increasing cardiac output during anemia are contradictory. For instance, Glick (1964) reported that the increase in cardiac output caused by anemia was reduced approximately 35 per cent by denervation of the heart. Similar results have been found by Escobar (1966). On the other hand, Gowdey (1962), Lovegrove (1957), and Neill (1969) have shown that anemia-induced changes in cardiac output are hardly affected by adrenergic blocking agents. In spite of the discrepancy in the results of these studies, it seems reasonable to assume, on the basis of general knowledge of chemoreceptor function, that chemoreceptor reflex stimulation of the heart in severe anemia might increase the heart's pumping ability to a small degree, perhaps as much as 15 to 20 per cent.

Decreased Contractility of the Heart in Very Severe Anemia

Finally, it must be recognized that in very severe anemia the heart can be weakened as a result of inadequate transport of oxygen to the myocardium itself (Case, 1955). This is borne out, particularly, by the fact that the heart becomes greatly dilated in many patients with very severe anemia. Indeed, in anemia patients approaching the lethal state, the heart often fails completely. Therefore, all degrees of weakening of the heart can occur in severe anemia (Roy, 1963; Engle, 1964).

If we summate (1) the effect of decreased resistive load on the heart, (2) the effect of reflex stimulation, and (3) the weakening effect of anemia, we can come to the conclusion that in mild cases of anemia the first two of these factors should dominate and might easily increase the cardiac output curve; in moderate anemia the factors might all cancel out; and in extremely severe anemia the cardiac output curve would almost certainly be diminished to an extremely low level.

ANALYSIS OF CARDIAC OUTPUT CHANGES IN VARIOUS DEGREES OF ANEMIA

Theoretical Effect of Viscosity Changes Alone

In Figure 22–3 the solid curves represent an analysis of normal cardiac output with equilibrium at point A. Now let us assume that the hematocrit is decreased to 12, almost to a lethal level of anemia. If we assume the hindlimb viscosity measurements to be correct, the theoretical effect that the change in blood viscosity alone should have on cardiac output is represented by the short dashed venous return and cardiac output curves. These curves equate at point B, showing about 35 per cent increase in cardiac output. If we assume the glass viscometer measurements of viscosity to apply to cardiac output dynamics, then the long dashed curves will apply, with equilibrium at point B', representing 100 per cent increase in cardiac output. The two dashed venous return curves represent the effect of decreasing the viscosity 25 and 50 per cent respectively, which are the respective measured values by the hindlimb and viscometer methods. The decreased resistance to venous return is represented by increases in the slopes of the curve to $1\frac{1}{3}$ times and 2 times normal. The cardiac output curve is also presumed to rise because of a decreased resistive loading effect on the heart, which explains the two dashed cardiac output curves.

Effect of Hypoxic Vasodilatation

As pointed out above, additional effects besides those caused by viscosity changes also occur in anemia. Let us assume, for instance, that reflexes further stimulate the heart while the anemia decreases the strength of the heart because of diminished nutrition. Furthermore, lack of oxygen

Figure 22–3. Theoretical effect on cardiac output of decreased viscosity caused by anemia. Explanation is found in the text.

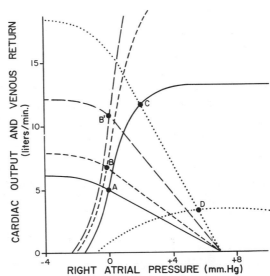

transport to the tissues undoubtedly will dilate the peripheral vessels and cause further increase in the slope of the venous return curve (Crawford, 1959; Ross, 1962). [See Chapter 19 for a discussion of this effect and see Hatcher (1954) for a discussion of other possible effects of anemic anoxia.]

If we assume that the reflex and unloading effects on the heart exactly balance the weakening effect of the anemia, then the cardiac output curve returns to the normal level, as represented by the solid curve in the figure, neither enhanced nor depressed. Let us assume that the anoxic vasodilatation increases the venous return curve to the dotted curve. This curve equates with the solid cardiac output curve at point C, which designates a cardiac output approximately $2\frac{1}{3}$ times normal and a right atrial pressure of 1 mm. Hg. This is approximately what one finds in severe anemia — that is, between a two and a three fold increase in cardiac output and sometimes a slightly elevated right atrial pressure (Sharpey-Schafer, 1944; Brannon, 1945; Sunahara, 1954; Fowler, 1956; Richardson, 1959; Roy, 1963; Cropp, 1969; Duke and Abelmann, 1969).

It is obvious from Figure 22–3 that most of the increase in cardiac output during anemia is caused by a decrease in the resistance to venous return. Therefore, at this point we must attempt to evaluate the relative importance of decreased viscosity and hypoxic vasodilatation in causing the decreased resistance to venous return. If we accept the hindlimb measurements of viscosity as shown in Figure 22–1, we must conclude that the decrease in resistance to venous return caused by a decrease in viscosity would be insufficient to account for the tremendous decrease in the resistance to venous return that occurs in anemia. On the other hand, if we accept the glass viscometer measurements of viscosity, we see that the decrease in resistance caused by a reduction in hematocrit would be nearly sufficient to cause the decrease in resistance to venous return actually observed. Thus, it is at least theoretically possible that the changes in viscosity alone are responsible for the changes in cardiac output during anemia. Any attempt to make a more conclusive statement is impossible, since definitive results from the necessary research studies are not available. However, studies have been directed toward this end, and the more important findings are reviewed below.

Several studies have been performed in which the viscosity and the oxygen transport capability of the blood were altered independently of each other. For instance, Murray and Escobar (1968) reduced the oxygen carrying capacity of blood without reducing the hematocrit in dogs by exchanging a portion of the normal blood in the animals with blood in which all of the hemoglobin had been converted to methemoglobin, a nonfunctional form of hemoglobin. They observed that in animals transfused with methemoglobin blood, the cardiac output was not increased nearly as much as in animals in which the oxygen carrying capacity of the blood had been reduced to the same degree by reducing the hematocrit. These results clearly indicate that it is the decrease in viscosity rather than a decrease in oxygen transport capability that is most responsible for the increase in cardiac output during anemia. Murray and Escobar also demonstrated that if anemia was produced in dogs by exchanging a portion of the blood for dextran solution, approximately a two-fold increase in cardiac output occurred. If methemoglobin and dextran were given simultaneously, the increase in cardiac output was only slightly greater than that observed with dextran alone. In additional studies, Murray and coworkers (Murray, 1966, 1969b) reduced both the viscosity and the oxygen transport capability of dogs' blood by transfusion with dextran solutions of various molecular weights and viscosities. They found that the increase in cardiac output was over twice as great in the animals transfused with low molecular weight dextran than in the animals transfused with a high molecular weight dextran. Results similar to this can be seen in the study of Fowler and Holmes (1964). Thus, all of these results imply that the reduction in viscosity is, indeed, a very important factor.

However, there have also been several studies which indicate that hypoxic vasodilatation may be a very significant factor in reducing the resistance to venous return. Barlett and Tenney (1963) estimated the oxygen tension of the tissues in anemic rats and observed that when the hematocrit was reduced to less than 25, the tissue P_{O_2} was substantially reduced. Furthermore, a substantially reduced venous oxygen tension (Cropp, 1969; Duke, 1969) during severe anemia also indicates that the tissues, indeed, are hypoxic. Putting these results together with the fact that hypoxia can cause up to a four-fold vascular dilatation (Carrier, 1964), one can see that, at least in very severe anemia, hypoxic vasodilatation should account for a substantial portion of the reduction in the resistance to venous return.

Effect of Lethal Anemia

Let us assume that the person of Figure 22–3 develops a degree of anemia that, if continued for a long period of time, will be lethal. This means a decrease in hematocrit down to perhaps 8 per cent. The decrease in hematocrit from 12 down to 8 does not further change the viscosity significantly and possibly does not cause much additional vasodilatation. Therefore, we might assume that the venous return curve remains approximately that shown by the dots in Figure 22–3. On the other hand, the lethal nature of the anemia would markedly depress the pumping ability of the heart so that after a few hours the cardiac output curve might well have decreased to the level shown by the dotted output curve. The dotted cardiac output and venous return curves equate with each other at point D, which denotes a cardiac output of 3 liters per minute and a right atrial pressure of about 6 mm. Hg. In other words, this analysis shows that in the terminal stages of anemia the cardiac output will fall below normal and eventually will approach zero, while the right atrial pressure approaches the mean systemic pressure. Somewhere along the line, extensive cardiovascular reflexes resulting from stimulation of the pressoreceptors and from excitation of the central nervous system ischemic reflex would undoubtedly cause the mean systemic pressure to rise, and this would shift the venous return curves far to the right. But at the same time the cardiac output curve would be decreasing very rapidly, which unfortunately would prevent the reflex increase in mean systemic pressure from benefiting the cardiac output significantly.

EFFECT OF POLYCYTHEMIA ON CARDIAC OUTPUT

In polycythemia we have a paradoxical situation in that acute polycythemia in animal experiments, without other complicating factors, reduces the cardiac output markedly (Richardson, 1959; Guyton, 1961a; Weisse, 1964, 1966; Murray, 1963b), while polycythemia in human patients or in long-term animal experiments hardly changes the cardiac output (Goldsmith, 1936; Altschule, 1940; Hovarth and Howell, 1964; Weisse, 1966). The difference is probably a reflection of the fact that polycythemia in human cases is a chronic condition associated with many compensatory changes. We will attempt to explain, though undoubtedly inadequately so, the difference between these two conditions.

BASIC MECHANISMS BY WHICH POLYCYTHEMIA CAN AFFECT CARDIAC OUTPUT

Polycythemia can affect cardiac output in almost exactly opposite ways to the effects of anemia on cardiac output. However, some of the factors that are relatively unimportant in anemia are highly important in polycythemia. The basic mechanisms by which polycythemia can affect cardiac output are the following:

Increase in Blood Viscosity

In anemia we noted that the viscosity can decrease 25 to 50 per cent; in polycythemia, within limits that are not lethal (up to a hematocrit of 80), the viscosity can increase, as illustrated in Figure 22–1, to 3½ times normal when measured by the glass viscometer or to 2½ times normal when measured in the hindlimb of the dog. Therefore, the *change* in viscosity can be considerably greater in polycythemia than in anemia. Obviously, therefore, the resistance to blood flow through the peripheral vessels is also changed by a greater percentage in polycythemia than in anemia.

Increased Resistive Loading of the Heart in Polycythemia

If the resistance to blood flow through the peripheral vessels increases, this adds increased resistive load on the heart and decreases the pumping ability of the heart. This factor could well be of more importance in polycythemia than in anemia, because the blood viscosity in polycythemia is, in terms of percentage, much more abnormal than it is in anemia. Fortunately, however, in *chronic* polycythemia, compensatory dilation of the peripheral vasculature partially offsets the increased resistance in the peripheral circulation (Goldsmith, 1936; Altschule, 1940; Weisse, 1966), which permits normal cardiac output, as will be explained in the following few sections.

Possibility of Vasoconstriction in Polycythemia

In the discussion of anemia earlier in the chapter it was pointed out that tissue oxygen lack could easily cause vasodilatation, which could be one of the factors that helps to increase the cardiac output in anemia. If we apply the reverse mechanism in polycythemia, an excess of oxygen would be expected to cause vasoconstriction. However, there is no evidence that vasoconstriction does truly occur in polycythemia. Therefore, we can assume that this mechanism is probably of no significance in the analysis of the effect of polycythemia on cardiac output.

Possibility of Reflex Inhibition of the Heart

It was also pointed out earlier that anemia might cause a slight degree of reflex excitation of the circulation because of decreased oxygen supply to the chemoreceptors. A reverse mechanism in polycythemia could be an excess oxygen supply to the chemoreceptors, causing inhibition of the heart. But several different studies have shown that *acute* polycythemia actually *reduces* oxygen transport to the tissues rather than increasing it, which results from the increased viscosity of the blood and the greatly slowed cardiac output (Crowell, 1959; Richardson, 1959; Guyton, 1961a; Smith and Crowell, 1963, 1967a).

COMPENSATIONS IN CHRONIC POLYCYTHEMIA

Increased Vascularization

A compensatory mechanism observed in chronic experimental polycythemia, but not found in acute experimental polycythemia, is a substantial increase in the size and number of blood vessels (Mercker and Schneider, 1949; Anthony and Kreider, 1961; Van Liere, 1963; Miller and Hale, 1970). Indeed, Anthony and Kreider observed a 60 per cent increase in the size of noncapillary blood vessels and a 25 per cent increase in the size of the capillary bed during chronic polycythemia. And Miller and Hale (1970) observed a 20 to 40 per cent increase in the number of capillaries of brain, heart muscle, and skeletal muscle of polycythemic rats. Obviously, such an increase in the number of vessels may be expected to cause a decrease in the resistance to venous return. This could easily help to compensate for the increased blood viscosity in polycythemia.

Possibility of an Increased Mean Systemic Pressure

Human beings or experimental animals with severe polycythemia often have blood volume increases to 40 to 60 per cent above normal (Altschule, 1940; Lawrence, 1952; Anthony and Kreider, 1961; Verel, 1961; Mylrea and Abbrecht, 1970; Rosenthal, 1970; Sanchez, 1970), which could easily increase the mean systemic pressure from its normal value of 7 mm. Hg up to several times this value. Such an effect would then cause a very high "pressure gradient for venous return," which could also help to offset the increased resistance to venous return caused by high blood viscosity. However, no measurements of mean systemic pressure have ever been made in patients with polycythemia. Therefore, this possible compensatory effect in polycythemia is yet to be studied.

Cardiac Hypertrophy

Another possible compensatory mechanism in chronic polycythemia is hypertrophy of the heart. Human beings and experimental animals with severe polycythemia often have substantially hypertrophied right ventricles, with much less hypertrophy of the left ventricle (Kerwin, 1944; Rotta, 1949; Valdiva, 1957; Swigart, 1965; Burton, 1967, 1969). This hypertrophy may be the result of a chronically elevated resistive load especially in the pulmonary circulation (Murray, 1969a). The importance of cardiac hypertrophy, primarily right ventricular hypertrophy, in compensating for the effects of chronic polycythemia, are uncertain. However, we might expect that this factor may be of some value in maintaining cardiac output despite the tremendously increased viscous resistance.

Though we are yet unsure of the roles played by increased vascularization, increased mean systemic pressure, and cardiac hypertrophy in compensating for the decreased cardiac output caused by acute polycythemia, we do know that they, plus perhaps other compensations, do return the cardiac output to normal in chronic polycythemia.

GRAPHICAL ANALYSIS OF THE EFFECTS OF POLYCYTHEMIA ON CARDIAC OUTPUT

Figure 22–4 illustrates the effects of polycythemia *per se* on venous return. In the experiments depicted by these venous return curves, the pumping ability of the heart was controlled by an external perfusion system, as explained in Chapter 6, and all circulatory reflexes were blocked by total spinal anesthesia. Furthermore, the mean circulatory pressure was kept exactly constant. To do this, whole blood was removed from the circulation and replaced by an equal volume of washed red blood cells to keep the blood volume normal. The average hematocrit was increased from 39 to 59 by this procedure. Note that the polycythemic venous return curve shows a very high resistance to venous return, 2.2 times the normal value, which is indicated by the 2.2 fold decrease in the slope. Higher levels of polycythemia reduce the venous return curve still more. However, it must be recognized that these were acute experiments and that the chronic effects of increased vascularization could not possibly have occurred during the course of the experiments. Also the compensatory effects of an increased blood volume, which is normally found in polycythemic patients, were prevented from occurring by the nature of the experiments.

Figure 22–5 illustrates a graphical analysis of cardiac output, showing by the solid curves an analysis for the normal circulation, with equilibrium

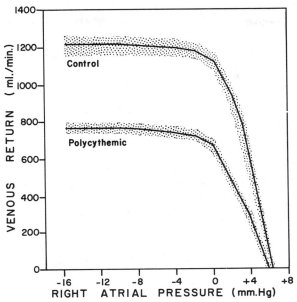

Figure 22–4. Effect on the venous return curve of changing the hematocrit from the control value of 39 up to a polycythemic value of 59. Results are averages from eight animals, and the shaded areas show the probable errors of the mean. [Modified from Guyton and Richardson (1961a).]

at point A. Now let us assume that the hematocrit is increased from the normal value of 40 or 45 up to approximately 80, which increases the viscosity of the blood about three fold (2½ fold by the hindlimb method and 3½ fold by the glass viscometer method) and likewise increases the resistance to venous return 3 fold. This would cause the venous return curve to fall to the dashed curve, and it would also increase resistance to flow through the systemic circulation enough to load the heart down to the dashed cardiac output curve. The new equilibrium is at point B, with a cardiac output of about two-fifths normal and a right atrial pressure hardly changed from the normal. This is almost the identical result that Richardson (1959) found in his animals made acutely polycythemic. That is, the cardiac output decreased approximately in proportion to the increase in viscosity of the blood.

However, in the human being with chronic polycythemia, the cardiac output is approximately normal (Goldsmith, 1936; Altschule, 1940; Hovarth, 1964). Furthermore, as pointed out above, there are reasons to believe that mean systemic pressure is increased considerably in polycythemia and that there is a considerable degree of increased vascularization which could decrease the high resistance to venous return caused by the greatly increased blood viscosity. Therefore, the dotted curve of Figure 22–5 is an estimate of the situation in chronic polycythemia. It is estimated that the mean systemic pressure is 13 mm. Hg and that the resistance to venous return is approximately two times the normal resistance to venous return. In other words, the resistance to venous return is about two times

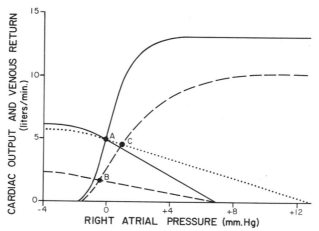

Figure 22–5. Graphical analysis of the effect of polycythemia on cardiac output both when the mean systemic pressure does not increase and when the mean systemic pressure does increase.

normal, but the pressure gradient for venous return has also been almost doubled by the increase in mean systemic pressure. The new equilibrium at point C shows a cardiac output of 4.6 liters per minute and a right atrial pressure slightly above normal. It may also be postulated that because of the lessened resistive load on the heart and the cardiac hypertrophy, the cardiac function curve shown by the dashed line in Figure 22–5 would tend to return to the normal curve shown by the solid line. However, we need far more information regarding the mean systemic pressure and the compensatory effects of increased vascularization and cardiac hypertrophy in polycythemia before a completely accurate analysis can be achieved.

Simulated Effects of Acute Anemia on Circulatory Dynamics

Figure 22–6 shows the simulated effects of acute anemia on circulatory dynamics. Beginning at time zero and for the next 20 minutes, the hematocrit was progressively reduced from its normal level of 40 to a near lethal level of 12. Illustrated in Figure 22–6 (from top to bottom) are the simulated effects of this reduction in hematocrit on cardiac output, arterial pressure, total peripheral resistance, heart rate, and the oxygen tension of the venous blood draining the muscles. In each case the solid curve represents the simulated effect when the sympathetic nervous system was functional, and the dashed curve represents the effect after removal of sympathetic influences.

Following the reduction in hematocrit, the muscle venous P_{O_2} was progressively reduced. Note, however, that the reduction in muscle venous oxygen tension was substantially greater in the absence of the sympathetic nervous system, indicating that during anemia the muscle blood flow was greater when the sympathetic nervous system was functional. Note also that throughout the reduction in hematocrit, the total peripheral resistance fell from its normal level to approximately one-half its normal level, and this reduction in total peripheral resistance was essentially the same before and after removal of the sympathetics. The decrease in total peripheral resistance was due both to a reduction in blood viscosity and to the hypoxic vasodilatation phenomenon which is present in nearly every tissue.

Almost simultaneously with the reduction in hematocrit and total peripheral resistance, cardiac output increased tremendously, both with and without sympathetic influences. However, note that the increase in cardiac output was somewhat greater when the sympathetic nervous system was functional. This greater increase in cardiac output may be attributed primarily to the chemoreceptors, the stimulation of which caused a substantially greater increase in heart rate. Also, not shown in Figure 22–6 is an increase in mean systemic pressure which occurred before the sympathetics were removed but not after functional sympathectomy. Thus, these simulated results support the experimental animal studies (cited earlier in this chapter) which indicate that the sympathetic nervous system is effective in increasing cardiac output during anemia.

Arterial pressure was reduced during anemia, both before and after removal of the sympathetics. However, arterial pressure was maintained at a substantially higher level when the sympathetic nervous system was functional. This maintenance of a higher arterial pressure was due solely to the greater cardiac output associated with a functional sympathetic nervous system.

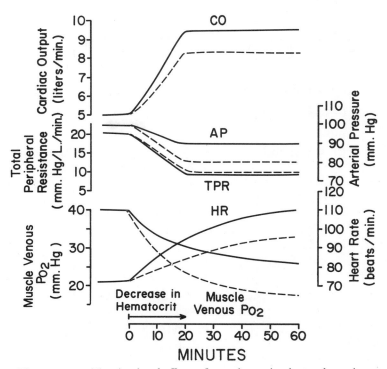

Figure 22–6.   The simulated effects of anemia on circulatory dynamics.

THE CONCEPT OF THE "OPTIMAL HEMATOCRIT"

Any discussion of the influence of the hematocrit on cardiac output would be incomplete without at least a brief description of the concept of the optimal hematocrit. The essentials of this concept are presented here.

The ability of the circulatory system to deliver oxygen to the tissues is determined by the product of two factors—the oxygen carrying capacity of the blood and the rate of blood flow to the tissues. Thus, from the previous discussions in this chapter we can see that the hematocrit has two opposing effects on the oxygen transportability of the circulatory system. First, as the hematocrit is increased, the oxygen carrying capacity of the blood is increased and, second, as the hematocrit is increased, the rate of blood flow to the tissues is decreased because of the increased blood viscosity. Experiments have illustrated that there is a hematocrit at which the ability of the circulatory system to transport oxygen is maximum, and this hematocrit has been termed the optimal hematocrit (Crowell, 1959, 1967; Smith and Crowell, 1963, 1967a).

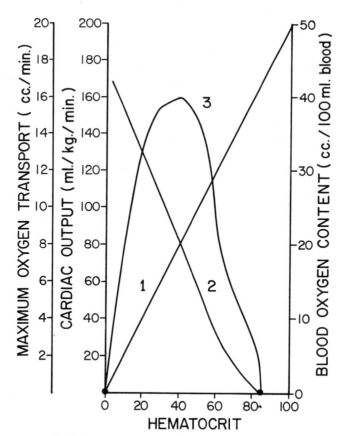

Figure 22–7. The influence of hematocrit on arterial oxygen content (curve 1) and cardiac output (curve 2). Curve 3 is the product of curves 1 and 2 and is the maximum quantity of oxygen that can be transported to the tissues at any given hematocrit.

The concept of the optimal hematocrit can be explained by referring to Figure 22–7. Curve 1 shows the relationship between hematocrit and the oxygen content of blood that is fully saturated with oxygen. When the hematocrit is zero the oxygen content of the blood is practically zero, since the quantity of oxygen dissolved in the plasma is negligible, and when the hematocrit is 100, the oxygen content of the blood is approximately 50 cc. per 100 ml. of blood. Curve 2 shows the relationship between the hematocrit and the cardiac output in the normal dog before any of the compensations discussed previously could occur (Richardson and Guyton, 1959). The opposing effects of hematocrit on blood flow and of oxygen content of the blood are obvious in curves 1 and 2. Curve 3 shows the product of curves 1 and 2 and is, therefore, the maximum quantity of oxygen that can be transported to the tissues at any hematocrit. It can be seen that as the hematocrit increases, the maximum oxygen transport capability also increases initially, but declines at very high hematocrits. Note also that the maximum quantity of oxygen that can be transported to the tissues is greatest at a hematocrit of approximately 40, which is the hematocrit of the normal animal and man. Thus, in normal man the optimal hematocrit for oxygen transport is approximately 40.

The factors involved in the regulation of the hematocrit such that it is normally maintained at its optimal level are almost completely unknown, but can be quite puzzling, especially since the oxygen consumption of the normal man is, under most conditions, far below the maximal amount of oxygen that can be made available to the tissues at the optimal hematocrit, or at hematocrits far removed from the optimal level. However, studies have demonstrated that animals having hematocrits at the optimal level tolerate certain stressful conditions, such as severe hemorrhage (Crowell, 1959) and high altitude (Smith and Crowell, 1967a), much better than animals having hematocrits above or below the optimal level.

OTHER CONDITIONS WHICH AFFECT CARDIAC OUTPUT BY CHANGING PERIPHERAL RESISTANCE

Some other conditions that affect cardiac output moderately by changing the systemic resistance include (1) beriberi (Keefer, 1930; Burwell, 1947; Lahey, 1953), febrile diseases (Hamrick, 1955), overheating of the body (Burch, 1957, 1959), and thyrotoxicosis (Liljestrand, 1925; Ernstene, 1938; Stead, 1950; Bishop, 1955; Graettinger, 1956), all of which reduce the peripheral resistance because of intense vasodilatation; (2) Paget's disease, which reduces the peripheral resistance because of markedly increased numbers of A-V shunts in the bone (Dexter, 1958); (3) pregnancy, because of the vascular shunt through the uterus (Hamilton, 1949); and (4) A-V fistulas, because of vascular shunts directly from the arteries to the veins (these will be discussed in detail in the next chapter). One can easily analyze the effect of beriberi or Paget's disease on cardiac output in much the same way that the effect of anemia was analyzed in Figure 22–3. Both these conditions increase the slope of the venous return curve and reduce the cardiac output curve slightly because of the reduced degree of resistive loading on the heart. Therefore, the equilibrium point can be increased to a cardiac output as much as two to three times normal, which explains why the cardiac output is so greatly increased in these conditions. In beriberi, the heart is usually also weakened by the avitaminosis so that the cardiac output curve is often reduced rather than elevated. If it is reduced enough, the cardiac output may be normal or even subnormal despite the greatly decreased peripheral resistance.

In the following chapter we will discuss in more detail the effect of A-V shunts, because these have been studied especially thoroughly by many separate investigators.

EFFECT OF INCREASED PULMONARY RESISTANCE ON CARDIAC OUTPUT

The normal pulmonary resistance is about one-ninth that in the systemic circulation and ordinarily offers very little impediment to the pumping action of the right heart. Indeed the resistance is so slight that elevations in left atrial pressure of only a few millimeters of mercury are reflected all the way back through the pulmonary circulation to the pulmonary artery (Cournand, 1950). Because of this normally low level of resistance in the lungs, even marked physiological changes in pulmonary resistance rarely have significant effects on cardiac output (Takaro, 1951; Taquini, 1960). However, in certain disease conditions, the pulmonary resistance is often increased as much as five to ten fold so that the loading effect on the right heart then becomes a major factor in affecting cardiac output.

Figure 22–8 illustrates a complex graphical analysis of the effect on cardiac output of a large acute increase in pulmonary resistance. In this figure, the solid curves represent an analysis of the normal circulation; to the left are the ventricular output and systemic venous return curves for the right heart, which equate at point A, and to the right and the ventricular output and pulmonary venous return curves for the left heart, equating at point B. Both points A and B show ventricular outputs of 5 liters per minute.

Now let us assume that the pulmonary resistance is increased four fold. Suddenly the solid pulmonary venous return curve passing through point B on the graph rotates to the right and becomes the dashed pulmonary venous return curve. This equates with the normal left ventricular output curve at point D, giving a left ventricular output of 2.8 liters per minute.

Another important effect of the increased pulmonary resistance is increased loading of the right ventricle, decreasing the right ventricular output curve from the solid curve to the dashed curve. Therefore, the output from the right ventricle immediately falls from 5 liters to approximately 4.2 liters per minute.

Thus, there now exists a disparity between left and right ventricular

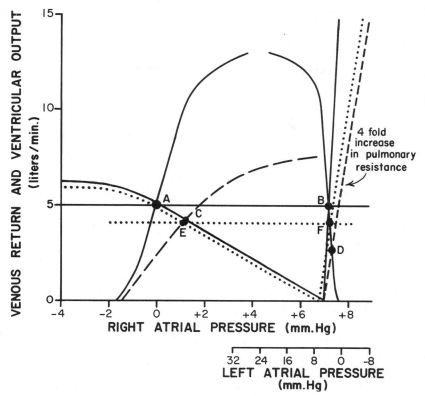

Figure 22–8. Complex analysis of the effect of a large acute increase in pulmonary resistance on cardiac output and other circulatory factors. The figure is explained in the text.

outputs (2.8 and 4.2 liters per minute), so that blood immediately shifts into the lungs from the systemic circulation, elevating the mean pulmonary pressure from its normal value of 5 mm. Hg up to 7 mm. Hg and decreasing the mean systemic pressure from 7 mm. Hg down to 6.7 mm. Hg. As a result, the pulmonary and systemic venous return curves now shift to the left to become the dotted curves. These two curves equate respectively with the loaded right ventricular output curve (dashed curve) and the normal left ventricular output curve at points E and F, at a cardiac output slightly greater than 4 liters per minute.

Thus, we see that a four fold increase in pulmonary resistance decreases the cardiac output slightly less than 20 per cent. However, if we should have considered a nine or ten fold increase in pulmonary resistance, then the loading effect on the right heart could have been so great that the cardiac output would have been decreased to levels as low as 40 to 50 per cent of normal. This analysis emphasizes, particularly, that pulmonary resistance must be increased by extreme amounts to affect cardiac output greatly. Yet such extreme increases in pulmonary resistance are known to occur on occasion.

Chapter 23

EFFECT OF A-V FISTULAS AND CARDIAC SHUNTS ON CARDIAC OUTPUT

The opening of an A-V fistula causes an *instantaneous* increase in cardiac output, which is the same effect observed when the blood viscosity is decreased, as discussed in the previous chapter. However, A-V fistulas deserve special comment because their effects on cardiac output and other circulatory dynamics are dramatic and have been studied extensively by many different investigators.

Another purpose of this chapter will be to analyze very briefly the effects of different types of cardiac shunts on cardiac output. Such shunts often have effects similar to those observed with A-V fistulas. However, since they involve only a single side of the heart, a complex type of analysis rather than the simplified type is required.

EFFECT OF A-V FISTULAS ON CARDIAC OUTPUT

BASIC CHANGES IN THE CIRCULATION ON OPENING AND CLOSING FISTULAS

As is true of almost all major circulatory changes, opening and closing A-V fistulas affect both the tendency for blood to return to the heart and the ability of the heart to pump blood, thus affecting greatly both the venous return curve and the cardiac output curve. Therefore, before analyzing the effect of A-V fistulas on cardiac output, we must first examine the effects of opening and closing fistulas on these respective curves.

Effect on the Venous Return Curve of Opening an A-V Fistula

Opening an A-V fistula affects the venous return curve in at least three different ways: (1) Immediately upon opening the fistula, the *resistance to venous return* decreases markedly, thereby allowing blood

412

to return to the heart with extreme ease (Guyton, 1961b). (2) Within 20 to 30 seconds following opening of the fistula, sympathetic reflexes increase the mean systemic pressure, which further promotes an increased flow of blood toward the heart (Guyton, 1961b). (3) Over a period of several days following the opening of a large fistula, the blood volume gradually rises (Frank, 1955; Hilton, 1955; Crawford, 1963; Davis, 1964; Taylor, 1968), which also increases the mean systemic pressure (Richardson, 1961). This in turn promotes further increased return of blood to the heart.

DECREASED RESISTANCE TO VENOUS RETURN. The cause of the decreased resistance to venous return on opening a fistula is, very simply, the establishment of a direct communication between the arteries and the veins, which allows the high pressure arterial system to empty directly into the veins and thence into the right atrium. Consequently, blood stored in both the arterial and venous capacitative chambers of the systemic circulation can flow almost directly into the right atrium, thereby allowing rapid filling of the heart and consequently an increased cardiac output. To emphasize the importance of this effect in altering the venous return we need to recall the following formula from Chapter 14:

$$\text{Venous return} = \frac{\text{Pressure gradient for venous return}}{\text{Resistance to venous return}}$$

That is, a decrease in resistance to venous return causes an almost equal and opposite increase in venous return.

REFLEX COMPENSATIONS. The principal effect of reflexes in the compensatory adjustments of the cardiac output following the opening of an A-V fistula is to increase the mean systemic pressure, the effect beginning to develop within a few seconds and reaching full development in less than a minute. When a fistula is opened in an animal with its reflexes completely abrogated by total spinal anesthesia, the mean systemic pressure does not change. However, when the reflexes are intact, the mean systemic pressure rises above 20 to 30 per cent when the fistula is large enough for the fistula flow to equal the systemic flow (Guyton, 1961b). If the fistula should be extremely large — several times the systemic flow — the mean systemic pressure could theoretically rise to at least double the normal as a result of sympathetic reflexes.

From a quantitative point of view, the reflexes are far less important in compensating for a *moderate sized* A-V fistula than is the decreased resistance to venous return discussed above (Guyton, 1961b). This is borne out in Figures 23–1, 23–2, and 23–3, and may be explained as follows: Figure 23–1 illustrates the effect on the venous return curve, in 10 dogs with all reflexes abrogated by total spinal anesthesia, of opening A-V fistulas that approximately doubled the cardiac output. The curve labeled "systemic flow — fistula closed" was the average venous return curve before the fistulas were opened. The curves labeled "total flow — fistula open" was the total venous return curve a minute after the fistulas were opened. The curve labeled "systemic flow — fistula open" was the venous return curve for that portion of the blood flowing through the systemic

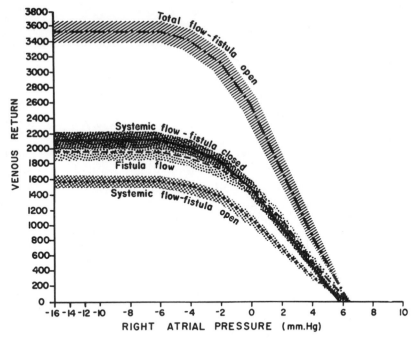

Figure 23-1. Studies in 10 dogs under total spinal anesthesia, showing the effects on the total venous return, the venous return through the fistula, and the venous return through the systemic circulation caused by suddenly opening a large A-V fistula. The shaded areas represent probable errors of the mean. [Reprinted from Guyton and Sagawa (1961b).]

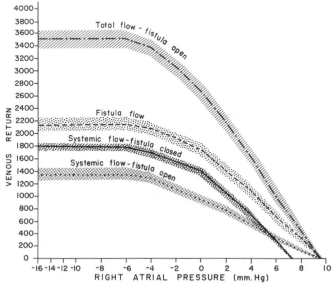

Figure 23-2. Studies in 10 dogs with normal circulatory reflexes, showing the effects on the total venous return, the venous return through the A-V fistula, and the venous return through the systemic circulation caused by suddenly opening a large A-V fistula. The shaded areas represent the probable errors of the mean. [Reprinted from Guyton and Sagawa (1961b).]

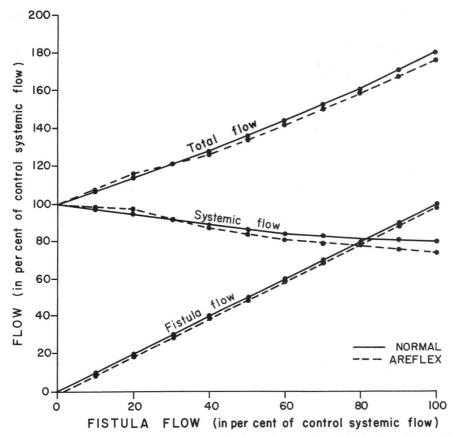

Figure 23–3. Stepwise opening of A-V fistulas in dogs under total spinal anesthesia and in dogs with normal reflexes, showing the comparative effects on the systemic blood flow of opening the fistulas to different degrees. [Reprinted from Guyton and Sagawa (1961b).]

circulation after the fistulas were opened. The curve labeled "fistula flow" represents that portion of the blood flowing through the fistula itself. Note especially from this figure that the mean systemic pressure (the point at which each curve crosses the zero flow level) did not change on opening the fistula. However, the resistance to venous return did decrease very markedly, as demonstrated by the steepened slope of the curve labeled "total flow — fistula open." Note also that the blood flow through the systemic circulation did not decrease greatly below the control value. It was the great decrease in *resistance to venous return* that allowed sufficient rise in the total venous return to prevent the flow through the systemic vessels from being greatly compromised.

Figure 23–2 illustrated exactly the same study with the reflexes intact. The difference between this study and the one in which the animals were under total spinal anesthesia was mainly the rise in mean systemic pressure of 2.2 mm. Hg. Essentially the same decrease in *resistance to venous return* occurred in these animals as in the spinal anesthesia animals, and the blood flow through the systemic vessels was still depressed slightly below the control value when the fistula was opened, but not quite so much so as in the spinal anesthesia animals. In other words, the reflexes were of some benefit, though not of great benefit, in preventing a significant decrease in systemic venous return after opening the fistulas.

Figure 23–3 illustrates a comparative study of the effect on blood flow through the systemic vessels of opening A-V fistulas to different degrees in ten total spinal anesthesia animals and in ten animals with intact reflexes. Note that when the fistula flow equaled 100 per cent of the previous control cardiac output, the blood flow through the systemic vessels in the spinal anesthesia animals fell to an average of 75 per cent of the original control value, while in the animals with reflexes intact the flow fell to 82 per cent of the original control value. This experiment illustrates that the instantaneous decrease in resistance to venous return caused a 75 per cent compensation for the flow through the fistula. Then, superimposed on this instantaneous effect of decreased resistance to venous return is the effect of the reflexes which increased the systemic venous return another 7 per cent. This 7 per cent represented a 28 per cent compensation of the remaining 25 per cent deficiency in systemic blood flow.

Unfortunately, these experiments do not tell the whole story of the value of reflexes, because reflexes can also increase the heart rate and the pumping ability of the heart, which are effects not reflected in the above venous return studies (Lewis, 1923; Ellis, 1930; Elkin, 1947; Cohen, 1948; Loo, 1949; Nickerson, 1951b; Murphy, 1958). Furthermore, when fistulas are extremely large, the reflex effects are undoubtedly far more important than the 28 per cent compensation that these experiments would indicate (Cohen, 1948; Murphy, 1958; Cowley and Guyton, 1971). The reflex changes in cardiac function will be discussed in more detail below.

BLOOD VOLUME CHANGES. The final factor of major importance in compensating for the deficiency in systemic flow is an increase in blood volume. This comes about as a result of at least two factors: First, when a large A-V fistula is opened, the reduction in arterial pressure causes a reduction in the quantity of the blood flowing to the kidneys (Davies, 1952). The decrease in renal blood flow causes the glomerular filtration rate to decrease and tubular reabsorption of fluid to increase, these two effects greatly reducing the urinary output and, therefore, increasing extracellular fluid volume and blood volume. Second, when the blood flow to the kidney becomes reduced, the ischemic kidney secretes increased quantities of *renin;* this causes the formation of the hormone *angiotensin* within the blood (Davis, 1964). The increased angiotensin in turn stimulates the adrenal glands to secrete aldosterone, which then enhances the reabsorption of sodium and water from the renal tubules.

The increase in blood volume after opening a large A-V fistula does not come about immediately but over a period of several days (Frank, 1955; Hilton, 1955). In human beings with chronic fistulas of significant size, the blood volume has been measured to be 4 to 20 per cent above normal (Warren, 1951a; Crawford, 1963). Obviously, an increase in blood volume can increase the mean systemic pressure, and this in turn can increase the venous return.

SUMMARY OF FACTORS AFFECTING THE VENOUS RETURN CURVE. Now let us summarize the changes in the venous return curve that occur upon opening a fistula. First, we find an instantaneous increase in the slope of the venous return curve caused by the decrease in resistance to venous return. Second, during the ensuing minute, the reflexes increase the mean systemic pressure as much as 20 to 30 per cent in the case of moderately large fistulas, which increases the *pressure gradient for venous return* and thereby further enhances venous return to the heart, shifting the venous return curve to the right and upward. On opening extremely large fistulas it is theoretically possible that the mean systemic pressure could increase as much as 100 per cent. Third, very large fistulas cause the blood volume to increase as much as 4 to 20 per cent within a few days after the fistula is opened, presumably by depressing the renal output and increasing the formation of blood. This can increase the mean systemic pressure and also would increase the *pressure gradient for venous return*, thereby aiding in compensating for the flow through an A-V fistula.

Effect on the Cardiac Output Curve of Opening an A-V Fistula

Opening an A-V fistula has at least three very distinct effects on the cardiac output curve: (1) instantaneous enhancement of the curve caused by reduction of the resistive load on the left ventricle (Nickerson, 1951b; Crawford, 1963), (2) reflex enhancement of cardiac function (Ellis, 1930; Elkin, 1947; Cohen, 1948; Loo, 1949; Murphy, 1958) with consequent enhancement of the cardiac output curve following within one minute after the fistula is opened, and (3) hypertrophy of the heart over a period of weeks to months caused by the increased work output of the heart (Harrison, 1924; Taylor, 1968).

UNLOADING OF THE LEFT VENTRICLE. The degree of enhancement of the cardiac output curve as a result of reducing the resistive load on the left ventricle when an A-V fistula is opened has not been studied enough for us to be certain of the effect. However, it was pointed out and discussed in Chapter 14 that the cardiac output curve of the entire heart is controlled mainly by the pumping action of the *right* heart, and this, within very wide limits, is almost independent of the load on the left ventricle (Markwalder, 1914; Sagawa, 1966, 1967; Herndon, 1969). Therefore, unloading the left ventricle as a result of decreased resistance in the systemic circulation would not be expected to enhance the cardiac output curve by more than 10 to 20 per cent. Yet, even so, this small effect enters into the compensations that occur when an A-V fistula is opened.

REFLEX ENHANCEMENT OF CARDIAC FUNCTION. Presumably the circulatory reflexes that occur when an A-V fistula is opened result mainly from stimulation of the pressoreceptor system, for when all reflexes are abrogated by total spinal anesthesia, the arterial pressure falls upon opening an A-V fistula considerably more than is true when the reflexes are intact (Loo, 1949; Guyton, 1961b). The reflex effects can probably enhance the cardiac output curve 10 to 25 per cent when the fistula flow approximately equals the systemic flow, or perhaps can enhance the cardiac output curve as much as 50 to 60 per cent when the fistula is so large that it is almost lethal (this is about the maximum amount of enhancement of the cardiac output curve that can be effected by sympathetic stimulation).

It is noteworthy that in contrast to the influence of heart rate on cardiac output under normal conditions, reflex changes in heart rate are extremely important in determining cardiac output under conditions of high venous return, such as prevail following the opening of a large A-V fistula. This was recently demonstrated in a study (Cowley and Guyton, 1971) in which the ventricles of dogs were paced at various rates following the opening of a large aorta-venacaval fistula. Results of this study are illustrated in Figure 23–4. Note that under normal conditions (curve C), increasing the heart rate from approximately 50 beats per minute to 200 beats per minute had very little effect on cardiac output, producing a maximum increase of only 10 per cent at a rate of approximately 100 beats per minute. However, after partially opening the large A-V fistula, varying heart rate over a wide range had a more substantial effect on cardiac output (curve PO). It may be noted that opening the fistula resulted in a 50 per cent rise in cardiac output even if the heart rate was maintained at 50 beats per minute, this increase in output being due to an increase in stroke volume alone. Increasing the heart rate to 200 beats per minute resulted in a 130 per cent increase in cardiac output within the range of 100 to 150 beats per minute. Thus, it may be surmised from curve PO

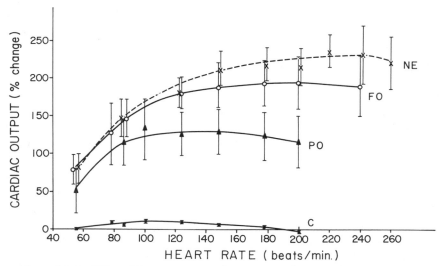

Figure 23–4. Effect of heart rate on cardiac output under control conditions (curve C); after partial opening of a large A-V fistula (curve PO); after fully opening a large A-V fistula (curve FO); and after fully opening the fistula and infusing norepinephrine (curve NE). Vertical bars indicate standard errors of the mean. [From Cowley and Guyton (1971).]

that a reflex increase in heart rate from the normal value of approximately 75 beats per minute to approximately 120 beats per minute would cause an increase in cardiac output of approximately 30 per cent. The influence of heart rate on cardiac output was even more profound when the large fistula was fully opened (curve FO). When heart rate was maintained at 50 beats per minute, fully opening the fistula caused an increase in cardiac output of 75 per cent. Increasing the heart rate to 240 beats per minute resulted in a rise in cardiac output to 190 per cent above the control value. The maximum increase in cardiac output under these conditions occurred between 150 and 200 beats per minute. Thus, when the fistula was fully open, a reflex increase in heart rate from the normal value of approximately 75 beats per minute to a rate of approximately 180 beats per minute resulted in an increase in cardiac output of 60 per cent. Curve NE shows the effects of infusing norepinephrine on the heart rate—cardiac output relationship when the fistula was fully open. In this case, the influence of heart rate on cardiac output was even more increased, most likely because of the increased mean systemic pressure and pressure gradient for venous return caused by the exogenous norepinephrine. Under all the conditions shown in Figure 23–4, the plateau and subsequent decline in cardiac output observed when heart rate was progressively increased were due to a compromise in stroke volume, probably caused by decreased diastolic filling period, incomplete ventricular relaxation, and increasing viscous resistance to ventricular distention (Buckley, 1955; Braunwald, 1960; Miller, 1962).

The importance of heart rate as a determinant of cardiac output under conditions of high venous return has also been demonstrated by the work of Sugimoto (1966), who used means other than an A-V fistula to increase venous return.

Unfortunately, most cardiovascular reflexes can maintain enhanced activity for only a few days. Gradually the reflex effects die out, even though the initiating stimulus of the reflex remains (Kubicek, 1953). For instance, if the arterial pressure in the region of the pressoreceptors remains very low for a long period of time, the pressoreceptor response gradually fades over a period of days. Therefore, even though reflex effects might be of particular value for the first few days after opening an A-V fistula, in the long run these reflex effects probably cannot be depended upon to continue their compensatory value. However, an increase in blood volume occurs which takes the place of the reflex constriction of the systemic vessels (Frank, 1955; Hilton, 1955; Warren, 1951a; Crawford, 1963; Davis, 1964). Also, the cardiac muscle hypertrophies (Harrison, 1924; Taylor, 1968), which could take the place of the reflex effects on the heart.

CARDIAC HYPERTROPHY. Hypertrophy of the heart is slow to occur, requiring several months to develop fully in response to cardiac strain. Nevertheless, if a very large A-V fistula is opened, detectable amounts of cardiac hypertrophy will appear within a few weeks (Harrison, 1924; Taylor, 1968). As pointed out in Chapter 9, hypertrophy of the heart can undoubtedly enhance the cardiac output curve very markedly, perhaps under some circumstances raising the curve to at least 100 per cent above the normal level.

GRAPHICAL ANALYSIS OF THE EFFECT ON CARDIAC OUTPUT OF OPENING A LARGE A-V FISTULA

The graphical analysis of the circulatory effects when a A-V fistula is opened depends upon the size of the fistula. Figure 23–5 illustrates a typical analysis when the fistula is large enough for approximately three times as much blood to flow through the fistula as through the systemic circulation. At this fistula size, the amount of cardiac output is reaching the upper limit that the heart can pump, which means that both cardiac and systemic circulatory compensations must take place simply to keep the person alive. In this analysis, the solid curves represent the normal circulation with equilibrium at point A, showing a cardiac output of 5 liters per minute and a right atrial pressure of 0 mm. Hg. Then the fistula is opened, which causes two immediate effects: (1) The slope of the venous return curves becomes very steep, as illustrated by the long-dashed venous return curve, and (2) the decreased load on the left ventricle causes the cardiac output curve to rise slightly, which is illustrated by the long-dashed cardiac output curve. These two curves equate at point B, which shows a cardiac output of approximately 13 liters per minute and a right atrial pressure of 2.5 mm. Hg.

Note that once the fistula is opened and the circulatory system is operating at point B, the pressure gradient for venous return then is equal

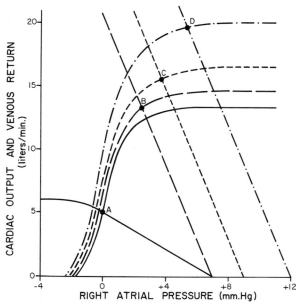

Figure 23–5. Analysis of the stages of compensation following the opening of a large A-V fistula.

to 4.5 mm. Hg instead of the normal 7 mm. Hg (7 mm. Hg minus 2.5 mm. Hg right atrial pressure). Therefore, one would expect the blood flow through the systemic circulation to be reduced to approximately 60 per cent of normal. As a consequence, the arterial pressure should fall, and reflexes should ensue. Within the next minute the circulatory reflexes would cause (1) an increased mean systemic pressure and (2) further enhancement of the cardiac output curve. The new venous return and cardiac output curves are illustrated by the short-dashed curves; these equilibrate with each other at point C, giving a cardiac output now of almost 16 liters per minute and a right atrial pressure of about 4 mm. Hg. Yet the pressure gradient for venous return is still only slightly greater than 5 mm. Hg, which means that the flow through the systemic circulation is still somewhat compromised ($5/7$, or 72 per cent, of normal).

Over a period of several weeks, the blood volume increases and the heart hypertrophies. As a result, one would expect the venous return and cardiac output curves to become approximately those represented by the dash-dot curves, equilibrating at point D with a cardiac output of approximately 20 liters per minute and a right atrial pressure about 5 mm. Hg. Note that by this time the mean systemic pressure is 12 mm. Hg, and the pressure gradient for venous return is almost back to its normal value of 7 mm. Hg. As a consequence, the flow of blood through the systemic circulation is essentially normal. At this time, the reflex adjustments of the circulation are no longer required, because by now there is an increased blood volume which gives an adequate pressure gradient for venous return and an enhanced cardiac output curve resulting from hypertrophy of the heart which allows the heart to pump the extra blood without the necessity of reflexes. Therefore, gradually, the effects of the circulatory reflexes disappear while these other two factors take over to aid in compensating for the fistula flow.

The above analysis obviously depends to a great extent on assumptions. Also, the effects have been dramatized by analyzing in this figure the effects of an extremely large fistula. The effect on right atrial pressure is especially great in this analysis in contrast to the very small increase when a smaller fistula is opened (Reid, 1938; Heringman, 1945; Stead, 1947b; Cohen, 1948; Warren, 1951b; Frank, 1955). However, this difference is to be expected because of the very *steep slope* of the cardiac output curve at low outputs and the *plateau* at higher outputs. It would be very fortunate if we had available at this time all the measurements needed to give more precision in this analysis. Nevertheless, the analysis is presented to show the general trends in the changes that follow the opening of an A-V fistula and also to provide a framework for further investigation into the quantitative aspects of these changes.

If the reader will now analyze for himself the effects of opening small A-V fistulas rather than the large one analyzed in Figure 23–5, he will see that the instantaneous decrease in resistance to venous return causes sufficient compensation entirely by itself to explain almost all the increased cardiac output which results when the fistula is opened. In other words, when a small fistula is opened, the decrease in resistance to venous return is probably by far the most important of all the compensatory effects, while on the other hand, when very large fistulas are opened, the reflex (Loo, 1949), blood volume (Hilton, 1955), and cardiac hypertrophy (Harrison, 1924) effects are also of major importance.

(Another compensatory effect that was not discussed in the above analysis is a probable shift of blood from the pulmonary circulation to the systemic circulation. To analyze this effect, the complex form of cardiac output analysis presented in Chapter 14 would be required. Though such a shift of blood has never been demonstrated experimentally, and even though the complex analysis shows this compensation to be much less important than those discussed above, it would nevertheless be a rewarding exercise for the reader to analyze this shift for himself, using the principles of the complex analysis as presented in Chapter 14.)

Simulation of Circulatory Dynamics Following the Opening of a Large A-V Fistula

Figure 23–6 shows the simulated effects on circulatory dynamics of opening a large A-V fistula. Illustrated (from top to bottom) are changes in extracellular fluid volume, blood volume, heart rate, cardiac output, total peripheral resistance, arterial pressure, angiotensin concentration in the blood, and urinary output. The complex computer model described in Chapter 17 was used to simulate these effects.

When the A-V fistula was opened, the initial event was a large reduction in total peripheral resistance to essentially one-half normal. This was followed within seconds by an increase in cardiac output to approximately 175 per cent of the normal level and a decrease in arterial pressure to approximately 88 mm. Hg. Also, because of the increased sympathetic activity, the heart rate immediately increased by approximately 50 per cent. As explained earlier in this chapter, the reduction in arterial pressure caused urinary output to decrease almost to zero. This decrease in urine output was due both to a decrease in renal blood flow, and to an increase in the rate of renin secretion by the ischemic kidneys with a consequent increase in the blood angiotensin concentration. The reduction in urinary output caused extracellular fluid volume and blood volume to increase during the ensuing day, and the increases in these volumes caused cardiac output to increase to exactly two times normal. This increase in cardiac output also returned arterial pressure to its normal level. Once arterial pressure returned to its normal level, the urinary output again returned to its control level, and all circulatory variables reached a steady state.

When the fistula was closed, essentially the opposite effects occurred. Cardiac output decreased to approximately 150 per cent of control, and arterial pressure rose abruptly to approximately 120 mm. Hg. The increase in arterial pressure caused urinary output to increase abruptly to approximately five times its normal level, and during the ensuing day, extracellular fluid volume and blood volume once again returned to their control levels. The decrease in these volumes led to a return of cardiac output and arterial pressure to normal.

The events illustrated in Figure 23–6 have also been demonstrated in studies of A-V fistulas in human beings and experimental animals as

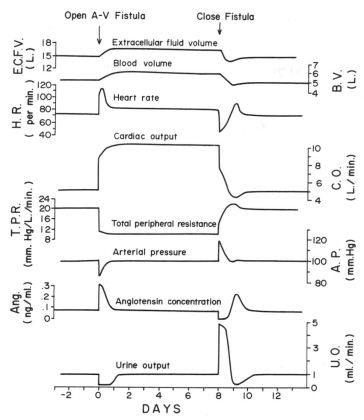

Figure 23–6. Simulation of changes in circulatory dynamics after opening a large A-V fistula. (From Guyton, to be published.)

discussed earlier in this chapter. The reader should attempt to correlate the events depicted in Figure 23–6 and the analysis illustrated in Figure 3–5 in order to be sure that he fully understands the effect on cardiac output of opening a large A-V fistula.

EFFECT OF CARDIAC SHUNTS ON CARDIAC OUTPUT

Discussion of the effect of cardiac shunts on cardiac output will necessarily be very brief because the analysis of each type of cardiac shunt is different from the analyses of all others, and, to be precise, each analysis would have to be even more complex than those already developed in this book. However, some types of cardiac shunts can be treated in a simplified way so that the effect on cardiac output can be estimated with reasonable accuracy.

Though congenital cardiac shunts are usually classified into (a) left to right shunts and (b) right to left shunts, these two categories cannot be used when discussing the effects of shunts on cardiac output, because more important than the category is the precise point in the heart or extracardiac circulation at which the shunt occurs. For instance, a right to left shunt *from the right to the left ventricle* gives a quite different analysis from the analysis for a right to left shunt *through a pulmonary A-V fistula.*

One of the ways in which cardiac shunts can be treated in analyzing their effect on cardiac output is simply to consider the entire heart and pulmonary circulation as a unit in the manner described in the simplified graphical analysis of Chapter 14. The effect of the shunt on the overall function of the entire unit can then be represented by a change in the cardiac output curve. Ordinarily, any type of shunt, whether it be a right to left shunt or a left to right shunt, will decrease the pumping effectiveness of the heart, thereby lowering the cardiac output curve. Using this fact, we can employ the simplified method for cardiac output analysis presented in Chapter 14 to give a typical analysis of the effect of a cardiac shunt on cardiac output. Since use of this type of analysis and its implications should be obvious to the reader by this time if he is familiar with the previous chapters, he will be left to prepare his own analysis of the effect on cardiac output of a hypoeffective heart caused by a cardiac shunt. In making this analysis, note especially that if the pumping effectiveness of the heart is decreased no more than 50 per cent below normal, the cardiac output ordinarily will be entirely normal and the right atrial pressure will be elevated only 1 to 2 mm. Hg. However, if the effectiveness of the heart is reduced to levels as low as 25 to 40 per cent of normal, one then finds that the cardiac output often falls below normal, and the right atrial pressure begins to rise markedly.

Analysis for a Patent Ductus Arteriosus

Certain types of cardiac shunts cause excessive pumping of blood by one of the ventricles but not by the other, and, therefore, affect the dynamics of one of the ventricles markedly without significantly affecting the dynamics of the other ventricle. A particular example of this is a patent ductus arteriosus (Leeds, 1943), the effects of which will be explained in the following paragraphs.

Figure 23–7 illustrates an analysis of the effect on cardiac output of a patent ductus arteriosus. The solid curves of this figure represent a normal complex analysis of the outputs of the two ventricles, with equilibrium points at A and B, respectively, for the right and left ventricles. Now, using this analysis as the beginning point for discussion, let us see what will happen if a ductus is opened. On opening the ductus, the extra pressure load in the pulmonary artery will cause the right ventricular output curves to decrease. However, over a period of time the right ventricle hypertrophies. Consequently, the cardiac output curve of the right ventricle eventually would be expected to become essentially normal if we assume that the hypertrophy fully compensates for the extra pressure load.

Opening the patent ductus also increases the work load on the left

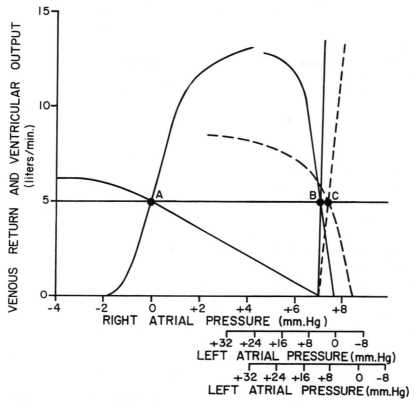

Figure 23-7.   Graphical analysis of cardiac output in patent ductus arteriosus.

ventricle but for different reasons: It increases the quantity of blood which must be pumped through the left ventricle per minute. In analyzing the net cardiac output, however, we are interested in the *quantity of blood which gets past the ductus into the systemic arterial tree* rather than the total amount which is pumped by the left ventricle itself. The amount that gets past the ductus is only a fraction of the total amount pumped by the left ventricle, and even though the left ventricle hypertropies, the "effective" pumping ability of the ventricle for pumping blood beyond the patent ductus is still decreased below normal. Therefore, in Figure 23-7, the "effective" pumping ability of the left ventricle (aside from the blood which returns through the ductus) is represented by the dashed cardiac output curve.

In determining what happens to the pulmonary venous return curve, we find two different volumes of blood passing through the lungs at the same time: the blood from the right ventricle and the blood from the patent ductus. The extra blood from the patent ductus increases the pressure gradient through the pulmonary system, thereby increasing the "effective" pulmonary resistance to venous return for that portion of the blood coming from the right ventricle. This would cause the pulmonary venous return curve to rotate to the right, as illustrated by the dashed curve.

In summary, then, the two primary effects in Figure 23-7 of a patent ductus arteriosus would be (1) a considerably reduced "effective" left ventricular output curve and (2) an "effective" pulmonary venous return curve rotated to the right. A third effect that would probably occur secondarily to these primary effects would be an increase in blood volume, particularly so when the heart is failing. If such an increase in blood volume did not occur, the changes in the pulmonary venous return curve and in the left ventricular output curve would be expected to decrease the cardiac output. This decrease in cardiac output would then be expected to decrease renal output and thereby raise the blood volume and cardiac output above normal. The effect of such an increase in blood volume is illustrated in Figure 23-7 by a shift of the left atrial pressure scale to the right.

Therefore, after all compensations have taken place, the analysis shows the right ventricular output (represented by point A) and the "effective" left ventricular output (represented by point C) both to be 5 liters per minute. The principal change from normal circulatory function, except for the recirculating fistula flow, is an increased left atrial pressure, especially if the left ventricle is failing.

Several of the steps in the changes in the circulation on opening a ductus arteriosus have been omitted from Figure 23-7. If the reader will think about this problem long enough to fill in the steps himself, his understanding of the analysis will be greatly enhanced.

An important fact that can be learned from the analysis in Figure 23-7 is that extreme exercise or any other extreme physical stress on the circulation will cause the left ventricle to fail because the "effective" left ventricular cardiac output curve does not plateau at a high enough level to allow the needed increase in systemic flow required in such conditions.

Another implication of this analysis is that an increase in blood volume is often a valuable compensation for decreased effectiveness of the heart as a pump. In this particular case, the mean systemic pressure is normal at a value of 7 mm. Hg, but the mean pulmonary pressure is 11 mm. Hg, representing an increase of 6 mm. Hg above the normal value of 5 mm. Hg. Thus, the increase in blood volume is entirely in the lungs and not in the systemic circulation. Furthermore, the total increase in blood volume is very slight because the capacitance of lungs is very slight. Indeed, if we remember that seven-eighths of the mean circulatory pressure is determined by the mean systemic pressure and that one-eighth is determined by the mean pulmonary pressure, we will see that in the analysis of Figure 23-7, the mean circulatory pressure has been increased by less than 1 mm. Hg; referring back to Figure 12-6 in Chapter 12, we see that the total blood volume increase required to cause this much rise in mean circulatory pressure is approximately 2 per cent. Actually this amount of blood volume increase is unmeasurable. Yet in very severe cardiac abnormalities, the blood volume is known to increase as much as 15 to 20 per cent, illustrating that at least under some circumstances blood volume increases are exceedingly important as compensations for cardiac ineffectiveness.

Chapter 24

EFFECT ON CARDIAC OUTPUT OF RESPIRATION, OPENING THE CHEST, AND CARDIAC TAMPONADE

Respiration, opening the chest, and cardiac tamponade all affect the cardiac output in almost exactly the same way—by altering the extracardiac pressure. Reference to the figures of Chapter 9 and of this chapter will illustrate that a rise in extracardiac pressure shifts the cardiac output curve to the right, while a decrease in extracardiac pressure shifts the curve to the left. Thus, Figure 24–1 shows that the cardiac output curve shifts 3 mm. Hg to the right of the mean during normal expiration, and 3 mm. Hg to the left during normal inspiration; Figures 24–2 and 24–3 illustrate the effects on the cardiac output curve of negative and positive pressure respiration respectively; Figure 24–4 illustrates the shift of the cardiac output curve to the right when the chest is opened; and Figure 24–6 illustrates the shift of the curve to the right, plus some depression of the curve, in cardiac tamponade. For a fuller discussion of these changes in the cardiac output curve caused by changes in extracardiac pressure, the reader is now referred to Chapter 9.

GRAPHICAL ANALYSIS OF THE EFFECT OF RESPIRATION ON CARDIAC OUTPUT

Effect of Normal Respiration

In normal respiration, the intrapleural pressure rises to approximately 3 mm. Hg above the normal mean value during expiration and falls to about 3 mm. Hg below the normal mean value during inspiration. As a result, the cardiac output curve shifts back and forth during each respiratory cycle, as is illustrated in Figure 24–1. The shaded areas of this figure denote the entire sequence of cardiac output curve shifts.

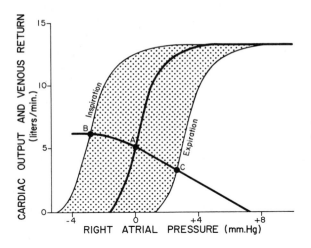

Figure 24–1. Analysis of the effect of normal respiration on cardiac output.

The normal mean cardiac output curve is represented by the very dark curve. The venous return curve equates with this curve at point A, at a cardiac output of 5 liters/minute and a right atrial pressure of 0 mm. Hg. During expiration, the intrapleural pressure rises 3 mm. Hg above normal, and the cardiac output curve shifts to the right, equating with the venous return curve at point C, which shows a cardiac output of 3 liters/minute and a right atrial pressure of 2.6 mm. Hg. During inspiration, the cardiac output curve shifts to the left, equating with the venous return curve at point B, which designates a cardiac output of 6.3 liters/minute and a right atrial pressure of −2.7 mm. Hg. Thus, the cardiac output rises and falls markedly during each respiratory cycle, as is well known (Burton-Opitz, 1902; Henderson, 1913; Rost, 1932; Eyster, 1933; Cahoon, 1941; Boyd, 1941; Shuler, 1942; Eckstein, 1947b; Alexander, 1951; Mixter, 1953; Brecher, 1953a; Knebel, 1958; Morgan, 1966; Moreno, 1967; Abel, 1969). These fluctuations are even more pronounced in the venous input to the heart than in the cardiac output because the pulmonary circulation partially damps the fluctuations in the left ventricular output. Brecher, as well as others, in his studies on the venous return to the heart during respiration showed that the venous return to the heart during inspiration is often two or more times the venous return during expiration (Brecher, 1952a, 1952b, 1952c, 1953a; Mixter, 1953; Moreno, 1967).

Figure 24–1 does not show any effect of respiration on the venous return curve. Actually this may not be true because contraction of the respiratory muscles during inspiration compresses the vascular reservoirs in the abdomen and thereby undoubtedly increases the mean systemic pressure during inspiration. On the other hand, contraction of the expiratory muscles, particularly the abdominal muscles, could also increase the mean circulatory pressure and thereby promote venous return during expiration (Eckstein, 1947b; Alexander, 1951; Brecher, 1952b; Mixter, 1953; Krug, 1960). Though these changes in mean circulatory pressure could cause transient changes in the venous return curve, not enough is known about these effects to consider them intelligently at the present time. In fact, studies by a number of investigators (reviewed by Krug, 1960) have indicated that in normal respiration the abdominal compressional effects are of little value in promoting venous return, because the compression effect on the vessels is offset by an increase in resistance in the large veins caused by the external pressure on the large veins. Yet when abdominal contractions are very strong, they undoubtedly aid venous return markedly, as will be discussed later in this chapter in relation to positive pressure breathing.

EFFECT OF NEGATIVE AND POSITIVE PRESSURE BREATHING ON CARDIAC OUTPUT

Many different investigators have studied the effects of negative (Rost, 1932; Holt, 1943, 1944a, 1959; Kilburn, 1960) and positive pressure breathing (Humphreys, 1938; Holt, 1943, 1944a; Otis, 1946a, 1946b; Carr, 1946; Cournand, 1948; Motley, 1948; Candel, 1953; Cain, 1953; Brecher, 1953a; Hubay, 1954; Maloney, 1954; Braunwald, 1957; Cathcart, 1958; Nealon, 1959; Kilburn, 1960) on cardiac output. In general, all students of the subject have found that negative pressure breathing causes either no effect or at most only a slight increase in cardiac output, while positive pressure breathing greatly decreases the output.

Effect of Negative Pressure Breathing on Cardiac Output

Figure 24–2 illustrates a graphical analysis of the effect of negative pressure breathing on cardiac output. The dark curves represent the normal cardiac output curve and the normal venous return curve, with equilibrium at point A. Now let us assume that the person suddenly begins to breathe against a continuous negative pressure of −3 mm. Hg. This will cause the average cardiac output curve to shift to the left 3 mm. Hg, and the new equilibrium point will be point B. This represents approximately 15 per cent increase in cardiac output and a right atrial pressure decrease from 0 mm. Hg to −3 mm. Hg. However, this 15 per cent increase in cardiac output is still only barely measurable by the usual methods for measuring cardiac output.

Now let us assume that the person breathes continuously against a negative pressure of −10 mm. Hg. This will shift the cardiac output curve to the far left, as illustrated by the short-dashed curve in Figure 24–2. This curve will equate with the venous return curve at point C, which also represents a cardiac output 15 per cent above normal. In other words, the initial negative pressure of −3 mm. Hg causes all the increase in cardiac output that is going to occur, and further negativity causes no further enhancement in cardiac output. The obvious reasons for this is that at right atrial pressures below −3 mm. Hg, the cardiac output curve equates with the venous return curve on its plateau, and any degree of change in the cardiac output curve within this range will have no effect on cardiac output. It will be remembered that the plateau of the venous return curve is determined by collapse of the veins entering the thorax (Holt, 1943, 1944a, 1959; Duomarco, 1945, 1946, 1950a, b, c, d; Guyton, 1954a, 1962a).

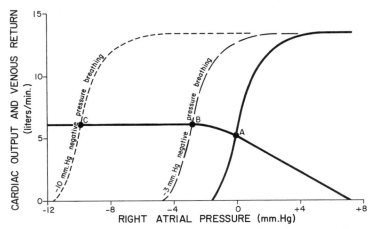

Figure 24–2. Analysis of the effect of negative pressure breathing on cardiac output.

Therefore, to summarize the effect of negative pressure breathing on cardiac output, the initial few millimeters of negative pressure probably can cause a very slight increase in cardiac output, but further decrease in negativity will not cause any additional increase in output.

Effect of Positive Pressure Breathing on Cardiac Output

In contrast to the very slight effect of negative pressure breathing on cardiac output, positive pressure breathing has a very serious effect, but this time decreasing the output rather than increasing it. Furthermore, the normal human being is far more likely to be subjected to positive pressure breathing than to negative pressure breathing, for example, in the use of various respiratory apparatuses including the anesthesia machine, the SCUBA diving apparatus, gas masks, and even musical instruments.

Figure 24–3 gives an analysis of cardiac output when a person suddenly begins to breathe against a positive pressure of $+80$ mm. Hg. Immediately after the beginning of breathing against this pressure, the cardiac output curve shifts from the solid curve (normal) to the right, as illustrated by the long-dashed curve. For the first second or so after exposure to the positive pressure, the venous return curve remains essentially the same, and the new cardiac output curve would equate with the normal venous return curve at point B, with a cardiac output of only 0.5 liter per minute.

However, within the first few seconds, two compensations occur that instantaneously help to compensate for the decrease in cardiac output. First, and probably the most important of these, is the very strong contraction of the expiratory muscles during expiration in order to force air out of the lungs against the positive pressure. The powerful contraction, principally of the abdominal muscles, increases the mean systemic pressure many millimeters of mercury—under maximal conditions to as high as 20 mm. Hg (Guyton, 1962b). Second, the positive pressure in the lungs forces a portion of the blood in the lungs and heart into the systemic circulation.

This, too, tends to increase the mean systemic pressure. Therefore, within the first few seconds after the person begins positive pressure breathing, the venous return curve shifts far to the right, as illustrated by the long-dashed curve, and this equates with the cardiac output curve at point C at a cardiac output of approximately 4 liters per minute.

A third compensation develops during the ensuing 20 to 40 seconds, that is, excitation of the autonomic reflexes, which further enhance the cardiac output in two ways: (1) by sympathetic stimulation of the peripheral vessels, this increasing the mean systemic pressure still further, and (2) by enhancing the cardiac output curve. The two new curves, after these effects take place, are represented by the short-dashed curves, which equate at point D, showing a cardiac output of 4.5 liters per minute and a right atrial pressure of 7 mm. Hg.

The analysis in Figure 24–3 shows that the strong contraction of expiratory muscles and the shift of blood from the chest into the systemic circulation are usually enough by themselves to cause most of the compensation required during breathing against a positive pressure of only 8 mm. Hg. In this case, the cardiovascular reflexes are not called on to a great extent. However, at higher positive pressures, all three of these compensations undoubtedly play major roles, the elevation of mean systemic pressure by the strong expiratory muscle contraction probably always playing the most important role. The normal animal can breathe continuously for several hours against a positive pressure of up to 15 to 25 mm. Hg without this causing death (Carr, 1946). However, at pressures that are not very much higher, the cardiac output falls so low that death ensues.

Since the normal person can breathe continuously against a positive pressure of 15 to 25 mm. Hg, which would also raise the right atrial pressure up to approximately these same values, we can assume that the three compensatory mechanisms discussed above can raise the mean systemic pressure to a value at least a few millimeters of mercury higher than the positive pressure in the lungs—that is, to perhaps 20 to 30 mm. Hg.

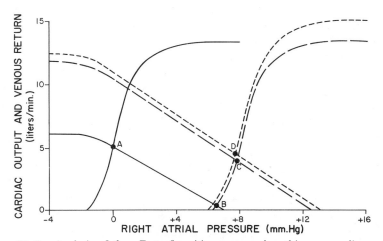

Figure 24–3. Analysis of the effect of positive pressure breathing on cardiac output.

Effect of Positive Pressure Breathing on the Pumping by the Left Ventricle

In the foregoing discussions of positive and negative pressure breathing, we have not mentioned their effect on blood flow through the lungs or on the function of the left heart, because both the pulmonary vessels and the left heart are subjected simultaneously to the same changes in external pressure. That is, an increase in intrapleural pressure of 5 mm. Hg increases the pressures in the left heart by 5 mm. Hg and also in the pulmonary vessels by 5 mm. Hg. Therefore, one would expect no significant net changes in the ability of blood to flow through the pulmonary circulatory circulation or of the left heart to fill during positive or negative pressure breathing. For reasons already explained the primary effect almost certainly is on the inflow of blood from the systemic vessels to the right heart.

EFFECT ON CARDIAC OUTPUT OF OPENING THE CHEST

The effect on cardiac output of opening the chest is similar to the effect of breathing against a positive pressure, though we shall see that the two are not exactly the same (Wiggers, 1947b; Fermoso, 1964). The normal intrapleural pressure averages about -4 mm. Hg (this is variable in different parts of the chest [Coleridge, 1954]). When the chest is opened, the intrapleural pressure rises from -4 mm. Hg to 0 mm. Hg. The initial effect, therefore, is a shift in the cardiac output curve to the right, as illustrated by the long-dashed curve of Figure 24–4. The cardiac output falls from the normal value at point A to point B or, in other words, it decreases to approximately one-half normal. Immediately thereafter, however, compensatory effects begin. These compensatory measures are somewhat different

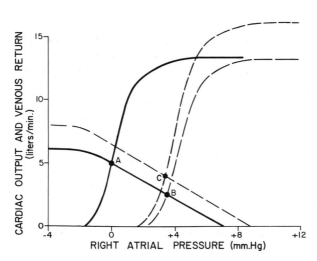

Figure 24–4. Analysis of the effect of opening the chest on cardiac output.

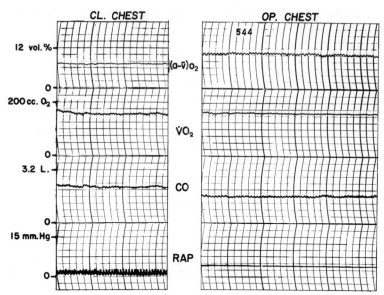

Figure 24–5. Record of changes in cardiac output, A-V oxygen difference, rate of oxygen consumption, and right atrial pressure when the chest is opened, showing decreased output, increased A-V O_2 difference, and increased right atrial pressure but no change in oxygen consumption. [From Fermoso (1964).]

from those that occur in positive pressure breathing because the animal does not have to expire with forceful expiratory movements. Instead, some artificial means must be provided to keep the lungs inflated and to provide artificial respiration.

During the ensuing 20 to 40 seconds, cardiovascular reflexes cause an increase in the mean systemic pressure, thereby shifting the venous return curve upward and to the right, as illustrated by the dashed curve. The reflexes also enhance the cardiac output curve, as is also illustrated by a dashed curve. Thus, the new equilibrium point becomes point C, giving a cardiac output of approximately 4.0 liters per minute, which is somewhat below the normal value. These figures are in accord with Fermoso's results (illustrated in Figure 24–5), showing that opening the chest of the dog decreases the cardiac output by an average of 19 per cent. However, this amount is not very great, and this could account for reports by Blalock (1933b) and Rost (1932) that opening the chest has little effect on cardiac output.

A particular lesson that one can learn from this type of analysis is that experiments in open chest animals are likely to be misleading, because the sympathetic reflexes are already very active and much of the reflex reserve is already used up simply in compensating for the effect of the opened chest. Therefore, *further* reflex response by the animal is likely to be very weak in comparison with that which would be observed in the animal with a closed chest.

EFFECT OF CARDIAC TAMPONADE (AND CONSTRICTIVE PERICARDITIS) ON CARDIAC OUTPUT

Referring to Chapter 9, we see that cardiac tamponade (or constrictive pericarditis) shifts the cardiac output curve to the right, as do all other factors that increase the extracardiac pressure, but in addition, tamponade also depresses the slope of the curve (Isaacs, 1954). This depression of the cardiac output curve is due to the limitation on ventricular filling imposed by the increased pericardial pressure. Thus, at any ventricular volume, the actual transmural pressure tending to stretch the ventricular muscle is reduced because of the greatly increased extracardiac pressure resulting from the tamponade (Sharp, 1960; Ferguson, 1963; Craig, 1968; Fowler and Holmes, 1969). The degree of depression of the curve is greater in the higher cardiac output ranges than in the lower ranges, because it is in the higher cardiac output ranges that the heart needs to expand greatly in order to pump an adequate amount of blood. Thus, as illustrated in Figure 24–6, cardiac tamponade not only shifts the curve to the right but also causes its slope to be greatly decreased. For other representative cardiac output curves that occur in cardiac tamponade the reader is referred to a more complete discussion of this problem in Chapter 9.

Figure 24–6 analyzes the effect of moderately severe cardiac tamponade on the cardiac output. The solid curves represent the analysis for the normal circulation. Let us assume that cardiac tamponade develops and that sufficient fluid fills the pericardial cavity to shift the cardiac output curve to the right and to depress it, as illustrated by the long-dashed curve. The instantaneous effect of this, if it could occur instantaneously, is represented by point B, which is the point at which this long-dashed curve equates with the normal venous return curve. The cardiac output, therefore, would fall instantaneously to approximately 1 liter, and the right atrial pressure would rise to about 6 mm. Hg. However, an instantaneous

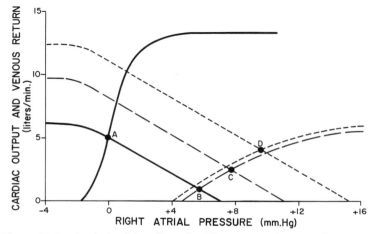

Figure 24–6. Analysis of the effect of cardiac tamponade on cardiac output.

compensatory effect is a shift of blood out of the cardiac chambers into the systemic circulation; that is, the pressure around the heart reduces the amount of blood stored in the heart. Also, expansion of the pericardial cavity against the lungs might compress additional small quantities of blood from the lungs into the systemic circulation. At any rate, one can calculate from Richardson's (1961) pressure-volume curves of the circulation that a severe degree of cardiac tamponade can be expected to increase the mean systemic pressure about 3 to 4 mm. Hg. In the human being this would represent a shift of approximately 350 ml. of blood out of the cardiac chambers into the systemic circulation. In Figure 24–6, this immediate compensation is shown to shift the venous return curve to the right, as illustrated by the long dashed curve, which equates with the new cardiac output curve at point C, giving a cardiac output of 2.5 liters/minute and a right atrial pressure of 8 mm. Hg.

At this point, the same cardiovascular reflex compensations occur as during positive pressure breathing. That is, the decreased cardiac output (and arterial pressure) elicits pressoreceptor reflexes and perhaps also other reflexes that stimulate the sympathetic nervous system (Post, 1951). This further enhances the mean systemic pressure, shifting the venous return curve further to the right, as illustrated by the short-dashed curve. It also enhances the cardiac output curve, which is also illustrated by a short-dashed curve. These two new curves now equate at point D, which represents a cardiac output of 4 liters/minute and a right atrial pressure of 10 mm. Hg.

In prolonged cardiac tamponade or chronic constrictive pericarditis (Boucek, 1952b), the blood volume often increases, further increasing the mean systemic pressure and thereby further overcoming the filling impediment produced by the extracardiac pressure. The important feature of all the compensations is that they keep the mean systemic pressure enough above the right atrial pressure to keep blood flowing into the heart (Fletcher, 1945; Nerlich, 1951; Metcalfe, 1952; Boucek, 1952b; Isaacs, 1954).

In very severe cardiac tamponade, another factor that could possibly affect cardiac output is a reduction in coronary blood flow. Recent work (O'Rourke, 1967) has indeed demonstrated that coronary blood flow is reduced in severe experimental tamponade. This reduction in coronary blood flow presumably results from compression of the myocardial vasculature by the greatly increased pericardial pressure. Although it has not been proved, it might be expected that such a retarded coronary blood flow would cause a decrease in cardiac contractility. This would cause the cardiac output curve during cardiac tamponade to be shifted even further to the right, resulting in further diminution of cardiac output.

Chapter 25

CARDIAC OUTPUT IN MUSCULAR EXERCISE

The most stressful to the circulatory system of all normal physiological conditions is severe muscular exercise. The cardiac output increases almost linearly with the degree of exercise, as was illustrated in Figure 1–1 of Chapter 1, and outputs have been recorded as high as six to seven times normal in athletes (Christensen, 1931; Ekblom and Hermansen, 1968). In the normal young adult, the cardiac output increases to about double the normal when the person is walking up a moderate grade and can increase to four to five times normal during heavy exercise (Chapman, 1954, 1960; Wang, 1960; Theilen, 1955b; Stydom, 1952; Musshoff, 1959; Dexter, 1951; Kowalski, 1954; Widimsky, 1963; Tabakin, 1964; Astrand, 1964; Khouri, 1965; Damato, 1966; Faulkner, 1971; Gilbert, 1971). Almost all the other physiological conditions that we have discussed in previous chapters alter the cardiac output about one-third to one-half as much as does severe exercise. The purpose of the present chapter, therefore, will be to analyze the basic factors in exercise that can cause the tremendous increase in cardiac output.

BASIC MECHANISMS BY WHICH EXERCISE CAN AFFECT CARDIAC OUTPUT

Exercise affects cardiac output in at least three major ways, as follows: (1) Instantaneous tensing of the muscles, especially of the abdominal muscles, can quadruple the mean systemic pressure, thereby increasing the pressure gradient for venous return (Guyton, 1962b). (2) Autonomic effects increase the mean systemic pressure (Guyton, 1954c; Richardson, 1964) and also strengthen the heart as a pump (Krogh, 1913; Meek, 1923; McCrea, 1928; Sarnoff, 1954a; Franklin, 1959; Epstein, 1965; Donald, 1968a,b). (3) The tremendous increase in metabolism in the muscles causes local vasodilatation, which *decreases the resistance to venous return* and thereby increases the cardiac output (Guyton, 1962b; Barcroft, 1953; Skinner and Powell, 1967b).

Instantaneous Increase in Mean Systemic Pressure at the Onset of Exercise

Everyone is familiar with the fact that at the onset or sometimes even before the onset of exercise essentially all the muscles in the entire body become tensed; this generalized tensing of muscles occurs in addition to contraction of the specific muscles which are used to perform the exercise. Measurements in our laboratory have shown that sudden tensing of the abdominal muscles and muscles of the lower leg can increase the mean systemic pressure from the normal of 7 mm. Hg up to 18 to 20 mm. Hg in less than 1 second (Guyton, 1962b). The method used to show this was to cut the spinal cord in the midthoracic region and then to stimulate the distal portion of the cord. The transection of the cord prevented reflex effects from taking place. Furthermore, sympathetic blocking agents were given to the animal to prevent direct stimulation of the sympathetic nerves to the periphery. And still the effect occurred, the mean circulatory pressure rising instantaneously from the normal value of 7 mm. Hg up to 18 to 20 mm. Hg.

It was pointed out in Chapter 12 that seven-eighths of the mean circulatory pressure is determined by the mean systemic pressure and one-eighth by the mean pulmonary pressure. Therefore, it is readily evident that when the mean circulatory pressure rises instantaneously to 18 to 20 mm. Hg, the mean systemic pressure also rises almost proportionately.

A rise in mean systemic pressure such as this up to two to three times normal obviously will increase the *pressure gradient for venous return* almost the same amount. Thus, one would expect an instantaneous increase in cardiac output. Our experiments have, indeed, shown that this instantaneous increase in output occurs just as soon as muscular activity begins; this is illustrated in Figure 25–1. However, the instantaneous increase in output has been approximated 40 per cent rather than the 150 per cent which one would have predicted from the great increase in pressure gradient for venous return (Guyton, 1962b). Present evidence indicates that the reason

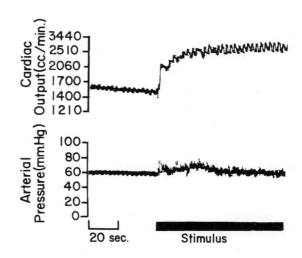

Figure 25–1. Instantaneous increase in cardiac output caused by sudden intermittent stimulation (2 times per second) of the lower half of the spinal cord. The mean systemic pressure rose simultaneously from 7 to 18 mm. Hg. [Reprinted from Guyton, Douglas, Langston, and Richardson (1962b).]

for this disparity is that muscular compression not only increases the mean systemic pressure but also simultaneously compresses the intramuscular and intra-abdominal vessels, thereby increasing the *resistance to venous return*, which partially opposes the expected rise in cardiac output (Anrep, 1935). This will be discussed later in the Chapter.

Autonomic Changes That Enhance Cardiac Output During Muscular Exercise

Rushmer and his colleagues (1959) have emphasized the importance of autonomic effects in enhancing cardiac output following the onset of exercise. They have demonstrated that within a second or so after the onset of exercise, the heart rate begins to increase, and within 10 to 20 seconds it will have doubled, or perhaps even become 2.5 times normal. This effect results from decreased vagal impulses and enhanced sympathetic impulses to the heart (Warner, 1960). Other studies, particularly by Sarnoff (1955), Sonnenblick (1965b), and Keroes (1969), have shown that sympathetic stimulation of the heart increases cardiac contractility. Therefore, in two ways the heart becomes a much better pump: first, by increasing its rate (Meek, 1923; Krogh, 1913; Rushmer, 1959; Franklin, 1959; Donald and Shepard, 1963; Cerretelli, 1964; Tabakin, 1964; Ashkar, 1966; Damato, 1966; Braunwald, 1967; Van Clitters and Franklin, 1969; Hermansen, 1970; Faulkner, 1971), and, second, by increasing its strength of contraction (Sarnoff, 1955; Sonnenblick, 1965b; Keroes, 1969). Both these effects elevate the cardiac output curve, as is shown in the graphical analyses of Figures 25–3 and 25–4.

Many recent studies have attempted to evaluate the importance of autonomic stimulation of the heart in elevating cardiac output during exercise (Kahlar, 1962a; Ashkar, 1963; Bishop and Segel, 1963; Bruce, 1963; Chamberlain and Howard, 1964; Epstein, 1965; Schroder and Werkö, 1965; Donald, 1964a,b, 1968a,b; Cronin, 1967). The results of these studies on experimental animals have, in general, been conflicting, but a thorough examination of the data reveals the following facts: First, total denervation of the heart causes only a slight depression of cardiac output at near maximum levels of exercise. However, dogs with denervated hearts require approximately 20 to 30 seconds longer than normal animals to reach peak values of cardiac output following the onset of exercise. Second, the autonomic stimulation of the heart occurs both through the actions of the cardiac nerves and through the action of the adrenal catecholamines. The performance of the heart during exercise is little impaired if either of these mechanisms of autonomic stimulation is removed. Third, following denervation of the heart and inhibition of adrenal catecholamines, the heart is still able to increase its output two to three times above the resting level, this increase in output being due solely to the classic Starling's law of the heart. Thus, the performance of the heart is only slightly impaired by this procedure at submaximal levels of exercise. Fourth, following cardiac denervation and inhibition of adrenal catecholamines, the cardiac output is substantially curtailed at maximum levels of exercise. This is particularly shown in the studies of Donald (1968a), who compared the cardiovascular responses to racing in greyhound dogs before and after total cardiac denervation and inhibition of adrenal catecholamines. In contrast to normal dogs, denervated greyhounds treated with an adrenergic blocking agent were often unable to complete a five-sixteenth mile course. Of those animals completing the course, most had slowed to a walk in the last third of the race or collapsed from total exhaustion immediately upon completion of the race. As we shall see, these results are exactly what one would expect on the basis of the graphical analyses of cardiac output during exercise, which appear later in this chapter.

The autonomic effects are not limited to the heart, however, for at the same time that the effectiveness of the heart as a pump is being increased, the sympathetic stimuli also cause peripheral vasoconstriction (Herrick, 1940; Merritt, 1959; Rowlands and Donald, 1968; Bevegard and Shepherd, 1965; Shepherd, 1967), thereby further increasing the mean systemic pressure (Guyton, 1962). Very powerful sympathetic stimulation can increase the mean systemic pressure approximately 12 mm. Hg, up to about 19 mm. Hg (Richardson, 1964). This increase in mean systemic pressure is about three-fifths as great as that caused by muscular compression (Guyton, 1962b). If we add this additional increase to the instantaneous increase resulting from tensing of all the musculature of the body, we find that it can rise to as high as 30 or more mm. Hg.

In addition to the sympathetic constriction of the peripheral vessels during exercise, the heart also usually constricts, which displaces blood into the peripheral vessels and thereby undoubtedly adds another few millimeters of mercury to the mean systemic pressure (Gauer, 1955; Rushmer, 1959; Braunwald, 1963b, 1967).

The causes of the autonomic stimulation in exercise are not well known. However, studies for over half a century have indicated that the autonomic centers of the nervous system are not stimulated significantly by impulses from peripheral receptors during exercise but instead are stimulated by collateral fibers coming from the motor areas of the brain (Krogh, 1913; Rushmer, 1959). That is, not only do impulses travel from the motor areas of the brain to the skeletal muscles during exercise, but collateral impulses also go to diencephalic and medullary vasomotor centers, resulting in the autonomic effects observed during exercise, as discussed above. Smith, in particular, has implicated the fields of Forel in these autonomic reactions (Rushmer and Smith, 1959), for electrical stimulation in this region of the brain stem causes reactions in the circulatory system similar to those observed during exercise.

NEUROGENIC VASODILATION OF THE MUSCULAR VESSELS AT THE ONSET OF EXERCISE. Another autonomic effect that occurs in muscular exercise is stimulation of vasodilator nerve fibers to the active muscles at the onset of exercise. This effect has been studied principally by Uvnas and Folkow (Folkow, 1956), who have shown that at the instant a muscle becomes active, or in some instances even before it becomes active, blood flow increases in the muscle. This increased flow is blocked by atropine or by denervation of the sympathetic nerves to the muscle. Therefore, it is assumed to be mediated by sympathetic cholinergic vasodilator nerve fibers. The effects seem to result from parallel excitation by the motor cortex of vasodilator fibers leading to the muscles at the same time that the skeletal muscle fibers are activated.

The importance of this vasodilating effect is yet unknown, because after a few seconds' time the muscle vessels dilate anyway as a result of local muscle metabolism, as will be discussed below. It is quite possible that this nervous vasodilatation is an anticipatory reaction which increases the nutrient supply to the muscle even before the muscle reaches a state of extra nutritional need. Obviously, this would enhance the effectiveness of muscle contraction.

Decrease in Intramuscular Resistance to Blood Flow Resulting from Muscular Metabolism

From the earliest studies on muscular blood flow, it has been known that muscular activity increases the rate of blood flow through the active muscles (Tichy, 1948; Stainsby, 1962; Guyton, 1962b; Coffman, 1963; Hyman, 1963; Corcondilas, 1964; Jones and Berne, 1964; Bevegard and Shepherd, 1967; Costin and Skinner, 1971). Indeed, local blood flows as great as 12 to 15 times normal have actually been recorded immediately following intense muscular activity (Barcroft, 1953), and this occurs even when the nervous vasodilator effect of Uvnas and Folkow, which was discussed above, is completely blocked. Therefore, one of the most important factors affecting cardiac output in muscular exercise is undoubtedly the greatly reduced resistance to blood flow in the muscles themselves. This metabolic decrease in resistance begins about 5 to 10 seconds after the onset of exercise and becomes maximal only after a minute or more (Guyton, 1962). Therefore, it is a lagging response.

The precise cause of the metabolic vasodilatation in active muscles is yet unknown. Many different suggestions have been offered, such as the release of various vasodilator substances from the muscles, including acetylcholine, histamine, various cellular electrolytes such as potassium, breakdown products of adenosine triphosphate, and other proteolytic substances (Anrep, 1944; Barsoum, 1936; Skinner, 1967a,b, 1969, 1970; Kontos, 1968; Stainsby and Fregly, 1968; Wildenthal, 1968; Overbeck and Grega, 1970; Scott, 1970; Dobson, 1971; see also references in Chapter 19). Although all of these substances have vasodilating properties, their actual importance in regulating blood flow in exercise is still in question.

Another suggestion that one frequently hears, but which lacks support, has been that the increased metabolism of muscular activity causes reflex vasodilatation in the muscles. However, experiments in persons in whom the autonomic nerves to the muscles have been completely removed have demonstrated that vasodilatation still occurs equally as much as when the nerves are intact (Barcroft, 1952), except perhaps for the initial vasodilating effect studied by Uvnas and Folkow and which was discussed above. Consequently, this shows that, even if reflexes do occur, they are of minor importance in comparison with the metabolic vasodilatation.

Finally, a number of different investigators, including workers in our laboratory, have suggested that the vasodilatation might result from a relative lack of oxygen in the vascular smooth muscle during skeletal muscle activity (Jalavisto, 1948; Crawford, 1959; Ross, 1962; Guyton, 1964; Carrier, 1964, 1966; Fairchild, 1966; Walker and Guyton, 1967). Certainly it is well known that the oxygen saturation of the venous and capillary blood falls drastically during exericse (Donald, 1957; Barger, 1961). It is suggested, therefore, that the muscle fibers utilize oxygen so rapidly during muscular activity that the amount of oxygen available to the vascular walls themselves is reduced. To express this still another way, the active skeletal muscle fibers are presumed to be in competition with the vascular elements for the available oxygen, so that when the muscle uses an excess of oxygen, one would also expect a deficiency of oxygen in the vascular smooth muscle, this perhaps causing vasodilatation simply because of lack of adequate nutrition of the smooth muscle. This subject was discussed in far more detail in Chapter 19, which took up specifically the effect of oxygen lack on cardiac output. At any rate, many studies correlating cardiac output with the increase in rate of oxygen consumption during muscular exercise have demonstrated an almost linear relationship between these two factors (Boothby, 1915; Douglas, 1922; Asmussen, 1941, 1955a, 1955b; Sleator, 1951; Kao, 1954; Bishop, 1954; Donald, 1955; Freedman, 1955; Barger, 1956; Barratt-Boyes, 1957; Astrand, 1964; Tabakin, 1964; Smulyan, 1965; Wright and Sonnenschein, 1965; Ekelund and Holmgren, 1967; Douglas and Becklake, 1968; Ouellet and Becklake, 1969).

Other Effects of Muscular Contraction on Blood Flow

Two other effects of muscular contraction on blood flow are: activation of the "venous pump" during muscular activity and occlusion of blood vessels in the muscles during tetanic contraction.

THE VENOUS PUMP. The function of the venous pump has already been discussed in Chapter 10. It is important only when the person is in the upright position; ordinarily only a slight amount of muscular activity in the lower limbs is sufficient to activate the venous pump almost fully (Pollack, 1949a, 1949b; Hickam, 1949; Walker, 1950; Hojensgard, 1952; Stegall, 1966). Yet if a person stands absolutely still in the upright position, so much blood often "pools" in the lower part of the body that the cardiac output falls drastically, and the person faints. However, if he occasionally moves from side to side or walks slowly, even this very slight amount of exercise is usually sufficient to activate the venous pump almost entirely, and further degrees of exercise have little additional effect on the effectiveness of the pump.

OCCLUSION OF MUSCLE VESSELS DURING TETANIC CONTRACTION. Occlusion of blood vessels during tetanic muscular contraction can be a serious detriment to blood flow in the muscles (Anrep, 1935; Barcroft, 1953). For instance, one can demonstrate this effect simply by closing the fists extremely tightly for 20 to 30 seconds. The lack of blood flow through the muscles causes both pain and muscle weakness.

In the experiments quoted earlier in the chapter in which the spinal cord was sectioned in the mid-thoracic region (Guyton, 1962b), *tetanic* stimulation of most of the muscles of the lower body at first caused as much as a 30 to 40 per cent increase in cardiac output, but this lasted only for a few seconds before the cardiac output returned almost back to normal even though the pressure gradient for venous return remained as much as two times the normal. In other words, the strong tetanic contraction of the abdominal muscles and muscles of the legs caused so much compression of the vessels that the *resistance to venous return* had risen as much as had the pressure gradient for venous return. The two effects therefore nullified each other and prevented any permanent increase in cardiac output. On the other hand, *intermittent* contraction of the same muscles caused an immediate and sustained increase in cardiac output. These results have been further borne out in experiments by others in which tetanic contraction has been shown to decrease the blood flow through muscles very greatly in comparison with intermittent contraction (Anrep, 1935; Barcroft, 1953; see also Figure 19–1, which is reproduced from Barcroft).

GRAPHICAL ANALYSIS OF CHANGES IN CARDIAC OUTPUT AFTER THE ONSET OF EXERCISE

Time Course of the Changes That Affect Cardiac Output Following the Onset of Exercise

Figure 25–2 illustrates how each of the major factors that affect cardiac output changes following the onset of exercise; these time values are based on studies of mean systemic pressure, resistance to venous return, and cardiac output that we have carried out recently in our department (Guyton, 1962b), on heart rate studies reported by Rushmer (1954) and Warner (1960a), and on cardiac output studies by Wang (1960) and Chapman (1960). The solid curve represents the changes in mean systemic pressure, showing that when very heavy exercise begins, this can rise instantaneously from the normal resting value of 7 mm. Hg up to as high as 18 mm. Hg. During the ensuing 7 to 8 seconds the mean systemic pressure remains at this level, but by then sympathetic stimulation begins, increasing the vasomotor tone throughout the body, which in turn further increases the mean systemic pressure up to as high as 25 mm. Hg or more. After about 20 to 40 seconds, the mean systemic pressure has reached a new plateau. Obviously, the *pressure gradient for venous return* (mean systemic pressure minus right atrial pressure) increases simultaneously with this increase in mean systemic pressure.

The dashed curve of Figure 25–2 illustrates the changes in heart rate, showing that after approximately 1½ to 2 seconds the heart rate begins to rise and within approximately 20 seconds has become over 2½ times normal. (These data are based on published records by Rushmer and his colleagues, 1954.) It is reasonable to expect, on the basis of Sarnoff's (1954) demonstration that sympathetic stimulation greatly enhances cardiac contractility, that the strength of contraction of the heart has also greatly increased during this same period of time.

The dash-dot curve shows the changes in resistance to venous return during the course of the muscular exercise. Immediately after the onset of

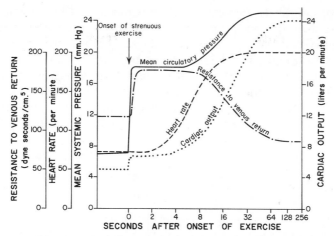

Figure 25–2. Time course of the major changes that affect cardiac output following the onset of very strenuous exercise.

very strenuous exercise, the clamping of the muscles around the vessels, particularly around the veins in the abdomen, tends to block blood flow from the peripheral vessels back to the heart, thereby immediately increasing the resistance to venous return at the onset of muscular exercise. However, this increase in resistance is more than outweighed by the increased mean systemic pressure. Consequently, as much as a 40 to 60 per cent instantaneous increase in cardiac output still occurs despite this rise in resistance to venous return.

Approximately 5 to 10 seconds after the onset of the exercise, the metabolism in the muscles begins to cause vasodilatation, the blood vessels dilating progressively during the next minute. This offsets the increase in resistance to venous return caused by muscular compression of the vessels and eventually reduces the resistance to venous return down to a value about three-fourths the normal value after a minute and a half.

[It must be noted that these effects on the resistance to venous return are somewhat different from the effects of exercise on the total peripheral resistance, because the resistance to venous return is determined mainly by the resistance in the veins rather than in the arterial side of the vascular tree, whereas total peripheral resistance is determined mainly by arterial and arteriolar resistance (see Chapter 13 for a discussion of this difference). The total peripheral resistance normally remains almost constant during the first 10 to 15 seconds of exercise and then, if the exercise is extremely severe, falls down to as low as one-third to one-half normal.]

The dotted curve of Figure 25–2 illustrates the net effect on cardiac output. The two instantaneous effects that occur at the onset of exercise—the rise in mean systemic pressure and the rise in resistance to venous return—cause opposite effects on cardiac output. The first of these tends to increase the cardiac output, while the second tends to reduce it. Yet ordinarily the increase in the first is sufficiently greater than that of the second that cardiac output rises within the first second after the onset of hard exercise an average of 40 per cent or a maximum of 70 per cent (Guyton, 1962b). Then, as the exercise continues, sympathetic stimulation further elevates the mean systemic pressure and increases the strength of the heart as a pump. Consequently, the cardiac output rises still more. At about this same time, metabolic dilatation of the muscle vessels begins, increasing the venous return still more and allowing the cardiac output to rise much higher. Thus, Figure 25-2 shows that by the end of 40 seconds, the cardiac output has risen to approximately 24 liters per minute, which is almost five times normal.

Graphical Analysis of the Effect of Moderate Exercise on Cardiac Output and Right Atrial Pressure

Figure 25-3 illustrates an analysis of the sequential changes in cardiac output and right atrial pressure at different time intervals after the onset of moderate exercise. The solid curves of the figure are an analysis of the normal resting circulation, the normal operating state being represented by point A. Now assume that there is a sudden onset of moderate exercise. Tensing of the muscles throughout the body immediately causes the mean systemic pressure to rise from 7 mm. Hg to 10 mm. Hg. However, contraction of the muscles around the vessels, particularly of the abdominal muscles around the veins leading to the heart, simultaneously increases the resistance to venous return. Therefore, the venous return curve becomes that represented by the long dashed curve, which illustrates a mean systemic pressure of 10 mm. Hg and a slightly increased resistance to venous return, as denoted by the decreased slope. This venous return curve repre-

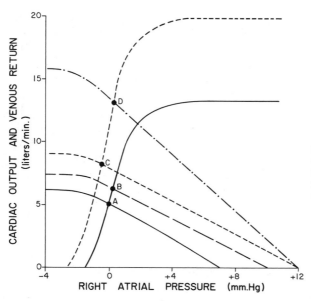

Figure 25-3. Graphical analysis of the changes in cardiac output and right atrial pressure at various time intervals following the onset of moderate exercise.

sents the function of the systemic circulation during the first few seconds after the onset of the moderate exercise. During this same period of time the heart still has not increased its pumping ability. Therefore, the normal cardiac curve is still applicable. The new venous return curve, therefore, equates with the cardiac output curve at point B, which shows that the cardiac output has instantaneously increased from 5 liters to 6 liters per minute and that the right atrial pressure has risen a fraction of a millimeter of mercury.

During the next 15 to 20 seconds, sympathetic stimulation of the circulation will have developed significantly, causing major effects both on the heart and on the peripheral circulation. The short-dashed cardiac output curve shows the effect on cardiac pumping resulting from reflex stimulation of the heart, and the short-dashed venous return curve shows the new venous return curve, which has risen and shifted to the right because of sympathetic enhancement of the mean systemic pressure from 10 to 12 mm. Hg. These two curves equilibrate with each other at point C, which represents a cardiac output of 8 liters per minute and a right atrial pressure slightly less than 0 mm. Hg.

However, even before the autonomic effects become fully developed, metabolic vasodilatation in the active muscles begins, which reduces the resistance to venous return. As a consequence, the venous return curve rotates toward the right and, approximately a minute after the onset of exercise, becomes the dashed-dot curve of Figure 25–3. If we assume that the heart is not further stimulated, the cardiac output curve remains the short-dashed. The new venous return curve equates with the cardiac output curve at point D, which depicts a cardiac output of 13 liters per minute and a right atrial pressure still essentially zero.

The analysis of Figure 25–3 gives essentially the same results that Franklin and Rushmer found in their studies of moderate exercise in dogs on the treadmill, showing a moderate increase in cardiac output with essentially no change in right atrial pressure (Franklin, 1959). Similar results have been observed in human subjects during moderate exercise (Braunwald, 1963b; Ekelund, 1967). Rushmer (1959) used these studies to disclaim the importance of cardiac function curves in the analysis of cardiac output. However, he failed to consider the changes in the venous return curves as well as changes in the cardiac output curves. It is obvious from this analysis that had he considered the changes in the peripheral circulation as well as in the heart, his experiments would have explained beautifully the conditions observed, and, instead of disproving the importance of cardiac function curves, his experiments actually confirm their importance more than ever.

Graphical Analysis of Changes in Cardiac Output and Right Atrial Pressure in Strenuous Exercise

Figure 25–4 illustrates an analysis of the changes in cardiac output and right atrial pressure in strenuous exercise at various time intervals after the onset of exercise. The solid curves with equilibrium at point A represent the normal circulatory conditions. Now let us assume that this normal,

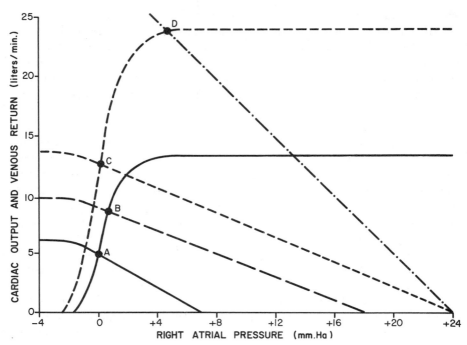

Figure 25–4. Graphical analysis of the changes in cardiac output and right atrial pressure at various time intervals following the onset of very strenuous exercise.

healthy, but not especially athletically trained person suddenly begins the most strenuous exercise that he can attain. Two immediate effects result from instantaneous tensing of all the muscles in his body—a great increase in mean systemic pressure and an increase in resistance to venous return as discussed above. Thus, the long-dashed venous return curve of Figure 25–4 shows a mean systemic pressure of 18 mm. Hg and a decreased slope denoting increased resistance to venous return. During the first few seconds, the strength of the heart as a pump has not increased; therefore, this new venous return curve equates with the normal cardiac output curve at point B, showing an instantaneous increase in cardiac output of approximately 70 per cent, or, in other words, an increase up to a value slightly greater than 8 liters per minute. The right atrial pressure at the same time rises about 0.7 mm. Hg.

During the next 15 to 20 seconds, considerable sympathetic activity begins, causing the venous return and cardiac output curves to become those designated by the short-dashed curves. These equate with each other at point C, showing that by this time the cardiac output has increased to 12.5 liters per minute and that the right atrial pressure is now essentially zero.

Beginning in about 10 seconds, and continuing on for at least the first minute, the resistance to blood flow through the muscles progressively decreases because of metabolic vasodilatation. As a consequence, the venous return curve rotates upward, causing a new point of equilibrium at point D, designating a cardiac output of slightly less than 24 liters per minute and a right atrial pressure of almost 5 mm. Hg. Note particularly in Figure 25-4 that during very strenuous exercise, the heart is operating on the plateau of the cardiac output curve. That this is, indeed, true is demonstrated by the study of Robinson and coworkers (1966), who compared the effect of acute blood volume expansion on cardiac output in human subjects both at rest and during severe exercise. They observed that the acute expansion of blood volume by approximately 1 liter at rest produced only a small increase in central venous pressure but a substantial increase in cardiac output, the output rising approximately one and one-half liters per minute. During maximum exercise, however, the same expansion of the blood volume resulted in a much larger increase in central venous pressure but no increase in cardiac output. Upon examination of Figure 25-4, we see that this is exactly what one would expect.

These are all relatively typical findings during very strenuous exercise in the nonathlete. Even though the right atrial pressure usually remains almost exactly normal in moderate exercise, it often rises a small amount in very strenuous exercise.

If the person had been a well trained athlete, his cardiac output curve might have risen considerably higher than that shown in Figure 25-4 and might have shifted further to the left (Schneider, 1940; Musshoff, 1957, 1959; Epstein, 1965; Donald, 1968a,b). Therefore, the venous return curve would have equated with the cardiac output curve quite a bit further to the left, giving a right atrial pressure much closer to normal. This too is a common finding in exercise, that the right atrial pressure remains closer to zero in the well trained athlete than in the untrained person.

On the other hand, the cardiac output curve in patients with cardiac debility would be expected to shift to the right and to plateau at much lower levels than those shown in Figure 25-4. This obviously would result in both a low cardiac output response to exercise and a markedly rising right atrial pressure, effects that have been observed many times when a person or animal with cardiac insufficiency exercises (McGuire, 1939a; Simonson, 1942; Hickham, 1948a; Barger, 1952; Bishop, 1955; Taylor, 1957; Jones and Reeves, 1968b).

COMPUTER SIMULATION OF CHANGES IN CARDIAC OUTPUT AND OTHER CIRCULATORY FACTORS DURING EXERCISE

Figure 25-5 shows simulated changes in circulatory dynamics during one and one-half minutes of severe exercise, and for three minutes following cessation of exercise. For this simulation the complex computer model described in Chapter 17 was used. Shown in Figure 25-5 (from top to bottom) are changes in the rate of metabolic activity in all of the skeletal muscles of the body, blood flow through these skeletal muscles, cardiac output, degree of sympathetic stimulation, systemic arterial pressure, the oxygen tension of mixed venous blood, the intracellular oxygen tension of the muscles, and urinary output.

Immediately after the onset of exercise, the metabolic rate of the

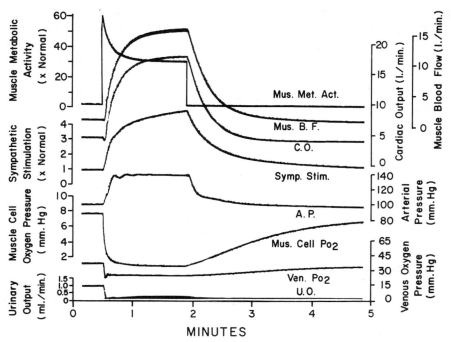

Figure 25-5. Simulation of circulatory dynamics during muscular exercise. At the initial break in the curves the muscles aere activated to a level 60 times their normal value, and their degree of activation was returned to normal at the second break in the curve. [From Guyton, Coleman, and Granger (1972).]

muscles rose to approximately 60 times its resting value, and there was a subsequent rapid increase in the activity of the sympathetic nervous system. These two events were followed within seconds by (1) a rapid reduction in the intracellular oxygen tension of the muscles and in mixed venous oxygen tension, and (2) substantial increases in muscle blood flow and cardiac output. The increase in cardiac output was accounted for entirely by the increase in the rate of blood flow through the skeletal muscles. Note that the simulated increase in cardiac output is very close to that predicted by the graphical analysis of Figures 25-3 and 25-4. Note also in Figure 25-5 that even though cardiac output increased tremendously, the arterial pressure rose only moderately, indicating a drastic reduction in total peripheral resistance. This decrease in total peripheral resistance, despite an increase in the sympathetic stimulation of the cardiovascular system, was due to the intrinsic system for regulating local blood flow in the muscles. That is, any time the muscle blood flow is insufficient to meet the metabolic requirements of the muscle, the arterioles dilate in an effort to increase the local blood flow. This phenomenon was discussed at length in Chapter 19.

The decrease in urinary output to approximately one-third normal following the onset of increased muscular activity is explained as follows: During muscular exercise, the degree of sympathetic stimulation of the cardiovascular system increases markedly. This increase in a sympathetic stimulation causes the afferent arterioles of the kidney to constrict, thus reducing renal blood flow, glomerular filtration, and, consequently, urinary output.

Despite neurogenic driving of the muscles at the same continuous level, the metabolic activity of the muscles decreased considerably from its peak level. This reduction in metabolic activity was due to the development of a metabolic deficit in the muscles. When muscular exercise was abruptly stopped after one and one-half minutes, the metabolic activity of the muscles instantly decreased essentially to normal, but blood flow through the muscles continued at an elevated level for the next several minutes as did cardiac output and arterial pressure. The continued elevations of cardiac output and muscle blood flow resulted from the oxygen debt accumulated in the muscle during the period of increased activity. Thus, muscle blood flow and cardiac output returned to normal only when the oxygen debt within the muscle was repaid, and the intracellular oxygen tension of the muscle returned to normal.

Not shown in Figure 25–5 is the effect of exercise on heart rate. This increased during extreme exercise to approximately 170 beats per minute and returned to normal along a curve similar to that for arterial blood pressure, but slightly less rapidly.

The simulation shown in Figure 25–5 again demonstrates that by using established data the computer may be used to predict changes in many circulatory variables, some of which have been only slightly studied in the past.

STROKE VOLUME VERSUS HEART RATE CHANGES DURING EXERCISE

This chapter would not be complete without mention of the controversy that has raged in the past few years as to whether the increased cardiac output in exercise results from a stroke volume increase or a heart rate increase. Many investigators have provided evidence that the increase in cardiac output results primarily from an increase in heart rate and that stroke volume increases relatively little, approximately 25 to 40 per cent (Meek, 1923; Henderson, 1927b; Rushmer, 1959; Cerretelli, 1964; Tabakin, 1964; Damato, 1966; Grimby, 1966; Erikson, 1971; Faulkner, 1971). Furthermore, Rushmer has collected a large amount of convincing evidence that in *mild to moderate exercise* an increase in heart rate is far more important than the increase in stroke volume. On the other hand, well-controlled experiments by Wang (1960) have shown that the stroke volume output can increase as much as 100 per cent in some persons during *extremely severe exercise*. Results similar to this can be seen in the studies of Smith (1964), who demonstrated that at moderate levels of exercise, increases in heart rate were sufficient to account for the increases in cardiac output, but at maximum levels of exercise, increases in stroke volume became predominant and were often as great as 100 per cent. The importance of an increase in stroke volume during very severe exercise becomes apparent when one recalls that under these conditions, cardiac output can increase to four to five times normal while heart rate increases, at most, to two and one-half times normal.

However, far more significant than the question of whether heart rate or stroke volume is the more important cause of the increased cardiac output is the fact that *either* of these two mechanisms can increase the output if the other fails to do so. Particularly significant studies showing this have been those by Warner (1960b), Miller (1962), Snyder (1962), Donald and Shepherd (1963), and Smulyan (1965), all of whom have shown that when the heart rate mechanism is prevented from operating, the stroke volume mechanism will then operate enough, within its physiological range, to make up for the difference. However, in severe exercise its physiological range is not great enough to supply the demand. Results similar to those in experimental animals can be seen in studies of human patients with complete heart block in whom the hearts were paced at constant rates during periods of exercise (Benchimol, 1964, 1965b).

Therefore, we can conclude (1) that both of these mechanisms are valuable, (2) that either can do the job during light to moderate exercise, and (3) that both are needed to their fullest extent during strenuous exercise.

Furthermore, when the heart rate increases in exercise without an increase in stroke volume output, it still is not the heart rate increase alone that is increasing the output, for we know that increasing the heart rate *per se* above about 125 beats per minute not only fails to increase the pumping effectiveness of the heart but actually decreases it (Miller, 1962; Snyder, 1962; Braunwald, 1967). In addition to the heart rate increase, the heart simultaneously is made a much stronger pump by the same sympathetic stimulation (Sarnoff, 1955) that increases the rate, and several different peripheral factors also work together, as discussed earlier in this chapter, to make the blood in the peripheral circulation flow into the heart with much greater ease, thereby increasing the output. Indeed, without these peripheral factors, however much the heart is stimulated, the output still will not increase because of venous collapse caused by the heart trying to suck blood from the peripheral vessels (Holt, 1959; Guyton, 1962a; see also Chapter 11).

Therefore, it is hardly worth-while to argue which is more important in exercise, increased heart rate or increased stroke volume, because both are necessary and because there are many other equally important factors to consider in the regulation of cardiac output in exercise.

Chapter 26

CARDIAC OUTPUT IN HEART FAILURE: I. BILATERAL FAILURE

A PHYSIOLOGICAL DEFINITION OF HEART FAILURE

Both the words "heart" and "failure" are quite explicit; therefore, the term "heart failure" should mean very simply failure of the heart to pump blood as well as it does normally. If we accept this definition of heart failure, our discussions in this chapter and in the following chapter will be quite simple. Unfortunately, heart failure has too often been defined in terms of the *results* of heart failure rather than in terms of failure of the heart itself. For instance, one type of heart failure is frequently called "backward failure," which means failure with peripheral or pulmonary congestion; another type is called "forward failure," which means failure with low cardiac output. Yet both these types can be traced back to failure of the heart as a pump. The discussions in this and the following chapter will show how the different results can develop from bilateral or unilateral heart failure.

Causes of Heart Failure

Whatever the cause of heart failure, whether it be myocardial damage (Gilbert, 1954; Gammill, 1955; Stone, 1964, 1966; Salisbury, 1965; Kuhn, 1966; Pentecost, 1966; Bradley, 1970; Loeb, 1969; Mueller, 1970), valvular damage (Wiggers, 1922a; Little, 1948; Ferrer, 1953; Hamilton, 1954; McMichael, 1957; Braun, 1959; Jones, 1964a; Miller, 1965; McCredie, 1967; Dodge, 1968; Genest, 1968), toxic damage of the heart (Besterman, 1954), arrhythmia (Wegria, 1950; Holmgren, 1959), or any other cardiac abnormality, the effect on the cardiac output is the same. Some clinicians reserve the term "heart failure" for use only when there is myocardial failure. However, if we accept the above simple definition of heart failure—that failure of the heart means failure to pump blood normally—

then the heart can fail as a result of serious valvular damage, toxicity, or serious arrhythmias equally as much as from myocardial damage. Therefore, in this present discussion, we will consider any pathological diminishment of pumping effectiveness by the heart to be heart failure.

Quantitation of Heart Failure

Heart failure can be quantitated very easily in terms of cardiac output curves (Sarnoff, 1955; Guyton, 1962c; Crowell, 1962; Stone, 1966). In Chapter 9 it was pointed out that any condition that depresses the effectiveness of the heart as a pump depresses the cardiac output curve and shifts it to the right. Such depression is shown in Figures 26–1 to 26–7, though a more complete discussion of this effect and its causes, along with appropriate illustrations, was presented in Chapter 9.

COMPENSATORY MECHANISMS IN HEART FAILURE

When the heart fails, at least three important compensatory mechanisms help to keep the cardiac output from falling too low. These are: (1) cardiovascular reflexes; (2) retention of fluid, which increases blood volume and consequently further increases the mean systemic pressure; and (3) hypertrophy of those portions of the heart that are not damaged.

Reflexes in Heart Failure

Several different cardiovascular reflexes become excited automatically whenever the cardiac output falls. Perhaps the most important of these is the pressoreceptor reflex which is initiated by a decrease in systemic arterial pressure (Charlier, 1947a,b, 1948a; Vleeschhouwer, 1950; Page, 1955; Leusen, 1956b; Sagawa, 1965; Allison, 1969). It is possible, also, that pressoreceptors in the pulmonary circulation enter in the elicitation of this reflex, though the importance of these in heart failure has not been studied.

In addition to the pressoreceptor reflex, depressed blood flow to the brain can initiate the central nervous system ischemic reflex. Most studies of this reflex have indicated that it is not initiated until the arterial pressure falls below approximately one-half normal (Sagawa, 1961a, 1961b, 1967b). However, these experiments were all performed under acute ischemia, and at least some evidence has accumulated recently which indicates that chronic ischemia can elicit the reflex even when the arterial pressure is depressed only slightly below normal (Dickinson, personal communication). Finally, we also know that some reflexes can be initiated in the myocardium itself when it becomes damaged or is stimulated in other ways (Doutheil, 1959; Frye, 1960; Gupta, 1966). Unfortunately, we know almost nothing about the value of these in cardiac failure.

Regardless of which reflexes participate in the reflex compensations to cardiac failure, the efferent limb of all the reflexes is the autonomic nervous system; within less than a minute after the onset of serious acute heart failure, the entire sympathetic nervous system becomes very strongly excited (Guyton, 1954c) and the parasympathetics to the heart presumably become inhibited. The outward signs of these effects are cold, clammy skin with sweating and a very rapid heart rate.

The reflexes cause two different effects which can be highly beneficial to the cardiac output: (1) They enhance the effectiveness of the heart as a pump (Sarnoff, 1954a; Folkow, 1956; Braunwald, 1963a; Randall, 1967) and (2) they enhance the mean systemic pressure (Guyton, 1958c; Richardson, 1964). The first of these two effects, the increase in cardiac pumping effectiveness, is known by everyone, but the increase in mean systemic pressure, except for a few notable exceptions (Weber, 1850; Starling, 1897; Bolton, 1903, 1917; De Burgh Daly, 1925; Starr, 1940a, 1940b), has been almost completely neglected in the study of heart failure. Studies in our laboratory have shown that maximal sympathetic stimulation can increase the mean systemic pressure from 7 mm. Hg up to 19 mm. Hg (Guyton, 1954c; Richardson, 1964), which represents about a 2½ fold increase. This obviously increases the pressure gradient for venous return. Thus, not only do the reflexes make the heart a better pump, they also force additional quantities of blood from the systemic circulation into the heart, thereby priming the chambers of the heart to greater volumes and, in accordance with Starling's law of the heart, enhancing the force of contraction up to the physiologic limit of the heart. Therefore, this increased pressure gradient for venous return resulting from the increased mean systemic pressure is undoubtedly one of the most important of all the cardiac output compensatory measures in heart failure—particularly in acute failure.

Reflexes begin to develop about 2 to 7 seconds after sudden acute failure of the heart and ordinarily become maximally developed within approximately a minute (Guyton, 1954c). They continue to be active at least for several days or until some other compensatory mechanism returns the cardiac output back to its normal level.

Most, though not all (Lewis, 1959), of the reflex compensations probably disappear in chronic heart failure. One of the reasons for this is that the pressoreceptors almost always adapt to the new pressure conditions over a period of several days, and the reflex fades away (Kubicek, 1953; Ueda, 1966; Alexander, 1967; Aars, 1968; Krieger, 1970). Also, as other compensatory mechanisms become active in heart failure, such as fluid retention to increase the mean systemic pressure or hypertrophy of undamaged portions of the heart, the cardiac output rises, and as a result, the reflexes lose their initiating stimulus. Another reason for the disappearance of reflex compensation of cardiac contractility, one that has only recently been recognized, is that the catecholamine stores of the heart become almost completely depleted in chronic heart failure (Chidsey, 1964; Spann, 1965, 1967; Covell, 1966; Pool, 1968). It is not certain whether this depletion of the catecholamine stores results from an increased utilization of the catecholamines because of the increased cardiac stimulation or from a depressed synthesis of these compounds, but the overall result is a loss of reflex stimulation of cardiac function (Covell, 1966). Thus, we see that the cardiovascular nervous reflexes are extremely important in compensating for the depressed cardiac output almost instantly after the onset of acute failure, and they probably play a major compensatory role during the next few days, but beyond that time other compensations are probably by then far more important.

We can illustrate the importance of cardiovascular reflexes in acute heart failure by alluding to experiments that we performed several years ago in which standard degrees of pulmonary constriction were applied in control animals and in animals whose reflexes had been blocked by spinal anesthesia. In the animals with intact reflexes, the cross-sectional area of the pulmonary artery could be reduced to less than one-half that in the total spinal anesthesia animals without causing death (Guyton, 1954b). In other words, the reflexes were exceedingly important in overcoming the depressed ability of the heart to pump blood under these conditions.

Fluid Retention in Heart Failure

Later in this and the next chapter we will see that intravenous administration of fluid to a patient in the late stages of heart failure can cause serious harm and can actually lead to reduction in cardiac output. Yet experiments have demonstrated that in the early stages of heart failure the retention of fluid is almost certainly an important compensatory mechanism in preventing the cardiac output from falling too low. The retention of fluid increases the mean systemic pressure, which in turn increases the pressure gradient for venous return (Guyton, 1955b). As a result, the heart's chambers became primed with larger than normal quantities of blood; if the heart has any intrinsic compensatory ability left, then this will benefit the cardiac output. Unfortunately, by the time many cases of heart failure are seen by the physician, the intrinsic compensatory ability of the heart has already been taxed to its maximum so that additional priming of the heart with blood will not cause the heart to pump extra amounts of blood. Under these conditions it is obvious that further retention of fluid cannot be of value but instead will only cause additional edema with eventual demise of the patient (Gilbert, 1944). Yet before the patient arrives at this serious stage, he often retains an amount of fluid equal to almost 50 per cent of his normal extracellular fluid volume (Seymour, 1942). Animal experiments have convinced us that this increase in fluid is of major compensatory value in preventing death from low cardiac output (Guyton, 1955a).

Causes of Fluid Retention in Cardiac Failure. Retention of fluid in heart failure is caused by at least two different mechanisms, one of which is entirely hemodynamic and the other of which is hormonal. The hemodynamic mechanism is simply the following: When the cardiac output falls below normal as a result of cardiac damage, the amount of blood flowing to the kidneys becomes reduced, partly because of reduced arterial pressure and partly because of cardiovascular reflexes which constrict the renal arterioles (Warren, 1944; Borst, 1948; Berne, 1950, 1952;

Levy, 1951; Davies, 1952). In addition, the back pressure in the veins resulting from cardiac failure might cause further reduction in renal function (Blake, 1949). The compounding of all these factors causes the glomerular filtration rate to decrease and tubular reabsorption to increase, these two effects greatly reducing the urinary output and causing fluid retention (Briggs, 1948; Davis, 1965; Baumber, 1970). In moderate cardiac failure the enhancement of tubular reabsorption seems to be the predominant factor (Briggs, 1948), but in severe failure both effects probably play a major role.

The hormonal mechanism results from the secretion of aldosterone by the adrenal cortex (Davis, 1958), perhaps initiated as follows: diminished cardiac output causes ischemia of the kidneys, which then release large quantities of the enzyme *renin* into the blood. Within the blood, renin causes formation of the hormone *angiotensin,* which in turn stimulates the zona glomerulosa of the adrenal glands to secrete aldosterone (Davis, 1962). Once aldosterone is released by the adrenal glands, it passes by way of the blood to the kidneys, where it enhances the reabsorption of sodium by the renal tubules. Sodium reabsorption then promotes water reabsorption from the tubules by two mechanisms. First, as the sodium is reabsorbed, it increases the osmotic pressure of the peritubular fluids while decreasing the osmotic pressure of the tubular fluids, thereby developing an osmotic gradient that causes very large quantities of water to pass through the tubular walls. Second, the large quantity of sodium accumulating in the body fluids increases the osmotic pressure of the body fluids, initiating the release of antidiuretic hormone by the supraoptico-neurohypophyseal axis; the anti-diuretic hormone in turn enhances the reabsorption of water by the kidneys (Harris, 1955).

That this hormonal mechanism plays a significant role in causing fluid retention during heart failure is evidenced by several findings. For example, following cardiac failure in dogs, there is marked retention of sodium and water (Barger, 1952; Davis, 1955, 1957, 1964; Hamilton, 1954; Wolff, 1957; Yagi, 1968). Coincident with the retention of water and sodium, the blood concentrations of renin (Johnston, 1968; Yagi, 1968; Baumber, 1969, 1970; Schneider, 1969), angiotensin (Genest, 1968), and aldosterone (Davis, 1957, 1965; Wolff, 1957) are all increased.

In summary, both hemodynamic and hormonal mechanisms promote marked retention of fluids and electrolytes when the cardiac output falls significantly below normal. However, as the cardiac output returns back toward normal during the course of compensation, the retention of fluids ceases, and renal output once again becomes essentially normal.

To exacerbate further the accumulation of fluid and electrolytes in heart failure, a decrease in cardiac output also causes thirst and a desire for salt, this presumably resulting from stimulation of the thirst center and the salt appetite center of the hypothalamus when the cardiac output falls below normal (Wolf, 1958). Therefore, if water and salt are available, the person's natural inclinations can, at least theoretically, further increase the amount of retained fluids and electrolytes in the body.

The buildup of body fluids increases the mean systemic pressure in two different ways: first, by increasing the interstitial fluid volume and, second, by increasing the blood volume (Warren, 1943). The increase in interstitial fluid volume increases the mean systemic pressure by compressing the outsides of the blood vessels (Guyton, 1952c), whereas the increase in blood volume increases the mean systemic pressure by enhancing the filling of the blood vessels (Guyton, 1954c; Richardson, 1961). Observations in our laboratory indicate that increasing the interstitial fluid volume increases the mean systemic pressure about one-eighth as much as does a similar increase in blood volume.

Hypertrophy of Undamaged Portions of the Heart

One of the principal long-term mechanisms of compensation for cardiac stress of many types is hypertrophy of the undamaged cardiac musculature (Friedberg, 1956; Katz, 1960; Linzbach, 1960; Badeer, 1964a,b; Zuehlke, 1966; Bing, 1968; Dodge and Baxley, 1968). The precise mechanism by which undamaged myocardial muscle is stimulated to hypertrophy is uncertain, but Badeer (1964a, 1968) has emphasized that all conditions which cause cardiac hypertrophy have one factor in common: these conditions cause an increase in the metabolic rate per heart beat of the myocardium. Thus, following acute damage to a portion of the heart, the remaining portions of the heart must work more strenuously with each contraction in an attempt to pump all the blood returning to the heart. Thus, the metabolic rate per beat of the undamaged heart muscle is increased. Furthermore, when fluid retention occurs, the tendency for venous return becomes even greater, and the undamaged myocardial muscle must now work even harder to pump all of the blood returning to it. As a result of this increased workload, the undamaged portions of the heart begin to hypertrophy. The clinical course of patients after a myocardial infarction indicates that the usual time course of the hypertrophy lasts over a period of several months, the hypertrophy becoming measurable within a few weeks and perhaps reaching maximum in five to eight months.

In some patients, the remaining musculature probably hypertrophies enough after a myocardial infarction to make the heart almost as strong a pump as it had been previously (Friedberg, 1956). Unfortunately, however, almost no quantitative information is available concerning this. Recent evidence, however, does indicate that the increase in contractile strength of the myocardium following hypertrophy is due to an increase in muscle mass alone, the contractile strength of the individual muscle fibers being unchanged or possibly even decreased slightly (Grimm, 1963; Sandler and Dodge, 1963; Meerson, 1965; Spann, 1966, 1967; Badeer, 1967).

Other types of cardiac damage besides infarction can also be compensated by hypertrophy of the musculature. This is particularly true for the different types of valvular disorders. For instance, the muscular mass of the left ventricle can hypertrophy to as much as six times normal size in serious aortic stenosis of regurgitation, and similar degrees of hypertrophy are also often found in some types of congenital heart disease.

GRAPHICAL ANALYSIS OF CARDIAC OUTPUT AND OTHER CIRCULATORY EFFECTS IN HEART FAILURE

In this chapter, we will analyze graphically the changes in cardiac output and other circulatory functions in bilateral heart failure, and in the following chapter we will analyze the effects of unilateral failure, especially the effects on the pulmonary circulation.

Initial Effect of Acute Bilateral, Moderate Heart Failure on Cardiac Output

The dark solid curves of Figure 26–1 illustrate an analysis of cardiac output and right atrial pressure for the normal circulation, with equilibrium at point A. Now let us assume that a moderate myocardial infarction suddenly develops that decreases the pumping effectiveness of the heart to approximately one-fourth normal, which is represented by the long-dashed cardiac output curve of the figure. The venous return is not altered during the first few seconds after this sudden diminishment of the pumping ability of the heart because the blood volume and the vasomotor tone are still the same. Therefore, the normal venous return curve is still operative in the circulation. The new cardiac output curve—the long-dashed curve—therefore equates with the normal venous return curve at point B, showing a cardiac output of approximately 2 liters per minute and a right atrial pressure of 4 mm. Hg. At this level of cardiac output, the person will either faint, or at least appear to be in shock.

Effect of the Cardiovascular Reflexes

The depression of the cardiac output down to 2 liters per minute in the example of Figure 26–1 lasts for only a few seconds, because within 2

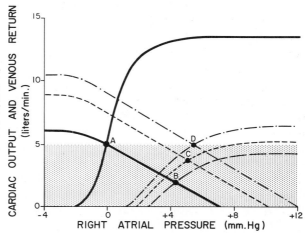

Figure 26–1. Analysis of the changes in cardiac output and right atrial pressure following acute onset of cardiac failure, showing complete compensation at equilibrium point D after a week or so of recovery.

to 7 seconds after the diminishment of the output, cardiovascular reflexes begin to develop (Rushmer, 1959; Guyton, 1954c). For instance, a cardiac output of only 2 liters per minute would lead to depressed arterial pressure, which in turn would elicit the pressoreceptor reflex. Then during the next 20 seconds to a minute, very powerful sympathetic stimulation will occur throughout the body. As a consequence, the heart becomes a more powerful pump, as depicted by the short-dashed cardiac output curve in Figure 26–1. And simultaneously the sympathetic reflexes increase the vasomotor tone throughout the body, which increases the mean systemic pressure and correspondingly increases the venous return curve. This is depicted in the figure by the short-dashed venous return curve, which shows a shift of the venous return curve to the right and upward, the mean systemic pressure also increasing from 7 mm. Hg up to 10 mm. Hg. This curve equates with the new cardiac output curve at point C, which indicates a cardiac output of 3.75 liters per minute and a right atrial pressure of 7 mm. Hg. Thus, within a few seconds, the cardiovascular reflexes play a major role in returning the cardiac output back toward normal; these reflexes are fully developed within approximately one minute after the onset of acute cardiac depression. Note especially that this acute cardiac failure causes the right atrial pressure to rise only a few millimeters of mercury, which is an effect observed both in human patients and in dogs (Starr, 1940b; Roos, 1948; Guyton, 1954b).

Chronic Compensation of the Failure

At equilibrium point C in Figure 26–1, with a cardiac output of 3.75 liters per minute, the person can live quite satisfactorily as long as he lies in bed and performs no exercise. However, at this low cardiac output level, the renal output of urine will probably be reduced (indicated in Figure 26–1 by the shaded area). That is, as long as the cardiac output is within this shaded area, the urinary output is ordinarily depressed below normal and, for reasons which were discussed earlier in the chapter, fluid accumulates in the body, causing both the interstitial fluid volume and the blood volume to increase. All these factors increase the mean systemic pressure, in this instance up to 12 mm. Hg, and after a few days the new venous return curve becomes that represented by the dots and dashes.

While fluid is being retained, some recovery from the damage to the heart might also occur, or in some instances the heart might become weaker because of further extension of the damage. In Figure 26–1 we have assumed that a small amount of recovery takes place either as a result of hypertrophy of undamaged portions of the heart or as the result of repair of some of the damage that had been sustained. Thus, the new cardiac output curve becomes that illustrated by the dots and dashes.

Therefore, after a week or more of compensation, one finds that the cardiac output has usually increased considerably (Grishman, 1941); the new cardiac output and venous return curves equate at point D, with an almost normal cardiac output and a right atrial pressure between 5 and 6 mm. Hg.

Once the cardiac output has risen to the level designated by point D in Figure 26–1, the renal retention of fluid ceases and normal urinary output returns. However, the urinary output rises only back to normal and not above normal. Therefore, the fluid that has already accumulated in the body will remain, and the patient will retain the extra fluid until some later date when either the heart becomes more effective as a pump or the patient is treated with diuretics (Borst, 1948).

DECREASE OF REFLEXES IN THE CHRONIC STAGE OF COMPENSATION. By the time the chronic stage of compensation has been reached, the cardiac output has returned essentially to normal, an effect that has been borne out by studies during recovery from acute myocardial infarction (Gilbert, 1954; Gammill, 1955). Also, for reasons discussed earlier, the cardiovascular reflexes lose most of their effect on cardiac output. The venous return curve is now shifted far to the right, mainly because of fluid accumulation and not because of increased vasomotor tone, and the cardiac output curve has become elevated mainly as a result of recovery of the heart and not as a result of autonomic stimulation. Thus, in this chronic state of compensation, the two major compensatory mechanisms are probably fluid retention and hypertrophy of the undamaged portions of the heart.

DECOMPENSATED HEART FAILURE

In the analysis of Figure 26–1, the degree of heart failure, though moderately severe, was not severe enough to prevent the cardiac output from coming back to normal after a reasonable period of compensation. Often, however, the heart is so severely damaged that the highest point on the cardiac output curve, even after all compensations have taken place, falls too low even to allow normal cardiac output. Let us assume in Figure 26–2, for instance, that acute cardiac failure causes the cardiac output curve to fall instantaneously down to the long-dashed curve; this equates with the normal venous return curve at point B, giving an instantaneous cardiac output of only 200 cc./min. Obviously, this person would come very near to death during the first few seconds before his cardiovascular reflexes could save him. However, after the cardiovascular reflexes have taken effect, the cardiac output curve becomes the light solid output curve. Furthermore, the reflexes cause the mean systemic pressure to rise to some value which we will assume to be about 11 mm. Hg. This gives us a new venous return curve, designated by number I, which equates with the new cardiac output curve at point C, indicating a cardiac output of 2.25 liters per minute. This is barely enough to keep the person alive if he remains absolutely quiet.

If we assume that the heart does not recover at all, or that the cardiac recovery is approximately equal to the gradual fading away of the reflexes, which was discussed earlier in the chapter, then during the ensuing days fluid will accumulate indefinitely because the cardiac output curve never rises out of the shaded area of the graph. Thus, during the first day, fluid and electrolyte retention causes the venous return curve to shift further

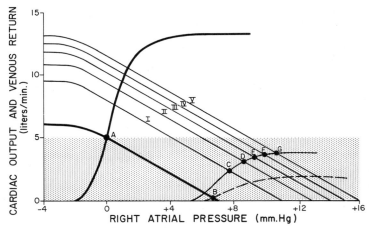

Figure 26–2. Analysis of cardiac output and right atrial pressure changes following the onset of heart failure that was too severe for complete compensation to be achieved, demonstrating decompensated heart failure.

to the right with the mean systemic pressure rising to 13 mm. Hg. This curve equates with the cardiac output curve at point D. On the second day, the cardiac output will be represented by point E, on the third day by point F, and on the fourth day by point G. Once point G is reached, the cardiac output has risen to its highest value, and by now the right atrial pressure is 11 mm. Hg.

Any further retention in fluid will cause no beneficial effect whatsoever as far as the cardiac output is concerned, but it will cause the right atrial pressure to rise to still higher values, causing increasingly severe peripheral edema. Thus, we now have a state of *decompensation*, in which the cardiac output is too low to meet the requirements of the body and in which the fluid volume of the body never reaches a steady compensated level. This is a situation from which the circulatory system usually does not recover without complete body rest or other therapy. The continued increase in accumulated fluid alone could eventually lead to such an edematous state that the person could die of the edema itself. However, in addition to this, in the later stages of fluid accumulation, the cardiac output itself begins to fall; this will be analyzed in the following section.

The Decrease in Cardiac Output in Decompensation

The precise cause of the decrease in cardiac output in decompensation has not been determined. Most frequently it is stated that the output decreases because of the "descending limb of the cardiac output curve" or the "descending limb of Starling's curve" (Howarth, 1948; Judson, 1955; Pickering, 1960; Katz, 1965). If this is the cause of the decreased cardiac output in the later stages of decompensation, the analysis would be that represented in Figure 26–3.

Point G in Figure 26–3 is exactly the same as point G in Figure 26–2, and the cardiac output and venous return curves intersecting at point G are also the same as in Figure 26–2. However, in Figure 26–3 we have

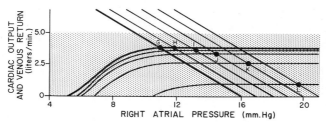

Figure 26-3. Deterioration of cardiac output in the late stages of decompensated heart failure explained by a descending limb in the cardiac output curve.

extended the cardiac output curve so that it has a descending limb as it proceeds toward the right. Since the cardiac output at point G is only 3.75 liters per minute, this is still far less than the 5 liters per minute required to make the kidneys function satisfactorily enough to maintain normal fluid balance. Consequently, fluid is retained until the mean systemic pressure has risen from 16 to 17 mm. Hg by the next day, and the new equilibrium point becomes point H. Then, by the following day, further fluid retention produces equilibrium at point I and the ensuing days, at points J, K, and L. Finally death follows because of the very low cardiac output. From this figure we see that progressive retention of fluid causes the right atrial pressure to rise extremely rapidly during the terminal phases of decompensated heart disease.

However, experiments in our laboratory have made us doubt the existence of this mechanism of the decrease in cardiac output in decompensated heart disease. The principal reason for this doubt is the following observation: In over 200 different experiments in which we have recorded cardiac output continuously and in which the heart has reached a state of depressed function approximately equal to that illustrated by the cardiac output curve in Figure 26-2, a sudden increase in right atrial pressure induced by transfusion has never caused an immediate decrease in cardiac output, even when the right atrial pressure was already high. If the cardiac output curve does have a descending limb, such as that illustrated in Figure 26-3, then an instantaneous rise in the atrial pressure, when the atrial pressure is already high, should decrease the cardiac output immediately, which it does not.

In these same experiments, we have often noted that a rise in atrial pressure sometimes causes the cardiac output to fall *5 to 10 minutes later* rather than immediately. This indicates that the increase in atrial pressure caused a depression in the ability of the heart to pump blood *a few minutes after the pressure had been increased,* which could easily result from an effect that Salisbury and Cross (Salisbury, 1961; Cross, 1961) have emphasized, namely, rapid development of edema in hearts under abnormal coronary perfusion states; or the depression could result from other diverse effects, such as progressively developing pulmonary edema or slow diastolic stretch of the heart. If this is the case, the analysis of the decrease in cardiac output in the late stages of decompensated heart disease would be that illustrated in Figure 26-4, which shows the same point G as that illustrated in Figure 26-2 and 26-3. However, this time the cardiac out-

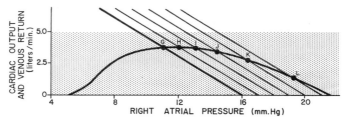

Figure 26–4. Another possible analysis of the deteriorating cardiac output in the late stages of decompensated heart disease, this time caused by progressive deterioration of the heart.

put curve reaches a plateau, which is what we have found to be the case in all the experiments in which we have suddenly increased the blood volume (Stone, 1963).

Let us assume that the person retains fluid for a day and that his venous return curve shifts to the right, giving us a new equilibrium point H. Then on the second day, further retention of fluid shifts the venous return still farther to the right, but by now this retention of fluid has begun to damage the heart itself, perhaps causing cardiac edema or overstressing the heart because of increased ventricular diastolic pressure. Whatever the cause, the weakened heart now has a lowered cardiac output curve, and the new equilibrium point becomes point I. Then during the next day, further retention of fluid shifts the venous return curve still farther to the right and also causes the cardiac output curve to fall a second time, giving the equilibrium point J. On the fourth day, the venous return curve shifts still farther to the right, and the cardiac output curve falls still more, giving point K. On the fifth day, additional changes give point L.

If we observe Figures 26–3 and 26–4 carefully, we will see that points G to L are the same in the two analyses. In Figure 26–3, we have assumed that the pumping ability of the heart has not changed at all but simply that there is a descending limb in the cardiac output curve. In the analysis of Figure 26–4, we have assumed that at the same time that fluid is being retained, the heart is becoming weaker. This makes it appear that there is a descending limb in the cardiac output curve, but actually this need not be the case. The selection of one of these two possible mechanisms of the decreasing cardiac output in the terminal stages of decompensation will require some very critical experiments, because studies thus far available on this point are consistent with either of the two mechanisms (Resnik, 1935; Howarth, 1948; Judson, 1955; Klepzig, 1955; Taquini, 1961; Monroe, 1970).

Sarnoff (1955) has found a descending limb in *stroke work output curves* in severely damaged hearts, but descending limbs often exist in stroke work curves without appearing in the cardiac output curves (Stone, 1963). This effect results from a rising atrial pressure, which reduces the work output but does not reduce the cardiac output. Furthermore, since the entire curve is determined never instantaneously but as a sequence of successfully determined points, the descending limb could be a time-dependent effect (discussed in Chapter 8) rather than a true descending limb. Regardless of which is the truth, one would still have essentially the same effects in decompensated heart disease, namely, a progressive decrease in cardiac output, rising fluid volume, and rising venous pressure in the terminal stages (McGuire, 1938, 1939b; Stewart, 1940; Espersen, 1941b; Suárez, 1946; Stead, 1948, 1949; Threefoot, 1947; McKee, 1959; Richards, 1942; Gibbons, 1948; Katz, 1960). Therefore, a descending limb is not a necessity for decompensated failure to occur, though the descending limb would exacerbate the condition.

SIMULATION OF CIRCULATORY DYNAMICS DURING BILATERAL HEART FAILURE

Figure 26–5 shows simulated changes in several circulatory variables following bilateral heart failure. Illustrated (from top to bottom) are changes in plasma volume, left atrial pressure, right atrial pressure cardiac output, free fluid volume in the lungs, arterial pressure, extracellular fluid volume, and urinary output. At the first break in the curves, the pumping capabilities of both ventricles were reduced to 30 per cent their normal values; that is, all segments of both ventricular function curves were reduced to 30 per cent normal. At each subsequent break in the curves,

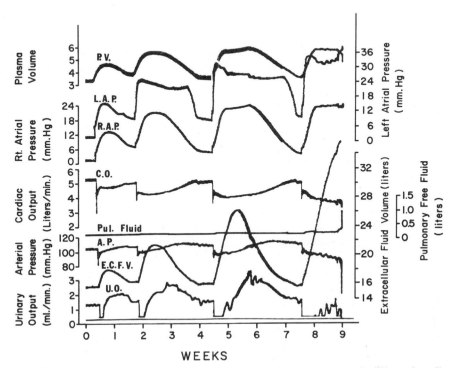

Figure 26–5. Simulation of circulatory dynamics following progressive bilateral cardiac failure. [From Guyton, Coleman, and Granger (1972).]

the pumping capabilities of both ventricles were decreased approximately another 10 to 15 per cent below their values immediately before the break.

Note the instantaneous decrease in urinary output at the onset of the first heart attack, with urinary output remaining for approximately one day at about 20 per cent of its normal level. Note also the instantaneous marked decrease in both cardiac output and arterial pressure, with recovery within minutes of both of these to levels only 10 to 20 per cent below normal, despite the severe reduction in the capability of the cardiac pump. These initial events were followed rapidly by increasing extracellular fluid and plasma volumes, and the initial slight increases in atrial pressure increased still more as fluid accumulated. However, during subsequent days, as the heart recovered from the attack, all the abnormal effects returned toward normal.

With additional reductions in the pumping capabilities of the heart, the simulated person went through repeated episodes until, finally, recovery was insufficient to return the person to a compensated state. The left atrial pressure eventually became so high that the volume of free fluid in the lungs began to rise drastically during the last hours of life. Not shown in Figure 26–5 are changes in the oxygen saturation of arterial blood. As long as no free fluid accumulated in the lungs, the oxygen saturation remained 100 per cent. However, following the final attack, when the lungs became progressively more edematous, the arterial oxygen saturation began to fall, and at the time of death was only 30 per cent.

The events depicted in Figure 26–5 are very similar to those which actually occur in cases of progressive bilateral cardiac failure, with transient episodes of edema following acute attacks and final entry into a severe stage of congestion in cardiac decompensation, followed by typical pulmonary congestive death. As will be pointed out in the following chapter, death due to pulmonary congestion is also typical of unilateral left heart failure.

TREATMENT OF DECOMPENSATED HEART DISEASE

In the above description of the state of decompensation, it was pointed out that in this condition the circulation is in a deteriorating state from which the normal control systems usually cannot extricate it without therapeutic aid. Decompensation has been treated empirically for several hundred years by two principal procedures: digitalization and the use of diuretics plus fluid and salt restriction. Obviously, also, the patient is always kept very quiet, which further aids in his recovery from the decompensation. In this present section we will attempt to explain graphically how both digitalization and the use of diuretics can revert the condition of decompensation to a state of compensation.

Treatment with Digitalis

Though digitalis has no beneficial effect on the strength of contraction of the normal heart muscle, in the greatly fatigued cardiac muscle, particularly in the heart that has been subjected to poor nutrition as a result of ischemia, digitalis usually increases the strength of cardiac contraction (Ringer, 1930; Cohn, 1932; Stewart, 1932a, 1932b; Hitzig, 1935; Seymour, 1942; Reichsman, 1946; Harvey, 1951; Gold, 1953; Blumgart and Zoll, 1960; Ferrer, 1960; Ross, 1967b), sometimes almost doubling the strength. Therefore, it is reasonable to expect that in many cases of decompensated heart disease, though not in all, digitalization of the patient will elevate the cardiac output curve.

Let us return to Figure 26-4 and assume that the patient has advanced in his state of decompensation to point K. Also observe Figure 26-6 in which the two curves that intersect at point K are the same ones that intersect at point K in Figure 26-4. Now let us digitalize the patient, which elevates the cardiac output curve to the upper one in Figure 26-6. The digitalization process, however, probably does not affect the venous return curve because digitalis has no proved *direct* effect on either the fluid volumes of the body or the vasomotor tone. Therefore, the new cardiac output curve equates with the venous return curve at point M, giving a cardiac output of 5.6 liters per minute. This is well above the shaded area of the diagram, which means not only that urinary output is normal but that it is actually above normal for reasons opposite to those (discussed earlier) that cause fluid retention in cardiac failure. That is, this greater than normal cardiac output results in diuresis. After one day of diuresis, we might expect the mean systemic pressure to have fallen from 20 mm. to 18 mm. Hg and the new venous return curve to equate with the cardiac output curve at point N. At this point, the cardiac output is still 5.5 liters per minute, which is greater than normal and therefore still causes diuresis. On the second day the mean systemic pressure falls to 16.6 mm. Hg, and the resulting venous return curve then equates with the cardiac output curve at point 0. This too is slightly above normal cardiac output so that diuresis continues, though at a slower rate. Then during the ensuing days the mean systemic pressure eventually falls to 15.7 mm. Hg, and the venous return curve then equates with the cardiac output curve at point P. This gives a cardiac output of 5 liters per minute, which is exactly the amount required for normal urinary output. In other words, at this point the fluid intake becomes equilibrated with the fluid output. Therefore, there is no further reduction in the fluid volume in the body. The mean systemic pressure remains at 15.7 mm. Hg, and the

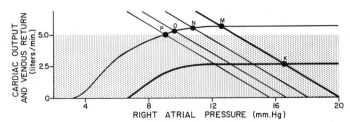

Figure 26-6. Treatment of decompensated heart disease with digitalis, showing the eventual state of compensation at equilibrium point P.

cardiac output remains at 5 liters per minute. At this high level of mean systemic pressure, there might be edema, at least dependent edema, but nevertheless there are no longer the progressive deteriorating effects observed in the state of cardiac decompensation—the progressive retention of fluid and the progressive decrease in cardiac output. Thus, we can say that the patient is in a compensated state, having been returned from the decompensated state to the compensated state by digitalization.

Note particularly in Figures 26–1 and 26–6 that the state of compensation occurs when the cardiac output curves and the venous return curve equate with each other at a cardiac output exactly equal to that required for normal urinary output. In other words, when the cardiac output is below this level, fluid will be retained until the venous return shifts enough to the right to raise the cardiac output up to the required level for normal urinary output. On the other hand, if the cardiac output is above this level, fluid will be lost from the body until the cardiac output falls back to the value just sufficient for normal urinary output. The basic mechanism of this diuresis has been studied in our laboratory by Langston (1959, 1961), who has shown especially that the urinary output is highly responsive to very slight changes in arterial pressure. Presumably the diuresis which occurs when digitalis is administered results mainly from a slight increase in arterial pressure when the cardiac output rises.

Treatment of Decompensated Heart Failure with Diuretics

Figure 26–7 illustrates one of the possible mechanisms by which diuretics could benefit decompensated heart disease and thereby return the circulation to a state of compensation. Let us assume that the cardiac output curve, even after all recovery of the heart has occurred, is that illustrated in Figure 26–7. Furthermore, let us assume that fluid retention has occurred until the venous return curve is the one illustrated at the far right. The equilibrium point will be point A with a cardiac output of 4.6 liters per minute and a right atrial pressure of 13 mm. Hg. A cardiac output of 4.6 liters per minute is sufficient in the normal person to cause almost, but not quite normal renal output; one might expect a few milliliters of fluid to be retained in the body each day. Thus, the person would become progressively more edematous, the edema eventually either itself killing the person or causing the heart to become weaker, thereby allowing the terminal stages of decompensation to proceed very rapidly.

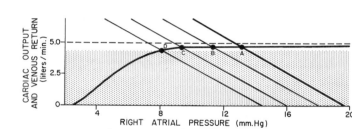

Figure 26–7.   Treatment of decompensated heart disease by use of a diuretic, showing final compensation at equilibrium point D.

Let us suppose, however, that once the patient has reached equilibrium point A, he is treated with a sufficient quantity of diuretics to cause a greater than normal urinary output even though the cardiac output is less than normal. Let us assume, for instance, that the diuretic causes the urinary output to be above normal until the cardiac output is reduced to 4.4 liters per minute. This is illustrated by the fact that the upper border of the shaded area in Figure 26–7 has been lowered to the 4.4 liter level instead of to the usual level of 5 liters. As long as the cardiac output is above this value, the urinary output will be above normal. When the cardiac output falls to 4.4 liters, however, the urinary output will be normal, and below 4.4 liters the output will be less than normal. Therefore, the first day of diuresis might reduce the mean systemic pressure sufficiently to shift the venous return curve to the second one from the right. This equilibrates with the cardiac output curve at point B; then another day of diuresis will have shifted the equilibrium point to point C, and a third day to point D. Once equilibrium point D has been reached, the fluid output from the body will have become equal to the fluid intake. Therefore, the mean systemic pressure now remains constant at a value of 14.3 mm. Hg, as depicted by the point at which the venous return curve reaches the zero cardiac output level. Once again, the patient has reached a state of compensation in which the cardiac output neither increase nor decreases, and the fluid volumes of the body are at a stationary level. Note again that this "compensation point" is reached only when the equilibrium point of the cardiac output and venous return curves coincides with the level required for normal renal output. Furthermore, it is especially interesting that in this case the patient is compensated at a lower than normal cardiac output, an effect that Stead (1948, 1949) found often to be the case in intractable cardiac failure that requires diuretics to cause compensation.

Another mechanism by which diuretics could benefit the cardiac output in the late stages of decompensation would be to reverse the detrimental effects of fluid retention on cardiac function, as depicted in Figures 26–3 and 26–4. In both these cases, reversing the fluid retention would reduce the mean systemic pressure and thereby shift the venous return curve to the left. In Figure 26–3, this would cause the equilibrium point to re-ascend the descending limb of the cardiac output curve, and in Figure 26–4, the reduction in fluid presumably would reduce the edema or some other factor depressing heart function and thereby make the heart a stronger pump, in this way also raising the level of the equilibrium point.

Regardless of whether diuretics can make the heart a stronger pump, they are invaluable in preventing the deteriorating effects of further fluid retention (Barger, 1960; Blumgart and Zoll, 1960; Nadas and Hauck, 1960; Rubin, 1960). Basically, therefore, the effect of diuretics is to make the body's daily fluid output equal the input. Once such a state of fluid equilibrium develops, the cardiac output will also be reasonably stable even though its mean level may be less than that normally required to maintain completely normal renal function.

Chapter 27

CARDIAC OUTPUT IN HEART FAILURE: II. HIGH OUTPUT FAILURE, PARTICIPATION OF THE PULMONARY CIRCULATION IN FAILURE, AND EFFECT OF EXERCISE IN FAILURE

HIGH OUTPUT FAILURE

Cardiac Overloading

Occasionally a person develops symptoms of cardiac failure even though the cardiac output is as great as two to three times normal. This condition is sometimes called "high output failure" even when the heart itself is completely normal and even though other factors besides a failing heart may be causing this simulated failure. This condition would be more properly called "cardiac overloading" rather than failure.

Some of the conditions that often cause cardiac overloading are: A-V fistulas (see Chapter 23), anemia (see Chapter 22), Paget's and Albright's diseases of the bones (Charlier, 1946; Bopp, 1962), thyrotoxicosis (Kattus, 1955; Charlier, 1946; Stead, 1950; Bishop, 1955), and occasionally excessive blood volume following transfusion (see Chapter 20). The characteristic symptoms are high right or left atrial pressure and sometimes edema, either peripheral or pulmonary. These are essentially the same findings as those found in many cases of true cardiac failure. Overloading the heart can be explained by the analysis in Figure 27–1.

The dark curves of Figure 27–1 are the standard analysis for the normal circulation, with equilibrium between venous return and cardiac output at point A. Let us assume that the total peripheral resistance decreases an extreme amount, such as might result from opening a large A-V fistula, even though the heart itself does not fail at all. The venous

469

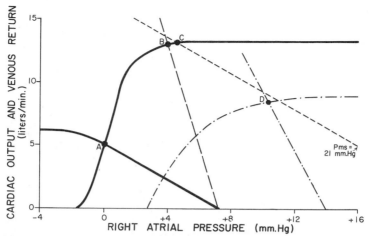

Figure 27-1. Analysis of "cardiac overloading" and "high output failure."

return curve rotates to the right, as illustrated by the long-dashed curve, and it equates with the normal cardiac output curve at point B. This gives a cardiac output of almost 13 liters/minute and a right atrial pressure of 4 mm. Hg. Such an increase in cardiac output would simultaneously increase the left atrial pressure up to approximately 16 mm. Hg, as one can readily deduce by studying the normal left ventricular output curve in Figure 27-2. Thus, we have both high left and right atrial pressures, which are characteristic of cardiac failure. Yet actually there is no failure of the heart as a pump; the only problem is that the amount of blood returning to the heart is more than the heart can handle satisfactorily. Thus, this condition should be called cardiac overloading rather than high output failure.

A second example of cardiac overloading is illustrated by the short-dashed venous return curve of Figure 27-1. In this case, the blood volume has been greatly increased, which results in a mean systemic pressure of 21 mm. Hg and a new equilibrium point at point C. This again gives a cardiac output of 13 liters per minute and a right atrial pressure of 4.5 mm. Hg. Furthermore, because of the very high mean systemic pressure, there might also be an excessively high capillary pressure and peripheral edema. Here again, we have some of the typical conditions of cardiac failure, yet the heart is not failing at all—it is simply overloaded.

True High Output Failure

There do exist certain instances of true high output failure. Particular instances of this occur in beriberi heart disease (Keefer, 1930; Burwell, 1947; Lahey, 1953), in heart failure patients residing in hot and humid climates (Burch, 1957), or in heart failure resulting from systemic anoxia (Gorlin, 1953; Öberg, 1961). In all these, the heart is actually failing, and yet the output is greater than normal. Such a condition is illustrated in Figure 27-1 by the dashed-dot cardiac output and venous return curves, which equilibrate with each other at point D, with a cardiac output of 8.4 liters/minute and a right atrial pressure of 10 mm. Hg. In this condition the cardiac output curve is depressed well below normal, indicating that the permissive level of cardiac pumping is greatly reduced, but at the same time two peripheral conditions have also been changed. First, large amounts of fluid have collected peripherally which increase the mean systemic pressure, and, second, peripheral vasodilatation has rotated the venous return curve upward. The high cardiac output is caused by the peripheral vascular changes and not by the failure of the heart; on the other hand, the heart failure results from the weakened heart itself.

In summary, many of the conditions called high output failure are not failure at all, but should be called "cardiac overloading." In occasional instances, true high output failure does occur, though the high output is not caused by the failure. Indeed the failing heart tends to decrease the output, but peripheral conditions have changed sufficiently that they more than overcome the depressant effect of the failing heart on the output. Therefore, the term "failure" should be separated from the high output. It simply happens that more than one condition is present at the same time. It would probably be better never to use the term "high output failure" but simply to call the condition heart failure in which there happens to be a high output because of other circulatory changes aside from the heart failure.

PARTICIPATION OF THE PULMONARY CIRCULATION IN CARDIAC FAILURE

In our discussions of cardiac failure up to this point, we have discussed principally the participation of the systemic circulation in failure. Now we would like to show how the pulmonary circulation is also affected. To do this, part of our discussion will require the complex form of graphical analysis.

The Pulmonary Circulation in Bilateral Cardiac Failure

Figure 27–2 illustrates an analysis of the changes in both the peripheral and pulmonary circulations in cardiac failure. The two solid curves are the right and left ventricular output curves of the normal heart, which were discussed in detail in Chapter 14. The two short-dashed curves are the right and left ventricular output curves in serious heart failure. Points A and B on the normal ventricular output curves represent respectively the ventricular output levels of the right and left ventricles. Now if both ventricles suddenly become greatly weakened, points C and D will represent the outputs of the respective left and right ventricles. Because of the low output, fluid will be retained, and this and other compensatory measures will cause the cardiac output level to rise progressively back up toward normal. After approximately a week's time we might expect the ventricular outputs to be represented respectively by points E and F for the right and left ventricles.

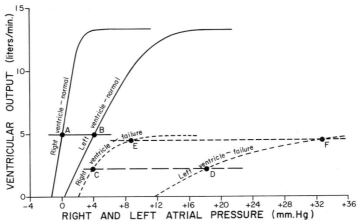

Figure 27-2. Effect of bilateral heart failure on right and left ventricular outputs and on right and left atrial pressures.

Thus, we see the following sequence of events in this example of bilateral heart failure. Immediately after the failure occurs, the cardiac output falls to 2.2 liters/minute, with the right atrial pressure rising to +4 mm. Hg (point C) and the left atrial pressure rising to 18 mm. Hg (point D). Then as the various compensations occur, particularly the retention of fluid, the cardiac output rises back to 4.5 liters/minute, while the right atrial pressure rises to 9 mm. Hg (point E) and the left atrial pressure rises to 34 mm. Hg (point F).

The principal point of this analysis is the following: Bilateral cardiac failure causes both atrial pressures to rise (Reiss, 1948; Katz, 1960) but causes a far greater rise in left atrial pressure than in right atrial pressure. Indeed, a 9 mm. Hg right atrial pressure can be tolerated almost indefinitely, whereas a 34 mm. Hg left atrial pressure would probably be lethal in a few hours because of the development of pulmonary edema, for experiments in dogs indicate that a left atrial pressure remaining above approximately 25 mm. Hg for more than a few hours at a time will always produce sufficient pulmonary edema to cause death (Guyton, 1959c; Gaar, 1967). Figure 27-2, therefore, demonstrates that unilateral left sided heart failure is not necessary for the development of pulmonary congestion and pulmonary edema. One can readily understand, then, why pulmonary edema is usually one of the earliest and most serious of the developments in cardiac failure (Blumgart and Zoll, 1960; Katz, 1960; Mauck, 1963; Bradley, 1970).

The Pulmonary Circulation in Left Sided Heart Failure

Figures 27-3 and 27-4 illustrate a complex analysis of the effect of pure left sided heart failure on the circulatory system. The point of these two figures is to show that even more extreme pulmonary congestion can occur in pure left sided failure than in generalized failure; also pulmonary congestion sometimes occurs with relatively little decrease in cardiac output (Boucek, 1952a; Wegria, 1958; Guyton, 1959c; Lindsey, 1959; Bradley, 1970).

The solid curves of Figure 27–3 represent the analysis of right and left ventricular outputs in the normal circulation. Then suddenly the left ventricular output curve decreases to that illustrated by the short dashes. Since this curve does not cross the normal pulmonary venous return curve at all, theoretically there will be no left ventricular output for an instant. Yet the right ventricular output will still be that illustrated by point A in the figure, namely, 5 liters per minute. As a consequence, blood continues to flow into the lungs without any being removed from the lungs back to the systemic circulation. This causes the mean pulmonary pressure to rise, while the mean systemic pressure falls, the sequence of events continuing until the new venous return curves become those represented by the short dashes. At the same time, the left atrial pressure is rising and is reflected back through the pulmonary circulation to the pulmonary artery to increase the load against which the right ventricle must pump. This increased load reduces the right ventricular output curve to that also illustrated by short dashes. The eventual equilibrium point between right and left ventricular outputs is represented by points C and D, with a cardiac output of about 3 liters/minute, a right atrial pressure of 0 mm. Hg and a left atrial pressure of 28 mm. Hg. In other words, the right atrial pressure is essentially unchanged while the left atrial pressure has risen from 4 mm. Hg to 28 mm. Hg, or a rise of 24 mm. Hg within a few heart beats. Since the left atrial pressure of 28 mm. Hg is about equal to the colloid osmotic pressure of the blood, and since the capillary pressure in the lungs must be slightly above 28 mm. Hg, one would expect fluid to exude out of the capillaries into the interstitial and alveolar spaces of the lungs, thus resulting in serious pulmonary edema and eventuating in death within a few hours (Guyton, 1959c; Gaar, 1967).

The analysis in Figure 27–3 assumes that there are no reflex compensations. However, reflex compensations do almost always occur after

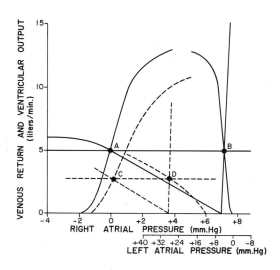

Figure 27–3. A complex graphical analysis of the effects of acute left sided heart failure on right and left ventricular outputs and on right and left atrial pressures.

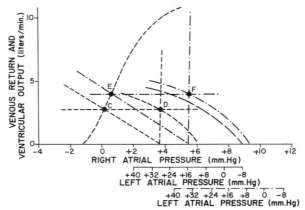

Figure 27-4. The same analysis as in Figure 27-3 but after reflex compensations have taken place approximately one minute later.

acute heart failure. Figure 27-4 illustrates the approximate reflex compensations which might occur within the next 60 seconds after the events of Figure 27-3 have taken place. The short-dashed curves of Figure 27-4 are identical with the short-dashed curves of Figure 27-3. One would then expect circulatory reflexes to change the conditions essentially to those illustrated by the dashed-dot curves of the figure. These can be explained as follows:

1. The reflexes increase the mean systemic pressure. In this example, the increase is from 7 to 9 mm. Hg, which causes the left atrial pressure axis to be shifted to the right as shown by the lowest abscissal scale of the figure. In shifting the left atrial pressure axis to the right, we also shift the left ventricular output curve to the right, as illustrated by the long-dashed curve.

2. Another reflex effect would be a direct effect on the ventricular output curves; the left ventricular output curve becomes elevated as illustrated by the shift of the curve from the long-dashed curve to the dashed-dot curve. The right ventricular curve would also be elevated, but at the same time the left atrial pressure is rising and this is increasing the pressure load in the pulmonary artery against which the right ventricle must pump blood. Therefore, in Figure 27-4 we will assume that the increased load depresses the right ventricular output curve by an amount exactly equal to the amount that the reflexes enhance the curve. Therefore, the right ventricular curve would remain the same.

3. Now to analyze what happens to the cardiac output and the atrial pressures, we shift the venous return curves along the atrial pressure axis until they equilibrate with the right and left ventricular output curves at the same output level (see Chapter 14 for explanation). Thus, we find the new equilibrium points to be, respectively, E and F for the right and left ventricles.

From this analysis, we see that the right atrial pressure has now risen to almost 1 mm. Hg, and the left atrial pressure has risen to 33 mm. Hg, and the cardiac output is up to 4 liters per minute. Immediately the patient would be in reasonably good condition, but pulmonary edema would develop very rapidly until death ensues. Here again, therefore, it is evident that pure left sided heart failure can result in serious pulmonary congestion and death, even though the cardiac output level is adequate to sustain life.

Another analysis of less severe left ventricular failure was given in Figure 14–12 of Chapter 14, and a general discussion of this complex method of analysis was also presented.

Effects of Pure Right Sided Failure on the Circulation

In this type of failure, blood shifts from the lungs into the systemic circulation, often reducing the pulmonary pressures considerably (Harrison, 1938; Boucek, 1952a; Kenner and Wood, 1966). However, since the capacitance of the systemic circulation is about seven times as great as that of the lungs (calculated from data in Lindsey, 1957, 1959) and the blood volume of the systemic circulation is also about seven times as great, a shift of 50 per cent of the blood from the pulmonary circulation into the systemic circulation causes 49 times less effect on the systemic pressures than a shift of 50 per cent of the systemic blood into the pulmonary circulation would cause on the pulmonary pressures. Because of this vast difference in effect, we find that very serious right sided failure causes very little *immediate* systemic congestion, though it does remove a large percentage of the blood from the pulmonary circulation. The typical *immediate* effect of pure right sided failure is a decrease in cardiac output without any serious congestive symptoms. This is followed by fluid retention and developing peripheral edema during the succeeding days because of renal retention of fluid (discussed in the previous chapter). Therefore, the analysis of the circulation in bilateral cardiac failure, as given in the previous chapter, holds almost precisely for pure right sided failure, namely, an initial decrease in cardiac output followed by a return of the cardiac output back toward normal as the various compensatory measures occur. In this connection, it is interesting that total coagulation of the right ventricular myocardium does not cause death of a dog (Starr, 1943; Kagan, 1952).

Simulation of Circulatory Dynamics Following Left and Right Unilateral Heart Failure

Figure 27–5 shows simulated effects of pure left sided heart failure. At zero time, the pumping capability of the left ventricle was reduced to 25 per cent of normal. Illustrated (from top to bottom) are the effects of such left heart failure on cardiac output, mean pulmonary pressure, left atrial pressure, mean systemic pressure, right atrial pressure, arterial pressure, free fluid volume in the lungs, extracellular fluid volume, and arterial oxygen saturation.

Note that immediately after the reduction in left ventricular pumping capability, cardiac output and arterial pressure decreased to approximately 50 per cent of their control values, but because of circulatory reflexes,

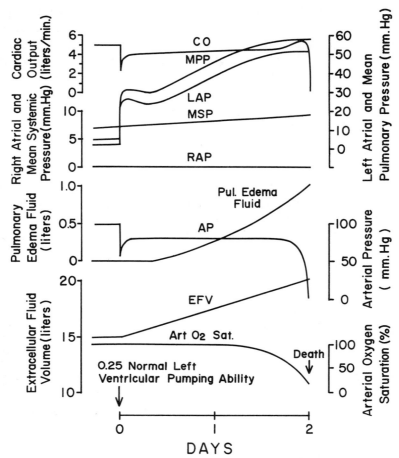

Figure 27–5. Simulation of circulatory dynamics following pure left sided heart failure.

both of these variables returned in minutes to within 20 per cent of normal. The reduction in left heart pumping ability caused blood to accumulate in the lungs such that left atrial pressure and mean pulmonary pressure increased drastically within seconds. There were no immediate changes in mean systemic pressure and right atrial pressure. The reduction in arterial pressure caused urinary output (not shown) to decrease almost to zero, and this in turn caused retention of fluid and a consequent increase in extracellular fluid volume. The accumulation of fluids, coupled with the reduced pumping capability of the left ventricle, caused mean pulmonary and left atrial pressures to increase even further during the ensuing two days. Note particularly that within hours after left ventricular failure, the volume of free fluid in the lungs began to rise drastically, and this simulated person eventually died in pulmonary congestion. At the time of death, the arterial oxygen saturation had been reduced 20 per cent.

The events depicted in Figure 27–5 approximate very closely those which actually occur. Note particularly that in the simulated person of

Figure 27–5, the cause of death was pulmonary congestion, and at the time of death the cardiac output had risen almost fully back to its control level.

Figure 27–6 shows the simulated effects of pure right sided heart failure. At zero time the pumping capability of the right ventricle was reduced to 20 per cent of normal, and illustrated in Figure 27–6 are the effects of such right sided heart failure on cardiac output, mean systemic pressure, right atrial pressure, mean pulmonary pressure, left atrial pressure, extracellular fluid volume, plasma volume, urine output, and arterial pressure.

The instantaneous effects of right sided heart failure were a drastic reduction in cardiac output and arterial pressure, with a partial return of these variables toward normal within minutes. Immediately following the right heart failure, both mean systemic pressure and right atrial pressure increased approximately 5 mm. Hg. However, because of the

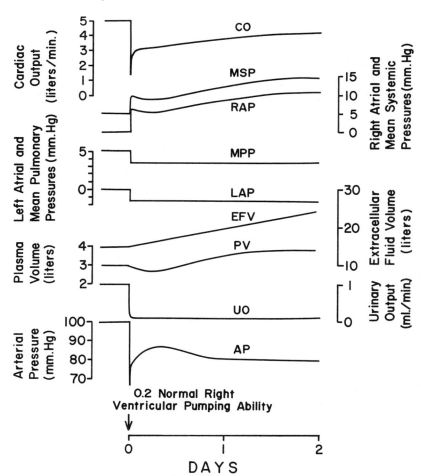

Figure 27–6. Simulation of circulatory dynamics following pure right sided heart failure.

shift of blood from the pulmonary circulation to the systemic circulation, the mean pulmonary and left atrial pressures decreased approximately 1.5 mm. Hg. Here again, the drop in arterial pressure caused urine output to decrease to nearly zero, which, in turn, caused a progressive rise over the ensuing two days in extracellular fluid and plasma volumes. Because of the retention of fluids, the mean systemic and right atrial pressure increased even further over the next several hours. In addition, the right ventricle partially recovered from its injury, such that two days following the right sided heart failure, cardiac output had stabilized at a level only approximately 15 per cent below normal. This level of cardiac output can sustain life if the person remains quiescent. Not shown in Figure 27-6 is a gradual return of urinary output toward normal with a consequent stabilization of extracellular fluid volume at a very high, but not lethal, level. Thus, the net result of the severe right unilateral heart failure in the simulated person of Figure 27-6 was a complete loss of all cardiac reserve and the development of a very severe peripheral edema. Theoretically, this person would live if he remained completely bedridden.

EFFECT OF EXERCISE IN HEART FAILURE

In general, exercise exacerbates the detrimental effects of cardiac failure (Harrison, 1932; Smirk, 1936; Nielsen, 1937; McGuire, 1939a; Hickam, 1948a; Barger, 1952; Bishop, 1955; Taylor, 1957; Holmgren, 1957; Lequime, 1958; Mauck, 1963; Schreiner, 1963; Lewis, 1964; Parker, 1969); this is true whether the cardiac failure is unilateral or bilateral.

Figure 27-7 illustrates a graphical analysis of the effects of exercise in bilateral cardiac failure. The dark curves depict the usual analysis for the normal circulation, with equilibrium at point A. Let us assume that the cardiac output curve becomes depressed to the short-dashed curve of the figure and that compensations take place until the venous return curve is that also illustrated by the short dashes. These two curves equilibrate at point B, giving a normal cardiac output but an elevated right atrial pressure of +6 mm. Hg. This represents a state of compensated failure. Now let us assume that the person exercises very strenuously. In Chapter 25 it was noted that during exercise two major effects occur in relation to the venous return curve. First, the mean systemic pressure rises markedly and, second, the resistance to venous return decreases moderately. Therefore, the venous return curve becomes that illustrated by the long dashes in Figure 27-7. We can also assume that the short-dashed cardiac output curve already represents the maximal degree of compensation that the heart can achieve and that reflex stimulation of the heart cannot achieve any extra compensation. Therefore, equilibrium occurs at point C, with a cardiac output of 7 liters per minute and a right atrial pressure of 15 mm. Hg. Because of this high right atrial pressure, one can reasonably expect that the capillary pressure throughout the systemic circulation also increases to a level far above its normal value and that fluid filtration into the tissue spaces would begin.

If we refer to the discussion of the pulmonary circulation in cardiac

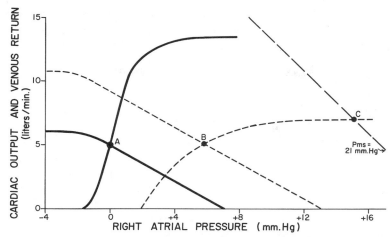

Figure 27–7.   Effect of exercise on cardiac output and right atrial pressure in compensated heart failure.

failure earlier in the chapter, we will see that not only does the right atrial pressure rise, but an even greater rise will occur in left atrial pressure during exercise because the left ventricular output curve slopes upward much more gently than does the right ventricular curve (see Figure 27–2). Consequently, as the cardiac output rises in exercise, the left atrial pressure can become tremendous, even in bilateral cardiac failure, and this can precipitate a serious bout of acute pulmonary edema.

Figure 27–8 illustrates even more impressively the effect of exercise on left atrial pressure when the heart failure is unilaterally left sided. In this figure, the two solid curves represent the normal right and left ventricular output curves, and the normal ventricular outputs are represented by points A and B. Then the left ventricle fails, reducing the left ventricular output curve to that represented by the short dashes, and backloading of the right ventricle as a result of high pulmonary pressures cause the right ventricular output curve to fall slightly. However, various compensatory mechanisms, explained earlier in the chapter, eventually return the cardiac output to its normal level of 5 liters per minute even though the left ventricle is still weak. The ventricular outputs and atrial pressures now are represented by points C and D, with a normal cardiac output of 5 liters per minute, a right atrial pressure of 0.5 mm. Hg and a considerable rise in left atrial pressure. Yet the left atrial pressure is still not high enough to cause significant congestion or any pulmonary edema.

Let us assume that the person then performs strenuous exercise. In doing so, there is an attempt to adjust the cardiac output to a much higher level, as explained in Chapter 25. Yet the approximate upper limit of the capacity of the left ventricle to pump blood is now about 8 liters per minute. Therefore, the ventricular outputs during the exercise become those represented by points E and F—that is, a cardiac output of 8 liters per minute, a right atrial pressure of 2 mm. Hg, and a left atrial pressure of 36 mm. Hg. It can readily be seen that this very high left atrial pres-

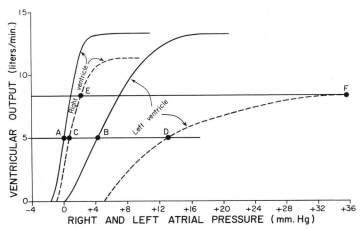

Figure 27-8. Effect of exercise on right and left ventricular outputs and right and left atrial pressures in a patient with compensated unilateral left sided failure.

sure is far above the normal colloid osmotic pressure of the blood. Therefore, fluid would be expected to transude rapidly into the interstitial spaces and alveoli of the lungs, causing very serious pulmonary edema, and possibly even death if the exercise is continued long.

Another interesting effect that occurs in exercise when the upper level of cardiac output is limited is that the active muscles usually obtain the needed blood flow to perform the exercise despite the limited output. This is accomplished by translocation of flow from other tissues, such as the skin, liver, and kidneys (Donald, 1959). This translocation presumably results from powerful sympathetic stimulation of the vessels in these extramuscular tissues. Donald has suggested that the other tissues might actually be harmed by the paucity of flow.

To summarize the effects of exercise in cardiac failure, exercise adds a greatly increased load on the heart. If the heart is already failing as a pump, one can expect markedly increased symptoms of failure during the exercise. Because of the relative shapes of the right and left ventricular output curves, exercise by a person with bilateral failure causes the left atrial pressure to rise more than the right atrial pressure, and if the failure is predominantly left sided, exercise often causes the left atrial pressure to rise as much as ten times as much as the right atrial pressure rises. In either instance, it is possible for the left atrial pressure to rise far above the colloid osmotic pressure of the blood and thereby result in serious acute pulmonary edema.

THE THREE BASIC PHYSIOLOGICAL EFFECTS OF CARDIAC FAILURE

If we review the analyses of the previous and present chapters, we find that there are only three *basic* physiological effects that occur in the different types and different stages of cardiac failure—not all, however, necessarily occurring at the same time. These are the following:

1. Decreased cardiac output.
2. Increased left atrial pressure with resulting pulmonary congestion.
3. Increased right atrial pressure with resulting systemic congestion.

At certain stages of bilateral or unilateral cardiac failure, each of these basic effects can be observed without the other two effects. For instance, in acute cardiac failure, particularly acute right side failure, one occasionally finds no demonstrable pulmonary or systemic congestion but only low cardiac output. In chronic left sided heart failure, one often finds normal cardiac output and no systemic congestion but marked pulmonary congestion. Finally, in chronic right sided heart failure one can find completely normal cardiac output, no pulmonary congestion, but serious systemic congestion.

On the other hand, patients in cardiac failure usually exhibit some combination of these three effects. For instance, in serious chronic bilateral cardiac failure there may be pulmonary congestion, systemic congestion, and low cardiac output at the same time. At other times, the cardiac output may be normal but there may be varying degrees of both pulmonary and systemic congestion. And so forth.

Therefore, if we should wish to divide cardiac failure into its different types, a physiological classification of the types would be simply:

1. Cardiac failure with low output.
2. Cardiac failure with pulmonary congestion.
3. Cardiac failure with peripheral congestion.

It should be noted that in this classification we have left "high output failure" out because the high output portion of high output failure is not one of the effects of failure. Occasionally failure does occur, even though the cardiac output is high, but the failure under these conditions falls into category 2 or 3 listed above. For instance, in beriberi heart disease there is often true failure of the heart and also high cardiac output, but even so, the failure is represented by pulmonary or systemic congestion or both, whereas the high output is not a result of the failure but occurs *in spite of* the failure, resulting from extracardiac changes in the circulation instead of from changes in the heart.

Forward Failure Versus Backward Failure

Though the terms "forward failure" and "backward failure" played their part in the days when the dynamics of heart failure were less well understood, further use of these terms can now only promote confusion rather than understanding. Actually forward failure means failure of the heart to pump blood forward, whereas backward failure means damming up of blood behind the heart. However, whenever the heart fails to pump blood forward, it also dams up blood behind it, and whenever the heart dams up blood behind it, it also fails to pump blood forward. Therefore, as far as the heart itself is concerned, forward failure and backward failure are identical; that is, the heart is simply failing to pump blood. These two terms, therefore, do not describe separate types of *heart failure* but describe separate types of *symptoms* resulting from heart failure. Forward failure is the same as cardiac failure with low output, or category 1 in the above physiological classification. Backward failure is cardiac failure with either pulmonary congestion or systemic congestion or both (categories 2 and 3 in the above physiological classification). It is far simpler to speak in physiological terms rather than to use archaic descriptions of cardiac failure, terms which are often poorly understood because they give the impression that the heart itself is failing in different ways in forward failure and backward failure, a concept that is entirely untrue.

Chapter 28

REGULATION OF CARDIAC OUTPUT FROM AN ARTIFICIAL HEART

The recent increase in interest in artificial hearts makes it important to understand the manner by which the body regulates cardiac output when such a device has been installed. Even more important, some of the problems that have been encountered in artificial heart research, and the solutions to these problems, are important reminders of the basic logic used by the body for normal cardiac output regulation.

In this chapter we will briefly describe some of the basic principles of artificial hearts that are being used and discuss the theory and practice of cardiac output control by these artificial hearts.

TYPICAL TYPES OF ARTIFICIAL HEARTS

The Air-Driven Artificial Heart

Though many types of artificial hearts have been used, having different shapes, different principles of pumping, and different types of motive power, the type that is most widely used at present is the air-driven heart, which uses the principle illustrated in Figure 28–1 (Seidel, 1961; Akutsu, 1963, 1964, 1966, 1970a; Bernard, 1968; and many others). This figure shows a typical ventricle with inlet and outlet valves. It consists of a rigid or semirigid outside chamber and a compressible internal sac. Pulsatile air pressure in the space between the outside chamber and the sac provides the motive power for pumping blood.

Among the most widely used materials for constructing artificial hearts are Silastic rubber and polyurethane rubber. The outside chamber usually has Dacron mesh embedded in the rubber matrix, so that air pressure in the chamber will not cause excessive outward ballooning. The inner sac, on the other hand, is constructed of a more flexible rubber or plastic material, so that air pressure applied on the outside of the sac can squeeze almost all of the blood from the sac. Figure 28–2 illustrates a

483

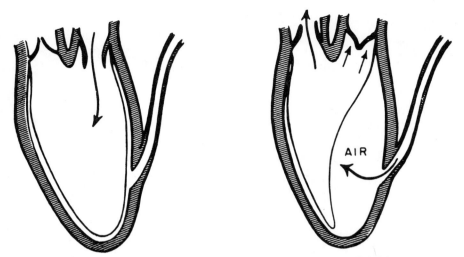

Figure 28–1. The sac principle utilized by most air-driven artificial hearts. [From Akutsu (1966).]

complete two-ventricle heart constructed of Dacron-reinforced Silastic rubber (Akutsu, 1966). To implant this heart, both ventricles of the animal's own heart are removed, but the right atrium is left intact. Surgical connections are then made between the right atrium and the inlet to the right heart, between the two pulmonary veins and the two inlets to the left heart, and between the two ventricular outputs and the pulmonary artery and aorta.

Once implanted, the artificial heart is driven by pulsatile air pressure, usually with a positive pressure cycle of 150 mm. Hg or greater, and a negative pressure cycle of a few mm. Hg to aid in filling of the ventricles. The exact values depend on the specific design of the artificial heart. The wave form of the pulsatile air pressure is adjusted to give an almost normal ventricular output pressure pulse. Therefore, use of an artificial heart of this type provides pumping characteristics similar to those of the natural heart.

Artificial hearts of this general design have maintained the lives of calves in several instances as long as 10 days, and in one instance for 15 days.

The Totally Implanted Artificial Heart

The artificial heart shown in Figure 28–2 requires an outside power source, which is not satisfactory for long-term heart replacement. Figure 28–3 illustrates an alternate system which might be used in future years for totally implanting an artificial heart in the human being (Harmison, 1972). It shows a hydraulically driven artificial heart implanted in the chest, and a nuclear thermal engine implanted in the abdomen. The nuclear engine is fueled by plutonium-238, which will last for the remaining lifetime of the person. The engine is designed to provide hydraulic pulses to the artificial heart, and it is these pulses that pump the blood.

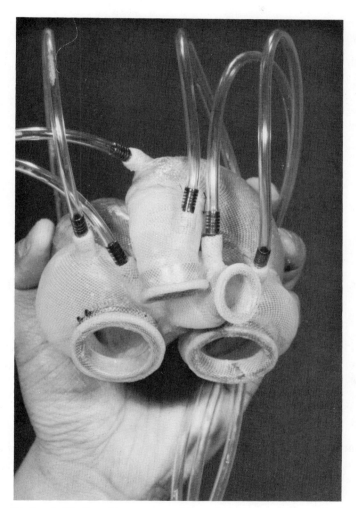

Figure 28–2.   A Silastic rubber two-ventricle artificial heart which can be implanted in the pericardium and which simulates the outlines of the natural heart. (Courtesy of Dr. J. Akutsu.)

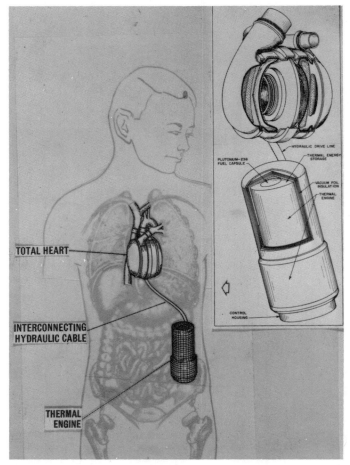

Figure 28–3. A totally implanted artificial heart proposed for implantation in the human being. The heart is driven hydraulically by a nuclear engine. [From Harmison (1972).]

A nuclear engine of this type will weigh approximately 5 pounds and will give off a reasonable amount of heat. However, the heat generated is not so great that it cannot be dissipated in the body. An artificial heart of this type is now being tested in lower animals.

PROBLEMS IN THE DESIGN OF THE ARTIFICIAL HEART

Blood Clotting

Obviously, one of the most important problems in use of an artificial heart is the tendency for blood to clot when it comes in contact with a foreign object (Mirkovitch, 1961; Akutsu, 1964, 1969; Okura, 1967;

Takano, 1971). Clotting in the artificial heart occurs at two points: (1) At points of abrupt changes in surface contour, such as around valves and at the junction between the artificial heart and the vessels to which it is attached, and (2) in recesses in the artificial heart where the blood does not flow significantly. Therefore, one of the most important phases of artificial heart development has been to design the hearts with as smooth contours as possible and with a flow design such that blood will "rub" all the surfaces of the heart as much as possible, thereby preventing no-flow nidi where small clots can begin to develop.

Other research has gone into developing artificial heart material that will not cause clotting. Though Silastic rubber has thus far proved to be one of the best materials from this point of view (Akutsu, 1967), many other materials are undergoing tests, and it is likely that better ones will be developed soon. In addition, special types of surfaces have been prepared that are relatively resistant to the development of clots. One of these is a graphite-coated surface that has also been soaked in heparin solution prior to implantation (Gott, 1964). Such surfaces have been resistant to clotting for as long as several months, but eventually the clot-resistance wears away. Another type of surface is Dacron velour, which traps fibrin from the flowing blood and builds up a fibrin layer that later becomes organized with fibrous tissue cells, thus forming a tissue lining of the inner surface of the artificial heart itself. The lining is not covered with the usual intravascular endothelial cells, but it is reasonably resistant to blood clotting and is called an "artificial intima." Unfortunately, even with this type of surface, it has been difficult to prevent clotting, especially at the junctions between the heart prosthesis and the natural blood vessels.

Hemolysis

A problem closely allied to that of blood clotting in artificial hearts has been hemolysis. This, too, is often a function of the types of material from which the artificial heart is made and also of the surface contours of the heart. In general, the less traumatizing the action of the valves and of the pulsating walls of the heart, and the less wettable the inner surface of the heart, the less hemolysis there will be. Silastic rubber is one of the better materials thus far used to prevent hemolysis, but other materials are being developed which should be superior.

Application of Power

To provide air power for the air-driven artificial heart, a tube must protrude through the chest wall, and this is a source of infection as well as other problems. However, to make the tube as small as possible, some investigators have resorted to driving the artificial heart with helium instead of air (Seidel, 1961; Akutsu, 1966). The helium moves through the tube with sufficient ease, in comparison with air, so that the internal diameter of the tube can be reduced to as little as one-third to one-fourth that required when using air. Some investigators have driven their artificial hearts with water (Hastings, 1961; Liotta, 1961; Atsumi, 1963), but this obviously requires an even much larger tube protruding through the chest wall.

A few artificial heart designs have employed implanted electromagnets to compress artificial ventricles (Kolff, 1959) or have employed implanted motors that either operate a roller (Akutsu, 1960; Atsumi, 1963), a bellows (Liotta, 1961; Atsumi, 1963), or a pendulum pressing against artificial ventricles (Houston, 1960; Akutsu, 1961). Unfortunately, the electrically driven devices thus far developed have all been excessively heavy and have also produced far too much heat to be dissipated, thus making the electrical models unpalatable. Indeed, the same two problems still plague the nuclear engine models; namely, excess weight and excess heat.

Bleeding at the Junctions Between the Heart Prosthesis and the Natural Vessels

Many experiments using the artificial heart have been self-terminated by bleeding at the junctions between the heart prosthesis and the natural blood vessels. However, with improved construction of the inlet and outlet orifices of the artificial heart, plus improved surgical technique, this is becoming less of a problem and probably will not be a limiting factor in practical use of artificial hearts.

Inlet Resistance to the Artificial Ventricles

One of the most serious problems in developing practical artificial hearts has been to devise inlet valves and inlet structural details so that blood can flow easily from the veins into the ventricles during diastole. The very filmy, thin, and almost zero-resistance atrioventricular valves of the natural heart have never been duplicated in artificial hearts. Instead either thick elastic vane valves or solid valves have been used (Burns, 1965; Wieting, 1969; Akutsu, 1970b). Both of these types have considerable inertia and resistance. Therefore, it has been difficult for the ventricles to fill rapidly in response to the very low venous pressures of both the systemic and pulmonary circulations. To overcome this difficulty, many users of artificial hearts provide a negative suction cycle on the ventricles to pull blood into the ventricles rather than allowing passive entry of the blood. In general, when negative suction has not been used, high venous return to the heart causes excessively high right atrial pressure and, consequently, moderate to marked venous congestion, often associated with marked loss of fluid out of the capillaries into the tissue spaces.

THEORY OF CARDIAC OUTPUT CONTROL BY THE ARTIFICIAL HEART

History

The theory of cardiac output control by the artificial heart has gone through almost the identical phases of thinking as has the theory of cardiac output control by the normal heart. One phase of this history was that of "cardiac control" of cardiac output, and the other has been the phase of "peripheral circulatory control" of cardiac output.

In the early development of artificial hearts, many investigators were concerned that the pumping cycle of the heart should be controlled very precisely, so that the cardiac output would be precisely that level that would be required by the body. Therefore, special sensors were often provided which monitored systemic arterial pressure, pulmonary arterial pressure, and inlet pressures to the artificial heart. The information from these sensors was in turn used to control, either manually or through the intervention of a servo mechanism, the pumping cycles of the artificial heart. This type of approach to the control of the artificial heart was based on the concept that the heart itself controls blood flow through the normal circulation; therefore, it was supposed that the only proper way for cardiac output to be controlled by the artificial heart was for the artificial heart itself to have very elaborate controls.

However, it has been noted throughout this text on cardiac output and its regulation that under normal conditions, the heart plays little role in cardiac output regulation. Instead, the heart simply responds to the demands of the peripheral circulation. Furthermore, the heart interprets these demands almost entirely in response to the amount of blood that flows from the peripheral circulation into the right atrium. Increased inflow expands the heart and this, in accordance with the Frank-Starling principle, causes the heart to pump the increasing amounts of venous return. Consequently, whenever peripheral blood vessels become dilated, thereby allowing extra quantities of blood to flow from the arteries into the veins, the heart simply acts as an automatic pump to propel the blood almost immediately back into the arteries. Thus, the peripheral tissues themselves normally control cardiac output. Fortunately, recent practitioners of the artificial heart cult have come to realize this basic principle by which the normal body controls cardiac output, and almost all investigators in the artificial heart field now utilize either input distention of the artificial heart or right atrial pressure as the index for control of the degree of pumping by the artificial heart. The result has been a much simpler design of the artificial heart, while at the same time greatly improving the animal's tolerance to the artificial heart.

THE IDEAL ATRIAL PRESSURE-VENTRICULAR FUNCTION CURVE FOR THE ARTIFICIAL HEART

The peripheral circulation is capable of controlling cardiac output only if the heart is capable of pumping with ease all the blood that flows from the peripheral vessels into the right atrium. For this to be achieved, the heart must pump maximum venous return without causing a significant rise in venous pressure, because a rise in venous pressure will cause back pressure on the peripheral circulation and limit the rate of blood flow into the ventricle, thus compromising the peripheral circulatory mechanism for control of output. That is, the response of right ventricular output

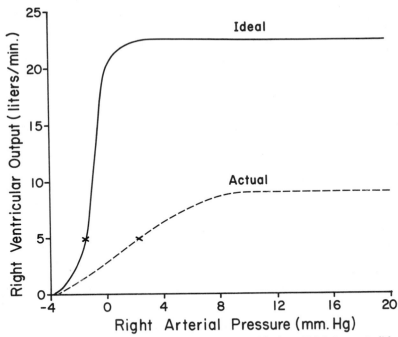

Figure 28–4. Ventricular output curves for the ideal artificial heart (solid curve) and for an artificial heart of good present design (dashed curve).

to input right atrial pressure must be approximately that illustrated by the curve labeled "Ideal" in Figure 28–4. This curve is almost the same as that of the normal human heart when it is stimulated maximally by the sympathetic nervous system. The normal resting heart does not have quite such an ideal curve, particularly in the upper portions of the curve. However, when one remembers that the normal human heart is vested with a special nervous control that can give an optimal curve when required, he can understand why it is not as important for the normal resting heart to have an ideal function curve as it is for the artificial heart to have such a curve. Furthermore, it must be remembered that the human heart lasts longer when it is not stimulated continually by the sympathetic nervous system, which means that it is advantageous to shift from the resting heart state to the stimulated state upon demand.

However, even without all the special controls of the human heart, if the design of the artificial heart were such that it obeyed the ideal curve from Figure 28–4, one can show theoretically that there would be no difficulty with cardiac output regulation. Indeed, output regulation would be equally as satisfactory under either resting conditions or high output conditions such as during exercise, because in both conditions the heart would be acting simply as a demand pump, responding to whatever amount of blood flows through the peripheral circulation into the right atrium – responding in exactly the same way as the normal heart responds.

METHODS FOR ACHIEVING THE IDEAL FUNCTION CURVE FOR THE ARTIFICIAL HEART

In artificial heart designs thus far, three general methods have been used to achieve as nearly as possible the ideal cardiac function curve. These are the following:

Provision of an Automatic Frank-Starling Mechanism in the Artificial Heart

If the inflow resistance to the artificial heart is very low, and if the artificial ventricle itself is compliant enough to stretch with ease, all the venous return can flow between successive heart beats from the periphery into the ventricle with ease. Then the pumping cycle of the heart can be arranged to pump all or most of the blood from the heart chamber with each pumping cycle. In this way, that amount of blood that returns to the ventricle will also be the amount of blood pumped into the outlet artery. Thus, the artificial heart obeys the Frank-Starling mechanism. Unfortunately, in practice, the inflow resistance to the ventricle has usually been too great for a completely satisfactory Frank-Starling mechanism to be achieved by the artificial heart (Akutsu, 1966). Furthermore, most artificial hearts have not had actively pumping atria. In the normal human heart, an actively pumping atrium functions as a negative resistance, which to a great extent helps overcome the inlet resistance to the heart. Perhaps with the development of active atria in the artificial heart, and with development of less resistance in the inlet valve system, an appropriate heart with an ideal ventricular output curve can be developed.

The lower curve (the dashed curve) of Figure 28–4 illustrates the actual Frank-Starling curve of one of the very good artificial hearts made for an animal approximately the size of a human being. It can be seen that the physical design of the artificial heart itself still needs considerable improvement.

Provision of a Suction Cycle for the Artificial Ventricle

Because of the problems of inlet resistance and ventricle compliance discussed above, some research workers provide negative pressure to suck blood into the ventricles during diastole (Hastings, 1961; Seidel, 1961; Norton, 1962; Rainer, 1963; Akutsu, 1966, 1972). To achieve reasonable success with the negative pressure, the outside chamber of the artificial heart needs at least a reasonable degree of rigidity, which, unfortunately, has the disadvantage that it then becomes less adaptable to the surrounding tissues. Nevertheless, use of such negative pressures makes it possible to prevent excess buildup of peripheral venous pressure when using the artificial heart.

Increase in Heart Rate

The third procedure for increasing the ability of the heart to accommodate increasing venous return is to increase the heart rate (Burney,

1963; Harmison, 1972). If there were excess power to spare, it would theoretically be better to maintain the optimal heart rate all of the time rather than to depend on the heart rate to increase with need. On the other hand, if power utilization by the heart is a function of heart rate, and if the supply of power is limited, as is true with the nuclear engine, it would obviously be advantageous to maintain a slow pumping rate under normal conditions but to increase the rate with increasing venous return. Indeed, this is one of the approaches that designers of the totally implanted artificial heart have used (Harmison, 1972). To provide the increase in rate, a sensor is built into the heart wall itself to sense the input pressure. This in turn operates through a minute solid state electronic servo controller to control the frequency of the pumping cycle provided by the nuclear engine.

Effectiveness of Cardiac Output Regulation by the Artificial Heart

Unfortunately, despite all efforts up to the present, the ideal ventricular output curve illustrated in Figure 28–4 has rarely, if ever, been realized, and the actual curves that have been achieved, as illustrated by the lower curve, leave much to be desired. For instance, this curve shows that even under normal conditions (with a cardiac output of 5 liters per minute) the right atrial pressure is approximately 2 mm. Hg. If the output should increase a significant amount above normal, as occurs in exercise, anemia, infection, fever, toxic states, and so forth, the right atrial pressure would rise very greatly—so much so that peripheral venous congestion would occur very easily and very rapidly. Furthermore, the increasing back pressure on the venous system would reduce the venous return and, thereby, reduce cardiac output to a level below that needed by the tissues. Thus, one can see that with the function curve illustrated by the dashed curve in Figure 28–4, regulation of cardiac output will be very inadequate, and this alone can easily lead to death of the animal within hours or days. This is analogous to the situation that occurs in cardiac failure, in which the ventricles simply do not have the necessary reserve to enhance cardiac output in response to excess tissue needs. To state this another way, most artificial hearts thus far used have operated mainly in a cardiac failure mode, a state in which a person or an animal can live for considerable periods of time but certainly cannot live in good health. With the development of increased pumping efficiency of the artificial hearts, one can expect the ventricular output curve of the artificial heart to approach the ideal illustrated in Figure 28–4, and he can also expect the survival times of animals with artificial hearts to increase markedly.

Chapter 29

EPILOGUE

Perhaps this chapter should best be entitled "Apologies and Defense" —apologies for attempting to write a monograph on cardiac output, a subject which has occupied such a tremendous portion of our literature, and defense for having done so. Particularly must we defend our attempts to present an "engineering schema" of the regulation of cardiac output, especially in the face of many physiologists' belief that we do not know enough about cardiac output regulation to discuss it in such quantitative terms. Yet our defense to this is that although our quantitative data regarding cardiac output regulation are still very meager, the facts are beginning to fit into place, as we have tried to show throughout this monograph.

It would be wrong to maintain that the graphical, the algebraic, or the computer analyses presented in this book are quantitatively accurate in their entirety, for we ourselves do not believe this. All these types of analyses are frameworks, which can be improved and improved again by future research workers. There are also other methods for analyzing cardiac output regulation, but each method, to be accurate, must include certain fundamental points, such as quantitative procedures for predicting the effect of each type of cardiac change on cardiac output and quantitative procedures for predicting the effect of each type of peripheral circulatory change on cardiac output. Paper after paper has been written on cardiac function alone, each of which has been claimed by the authors to describe cardiac output regulation; such papers might well describe dynamics of cardiac function, but if they leave out a simultaneous consideration of the peripheral circulation, then it is not possible for them to be discussing cardiac output regulation. Likewise, if anyone attempts to discuss cardiac output regulation entirely on the basis of the peripheral circulatory system without simultaneous consideration of cardiac function, too can not possibly be correct.

Fortunately, the mass of evidence points toward a few major factors that are especially important in cardiac output regulation. Let us review for a moment some of these and attempt to put them into their proper perspective.

First, there seems to be a central, basic, intrinsic system for cardiac output regulation which is entirely independent of reflexes, hormones, or fluid balance. This mechanism gears the cardiac output to the rate of metabolism and appears to be, very simply, the following: The degree of activity of each tissue determines the degree of local vasodilatation, always allowing just enough blood to flow through the tissue to supply the tissues' needs. The summated flow through all the tissues then determines how much blood flows to the heart. The heart in turn responds to this input by pumping whatever is demanded of it in accordance with the Frank-Starling law of the heart.

Yet this intrinsic mechanism for cardiac output regulation is modified by other factors, such as reflexes, blood volume changes, stress relaxation of the circulation, and still others. In fact, it is modified so much by these factors that many investigators have come to the point of denying the basic intrinsic mechanism. Yet instead of denying the intrinsic mechanism, it is much more valid to show how the other factors work together with it to make cardiac output regulation even more effective.

Let us consider, for instance, the regulation of cardiac output in exercise. Sympathetic stimulation of the heart greatly increases the heart rate and also increases the strength of heart contraction, making the heart a far more effective pump than normally. At the same time, compression of the intramuscular vessels by the contracting muscles as well as sympathetically induced contraction of the peripheral vessels increases the tendency for blood to translocate from the periphery into the heart, thereby making available more blood for the heart to pump. Therefore, one might conclude that cardiac output is regulated in exercise entirely through sympathetic stimulation and local mechanical factors. Yet the basic intrinsic mechanism is still there, hidden beneath these more overt effects, for the intrinsic mechanism still makes the adjustments in local tissue blood flow that are needed to keep cardiac output in step with the rate of metabolism.

The truth is that nervous factors, muscle compression of vessels, and shifts in fluid balance all work together to make the basic intrinsic mechanism a far better control system that it could possibly be by itself, but the effect of these other factors is *in addition to, rather than instead of,* the basic intrinsic mechanism. Certainly when the circulatory system is under severe stress, such as occurs in very heavy exercise, the intrinsic mechanism alone is not able to cope with the needed changes in cardiac output. Here the nervous factors play an exceedingly important part in helping to achieve the very high level of cardiac output necessary for massive work performance by the muscles. And when a person develops an A-V fistula, the heart hypertrophies and the blood volume increases so that in the long run these factors are the ones mainly responsible for maintaining the high cardiac output that is necessary to keep the person alive. These two control factors, like the nervous factors, are also superimposed on the intrinsic control mechanism, showing once again that we have several different parallel cardiac output control systems all working in unison, some called into play for one type of stress that alters cardiac output and others called into play for other types of stress.

Yet we do not mean to imply by this discussion that we know all there is to know about the basic mechanisms for cardiac output regulation. For instance, there is no agreement as to how oxygen lack causes peripheral vasodilatation. Many physiologists have postulated that oxygen lack causes the tissues to release a vasodilator substance, but thus far no such vasodilator substance has been proved to occur in enough quantity to be unequivocally important. Furthermore, experiments were presented in this monograph which actually indicate that there might not be a vasodilator substance, the vasodilatation instead possibly resulting simply from lack of sufficient oxygen to keep the metabolic systems of the vascular smooth muscle fully at work. This is an effect that we have attempted to demonstrate in our laboratory, but other investigators still hold to the view that a vasodilator substance must be present.

Another serious void in our knowledge of cardiac output regulation is the effect of blood volume changes on cardiac output. Anyone can demonstrate an acute and very marked rise in cardiac output when the blood volume is increased rapidly by only 10 to 15 per cent. Yet the cardiac output measured a few minutes later may be almost completely normal. Thus, we can say that an increase in blood volume *per se* increases the cardiac output, but an increase in blood volume *plus the subsequent compensatory effects* often does not increase the cardiac output. But why is this true? The stress relaxation mechanism must be important in moderating the effect of blood volume changes on cardiac output, but this possibility is only beginning to be studied. Several other mechanisms, such as the circulatory reflexes, readjustment of blood volume by the capillary fluid shift mechanisms, and perhaps still others, also begin immediately to readjust cardiac output after the blood volume is changed. Therefore, how do we separate out from among all of this melee of control systems that portion of the control which can be ascribed directly and only to the stress relaxation mechanism? No wonder researchers the world over have avoided this question. But still it must be answered before we can put together our final thoughts on the interrelationships between blood volume and cardiac output.

Finally, how much do we know about the relative quantitative values of the different cardiac output control mechanisms under different physiological conditions? For instance, how important are the circulatory reflexes following the opening of an A-V fistula? Are they more or less important when the fistula is small than when it is large? Do the reflex effects fade out as the chronic state develops?

How much is the cardiac output affected when increased vascularization occurs during prolonged hypoxia? Do anemia and polycythemia affect cardiac output mainly through changes in blood viscosity, through the oxygen-lack vasodilator mechanism, or through some other more obscure factor? For all these questions, we have only partial answers, and these are the same questions with which we began this book.

Therefore, please accept our apologies again for what we do not know and more particularly for the transgressions that we have made into the unknown, for the estimations that we have had to make in order to fit the pieces together, and for our temerity in calling this book a treatise on "cardiac output," when in reality it covers only a small segment of the vast literature that has been written on the subject.

BIBLIOGRAPHY

Aars, H. Aortic baroreceptor activity in normal and hypertensive rabbits. *Amer. J. Physiol.* 72:298, 1968.

Abbott, B. C., and W. F. H. M. Mommaerts. A study of inotropic mechanisms in the papillary muscle preparation. *J. Gen. Physiol.* 42:533, 1957.

Abbott, B. C., and R. J. Baskin. Volume changes in frog muscle during contraction. *J. Physiol.* 161:379, 1962.

Abel, F. L., and J. A. Waldhausen. Influence of posture and passive tilting on venous return and cardiac output. *Amer. J. Physiol.* 215:1058, 1968.

Abel, F. L., and J. A. Waldhausen. Respiratory and cardiac effects on venous return. *Amer. Heart J.* 78:266, 1969.

Abel, R. M., and R. L. Reis. Effects of coronary blood flow and perfusion pressure on left ventricular contractility in dogs. *Circ. Res.* 27:961, 1970.

Abramson, E. Die Rückstosskurve des Herzens (Kardiodynamogramm). *Skand. Arch. Physiol.* 66:191, 1933.

Adams, W., and I. Sandiford. Measurement of cardiac output; improvement of acetylene method providing inherent check. *J. Clin. Invest.* 20:87, 1941.

Adriani, J., and E. A. Rovenstine. Effects of spinal anesthesia upon venous pressure in man. *Proc. Soc. Exp. Biol. Med.* 45:415, 1940.

Akers, W. W., W. O'Bannon, C. W. Hall, and D. Liotta. Design and operation of a paracorporeal bypass pump. *Trans. Amer. Soc. Artif. Intern. Organs.* 12:86, 1966.

Akesson, S., E. Odelblad, and B. Selin. Circulation studies. II. Dilution curves after injection of Br 82 into the blood stream. *Acta Med. Scand.* 164:437, 1959.

Akutsu, T., C. S. Houston, and W. J. Kolff. Roller type of artificial heart within the chest. *Amer. Heart J.* 59:731, 1960.

Akutsu, T., W. Seidel, V. Mirkovitch, J. Feller, and W. J. Kolff. An electromotordriven pendulum-type artificial heart inside the chest. *Trans. Amer. Soc. Artif. Intern. Organs* 7:374, 1961.

Akutsu, T., V. Mirkovitch, S. Topaz, and W. J. Kolff. Silastic sac type of artificial heart and its use in calves. *Trans. Amer. Soc. Artif. Intern. Organs* 9:281, 1963.

Akutsu, T., V. Mirkovitch, S. Topaz, and W. J. Kolff. A sac type of artificial heart inside the chest of dogs. *J. Thorac. Cardiovasc. Surg.* 47:512, 1964.

Akutsu, T. Artificial hearts: available types. In A. N. Brest (Ed.). *Heart Substitutes.* Springfield, Illinois: Charles C Thomas, Publisher, 1966, Chapter 13.

Akutsu, T., and A. Kantrowitz. Problems of materials in mechanical heart systems. *J. Biomed. Mat. Res.* 1:33, 1967.

Akutsu, T., and H. Takagi. Thrombus formation in implanted blood pumps. *Trans. Amer. Soc. Artif. Intern. Organs* 15:55, 1969.

Akutsu, T., H. Takagi, and H. Takano. Total artificial heart with built in valves. *Trans. Amer. Soc. Artif. Intern. Organs* 16:392, 1970a.

Akutsu, T. Design criteria for artificial heart valves. *J. Thorac. Cardiovasc. Surg.* 60:34, 1970b.

Akutsu, T. Components of artificial hearts. *Bull. N.Y. Acad. Med.* 48:362, 1972.

Alexander, N., and M. Decur. Sinoaortic baroreflex system and early pressure rise in renal hypertensive rabbits. *Amer. J. Physiol.* 213:701, 1967.

Alexander, R. S. In vivo observations on distensibility of the femoral venous system. *Proc. Soc. Exp. Biol. Med.* 67:410, 1948.

Alexander, R. S. Influence of the diaphragm upon portal blood flow and venous return. *Amer. J. Physiol.* 167:738, 1951.

Alexander, R. S., W. S. Edwards, and J. L. Ankeney. The distensibility characteristics of the portal vascular bed. *Circ. Res.* 1:271, 1953.

Alexander, R. S. The participation of the venomotor system in pressure reflexes. *Circ. Res.* 2:405, 1954.

Alexander, R. S. Venomotor tone in hemorrhage and shock. *Circ. Res.* 3:181, 1955.

Alexander, R. S. Reflex alterations in venomotor tone produced by venous congestion. *Circ. Res.* 4:49, 1956.

Allen, S. C., C. L. Taylor, and V. E. Hall. A study of orthostatic insufficiency by the tiltboard method. *Amer. J. Physiol.* 143: 11, 1945.

Allison, J. L., K. Sagawa, and M. Kumada. An open-loop analysis of the aortic arch barostatic reflex. *Amer. J. Physiol.* 217: 1576, 1969.

Altman, R. Öber den Entstehungsmechanismus des systolischen Kollapses der Venenpulskurve. *Z. Kreislaufforsch.* 43: 738, 1954.

Altschule, M. D., M. D. Volk, and H. Henstell. Cardiac and respiratory function at rest in patients with uncomplicated polycythemia vera. *Amer. J. Med. Sci.* 200:478, 1940.

Anderson, R. A. Intrinsic blood pressure. *Circulation* 9:641, 1954.

Angenheister, G., and E. Law. Seismographische Aufnahmen der Herztätigkeit. *Naturwissenschaften* 16:513, 1928.

Anrep, G. V., and E. Saalfield. The blood flow through the skeletal muscle in relation to its contraction. *J. Physiol.* 85:375, 1935.

Anrep, G. V., G. S. Barsoum, S. Salama, and Z. Souidan. Liberation of histamine during reactive hyperaemia and muscle contraction in man. *J. Physiol.* 103:297, 1944.

Anthony, A., and J. Kreider. Blood volume changes in rodents exposed to simulated altitude. *Amer. J. Physiol.* 200:523, 1961.

Anzola, J. Right ventricular contraction. *Amer. J. Physiol.* 184: 567, 1956a.

Anzola, J., and R. F. Rushmer. Cardiac responses to sympathetic stimulation. *Circ. Res.* 4:302, 1956b.

Armstrong, G. G., P. L. Chipley, and A. C. Guyton. Simultaneous arterial and venous pressure-volume curves of the intact dog. *Amer. J. Physiol.* 179:616, 1954.

Arvidsson, H. Angiocardiograph determination of left ventricular volume. *Acta Radiol.* 56:321, 1961.

Aschoff, J., and R. Wever. Die Funktionsweise der Diathermie-Thermo-Stromuhr. *Pflüger's Arch. ges. Physiol.* 262:133, 1956.

Ashkar, E., and W. F. Hamilton. Cardiovascular response to graded exercise in the sympathectomized-vagotomized dog. *Amer. J. Physiol.* 204:291, 1963.

Ashkar, E. Heart rate and blood pressure during exercise and autonomic denervation. *Amer. J. Physiol.* 210:950, 1966.

Ashton, C. H., and G. J. R. McHardy. A rebreathing method for determining mixed venous Pco_2 during exercise. *J. Appl. Physiol.* 18:668, 1963.

Asmussen, E. Cardiac output in rest and work in humid heat. *Amer. J. Physiol.* 131:54, 1940.

Asmussen, E., and F. C. Consolazio. The circulation in rest and work on Mount Evans. *Amer. J. Physiol.* 132:555, 1941.

Asmussen, E., and M. Nielsen. The cardiac output in rest and work determined simultaneously by the acetylene and the dye injection methods. *Acta Physiol. Scand.* 27:217, 1952.

Asmussen, E., and M. Nielsen. The cardiac output in rest and work at low and high oxygen pressures. *Acta Physiol. Scand.* 35:73, 1955a.

Asmussen, E., and M. Nielsen. Cardiac output during muscular work and its regulation. *Physiol. Rev.* 35:778, 1955b.

Astrand, P., T. E. Cuddy, D. Saltin, and J. Stenberg. Cardiac output during submaximal and maximal work. *J. Appl. Physiol.* 19:268, 1964.

Atsumi, K., M. Hori, S. Ikeda, Y. Sakurai, Y. Fujimori, and S. Kimoto. Artificial heart incorporated in the chest. *Trans. Amer. Soc. Artif. Intern. Organs* 9:292, 1963.

Aub, R. Modellversuche zur Schlagvolumbestimmung. *Z. Biol.* 93:164, 1932.

Aviado, D. M., I. De Burgh Daly, C. Y. Lee, and C. F. Schmidt. The contribution of the bronchial circulation to the venous admixture in pulmonary venous blood. *J. Physiol.* 155:602, 1961.

Ayotte, B., J. Seymour, and M. B. McIlroy. A new method for measurement of cardiac output with nitrous oxide. *J. Appl. Physiol.* 28:863, 1970.

Bache, R. J., and H. E. Ederstrom. Reactive hyperemia in legs of dogs: effects of temperature and intravascular tension. *Circ. Res.* 16:416, 1965.

Bachofen, H. D., A. Bloom and L. E. Farhi. Determination of cardiac output by ether dilution. *J. Appl. Physiol.* 30:131, 1971a.

Bachofen, M., A. Gage, and H. Bachofen. Vascular response to changes in blood oxygen tension under various blood flow rates. *Amer. J. Physiol.* 220:1786, 1971b.

Badeer, H. S. The stimulus to hypertrophy of the myocardium. *Circulation* 30:128, 1964a.

Badeer, H. S. Biological significance of cardiac hypertrophy. *Amer. J. Cardiol.* 14: 133, 1964b.

Badeer, H. S. "Contractility" of the nonfailing hypertrophied heart. *Amer. Heart J.* 73:693, 1967.

Badeer, H. S. Metabolic basis of cardiac hypertrophy. Prog. Cardiovasc. Dis. 11: 53, 1968.

Baer, P. G., L. G. Navar, and A. C. Guyton. Renal autoregulation, filtration rate, and electrolyte excretion during vasodilatation. *Amer. J. Physiol.* 219:619, 1970.

Bailie, M. D., S. Robinson, H. H. Rostarfer, and J. L. Newton. Effects of exercise on heart output of the dog. *J. Appl. Physiol.* 16:107, 1961.

Baker, C. H., and H. D. Wycoff. Time-concentration curves and dilution spaces of T-1824 and I^{131}-labeled proteins in dogs. *Amer. J. Physiol.* 201:1159, 1961.

Baker, O., J. Khalaf, and C. B. Chapman. A scanner-computer for determining the volumes of cardiac chambers from cinefluorographic films. *Amer. Heart J.* 62:767, 1961.

Baldes, E. J., and J. F. Herrick. Thermostrumuhr with direct current heater. *Proc. Soc. Exp. Biol. Med.* 37:432, 1937.

Balent, P., E. Kiss, and J. Sturcz. Minutenvolumen und Nierendurchblutung im haemorrhagischen shock. *Pflüger's Arch. ges. Physiol.* 272:307, 1961.

Banet, M., and A. C. Guyton. Effect of body metabolism on cardiac output: role of the central nervous system. *Amer. J. Physiol.* 220:662, 1971.

Barcroft, H., and O. G. Edholm. Effect of temperature on blood flow and deep temperature in human forearm. *J. Physiol.* 102:5, 1943.

Barcroft, H., O. G. Edholm, J. McMichael, and E. P. Sharpey-Schafer. Post-hemorrhagic fainting; study by cardiac output and forearm flow. *Lancet* 1:489, 1944.

Barcroft, H., and O. G. Edholm. On the vasodilation in human skeletal muscle during posthemorrhagic fainting. *J. Physiol.* 104:161, 1945.

Barcroft, H., A. C. Dornhorst, H. M. McClatchey, and I. M. Tanner. On the blood flow through rhythmically contracting muscle before and during release of sympathetic vasoconstrictor tone. *J. Physiol.* 117:391, 1952.

Barcroft, H., and H. J. C. Swan. *Sympathetic Control of Human Blood Vessels.* London: Edward Arnold & Co., 1953.

Barcroft, J., and E. K. Marshall. Note on the effect of external temperature on the circulation in man. *J. Physiol.* 58:145, 1923.

Barcroft, J., L. B. Flexner, and T. McClurkin. Output of fetal heart in goat. *J. Physiol.* 82:498, 1934.

Bardeen, C. R. Determination of the size of the heart by means of the x-rays. *Amer. J. Anat.* 23:423, 1918.

Barger, A. C., B. B. Roe, and G. S. Richardson. Relation of valvular lesions and of exercise to auricular pressure, work tolerance, and to development of chronic congestive failure in dogs. *Amer. J. Physiol.* 169:384, 1952.

Barger, A. C., V. Richards, J. Metcalfe, and B. Günther. Regulation of the circulation during exercise; cardiac output (direct Fick) and metabolic adjustments in the normal dog. *Amer. J. Physiol.* 184:613, 1956.

Barger, A. C. The kidney in congestive heart failure. *Circulation* 21:124, 1960.

Barger, A. C., J. Metcalfe, V. Richards, and B. Günther. Circulation during exercise in normal dogs and dogs with cardiac valvular lesions. *Amer. J. Physiol.* 201:480, 1961.

Barlett, D., Jr., and S. M. Tenney. Tissue gas tensions in experimental anemia. *J. Appl. Physiol.* 18:734, 1963.

Barnett, G. O., J. C. Greenfield, Jr., and S. M. Fox, III. The technique of estimating the instantaneous aortic blood velocity in man from the pressure gradient. *Amer. Heart J.* 62:359, 1961.

Barr, J. W., and E. C. Bradley, A calibration device for the earpiece dichromatic densitometer. *J. Appl. Physiol.* 25:633, 1968.

Barratt-Boyes, B. G., and E. H. Wood. Hemodynamic response of healthy subjects to exercise in the supine position while breathing oxygen. *J. Appl Physiol.* 11:129, 1957.

Barratt-Boyes, B. G., and E. H. Wood. Cardiac output and related measurements and pressure values in the right heart and associated vessels, together with an analysis of the hemodynamic response to the inhalation of high oxygen mixtures in healthy subjects. *J. Lab. Clin. Med.* 51:72, 1958.

Barsoum, G. S., and F. H. Smirk. Observations on the increase in the concentration of a histamine-like substance in human venous blood during a period of reactive hyperaemia. *Clin. Sci.* 2:353, 1936.

Bartle, S. H., and M. E. Sanmarco. Comparison of angiocardiographic and thermal washout techniques for left ventricular measurement. *Amer. J. Cardiol.* 18:235, 1966.

Baskin, R. J., and P. J. Paolini. Volume change and pressure development in muscle during contraction. *Amer. J. Physiol.* 213:1025, 1967.

Baum, R., and M. J. Hosko, Jr. Response of resistance and capacitance vessels to central nervous system stimulation. *Amer. J. Physiol.* 209:236, 1965.

Baumber, J. S., J. O. Davis, E. G. Schneider, and J. A. Johnson. Plasma renin activity and the response to mineralocorticoid excess in dogs with chronic left ventricular overload. *Physiologist* 12:172, 1969.

Baumber, J. S., J. O. Davis, J. W. Mackenzie, E. G. Schneider, J. A. Johnson, and C. A. Robb. Chronic experimental left heart failure in the dog. *Amer. J. Physiol.* 219: 474, 1970a.

Baumber, J. S., J. O. Davis, E. G. Schneider, and J. A. Johnson. Plasma renin activity and the effects of deoxycorticosterone acetate in dogs with chronic left ventricular overload. *Circ. Res.* 27:1970b.

Baxter, I. G., and J. W. Pearce. Simultaneous measurement of pulmonary arterial flow and pressure using condensory manometers. *J. Physiol.* 115:410, 1951.

Baxter, I. G., D. J. C. Cunningham, and J. W. Pearce. Comparison of cardiac output determinations in the cat by direct Fick and flowmeter methods. *J. Physiol.* 118:299, 1952.

Bayliss, W. M. On the local reactions of the arterial wall to changes in internal pressure. *J. Physiol.* (London) 28:220, 1902.

Bazett, H. C. An analysis of the time-relations of electrocardiograms. *Heart* 7:353, 1920.

Bazett, H. C., F. S. Cotton, L. B. Laplace, and J. C. Scott. Calculation of cardiac output and effective peripheral resistance from blood pressure measurements, with appendix on size of aorta in man. *Amer. J. Physiol.* 113:312, 1935.

Bazett, H. C., J. C. Scott, M. E. Maxfield, and M. D. Blithe. Calculation of cardiac output from blood pressure measurements before and after meals. *Amer. J. Physiol.* 116:551, 1936.

Bazett, H. C., L. B. Laplace, and J. C. Scott. Estimation of cardiac output from blood pressure and pulse wave velocity measurements on subjects with cardiovascular disease other than aortic regurgitation. *Amer. Heart J.* 22:737, 1941.

Beard, E. F., J. W. Nicholson, III, and E. H. Wood. Application of an ear oximeter for estimation of cardiac output by the dye method in man. *J. Lab. Clin. Med.* 36:798, 1950.

Beard, E. F., and E. H. Wood. Estimation of cardiac output by the dye dilution method with an ear oximeter. *J. Appl. Physiol.* 4:177, 1951.

Beck, L., and A. S. Dontas. Vasomotor activity in hemorrhagic shock. *Fed. Proc.* 14:318, 1955.

Beck, L. Effect of the autonomic nervous system on arteriolar tone in the experimental animal. *Circulation* 17:798, 1958.

Becker, E. L., R. G. Cooper, and G. D. Hataway. Capillary vascularity in puppies born at a simulated altitude of 20,000 feet. *J. Appl. Physiol.* 8:166, 1955.

Becklake, M. R., C. J. Varvis, P. S. Kenning, M. McGregor, and P. V. Bates. Measurement of pulmonary blood flow during exercise using nitrous oxide. *J. Appl. Physiol.* 17:579, 1962.

Beecher, H. K., M. E. Field, and A. Krogh. Method of measuring venous pressure in human leg during walking. *Skand. Arch. Physiol.* 73:7, 1936a.

Beecher, H. K., M. E. Field, and A. Krogh. Effect of walking on venous pressure at ankle. *Skand. Arch. Physiol.* 73:133, 1936b.

Benchimol, A., E. G. Dimond, F. R. Carvalho, and M. W. Robertson. The forward triangle formula for calculations of cardiac output. *Amer. J. Cardiol.* 12:119, 1963.

Benchimol, A., Y. Li, and E. G. Dimond. Cardiovascular dynamics in complete heart block at various heart rates. *Circulation* 30:542, 1964.

Benchimol, A., P. R. Akre, and E. G. Di-

mond. Clinical experience with the use of computers for calculation of cardiac output. *Amer. J. Cardiol.* 15:213, 1965a.

Benchimol, A., T. Wu, and M. S. Liggett. Effect of exercise and isoproterenol on the cardiovascular dynamics in complete heart block at various heart rates. *Amer. Heart J.* 70:337, 1965b.

Benchimol, A., I. G. Maia, J. L. Gartlan, and D. Franklin. Telemetry of arterial flow in man with a Doppler ultrasonic flowmeter. *Amer. J. Cardiol.* 22:75, 1968.

Beneken, J. A mathematical analysis of cardiovascular function. To be published.

Beneken, J. E., A. C. Guyton, and K. Sagawa. Coronary perfusion pressure and left ventricular function. *Pflügers Arch.* 305:76, 1969.

Benis, A. M., S. Usami, and S. Chien. Effect of hematocrit and inertial losses on pressure-flow relations in the isolated hindpaw of the dog. *Circ. Res.*, 27:1047, 1970.

Benson, E. S., G. T. Evans, B. E. Hallaway, C. Phibbs, and E. F. Freier. Myocardial creatine phosphate and nucleotides in anoxic cardiac arrest and recovery. *Amer. J. Physiol.* 201:687, 1961.

Berconsky, I. El volumen circulatorio per minuto en el estado normal y patológico. Buenos Aires, 1930. Quoted by Grollman (1932).

Berglund, E. Ventricular function: VI. Balance of left and right ventricular output: relation between left and right atrial pressures. *Amer. J. Physiol.* 178:381, 1954.

Berglund, E. The function of the ventricles of the heart. *Acta Physiol Scand.* 33: Suppl. 119, p. 1, 1955a.

Berglund, E., S. J. Sarnoff, and J. P. Isaacs. Ventricular function: Role of the pericardium in regulation of cardiovascular hemodynamics. *Circulation Research* 3:133, 1955b.

Berglund, E., R. G. Monroe, and G. L. Schreiner. Myocardial oxygen consumption and coronary blood flow during potassium induced cardiac arrest and during ventricular fibrillation. *Acta Physiol. Scand.* 41:216, 1957.

Bergofsky, E. H., and T. Bertun. Response of regional circulations to hyperoxia. *J. Appl. Physiol.* 21:567, 1966.

Berkson, J., and W. M. Boothby. Studies of energy of metabolism of normal individuals. Comparison of estimation of basal metabolism from linear formula and "surface area." *Amer. J. Physiol.* 116:485, 1936.

Bernard, W. F., C. G. LaFarge, R. Robinson, I. Yun, and K. Shirahige. An improved blood-pump interface for left ventricular bypass. *Ann. Surg.* 168:750, 1968.

Berne, R. M., and M. N. Levy. Effects of acute reduction of cardiac output on the renal circulation of the dog. *J. Clin. Invest.* 29:444, 1950.

Berne, R. M., and M. N. Levy. Effect of acute

reduction in cardiac output on the denervated kidney. *Amer. J. Physiol.* 171:558, 1952.

Berne, R. M. Cardiodynamics and the coronary circulation in hypothermia. *Ann. N.Y. Acad. Sci.* 80:365, 1959.

Berne, R. M. Cardiac nucleotides in hypoxia; possible role in regulation of coronary blood flow. *Amer. J. Physiol.* 204:317, 1963.

Berne, R. M. Regulation of coronary blood flow. *Physiol. Rev.* 44:1, 1964a.

Berne, R. M. Metabolic regulation of blood flow. *Circ. Res.* 15:Suppl. I, 261, 1964b.

Berseus, S. Influence of heart glucosides, theophylline and analeptics on cardiac output in congestive heart failure, with remarks on acetylene methods for determination of arteriovenous oxygen difference. *Acta Med. Scand.* Supp. 145:1, 1943.

Berseus, S., H. Lagerlöf, and L. Werkö. A comparison between the direct Fick and the Grollman methods for determination of the cardiac output in man. *Acta Med. Scand.* Suppl. 239:258, 1950.

Besterman, E. M. The cardiac output in acute rheumatic carditis. *Brit. Heart J.* 16:8, 1954.

Bethea, H. L., C. E. Jones, and J. W. Crowell. Effect of pharmacologic coronary flow augmentation on cardiac function in hypotension. *Amer. J. Physiol.* 222:95, 1972.

Betticher, A., J. Maillard, and A. Müller. Un manomètre différentiel à transmission électrique entièrement alimenté sur le réseau alternatif, pour mesurer la vitesse d'écoulement dans des tuyaux et des vaisseaux sanguins. *Helv. Physiol. Pharmacol. Acta* 12:112, 1954.

Bevan, J. A., and J. V. Osher. Effect of potassium on the resting links of vascular smooth muscle of the rabbit aorta and its response to *l*-norepinephrine. *Circ. Res.* 13:346, 1963.

Bevegard, B. S., and J. T. Shepherd. Changes in tone of limb veins during supine exercise. *J. Appl. Physiol.* 20:1, 1965.

Bevegard, B. S., and J. T. Shepherd. Regulation of the circulation during exercise in man. *Physiol. Rev.* 47:178, 1967.

Bevegard, S., A. Holmgren, and B. Jonsson. The effect of body position on the circulation at rest and during exercise, with special reference to the influence on the stroke volume. *Acta Physiol. Scand.* 49:279, 1960.

Bickel, R. G., C. F. Diener, and H. L. Brammell. An analog computer program for cardiac output in humans, using mass spectrometer analysis of expired air. *Aerospace Med.* 41:203, 1970.

Bing, O. H. L., J. F. Keefe, M. J. Wolk, J. G. Lipana, K. M. McIntyre, and H. J. Levine. Cardiovascular responses to hypoxia and varying Pco_2 in the awake dog. *J. Appl. Physiol.* 27:204, 1969.

Bing, R. J., L. D. Vandam, and F. O. Gray, Jr. Physiological studies in congenital heart disease. *Bull. Hopkins Hosp.* 80:107, 1947.

Bing, R. J., M. M. Hammond, J. C. Handelsman, S. R. Powers, F. C. Spencer, J. E. Eckenhoff, W. T. Goodale, J. H. Hofkanschiel, and S. S. Kety. Measurement of coronary blood flow, oxygen consumption, and efficiency of left ventricle in man. *Amer. Heart J.* 38:1, 1949.

Bing, R. J., R. Heimbeckler, and W. Falholt. An estimation of the residual volume of blood in the right ventricle of normal and diseased human hearts in vivo. *Amer. Heart J.* 42:483, 1951.

Bing, R. J., D. Bottcher, and C. Gowan. What is cardiac failure? *Amer. J. Cardiol.* 22:2, 1968.

Bishop, J. M., K. W. Donald, and O. L. Wade. Minute to minute changes in cardiac output by the direct Fick method in normal subjects during exercise and recovery. *J. Physiol.* 123:12P, 1954.

Bishop, J. M., K. W. Donald, and O. L. Wade. Circulatory dynamics at rest and on exercise in the hyperkinetic states. *Clin. Sci.* 14:329, 1955.

Bishop, J. M., and N. Segel. The circulatory effects of intravenous pronethalol in man at rest and during exercise in the supine and upright positions. *J. Physiol.* (London) 169:112, 1963.

Bishop, V. S., H. L. Stone, and A. C. Guyton. Cardiac function curves in conscious dogs. *Amer. J. Physiol.* 207:677, 1964.

Blair, D. A., W. E. Glover, and I. C. Roddie. The abolition of reactive and post-exercise hyperemia in the forearm by temporary restriction of arterial inflow. *J. Physiol.* 148:648, 1959.

Blair, H. A., and A. M. Wedd. The action of cardiac ejection on venous return. *Amer. J. Physiol.* 145:528, 1946.

Blake, W. D., R. Wegria, R. P. Keating, and H. P. Ward. Effect of increased renal venous pressure on renal function. *Amer. J. Physiol.* 157:1, 1949.

Blalock, A. Mechanism and treatment of experimental shock. I. Shock following hemorrhage. *Arch. Surg.* 15:762, 1927.

Blalock, A. Effects of primary shock on cardiac output and blood pressure. *Proc. Soc. Exp. Biol. Med.* 31:36, 1933a.

Blalock, A. Exposure of heart to atmospheric pressure; effects on cardiac output and blood pressure. *Arch. Surg.* 26:516, 1933b.

Blumgart, H. L., and P. M. Zoll. The clinical management of congestive heart failure. *Circulation* 21:218, 1960.

Bock, J., and J. Buchholtz. *Arch. exp. Pathol. Pharmakol.* 88:192, 1920.

Böhme, W. Über den aktiven Anteil des Herzens an der Förderung des Venenblutes. *Ergeb. Physiol. u. exp. Pharmakol.* 38:251, 1936.

Bolton, C. The experimental production of uncompensated heart disease with especial reference to the pathology of dropsy. (Microfilm.) *J. Pathol. Bacteriol.* 9:67, 1903.

Bolton, C. The pathology of cardiac dropsy. *Brit. Med. J.* 1:642, 1917.

Bond, R. F., and C. A. Barefoot. Evaluation of an electromagnetic catheter tip velocity sensitive blood flow probe. *J. Appl. Physiol.* 23:403, 1967.

Boothby, W. M. A determination of the circulation rate in man at rest and at work. *Amer. J. Physiol.* 37:412, 1915.

Boothby, W. A., and I. Sandiford. Normal values of basal or standard metabolism; a modification of the Du Bois standards. *Amer. J. Physiol.* 90:258, 1929.

Bopp, P., E. F. Arnold, and F. Chatelanet. Cardiac output and Albright's syndrome. *Amer. Heart J.* 63:394, 1962.

Bornstein, A. Eine Methode zen vergleichenden Messung des Herzschlagvolumens beim Menschen. *Pflüger's Arch. ges. Physiol.* 132:307, 1910.

Borst, J. G. G. Maintenance of adequate cardiac output by regulation of urinary excretion of water and sodium chloride; essential factor in genesis of edema. *Acta Med. Scand.* 130:Suppl. 207, p. 1, 1948.

Boucek, R. J., J. H. Grindlay, and H. B. Burchell. Experimental constriction of inflow tracts in the heart: analysis of circulatory failure. *Amer. J. Physiol.* 169:442, 1952a.

Boucek, R. J., J. H. Grindlay, and H. B. Burchell. Experimental constrictive pericarditis: analysis of induced circulatory failure. *Amer. J. Physiol.* 169:434, 1952b.

Bounous, G., A. H. McArdle, and L. G. Hampton. Biosynthesis of intestinal mucin in shock: relationship to tryptic hemorrhagic enteritis and permeability to curare. *Ann. Surg.* 164:13, 1966.

Bousvaros, G. A., W. H. Palmer, P. Sekelj, and M. McGregor. Comparison of central and peripheral injection sites in the estimation of cardiac output by dye dilution curves. *Circ. Res.* 12:317, 1962.

Bove, A. A., and P. R. Lynch. Measurement of canine left ventricular performance by cineradiography of the heart. *J. Appl. Physiol.* 29:877, 1970a.

Bove, A. A., and P. R. Lynch. Radiographic determination of force-velocity-length relationship in the intact dog heart. *J. Appl. Physiol.* 29:884, 1970b.

Bove, A. A., R. E. Sturm, H. C. Smith, and E. H. Wood. Changes in left ventricular function during injection of opaque contrast medium. *Physiologist* 14:114, 1971a.

Bove, A. A. Radiographic evaluation of dynamic geometry of the left ventricle. *J. Appl. Physiol.* 31:227, 1971b.

Bowers, E., D. J. M. Campbell, and C. H. P.

Johnston. Factors promoting venous return from arm in man. *Lancet* 1:460, 1945.

Boyd, T. E., and M. C. Patras. Variations in filling and output of the ventricles with the phases of respiration. *Am. J. Physiol.* 134:74, 1941.

Bozer, J. M., and R. Gorling. Cardiac output measured by radioactive indicator. *Meth. Med. Res.* 7:70, 1958.

Braasch, W., S. Gudbjarnason, P. S. Puri, K. G. Ravens, and R. J. Bing. Early changes in energy metabolism in the myocardium following acute coronary artery occlusion in anesthetized dogs. *Circ. Res.* 23:429, 1968.

Bradley, R. D., B. S. Jenkins, and M. A. Branthwaite. The influence of atrial pressure on cardiac performance following myocardial infarction complicated by shock. *Circulation* 42:827, 1970.

Bramwell, J. C., and A. V. Hill. The velocity of pulse wave in man. *Proc. Roy. Soc. (London)* Series B, 93:298, 1922.

Brand, E. D., and A. M. Lefer. Myocardial depressant factor in plasma from cats in irreversible post-oligemic shock. *Proc. Soc. Exp. Biol. Med.* 122:200, 1966.

Brandfonbrener, M., M. Landowne, and N. W. Shock. Changes in cardiac output with age. *Circulation* 12:557, 1955.

Brannon, E. S., O. J. Merrill, J. V. Warren, and E. A. Stead, Jr. Cardiac output in patients with chronic anemia as measured by technic of right atrial catheterization. *J. Clin. Invest.* 24:332, 1945.

Branthwaite, M. A., and R. D. Bradley. Measurement of cardiac output by thermal dilution in man. *J. Appl. Physiol.* 24:434, 1968.

Brauer, R. W. Autoregulation of blood flow in the liver. *Circ. Res.* 15:Suppl. I, p. 213, 1964.

Braun, K., S. Z. Rosenberg, and A. Schwartz. A central blood volume, cardiac output, and pulmonary vascular pattern in mitral stenosis. *Amer. J. Cardiol.* 3:40, 1959.

Braunwald, E., J. T. Binion, W. L. Morgan, Jr., and S. J. Sarnoff. Alterations in central blood volume and cardiac output induced by positive pressure breathing and counteracted by metaraminol (aramine). *Circ. Res.* 5:670, 1957.

Braunwald, E., S. J. Sarnoff, R. B. Case, W. N. Stainsby, and G. H. Welch, Jr. Hemodynamic determinants of coronary flow: effect of changes in aortic pressure and cardiac output on the relationship between myocardial oxygen consumption and coronary flow. *Amer. J. Physiol.* 192:157, 1958.

Braunwald, E., R. L. Frye, and J. Ross, Jr. Studies on Starling's law of the heart: determination of the relationship between left ventricular end-diastolic pressure and circumference. *Circ. Res.* 8:1254, 1960.

Braunwald, E., E. C. Brockenkough, C. J.

Frohm, and J. Ross, Jr. Left atrial and left ventricular pressures in subjects without cardiovascular disease. *Circulation* 24:267, 1961a.

Braunwald, E., C. J. Frahm, and J. Ross, Jr. Studies on Starling's law of the heart. V. Left ventricular function in man. *J. Clin. Invest.* 40:1882, 1961b.

Braunwald, E., C. A. Chidsey, D. C. Harrison, T. E. Gaffney, and R. L. Kahler. Studies on the function of the adrenergic nerve endings in the heart. *Circ. Res.* 28:958, 1963a.

Braunwald, E., A. Goldblatt, D. C. Harrison, and D. T. Mason. Studies on cardiac dimensions in intact, unanesthetized man. III. Effects of muscular exercise. *Circ. Res.* 13:448, 1963b.

Braunwald, E., E. H. Sonnenblick, J. Ross, Jr., G. Glick, and S. E. Epstein. An analysis of the cardiac response to exercise. *Circ. Res.* 20:Suppl. I, p. 44, 1967.

Braunwald, E., J. Ross, J. H. Gault, D. T. Mason, C. Mills, I. T. Gabe, and S. E. Epstein. Assessment of cardiac function. *Ann. Intern. Med.* 70:369, 1969.

Brecher, G. A. Mechanism of venous flow under different degrees of aspiration. *Amer. J. Physiol.* 169:423, 1952a.

Brecher, G. A., and G. Mixter, Jr. Augmentation of venous return by respiratory efforts under normal and abnormal conditions. *Amer. J. Physiol.* 171:710, 1952b.

Brecher, G. A., G. Mixter, Jr., and L. Share. Dynamics of venous collapse in superior vena cava system. *Amer. J. Physiol.* 171:194, 1952c.

Brecher, G. A. Venous return during intermittent positive-negative pressure respiration studied with a new catheter flowmeter. *Amer. J. Physiol.* 174:299, 1953a.

Brecher, G. A., and G. Mixter, Jr. Effect of respiratory movements on superior cava flow under normal and abnormal conditions. *Amer. J. Physiol.* 172:457, 1953b.

Brecher, G. A., and J. Praglin. A modified bristle flowmeter for measuring phasic blood flow. *Proc. Soc. Exp. Biol. Med.* 83:155, 1953c.

Brecher, G. A. Cardiac variations in venous return studied with a new bristle flowmeter. *Amer. J. Physiol.* 176:423, 1954a.

Brecher, G. A., and C. A. Hubay. A new method for direct recording of cardiac output. *Proc. Soc. Exp. Biol. Med.* 86:464, 1954b.

Brecher, G. A. Experimental evidence of ventricular diastolic suction. *Circ. Res.* 4:513, 1956a.

Brecher, G. A. *Venous Return.* New York: Grune and Stratton, Inc., 1956b.

Brecher, G. A. Critical review of bristle flowmeter techniques. *I. R. E. Trans.* ME 6:294, 1959.

Brecker, G. H., and P. M. Galletti. Functional anatomy of cardiac pumping. In *Handbook of Physiology.* Baltimore. The Williams & Wilkins Co., 1963, Vol. II, No. II, p. 759.

Brendel, W., C. Albers, and W. Usinger. Der Kreislauf in Hypothermie. *Pflüger's Arch. ges Physiol.* 266:341, 1958.

Briggs, A. P., D. M. Fowell, W. F. Hamilton, J. W. Remington, N. C. Wheeler, and J. A. Winslow. Renal and circulatory factors in the edema formation of congestive heart failure. *J. Clin. Invest.* 27:810, 1948.

Brind, S. H., J. R. Bianchine, and M. N. Levy. Effect of bilateral occlusion of common carotid arteries on cardiac output and oxygen content of arterial and venous blood in the anesthetized dog. *Amer. J. Physiol.* 185:483, 1956.

Brodie, D. A., and D. M. Woodbury. Acid-base changes in brain and blood of rats exposed to high concentrations of carbon dioxide. *Amer. J. Physiol.* 192:91, 1958.

Broemser, P., and O. F. Ranke. Über die Messung des Schlagvolumens des Herzens auf unblutigem Weg. *Z. Biol.* 90:467, 1930.

Broemser, P., and O. F. Ranke. Die physikalische Bestimmung des Schlagvolumens des Herzens. *Z. Kreislaufforsch.* 25:11, 1933.

Brogdon, E., and F. A. Hellebrandt. Post-exercise orthostatic collapse. *Amer. J. Physiol.* 129:P318, 1940.

Bronk, D. W., L. K. Ferguson, R. Margaria, and D. Y. Solandt. The activity of the cardiac sympathetic centers. *Amer. J. Physiol.* 117:237, 1936.

Brotmacher, L., and D. C. Deuchar. The systemic blood flow in congenital heart disease, with an examination of the validity of the cardiac index. *Clin. Sci.* 15:441, 1956.

Brotmacher, L. Evaluation of derivation of cardiac output from blood pressure measurements. *Circ. Res.* 5:589, 1957a.

Brotmacher, L., and P. Fleming. Cardiac output and vascular pressures in 10 normal children and adolescents. *Guy's Hosp. Rep.* 106:268, 1957b.

Brown, G. S., and D. P. Campbell. *Principles of Servo-Mechanisms.* New York: John Wiley & Sons, Inc., 1948.

Brown, R., S. H. Rahmitoola, G. D. Davis, and H. J. C. Swan. The effect of angiocardiographic contrast medium on circulatory dynamics in man. Cardiac output during angiocardiography. *Circulation* 31:234, 1965.

Browse, N. L., J. T. Shepherd, and D. E. Donald. Differences in response of veins and resistance vessels in limbs to same stimulus. *Amer. J. Physiol.* 211:1241, 1966.

Bruce, T. A., C. B. Chapman, O. Baker, and J. N. Fisher. The role of autonomic and myocardial factors in cardiac control. *J. Clin. Invest.* 42:721, 1963.

Brücke, F., M. Loudon, and G. Werner. Durchblutungsänderungen der Hinterextremitäten bie Karotidenentlastung und zentraler Hypothalamusreizung. *Z. Kreislaufforsch.* 40:513, 1951.

Brutsaert, D. L., W. W. Parmley, and E. H. Sonnenblick. Effects of various interventions on the dynamic properties of the contractile elements of heart muscle of the cat. *Circ. Res.* 27:513, 1970.

Buccino, R. A., E. H. Sonnenblick, T. Cooper, and E. Braunwald. Direct positive inotropic effect of acetylcholine on myocardium. Evidence from multiple cholinergic receptors in the heart. *Circ. Res.*, 19: 1097, 1966.

Buckley, N. M., E. Ogden, and D. S. Linton, Jr. The effects of work load and heart rate on filling of the isolated right ventricle of the dog heart. *Circ. Res.* 3:434, 1955.

Burch, G. E., and W. A. Sodeman. Estimation of subcutaneous tissue pressure by direct method. *J. Clin. Invest.* 16:845, 1937.

Burch, G. E., and A. Hyman. Influence of a hot and humid environment upon cardiac output and work in normal man and in patients with chronic congestive heart failure at rest. *Amer. Heart J.* 53:665, 1957.

Burch, G. E., N. Depasquale, A. Hyman, and A. C. Degraff. Influence of tropical weather on cardiac output, work, and power of right and left ventricles of man resting in hospital. *Arch. Intern. Med.*, 104: 553, 1959.

Burdette, W. J. Studies on the metabolism of cardiac muscle from animals in shock. *Yale J. Biol. Med.* 23:505, 1950.

Burney, R. G., W. S. Pierce, K. R. Williams, M. H. Boyer, and C. K. Kirby. Studies on an artificial heart controlled by a venous pressure servomechanism. *Trans. Amer. Soc. Artif. Intern. Organs* 9:299, 1963.

Burns, W., J. Farlow, and R. Loubier. Two unique leaflet types of prosthetic heart valves. Digest of Sixth International Conference on Medical Electronics and Biology. *Japan Med. Elec. Bio.*, Tokyo, 1965, p. 346.

Burton, R. R., and A. H. Smith. Effect of polycythemia and chronic hypoxia on heart mass in the chicken. *J. Appl. Physiol.* 22:782, 1967.

Burton, R. R., A. H. Smith, J. C. Carlisle, and S. J. Sluka. Role of hematocrit, heart mass, and high altitude exposure in acute hypoxia tolerance. *J. Appl. Physiol.* 27:49, 1969.

Burton-Opitz, R. Flow of the blood in the external jugular vein. *Amer. J. Physiol.* 7:435, 1902.

Burwell, C. S., and G. C. Robinson. A method for the determination of the amount of oxygen and carbon dioxide in the mixed venous blood of man. *J. Clin. Invest.* 1:47, 1924a.

Burwell, C. S., and G. C. Robinson. The gaseous content of the blood and the output of the heart in normal resting adults. *J. Clin. Invest.* 1:87, 1924b.

Burwell, C. S., and L. Dexter. Beri-beri heart disease. *Trans. Ass. Amer. Physicians* 60:59, 1947.

Cahoon, D. H., I. E. Michael, and V. Johnson. Respiratory modification of cardiac output. *Amer. J. Physiol.* 133:642, 1941.

Cain, C. C., and D. I. Mahoney. The effect of high breathing pressure on cardiac output with and without counter pressure. *J. Aviation Med.* 24:308, 1953.

Caliva, F. S., R. Napodano, R. Zurek, T. Pombo, and R. H. Lyons. The effects on myocardial oxygen availability of hemorrhagic hypotension and its reversal by various agents, including l-norepinephrine. *Amer. J. Med. Sci.* 238:308, 1959.

Candel, S., and D. E. Ehrlich. Venous blood flow during the Valsalva experiment including some clinical applications. *Amer. J. Med.* 15:307, 1953.

Cander, L., and R. E. Forster. Determination of pulmonary parenchymal tissue volume and pulmonary capillary blood flow in man. *J. Appl. Physiol.* 14:541, 1959.

Carr, D. T., and H. E. Essex. Certain effects of positive pressure respiration on circulatory and respiratory systems. *Amer. Heart J.* 31:53, 1946.

Carrell, D. E., and H. T. Milhorn, Jr. Dynamic respiratory and circulatory responses to hypoxia in the anesthetized dog. *J. Appl. Physiol.* 30:305, 1971.

Carrier, O., J. Walker, and A. C. Guyton. Effect of sympathetic stimulation of the heart on cardiac output. Unpublished observations.

Carrier, O., J. Walker, and A. C. Guyton. Role of oxygen in autoregulation of blood flow in isolated vessels. *Amer. J. Physiol.* 206:951, 1964.

Carrier, O., J. Walker, and A. C. Guyton. Comparative effects of pH and hypoxemia on minute coronary, mesenteric and skeletal muscle arteries. *Angiology* 17:418, 1966.

Carsten, A., B. Folkow, and C. A. Hamberger. Cardiovascular effects of direct vagal stimulation in man. *Acta Physiol. Scand.* 41: 68, 1958.

Case, R. B., E. Berglund, and S. J. Sarnoff. Ventricular functions. II. Quantitative relationship between coronary flow and ventricular function with studies on unilateral failure. *Circ. Res.* 2:319, 1954.

Case, R. B., S. J. Sarnoff, and E. Berglund. Ventricular function. VII. Changes in coronary resistance and ventricular function resulting from acutely induced anemia and the effect thereon of coronary stenosis. *Amer. J. Med.* 18:397, 1955.

Cassin, S., R. D. Gilbert, C. E. Bunnell, and E. M. Johnson. Capillary development during exposure to chronic hypoxia. *Am. J. Physiol.* 220:448, 1971.

Cathcart, R. T., W. W. Field, and D. W. Richards. Comparison of cardiac output determined by the ballistocardiograph

(Nickerson apparatus) and by the direct Fick method. *J. Clin. Invest.* 32:5, 1953.

Cathcart, R. T., T. F. Nealon, Jr., W. Fraimow, L. J. Hampton, and J. H. Gibbon, Jr. Cardiac output under general anesthesia; effect of mean endotracheal pressure. *Ann. Surg.* 148:488, 1958.

Cerretelli, P., J. Piiper, F. Mangili, F. Cuttica, and B. Ricci. Circulation in exercising dogs. *J. Appl. Physiol.* 19:29, 1964.

Cerretelli, P., J. C. Cruz, L. E. Farhi, and H. Rahn. Determination of mixed venous O_2 and CO_2 tensions and cardiac output by a rebreathing method. *Resp. Physiol.* 1:258, 1966a.

Cerretelli, P., R. Sikand, and L. E. Farhi. Readjustments in cardiac output and gas exchange during onset of exercise and recovery. *J. Appl. Physiol.* 21:1345, 1966b.

Chalmers, J. P., P. I. Korner, and S. W. White. The effect of hemorrhage in the unanesthetized rabbit. *J. Physiol.* (London) 189:367, 1967.

Chalmers, J. P., and R. J. Wurtman. Participation of central noradrenergic neurons in arterial baroreceptor reflexes in the rabbit. *Circ. Res.* 28:480, 1971.

Chamberlain, D. A., and J. Howard. The haemodynamic effects of β-sympathetic blockade. *Brit. Heart J.* 26:213, 1964.

Chapman, C. B., H. L. Taylor, C. Baden, R. V. Ebert, A. Keys, and W. S. Carlson. Simultaneous determinations of the resting arteriovenous oxygen difference by the acetylene and direct Fick methods. *J. Clin. Invest.* 29:651, 1950.

Chapman, C. B., and R. S. Fraser. Studies on the effect of exercise on cardiovascular function. I. Cardiac output and mean circulation time. *Circulation* 9:57, 1954.

Chapman, C. B., O. Baker, J. Reynolds, and F. Bonte. Use of biplane cinefluorography for measurement of ventricular volume. *Circulation* 18:1105, 1958.

Chapman, C. B., J. N. Fisher, and B. J. Sproule. Behavior of stroke volume at rest and during exercise in human beings. *J. Clin. Invest.* 39:1208, 1960.

Chapman, C. B., O. Baker, J. H. Mitchell, and R. G. Collier. Experiences with a cinefluorographic method for measuring ventricular volume. *Amer. J. Cardiol.* 18:25, 1966.

Charlier, R. Measuring cardiac output in man; present status of problem; new direct method by right heart catheterization according to Fick principle: possibilities of application in circulatory disorders. *Acta Cardiol.* 1:136, 1946.

Charlier, R., and E. Philippot. Cardiac output and intraauricular pressure during carotid occlusion. *Compt. Rend. Soc. Biol.* 141:201, 1947a.

Charlier, R., and E. Philippot. Heart and carotid sinus; effect of endosinusal hypo-

tension on cardiac output. *Arch. Intern. Pharmacodynamie* 75:90, 1947b.

Charlier, R. Le role des regions sinusales et cardio-aortique dans la regulation reflexe du debit cardiaque. *Acta Cardiol.* 3:1948a.

Charlier, R., and E. Philippot. Reduction of cardiac and systolic output by chloroform inhalation; reestablishment of synephrin administration. *Arch. Intern. Pharmacodynamie* 77:233, 1948b.

Chidsey, C. A., H. W. Fritts, Jr., A. Hardewig, D. W. Richards, and A. Cournand. Fate of radioactive Krypton (Kr^{85}) introduced intravenously in man. *J. Appl. Physiol.* 14:63, 1958.

Chidsey, C. A., R. L. Frye, R. L. Kahler, and E. Braunwald. Influence of syrosingopine on the cardiovascular response to acute hypoxemia and exercise. *Circulation Research* 9:989, 1961.

Chidsey, C. A., G. A. Kaiser, E. H. Sonnenblick, J. F. Spann, Jr., and E. Braunwald. Cardiac norepinephrine stores in experimental heart failure in the dog. *J. Clin. Invest.* 43:2386, 1964.

Chien, S. A quantitative evaluation of the circulatory adjustments of splenectomized dogs to hemorrhage. *Amer. J. Physiol.* 193:605, 1958.

Chien, S., and S. Billig. Effect of hemorrhage on cardiac output of sympathectomized dogs. *Amer. J. Physiol.* 201:475, 1961.

Chien, S., R. J. Dellenback, S. Usami, D. Treitel, C. Chang, and M. I. Gregersen. Blood volume and its distribution in endotoxin shock. *Amer. J. Physiol.* 210:1411, 1966a.

Chien, S., S. Usami, H. Taylor, J. Lundberg, and M. I. Gregerson. Effects of hematocrit and plasma proteins on human rheology at low shear rates. *J. Appl. Physiol.* 21:81, 1966b.

Chiodi, H., D. B. Dill, F. Consolazio, and S. M. Horvath. Respiratory and circulatory responses to acute carbon monoxide poisoning. *Amer. J. Physiol.* 134:683, 1941.

Christensen, E. H., and V. Mitteilung. Minutenvolumen und Schlagvolumen des Herzens während schwerer körperlicher Arbeit. *Arbeitphysiologie* 4:470, 1931.

Christiansen, J., C. G. Douglas, and J. S. Haldane. The absorption and dissociation of carbon dioxide by human blood. *J. Physiol.* 48:244, 1914.

Clark, R. T., Jr., D. Criscuolo, G. Guy, G. Hataway, and H. M. Sweeney. Mechanisms of adaptation to chronic hypoxia within the tissues. Proc. XIX Intern. Physiol. Congress, 1953, p. 271.

Clausen, J. P., O. A. Larsen, and J. Trapensen. Cardiac output in middle-age patients determined with CO_2 rebreathing method. *J. Appl. Physiol.* 28:337, 1970.

Cleempoel, H., and A. Bertinchamps. Nouvelle technique de mesure du debit cardiaque par l'etude de la courbe de dilution arterielle de radiophosphore. *Acta Cardiol.* 12:675, 1957.

Clemedson, C. J., and H. Hultman. Cardiac output in early phase of blast injury in rabbits. *Amer. J. Physiol.* 194:601, 1958.

Clowes, G. H. A., and L. R. Del Guercio. Circulatory response to trauma of surgical operations. *Metabolism* 9:67, 1960.

Coffman, J. D., and D. E. Gregg. Reactive hyperemia characteristics of the myocardium. *Amer. J. Physiol.* 199:1143, 1960.

Coffman, J. D. Blood flow and oxygen debt repayment and exercising skeletal muscle. *Amer. J. Physiol.* 205:126, 1963.

Cohen, S. M., O. G. Edholm, S. Howarth, J. McMichael, and E. P. Sharpey-Schafer. Cardiac output and peripheral blood flow in arteriovenous aneurysm. *Clin. Sci.* 7:35, 1948.

Cohn, A. E., and J. M. Steele. Action of digitalis on output of dog's heart in heart-lung preparations. *J. Clin. Invest.* 11:871, 1932.

Cohn, J. D. A pump system for performing indicator-dilution curves without blood loss. *J. Appl. Physiol.* 26:841, 1969.

Coleman, T. G., and A. C. Guyton. Hypertension caused by salt loading in the dog. III. Onset transients of cardiac output and other circulatory variables. *Circ. Res.* 25:153, 1969.

Coleman, T. G., and F. J. Criddle, Jr. Computerized analysis of indicator-dilution curves. *J. Appl. Physiol.* 28:358, 1970a.

Coleman, T. G., J. D. Bower, H. G. Langford, and A. C. Guyton. Regulation of arterial pressure in the anephric state. *Circulation* 42:509, 1970b.

Coleman, T. G., H. J. Granger, and A. C. Guyton. Whole-body circulatory autoregulation and hypertension. *Circ. Res.* 28: Suppl. II, p. 76, 1971.

Coleridge, C. G., and R. J. Linden. The measurement of effective atrial pressure. *J. Physiol.* 126:304, 1954.

Collier, C. R. Determination of mixed venous CO_2 tensions by rebreathing. *J. Appl. Physiol.* 9:25, 1956.

Conn, H. L., Jr. Accuracy of a radiopotassium dilution (Steward principle) method for the measurement of cardiac output. *J. Appl. Physiol.* 7:542, 1955.

Conn, H. L., Jr., D. F. Heiman, and C. R. Joyner. Measurement of cardiac output and central volume by a modified decholin test of circulation time. *Circulation* 15:245, 1957.

Connolly, D. C., and E. H. Wood. Distensibility of peripheral veins in man determined by a miniature-balloon technic. *J. Appl. Physiol.* 7:239, 1954.

Conway, J. Hemodynamic consequences of induced changes in blood volume. *Circ. Res.* 18:190, 1966.

Cook, B. H., E. R. Wilson, and A. E. Taylor. Intestinal fluid loss in hemorrhagic shock. *Amer. J. Physiol.* 221:1494, 1971.

Corcondilas, A., D. E. Donald, and J. T. Shepherd. Assessment by two independent methods of the role of cardiac output in the pressor response to carotid occlusion. *J. Physiol.* 170:250, 1964.

Corcondilas, A., G. T. Koroxenidis, and J. T. Shepherd. Effect of a brief contraction of forearm muscle on forearm blood flow. *J. Appl. Physiol.* 19:142, 1967.

Cornell, W. P., E. Braunwald, and E. C. Brockenbrough. Use of krypton for the measurement of cardiac output by the single injection indicator-dilution technique. *Circ. Res.* 9:984, 1961.

Costin, J. C., and N. S. Skinner, Jr. Effects of systemic hypoxemia on vascular resistance in dogs' skeletal muscle. *Amer. J. Physiol.* 218:886, 1970.

Costin, J. C., and N. S. Skinner, Jr. Competition between vasoconstrictor and vasodilator mechanisms in skeletal muscle. *Amer. J. Physiol.* 220:462, 1961.

Cotton, F. S. Does the ventricle exert a suction action in diastole? *Amer. J. Physiol.* 107:178, 1934.

Cournand, A., and H. A. Ranges. Catheterization of the right auricle in man. *Proc. Soc. Exp. Biol. Med.* 46:462, 1941.

Cournand, A., H. A. Ranges, and R. L. Riley. Comparison of results of normal ballistocardiogram and direct Fick method in measuring cardiac output in man. *J. Clin. Invest.* 21:287, 1942.

Cournand, A. Measurement of cardiac output in man using right heart catheterization; description of technic, discussion of validity and of place in study of circulation. *Fed. Proc.* 4:207, 1945a.

Cournand, A., R. L. Riley, E. S. Breed, W. de F. Baldwin, and D. W. Richards, Jr. Measurement of cardiac output in man using the technique of catheterization of the right auricle or ventricle. *J. Clin. Invest.* 24:106, 1945b.

Cournand, A. H. L. Motley, L. Werkö, and D. W. Richards, Jr. Physiologic studies of effects of intermittent positive pressure breathing on cardiac output in man. *Amer. J. Physiol.* 152:162, 1948.

Cournand, A. Some aspects of the pulmonary circulation in normal man and in chronic cardiopulmonary diseases. *Circulation* 2:641, 1950.

Courtice, F. C., and C. G. Douglas. Ferricyanide method of blood-gas analysis. *J. Physiol.* 105:345, 1947.

Covell, J. W., C. A. Chidsey, and E. Braunwald. Reduction of the cardiac response to postganglionic sympathetic nerve stimulation in experimental heart failure. *Circ. Res.* 19:51, 1966.

Cowley, A. W., and A. C. Guyton. Heart rate as a determinant of cardiac output in dogs with arteriovenous fistula. *Amer. J. Cardiol.* 28:321, 1971.

Craig, R. J., R. E. Whalen, V. S. Behar, and H. D. McIntosh. Pressure and volume changes of the left ventricle in acute pericardial tamponade. *Amer. J. Cardiol.* 22: 65, 1968.

Crane, M. G., R. Adams, and I. Woodward. Cardiac output measured by injection method with use of radioactive material and continuous recording; results of circulation model studies. *J. Lab. Clin. Med.* 47:802, 1956.

Crawford, D. G., H. M. Fairchild, and A. C. Guyton. Oxygen lack as a possible cause of reactive hyperemia. *Amer. J. Physiol.* 197: 613, 1959.

Crawford, E. S., D. J. Turell, and J. K. Alexander. Aorto-inferior vena caval fistula of neoplastic origin. Hemodynamic and coronary blood flow studies. *Circulation* 27:414, 1963.

Cronin, R. F. P. Hemodynamic and metabolic effects of beta-adrenergic blockade in exercising dogs. *J. Appl. Physiol.* 22:211, 1967.

Cropp, G. J. A. Hemodynamic responses to oxygen breathing in children with severe anemia. *Circulation* 40:493, 1969.

Cross, C. E., P. A. Rieben, and P. F. Salisbury. Influence of coronary perfusion and myocardial edema on pressure-volume diagram of left ventricle. *Amer. J. Physiol.* 201:102, 1961.

Cross, K. W., A. C. Groom, R. F. Mottram, and S. Rowlands. Cardiac output in the cat; a comparison between the Fick method and a radioactive indicator dilution method. *J. Physiol.* 136:24P, 1957.

Cross, K. W., G. S. Dawes, and J. C. Mott. Changes in the cardiac output of the lamb after birth and during anoxia. *J. Physiol.* 144:16P, 1958.

Cross, K. W., G. S. Dawes, and J. C. Mott. Anoxia, oxygen consumption, and cardiac output in new-born lambs and adult sheep. *J. Physiol.* 146:316, 1959.

Crowell, J. W., and W. L. Read. In vivo coagulation—a probable cause of irreversible shock. *Amer. J. Physiol.* 183:565, 1955.

Crowell, J. W., S. H. Bounds, and W. W. Johnson. Effect of varying the hematocrit ration on the susceptibility to hemorrhagic shock. *Amer. J. Physiol.* 192:171, 1958.

Crowell, J. W., R. G. Ford, and V. M. Lewis. Oxygen transport in hemorrhagic shock as a function of the hematocrit ratio. *Amer. J. Physiol.* 196:1033, 1959.

Crowell, J. W. Digitalization as a treatment for irreversible hemorrhagic shock. *Circulation* 24:912, 1961a.

Crowell, J. W., and A. C. Guyton. Evidence favoring a cardiac mechanism in irreversible hemorrhagic shock. *Amer. J. Physiol.* 201:893, 1961b.

Crowell, J. W., and A. C. Guyton. Further evidence favoring a cardiac mechanism in irreversible hemorrhagic shock. *Amer. J. Physiol.* 203:248, 1962.

Crowell, J. W., and E. E. Smith. Oxygen deficit and irreversible hemorrhagic shock. *Amer. J. Physiol.* 206:313, 1964.

Crowell, J. W. Cardiac deterioration as the cause of irreversibility in shock. *In* L. C. Mills and J. H. Moyer (Eds.). *Shock and Hypotension.* New York, Grune & Stratton, Inc., 1965, p. 605.

Crowell, J. W., and E. E. Smith. Determinant of the optimal hematocrit. *J. Appl. Physiol.* 22:501, 1967.

Crowell, J. W. The heart. *In* H. G. Lasch and D. L. Heene (Eds.). *Microcirculation, Hemostasis and Shock.* Stuttgart and New York, F. K. Schattauer Verlag, 1969, p. 111.

Cruz, J. D., H. Rahn, and L. E. Farhi. Mixed venous P_{O_2}, P_{CO_2}, pH and cardiac output during exercise in trained subjects. *J. Appl. Physiol.* 27:431, 1969.

Daggett, W. M., G. C. Nugent, P. W. Carr, P. C. Powers, and Y. Harada. Influence of vagal stimulation on ventricular contractility, O_2 consumption, and coronary flow. *Amer. J. Physiol.* 212:8, 1967.

Daly, W. J., R. A. Krumholz, and J. C. Ross. The venous pump in the legs as a determinant of pulmonary capillary filling. *J. Clin. Invest.* 44:271, 1965.

Damato, A. N., J. G. Galante, and W. M. Smith. Hemodynamic response to treadmill exercise in normal subjects. *J. Appl. Physiol.* 21:959, 1966.

Danforth, W. H., S. Naegle, and R. J. Bing. Effect of ischemia and reoxygenation on glycolytic reactions and adenosinetriphosphate in heart muscle. *Cir. Res.* 8:965, 1960.

Daugherty, R. M., Jr., J. B. Scott, and F. J. Haddy. Effects of generalized hypoxemia and hypercapnia on forelimb vascular resistance. *Amer. J. Physiol.* 213:1111, 1967a.

Daugherty, R. M., Jr., J. B. Scott, J. M. Dabney, and F. J. Haddy. Local effects of O_2 and CO_2 on limb, renal, and coronary vascular resistances. *Amer. J. Physiol.* 213: 1102, 1967b.

Davies, C. E., J. Mackinnon, and M. M. Platts. Renal circulation and cardiac output in low-output heart failure and in myxoedema. *Brit. Med. J.* 2:595, 1952.

Davila, J. C., M. E. Sanmarco, and C. M. Phillips. Continuous measurement of left ventricular volume in the dog. I. Description and validation of a method employing direct external dimensions. *Amer. J. Cardiol.* 18:574, 1966a.

Davila, J. C., and M. E. Sanmarco. An analysis of the fit of mathematical models applicable to the measurement of left ventricular volume. *Amer. J. Cardiol.* 18:31, 1966b.

Davis, D. L. Effect of sympathetic stimulation on dog paw volume. *Amer. J. Physiol.* 205:989, 1963.

Davis, H. A. *Shock.* New York: Grune & Stratton, Inc., 1949, p. 52.

Davis, H. A., W. Al-Fadly, and L. H. Gibson. Use of dyes with rapid bloodstream clearance for serial determination of cardiac output. *Proc. Soc. Exp. Biol. Med.* 98:345, 1958.

Davis, J. O., R. E. Hyatt, and D. S. Howell. Right-sided congestive heart failure in dogs produced by controlled progressive constriction of the pulmonary artery. *Circ. Res.* 3:252, 1955.

Davis, J. O., M. M. Pechet, W. C. Ball, Jr., and M. J. Goodkind. Increased aldosterone secretion in dogs with right-sided congestive heart failure and in dogs with thoracic vena cava constriction. *J. Clin. Invest.* 36:689, 1957.

Davis, J. O., B. Kliman, N. A. Yankopoulos, and R. E. Peterson. Increased aldosterone secretion following acute constriction of the inferior vena cava. *J. Clin. Invest.* 37:1783, 1958.

Davis, J. O., P. M. Hartroft, E. D. Titus, C. C. J. Carpenter, C. R. Ayers, and H. E. Spiegel. The role of the renin-angiotensin system in the control of aldosterone secretion. *J. Clin. Invest.* 41:378, 1962.

Davis, J. O., J. Urquhart, J. T. Higgins, Jr., E. C. Rubin, and P. M. Hartroft. Hypersecretion of aldosterone in dogs with a chronic aortic-caval fistula and high output failure. *Circ. Res.* 14:471, 1964.

Davis, J. O. Physiology of congestive heart failure. In *Handbook of Physiology. Circulation.* Washington, D.C. Amer. Physiol. Soc. 1965, Sect. 2, Vol. III, Chap. 59, p. 2071.

Dawes, G. S. Vasodilator action of potassium. *J. Physiol.* (London) 99:224, 1941.

Dawson, P. M., and L. W. Gorham. The pulse pressure as an index of the systolic output. *J. Exp. Med.* 10:484, 1908.

De Burgh Daly, I. A closed circuit heart-lung preparation. I. Effects of alterations in blood volume. *J. Physiol.* 60:103, 1925.

De Burgh Daly, I. Blood velocity recorder. *J. Physiol.* 61:21, 1926.

Defares, J. G. Determination of P_{vco_2} from the exponential CO_2 rise during rebreathing. *J. Appl. Physiol.* 13:159, 1958.

Defares, J. G., M. E. Wise, and J. W. Duyff. New indirect Fick procedure for the determination of cardiac output. *Nature* 192:760, 1961.

De Geest, H., M. N. Levy, H. Zieske, and R. I. Lipman. Depression of ventricular con-

tractility by stimulation of the vagus nerves. *Circ. Res.* 17:222, 1965a.

De Geest, H., M. N. Levy, and H. Zieske. Carotid chemoreceptor stimulation of ventricular performance. *Amer. J. Physiol.* 209:564, 1965b.

De Geest, H., M. N. Levy, and H. Zieske. Reflex effects of cephalic hypoxia, hypercapnia, and ischemia upon ventricular contractility. *Circ. Res.* 17:349, 1965c.

Delaunois, A. L., and C. Vandenberghen. Influences of noradrenaline on cardiac output and metabolism of anesthetized dogs. *Arch. Int. Pharmacodyn.* 99:435, 1954.

Delaunois, A. L., and L. A. Rovati. A new method for continuous measurement of cardiac output. *Arch. Int. Pharmacodyn.* 116:228, 1958.

Delaunois, A. L. Continuous measurement of blood flow and cardiac output by means of a Cournand catheter equipped with thermistors. *Arch. Int. Pharmacodyn.* 134:245, 1961.

Denison, A. B., Jr., M. P. Spencer, and H. D. Green. Square-wave electromagnetic flowmeter for application to intact blood vessels. *Circ. Res.* 3:39, 1955.

Denison, A. B., Jr., and M. P. Spencer. Magnetic flowmeters. In Otto Glasser, *Medical Physics.* Chicago: Year Book Publishers, 1960, Vol. 3, p. 178.

Deppe, B., and E. Wetterer. Vergleichende tierexperimentelle Untersuchungen zur physikalischer Schlagvolumenbestimmung (1. Mitteilung). *Z. Biol.* 99:307, 1939.

Desliens, L. Contractions musculaires et circulation sanguine. Role des valvules veineuses. *Bull. Acad. Med.* 130:476, 1946.

Detar, R., and D. F. Bohr. Oxygen and vascular smooth muscle contraction. *Amer. J. Physiol.* 214:241, 1968.

Dexter, L., J. L. Whittenberger, F. W. Haynes, W. T. Goodale, R. Gorlin, and C. G. Sawyer. Effect of exercise on circulatory dynamics of normal individuals. *J. Appl. Physiol.* 3:439, 1951.

Dexter, L., and T. R. Harrison. Circulatory failure. In T. R. Harrison (Ed.). *Principles of Internal Medicine.* New York: McGraw-Hill Book Company, 1958.

Diemer, K. Capillarization and oxygen supply of the brain. In D. W. Lubbers, U. C. Luft, G. Thews, and E. Witzleb (Eds.). *Oxygen Transport in Blood and Tissue.* Stuttgart: George Thieme Verlag, 1968, p. 118.

Di Palma, J., S. Reynolds, and F. Foster. Quantitative measurements of reactive hyperemia in the human skin. *Amer. Heart J.* 23:377, 1942.

Dobbs, W. A., J. W. Prather, and A. C. Guyton. Relative importance of nervous control of cardiac output and arterial pressure. *Amer. J. Cardiol.* 27:507, 1971.

Dobson, J. G., R. Rubio, and R. M. Berne. Role of adenine nucleotides, adenosine, and inorganic phosphate in the regulation of skeletal muscle blood flow. *Circ. Res.* 29:375, 1971.

Dodge, H., H. Sandler, D. H. Ballew, and T. D. Lord. The use of biplane angiocardiography for the measurement of left ventricular volume in man. *Amer. Heart J.* 60:762, 1960.

Dodge, H. T., R. E. Hay, and H. Sandler. An angiocardiographic method for directly determining left ventricular stroke volume in man. *Circ. Res.* 11:739, 1962.

Dodge, H. T., H. Sandler, W. A. Baxley, and R. R. Hawley. Usefulness and limitations of radiographic methods for determining left ventricular volume. *Amer. J. Cardiol.* 18:10, 1966.

Dodge, H. T., and W. A. Baxley. Hemodynamic aspects of heart failure. *Amer. J. Cardiol.* 22:24, 1968.

Doi, Y. Studies on respiration and circulation in the cat. I. The influence of an acute anoxic anoxemia on respiration and circulation. *J. Physiol.* 55:43, 1921.

Dollery, C. T. Dynamic aspects of the retinal microcirculation. *Arch. Ophthal.* 79:536, 1968.

Donal, J. S., Jr., C. J. Gamble, and R. Shaw. Cardiac output in man; adaptation of katharometer for rapid determination of ethyl iodide in estimations of cardiac output by ethyl iodide method; study of effect of posture upon cardiac output and other circulatory and respiratory measurements. *Amer. J. Physiol.* 109:666, 1934.

Donald, D. E., and J. T. Shepherd. Response to exercise in dogs with cardiac denervation. *Amer. J. Physiol.* 205:393, 1963.

Donald, D. E., and J. T. Shepherd. Sustained capacity for exercise in dogs after complete cardiac denervation. *Amer. J. Cardiol.* 14:853, 1964a.

Donald, D. E., S. E. Milburn, and J. T. Shepherd. Effect of cardiac denervation on the maximal capacity for exercise in the racing greyhound. *J. Appl. Physiol.* 19:849, 1964b.

Donald, D. E., D. A. Ferguson, and S. E. Milburn. Effect of beta-adrenergic receptor blockade on racing performance of greyhounds with normal and with denervated hearts. *Circ. Res.* 22:127, 1968a.

Donald, D. E. Capacity for exercise after denervation of the heart. *Circulation* 38:225, 1968b.

Donald, K. W., J. M. Bishop, G. Cumming, and O. L. Wade. The effect of nursing positions on the cardiac output in man, with a note on the repeatability of measurements of cardiac output by the direct Fick method, and with data on subjects with a normal cardiovascular system. *Clin. Sci.* 12:199, 1953.

Donald, K. W., J. M. Bishop, G. Cumming, and O. L. Wade. The effect of exercise on the cardiac output and circulatory dynamics of normal subjects. *Clin. Sci.* 14:37, 1955.

Donald, K. W., P. N. Wormald, S. H. Taylor, and J. M. Bishop. Changes in the oxygen content of femoral venous blood and leg blood flow during leg exercise in relation to cardiac output response. *Clin. Sci.* 16:567, 1957.

Donald, K. W. Exercise and heart disease; a study in regional circulation. *Brit. Med. J.* 5128:985, 1959.

Doud, E. A., and E. A. Rovenstine. Changes in velocity of flow during spinal anesthesia. *Anesthesiology* 1:82, 1940.

Douglas, B. H., A. C. Guyton, J. B. Langston, and V. S. Bishop. Hypertension caused by salt loading. II. Fluid volume and tissue pressure changes. *Amer. J. Physiol.* 207:669, 1964.

Douglas, C. G., J. S. Haldane, Y. Henderson, and E. C. Schneider. VI. Physiological observations made on Pike's Peak, Colorado, with special reference to adaptation to low barometric pressures. *Phil. Trans. Roy. Soc. London.* Ser. B 203:185, 1913.

Douglas, C. G., and J. S. Haldane. The regulation of the general circulation rate in man. *J. Physiol.* 56:69, 1922.

Douglas, F. G. V., and M. R. Becklake. Effect of seasonal training on maximal cardiac output. *J. Appl. Physiol.* 25:600, 1968.

Doutheil, U., and K. Kramer, Über die Diffesensierung kreislaufregulierender Reflexe ans dem linken Herz. *Pflüger's Arch. ges. Physiol.* 269:114, 1959.

Dow, P., P. F. Hahn, and W. F. Hamilton. The simultaneous transport of T-1824 and radioactive red cells through the heart and lungs. *Amer. J. Physiol.* 147:493, 1946.

Dow, P. Dimensional relationships in dye-dilution curves from humans and dogs, with an empirical formula for certain troublesome curves. *J. Appl. Physiol.* 7:399, 1955.

Dow, P. Estimations of cardiac output and central blood volume by dye dilution. *Physiol. Rev.* 36:77, 1956.

Downing, S. E., J. H. Mitchell, and A. G. Wallace. Cardiovascular responses to ischemia, hypoxia, and hypercapnia of the central nervous system. *Amer. J. Physiol.* 204:881, 1963.

Downing, S. E., and E. H. Sonnenblick. Cardiac muscle mechanics and ventricular performance: force and time parameters. *Amer. J. Physiol.* 207:705, 1964.

Downing, S. E., N. S. Talner, and T. H. Gardner. Influences of hypoxemia and acidemia on left ventricular function. *Amer. J. Physiol.* 210:1327, 1966.

Doyle, J. T., J. S. Wilson, C. Lepine, and J. V. Warren. An evaluation of the measurement of the cardiac output and of the so-called pulmonary blood volume by the dye-dilution method. *J. Lab. Clin. Med.* 41:29, 1953.

Doyle, J. T., J. L. Patterson, J. V. Warren, D. E. Detweiler, and N. Reynolds. Hemodynamic observations on the cow. *Fed. Proc.* 17:38, 1958.

Drabkin, D. L. Spectroscopy: photometry and spectrophotometry. In Otto Glasser, *Medical Physics.* Chicago: Year Book Publishers, 1950, Vol. 2, p. 2.

Driscol, T. E., and R. M. Berne. Role of potassium in regulation of coronary blood flow. *Proc. Soc. Exp. Biol. Med.* 96:505, 1957.

Dubois, A. B., A. G. Brit, and W. O. Fenn. Alveolar CO_2 during the respiratory cycle. *J. Appl. Physiol.* 4:535, 1952.

Dubois, E. F.: *Basal Metabolism in Health and Disease.* Philadelphia: Lea and Febiger, 1936.

Duke, M., and W. H. Abelmann. The hemodynamic response to chronic anemia. *Circulation* 39:503, 1969.

Duling, B. R., and R. M. Berne. Longitudinal gradients in periarteriolar oxygen tension. *Circ. Res.* 27:669, 1970.

Duomarco, J., R. Rimini, and P. Recarte. La presión de los troncos venosos del torax. *Rev. Argent. Cardiol.* 11:129, 1945.

Duomarco, J., R. Rimini, and F. N. Predari. Sobre elestado de distensión o colapso de las venas cavas. Estudio radiológico. *Rev. Argent. Cardiol.* 12:333, 1946.

Duomarco, J., W. H. Dillon, and C. J. Wiggers. Comparison of cardiac output by direct method and Hamilton-Remington procedures. *Amer. J. Physiol.* 154:290, 1948.

Duomarco, J., and R. Rimini. La presión venosa en los miembros superiores, en condiciónes normales. *Rev. Argent. Cardiol.* 17:236, 1950a.

Duomarco, J., and R. Rimini. La presión veineuse des membres chez l'homme normal et chez l'insuffisant cardiaque. *Compt. Rend. Congr. Cardiol.* 3:1, 1950b.

Duomarco, J., R. Rimini, and J. P. Sapriza. Intento de apreciación de la presión venosa efectiva por medio de la angiocardiografía. *Rev. Argent. Cardiol.* 17:15, 1950c.

Duomarco, J., R. Rimini, J. P. Sapriza, and G. H. Surraco. A propósito del colapso yuxtadiafragmático de la vena cava inferior estudio angiocardiográfico. *Rev. Argent. Cardiol.* 17:220, 1950d.

Duomarco, J., and R. Rimini. Energy and hydraulic gradient along systemic veins. *Amer. J. Physiol.* 178:215, 1954.

Eckstein, J. W., and W. K. Hamilton. The pressure-volume response of human forearm veins during epinephrine and norepinephrine infusions. *J. Clin. Invest.* 36:1663, 1957.

Eckstein, R. W., G. R. Graham, I. M. Liebou, and C. J. Wiggers. Comparison of changes in inferior cava flow after hemorrhage and circulatory failure following transfusion. *Amer. J. Physiol.* 148:745, 1947a.

Eckstein, R. W., C. J. Wiggers, and G. R. Graham. Phasic changes in inferior cava flow of intravascular origin. *Amer. J. Physiol.* 148:740, 1947b.

Eckstein, R. W., M. Stroud, C. V. Dowling, R. Eckel, and W. H. Pritchard. Effects of over and under perfusion upon coronary arterial blood flow. *Fed. Proc.* 8:38, 1949a.

Eckstein, R. W., M. Stroud, C. W. Dowling, R. Eckel, and W. H. Pritchard. Response of coronary blood flow following stimulation of cardiac acceleration nerves. *Fed. Proc.* 8:38, 1949b.

Eckstein, R. W. Development of interarterial coronary anastomoses by chronic anemia. Disappearance following correction of anemia. *Circ. Res.* 3:306, 1955.

Eckstein, R. W. Effect of exercise and coronary artery narrowing on coronary collateral circulation. *Circ. Res.* 5:230, 1957.

Edwards, A. W., P. I. Kroner, and G. D. Thorburn. The cardiac output of the unanesthetized rabbit, and the effects of preliminary anesthesia, environmental temperature and carotid occlusion. *Quart. J. Exp. Physiol.* 44:309, 1959.

Edwards, W. S., A. Siegel, and R. J. Bing. Studies on myocardial metabolism. III. Coronary blood flow, myocardial oxygen consumption and carbohydrate metabolism in experimental hemorrhagic shock. *J. Clin. Invest.* 33:1646, 1954.

Eichna, L. W., W. M. Horvath, and W. B. Bean. Post-exertional orthostatic hypotension. *Amer. J. Med. Sci.* 213:641, 1947.

Ekblom, B., and L. Hermansen. Cardiac output in athletes. *J. Appl. Physiol.* 25:619, 1968.

Ekelund, L. G., and A. Holmgren. Central hemodynamics during exercise. *Circ. Res.* 20:Suppl. I, p. 33, 1967.

Eliasch, H., H. Lagerlöf, H. Bucht, J. Ek, K. Eriksson, J. Bergström, and L. Werkö. Comparison of the dye dilution and the direct Fick methods for the measurement of cardiac output in man. *Scand. J. Clin. Lab. Invest.* 7:Suppl. 20, p. 73, 1955.

Elkin, D. C., and J. V. Warren. Arteriovenous fistulas: their effect on the circulation. *J.A.M.A.* 134:1524, 1947.

Elkinton, J. R., and T. S. Danowski. *The Body Fluids.* Baltimore: The Williams & Wilkins Co., 1955.

Elliot, E. C. Controlled cardiac output studies in dogs. (Part I) Simple method for estimation of coronary return blood flow in dogs and its evaluation under conditions of controlled cardiac output. *Circ. Res.* 9:1357, 1961a.

Elliot, E. C. Controlled cardiac output studies in dogs. (Part II) Control canal return preparation for the purpose of varying the cardiac output in the closed-chest intact dog. *Cir. Res.* 9:1364, 1961b.

Ellis, L. B., and S. Weiss. The local and systemic effects of arterio-venous fistula on the circulation in man. *Amer. Heart J.* 5:635, 1930.

Elsberry, D. D., D. A. Bhoda, and W. R. Beisel. Hemodynamics of staphylococcal B enterotoxemia and other types of shock in monkeys. *J. Appl. Physiol.* 27:164, 1969.

Emanuel, D. A., J. B. Scott, and F. J. Haddy. Effect of potassium of small and large blood vessels of the dog forelimb. *Amer. J. Physiol.* 197:637, 1959.

Emmrich, J., H. Steim, H. Klepzig, K. Musshoff, H. Reindell, and B. Baumgarten. The effect of bloody examination methods on cardiac output. *Z. Kreislaufforsch.* 47:326, 1958.

Engle, M. A., M. Erlandson, and C. H. Smith. Late cardiac complications of chronic, severe, refractory anemia with hemochromatosis. *Circulation* 30:698, 1964.

Epstein, S. E., B. F. Robinson, R. L. Kahler, and E. Braunwald. Effects of beta-adrenergic blockade on the cardiac response to maximal and submaximal exercise in man. *J. Clin. Invest.* 44:1745, 1965.

Epstein, S. E., G. D. Beiser, R. E. Goldstein, M. Stampfer, A. S. Wechsler, G. Glick, and E. Braunwald. Circulatory effects of electrical stimulation of the carotid sinus nerves in man. *Circulation* 40:269, 1969.

Erickson, H. H., V. S. Bishop, M. B. Kardon, and L. D. Horowitz. Left ventricular internal diameter and cardiac function during exercise. *J. Appl. Physiol.* 30:473, 1971.

Erlanger, J., and D. R. Hooker. An experimental study of blood pressure and pulse pressure in man. *Johns Hopkins Hosp. Rep.* 12:145, 1904.

Ernstene, A. C.: The cardiovascular complications of hyperthyroidism. *Amer. J. Med. Sci.* 195:248, 1938.

Ershler, I., C. E. Kossmann, and M. S. White. Venous pressure and circulation time during acute progressive anoxia in man. *Amer. J. Physiol.* 138:593, 1943.

Escobar, E., N. L. Jones, E. Rapaport, and J. F. Murray. Ventricular performance in acute normovolemic anemia and effects of beta blockade. *Amer. J. Physiol.* 211:877, 1966.

Espersen, T. Modified acetylene method for determination of cardiac output and related circulatory functions based on recent views of ventilation of lungs. *Acta Med. Scand.* 106:108, 1941a.

Espersen, T. Studies on cardiac output and related circulatory functions, especially in patients with congestive heart failure. *Acta Med. Scand.* 108:153, 1941b.

Etsten, B., and T. H. Li. The determination of cardiac output by the dye dilution method: modifications, comparison with the Fick method, and application during anesthesia. *Anesthesiology* 15:217, 1954.

Etsten, B., and T. H. Li. Hemodynamic changes during thiopental anesthesia in

humans: cardiac output, stroke volume, total peripheral resistance, and intrathoracic blood volume. *J. Clin. Invest.* 34:500, 1955.

Evans, R. L. Cardiac output and central pressure data. *Nature* 181:1471, 1958.

Evonuk, E., C. J. Imig, W. Greenfield, and J. W. Eckstein. Cardiac output measured by thermal dilution of room temperature injectate. *J. Appl. Physiol.* 16:271, 1961.

Ewig, W., and K. Hinsberg. Kreislaufstudien I. *Z. Klin. Med.* 115:677, 1932.

Eyster, J. A. E., and W. F. Meek. Instantaneous radiographs of the human heart at determined points in the cardiac cycle. *Amer. J. Roentgenol.* 7:471, 1920.

Eyster, J. A. E., and E. V. Hicks. Effect of respiration on cardiac output. *Amer. J. Physiol.* 104:358, 1933.

Fahraeus, R., and T. Lindquist. The viscosity of the blood in narrow capillary tubes. *Amer. J. Physiol.* 96:562, 1931.

Fairchild, H. M., J. Ross, and A. C. Guyton. Failure of recovery from reactive hyperemia in the absence of oxygen. *Amer. J. Physiol.* 210:490, 1966.

Falholt, W., and J. Fabricius. Application of continuously recording dye colorimeter to determination of cardiac output by dye injection method. *Danish Med. Bull.* 3:55, 1956.

Falholt, W. The dye injection method for circulatory studies; a critical evaluation of the technique, apparatus and results. *Scand. J. Clin. Lab. Invest.* 10:Suppl. 35, p. 1, 1958.

Falsetti, H. L., R. E. Mates, C. Grant, D. G. Greene, and I. L. Bunnell. Left ventricular wall stress calculated from one-plane cineangiography: an approach to force-velocity analysis in man. *Circ. Res.* 26:71, 1970.

Falsetti, H. L., R. E. Mates, D. G. Greene, and I. L. Bunnell. V_{max} as an index of contractile state in man. *Circulation* 43:467, 1971.

Farber, S. J., J. D. Alexander, and D. P. Earle. Shock produced by obstruction of venous return to the heart in the dog. *Amer. J. Physiol.* 176:325, 1954.

Farhi, L. E., A. Chinet, and P. Haab. Pression partielle d'oxygene du sang veineux mele chez l'Homme en plaine et haute altitude. *J. Physiol.* (Paris) 58:516, 1966.

Farhi, L. E., and P. Haab. Mixed venous blood gas tensions and cardiac output by "bloodless method"; recent developments and appraisal. *Resp. Physiol.* 2:225, 1967.

Farrell, G. L. Regulation of aldosterone secretion. *Physiol. Rev.* 38:709, 1958.

Faulkner, J. A., D. E. Roberts, R. L. Elk, and J. Conway. Cardiovascular responses to submaximum and maximum effort cycling and running. *J. Appl. Physiol.* 30:457, 1971.

Fegler, G. Measurement of cardiac output

in anesthetized animals by a thermo-dilution method. *Quart. J. Exp. Physiol.* 39:153, 1954.

Fegler, G. The reliability of the thermo-dilution method for determination of the cardiac output and the blood flow in central veins. *Quart. J. Exp. Physiol.* 42:254, 1957.

Feigl, E. G., and D. L. Fry. Myocardial mural thickness during the cardiac cycle. *Circ. Res.* 14:541, 1964.

Feinburg, H., A. Gerola, and L. N. Katz. Effect of hypoxia on cardiac oxygen con-sumption and coronary flow. *Amer. J. Physiol.* 195:593, 1958.

Feldman, M., Jr., S. Rodbard, and L. N. Katz. Relative distribution of cardiac out-put in acute hypoxemia. *Amer. J. Physiol.* 154:391, 1948.

Fell, C. Plasma loss in dogs in irreversible hemorrhagic shock. *Amer. J. Physiol.* 211:885, 1966.

Fenn, W. O., and P. Dejours. Composition of alveolar air during breath holding with and without prior inhalation of oxygen and carbon dioxide. *J. Appl. Physiol.* 7:313, 1954.

Ferguson, R., D. Bristow, F. Mintz, and E. Rapaport. The effects of pericardial tamponade on left ventricular volumes and function as calculated from thermodilu-tion curves. *Clin. Res.* 11:100, 1963.

Ferguson, R., J. A. Faulkner, S. Julius, and J. Conway. Comparison of cardiac output determined by CO_2 rebreathing and dye dilution methods. *J. Appl. Physiol.* 25:450, 1968.

Ferguson, T. B., O. W. Shadle, and D. E. Gregg. Effect of blood and saline infusion on ventricular end diastolic pressure, stroke work, stroke volume and cardiac output in the open and closed chest dog. *Circ. Res.* 1:62, 1953.

Ferguson, T. B., D. G. Gregg, and O. W. Shadle. Effect of blood and saline infusion on cardiac performance in normal dogs and dogs with arteriovenous fistulas. *Circ. Res.* 2:565, 1954.

Fermoso, J. D., T. Q. Richardson, and A. C. Guyton. Mechanism of decrease in cardiac output caused by opening the chest. *Amer. J. Physiol.* 207:1112, 1964.

Ferrer, M. I., R. M. Harvey, M. Kuschner, D. W. Richards, Jr., and A. Cournand. Hemodynamic studies in tricuspid steno-sis of rheumatic origin. *Circ. Res.* 1:49, 1953.

Ferrer, M. I., R. J. Conroy, and R. M. Harvey. Some effects of digoxin upon the heart and circulation in man. *Circulation* 21:372, 1960.

Fick, A. Über die Messung des Blutquan-tums in den Herzventrikeln. *Sitz. der Physik-Med. ges. Würzburg.* 1870, p. 16.

Field, H., A. V. Bock, E. F. Gildea, and F. L. Lathrop. The rate of the circulation of the blood in normal resting individuals. *J. Clin. Invest.* 1:65, 1924.

Fine, J. Shock and electrolyte disturbances. Etiology and classification of shock. *Amer. J. Cardiol.* 12:587, 1963.

Fisher, E. W., and R. G. Dalton. Cardiac output in cattle. *Nature* 183:829, 1959.

Fishman, A. P., J. McClement, A. Hem-melstein, and A. Cournand. Effects of acute anoxia on the circulation and respira-tion in patients with chronic pulmonary disease studied during the "steady state." *J. Clin. Invest.* 30:770, 1952a.

Fishman, A. P., J. McClement, A. Hemmel-stein, and A. Cournand. Failure of the Fick method in anoxia. *J. Clin. Invest.* 30:937, 1952b.

Fitzhugh, F. W., Jr., R. L. McWhorter, Jr., E. H. Estes, Jr., J. V. Warren, and A. J. Merrill. The effect of application of tourniquets to the legs on cardiac output and renal function in normal human sub-jects. *J. Clin. Invest.* 32:1163, 1953.

Fleisch, A., and W. Tomaszewski. L'influ-ence de la Masse sanguine totale et de l'acide carbonique sur le débit cardiaque. *Arch. Internat. Physiol.* 42:367, 1936.

Fleming, J. W., and W. L. Bloom. Further observations on the hemodynamic effect of plasma volume expansion by dextran. *J. Clin. Invest.* 36:1233, 1957.

Fletcher, A. G., Jr., J. D. Hardy, C. Riegel, and C. E. Koop. Effects of intravenous infusion of gelatin on cardiac output and other aspects of circulation of normal persons, of chronically ill patients, and of normal volunteers subjected to large hemorrhage. *J. Clin. Invest.* 24:405, 1945.

Fog, M. Reaction of the pial arteries to a fall in blood pressure. *Arch. Neurol. Psychiat.* 37:351, 1937.

Folkow, B. Intravascular pressure as a factor regulating the tone of the small vessels. *Acta. Physiol. Scand.* 17:289, 1949.

Folkow, B. Nervous control of the blood vessels. In R. J. S. McDowall. *The Control of the Circulation of the Blood.* London: William Dawson and Sons, 1956a, p. 1.

Folkow, B., B. Lofving, and S. Mellander. Quantitative aspects of the sympathetic neuro-hormonal control of the heart rate. *Acta Physiol. Scand.* 37:363, 1956b.

Folkow, B. Autoregulation in muscle and skin. *Circ. Res.* 14:Suppl. I., p. 19, 1964.

Folkow, B., B. Lisander, and S. C. Wang. Changes in cardiac output in cats during stimulation of the hypothalamic defence area and the bulbar depressor area. *Acta Physiol. Scand.* 68:Suppl. 277, p. 50, 1966.

Folkow, B., B. Lisander, R. S. Tuttle, and S. C. Wang. Changes in cardiac output upon stimulation of the hypothalamic defence area and the medullary depressor area in the cat. *Acta. Physiol. Scand.* 72:220, 1968.

Folse, R., and E. Braunwald. Determination

of left ventricular volume ejected per beat and of ventricular end-diastolic and residual volumes. *Circulation* 25:674, 1962.

Folts, J. D. Electronic zero for chronic application of electromagnetic flowmeter probes. *J. Appl. Physiol.* 28:237, 1970.

Foltz, E. L., R. G. Page, W. F. Sheldon, S. K. Wong, W. J. Tuddenham, and A. J. Weiss. Factors in variation and regulation of coronary blood flow in intact anesthetized dogs. *Amer. J. Physiol.* 162:524, 1950.

Forrester, T., and A. R. Lind. Identification of adenosine triphosphate in human plasma and the concentration in the venous effluent of forearm muscles before, during and after sustained contractions. *J. Physiol.* 204:347, 1969.

Forssmann, W. Die Sondierung des rechten Herzens. *Klin. Wochschr,* 8:2085, 1929.

Forsyth, R. P. Hypothalamic control of the distribution of cardiac output in the unanesthetized rhesus monkey. *Circ. Res.* 26:783, 1970a.

Forsyth, R. P., and B. I. Hoffbrand. Redistribution of cardiac output after sodium pentobarbital anesthesia in the monkey. *Amer. J. Physiol.* 218:214, 1970b.

Foulger, J. H., P. E. Smith, Jr., and A. J. Fleming. Cardiac vibrational intensity and cardiac output. *Amer. Heart J.* 35:953, 1948.

Fourcade, J. C., L. G. Navar, and A. C. Guyton. Possibility that angiotensin resulting from unilateral kidney disease affects contralateral renal function. *Nephron* 8: 1, 1971.

Fowler, N. O., R. H. Franck, and W. L. Bloom. Hemodynamic effects of anemia with and without plasma volume expansion. *Circ. Res.* 4:319, 1956.

Fowler, N. O., C. Couves, and J. Bewick. Effect of inflow obstruction and rapid bleeding on ventricular diastolic pressure. *J. Thorac. Surg.* 35:532, 1958.

Fowler, N. O., and J. C. Holmes. Dextran-exchange anemia and reduction in blood viscosity in the heart-lung preparation. *Amer. Heart J.* 68:204, 1964.

Fowler, N. O., and J. C. Holmes. Hemodynamic effects of isoproterenol and norepinephrine in acute cardiac tamponade. *J. Clin. Invest.* 48:502, 1969.

Fox, I. J., L. Q. S. Brooker, D. W. Heseltine, H. E. Essex, and E. H. Wood. A tricarbocyanine dye for continuous recording of dilution curves in whole blood independent of variations in blood oxygen saturation. *Proc. Staff Meetings Mayo Clinic* 32:478, 1957.

Frank, C., H. Wang, J. Lammerant, R. Miller, and R. Wegria. An experimental study of the immediate hemodynamic adjustments to acute arteriovenous fistulae of various sizes. *J. Clin. Invest.* 34:722, 1955.

Frank, O. Die Grundform des arteriellen Pulses. *Z. Biol.* 37:483, 1899a.

Frank, O. Die Grundform des arteriellen Pulses. *Z. Biol.* 37:516, 1899b.

Frank, O. Theorie und Konstruktion eines optischen Strompendels. *Z. Biol.* 89:83, 1929.

Franklin, D. L., and R. M. Ellis. A pulsed ultrasonic flowmeter. *Fed. Proc.* 17:49, 1958.

Franklin, D. L., R. M. Ellis, and R. F. Rushmer. Aortic blood flow in dogs during treadmill exercise. *J. Appl. Physiol.* 14:809, 1959.

Franklin, D. L., W. Schlegel, and R. F. Rushmer. Blood flow measured by Doppler frequency shift of back-scattered ultrasound. *Science* 134:564, 1961.

Franklin, D. L., R. L. Van Citters, and R. F. Rushmer. Balance between right and left ventricular output. *Circ. Res.* 10:17, 1962.

Franklin, D. L., W. A. Schlegel, and N. W. Watson. Ultrasonic Doppler shift blood flowmeter: circuitry and practical applications. *Biomed. Sci. Instrum.* 1:309, 1963.

Franklin, D. L., N. W. Watson, and R. L. Van Citters. Blood velocity telemetered from untethered animals. *Nature* 203:528, 1964.

Franklin, D. L., N. W. Watson, K. E. Pierson, and R. L. Van Citters. Technique for radio telemetry of blood-flow velocity from unrestrained animals. *Amer. J. Med. Elec.* 5:24, 1966.

Franklin, K. J., and R. Janker. Effects of respiration upon the venae cavae of certain mammals, as studied by means of x-ray cinematography. *J. Physiol.* 81:434, 1934.

Franklin, K. J., and R. Janker. Respiration and the venae cavae—further x-ray cinematographic studies. *J. Physiol.* 86:264, 1936.

Franklin, K. J. *A Monograph on Veins.* Springfield, Illinois: Charles C Thomas, Publisher, 1937.

Freedman, M. E., G. L. Snider, P. Brostoff, S. Kimelblot, and L. N. Katz. Effect of training on response of cardiac output to muscular exercise in athletes. *J. Appl. Physiol.* 8:37, 1955.

Friedberg, C. K. *Diseases of the Heart,* 2nd Ed. Philadelphia: W. B. Saunders Company, 1956.

Frieden, J., and A. Shaffer. A simple method for repeated cardiac output determination in the unanesthetized dog using an indwelling cardiac catheter. *J. Lab. Clin. Med.* 39:968, 1952.

Friedlich, A., R. Heimbecker, and R. J. Bing. A device for continuous recording of concentration of Evans blue dye in whole blood and its application to determination of cardiac output. *J. Appl. Physiol.* 3:12, 1950.

Friedman, B., G. Clark, H. Resnik, Jr., and T. R. Harrison. Effect of digitalis on cardiac output of persons with congestive heart failure. *Arch. Int. Med.* 56:710, 1935.

Friesinger, G. C., J. Schaffer, J. M. Criley, R. A. Gaertner, and R. S. Ross. Hemodynamic consequences of the injection of radiopaque material. *Circulation* 31:730, 1965.

Fritts, H. W., Jr., P. Harris, C. A. Chidsey, III, R. H. Clauss, and A. Cournand. Validation of a method for measuring the output of the right ventricle in man by inscription of dye-dilution curves from the pulmonary artery. *J. Appl. Physiol.* 11:362, 1957.

Frohlich, E. D., R. C. Tarazi, M. Ulrych, H. P. Dustan, and I. P. Page. Tilt test for investigating a neural component in hypertension. Its correlation with clinical characteristics. Circulation 36:387, 1967.

Fry, D. L., A. J. Mallos, and A. G. Casper. A catheter tip method for measurement of the instantaneous aortic blood velocity. *Circ. Res.* 4:627, 1956.

Fry, D. L., D. M. Griggs, Jr., and J. C. Greenfield, Jr. Myocardial mechanics: tension-velocity-length relationships of heart muscle. *Circ. Res.* 14:73, 1964.

Frye, R. L., and E. Braunwald. Studies of Starling's law of the heart. I. The circulatory response to acute hypervolemia and its modification by ganglionic blockade. *J. Clin. Invest.* 39:1043, 1960.

Gaar, K. A., Jr., A. D. Taylor, L. J. Owens, and A. C. Guyton. Effect of capillary pressure and plasma protein on development of pulmonary edema. *Amer. J. Physiol.* 213:79, 1967.

Gabe, I. T., J. H. Gault, J. Ross, D. T. Mason, C. J. Mills, J. P. Schillingford, and E. Braunwald. Measurement of instantaneous blood flow velocity and pressure in conscious man with a catheter-tip velocity probe. *Circulation* 40:603, 1969.

Galdston, M., and J. M. Steele. Critique of area and height formulae for estimating cardiac output from the ballistocardiogram. *J. Appl. Physiol.* 3:229, 1950.

Gammill, J. F., J. J. Applegarth, C. E. Reed, and A. J. Antenucci. Hemodynamic changes following acute myocardial infarction using the dye injection method for cardiac output determination. *Ann. Intern. Med.* 43:100, 1955.

Gauer, O. H., Volume changes of the left ventricle during blood pooling and exercise in the intact animal. *Physiol. Rev.* 35:143, 1955.

Gazitua, S., J. B. Scott, B. Swindall, and F. J. Haddy. Resistance responses to local changes in plasma osmolality in three vascular beds. *Amer. J. Physiol.* 220:384, 1971.

Gebber, G., and D. W. Snyder. Hypothalamic control of the baroreceptor reflexes. *Amer. J. Physiol.* 218:124, 1969.

Genest, J., P. Granger, J. de Champlain, and R. Boucher. Endocrine factors in congestive heart failure. *Amer. J. Cardiol.* 22:35, 1968.

Gerlach, E., and B. Deuticke. Bildung und Bedeutung von Adenosin in dem durch Sauerstoffmangel geschädigten Herzmuskel unter dem Einfluss von 2, 6-bis(diaethanolamino)-4, 8-dipiperidino-pyrimido (5,4-d) pyrimidin. *Arzneimittelforschung* 13:48, 1963.

Gibbons, T. B.: The behavior of the venous pressure during various stages of chronic congestive heart failure. *Amer. Heart J.* 35:553, 1948.

Gilbert, N. C. Treatment of coronary thrombosis. *Med. Clin. N. Amer.* 28:1, 1944.

Gilbert, R., M. Goldberg, and J. Griffin. Circulatory changes in acute myocardial infarction. *Circulation* 9:847, 1954.

Gilbert, R., and J. H. Auchincloss, Jr. Comparison of single breath and indicator-dilution measurement of cardiac output. *J. Appl. Physiol.* 29:119, 1970.

Gilbert, R., and J. H. Auchincloss, Jr. Comparison of cardiovascular responses to steady- and unsteady-state exercise. *J. Appl. Physiol.* 30:388, 1971.

Gilfoil, T. M., W. B. Youmans, and J. K. Turner. Abdominal compression reaction: causes and characteristics. *Amer. J. Physiol.* 196:1160, 1959.

Gilmore, H. R., M. Hamilton, and H. Kopelman. The ear oximeter; its use clinically and in the determination of cardiac output. *Brit. Heart J.* 16:301, 1954a.

Gilmore, J. P., C. M. Smythe, and S. W. Handford. The effect of l-norepinephrine on cardiac output in the anesthetized dog during graded hemorrhage. *J. Clin. Invest.* 33:884, 1954b.

Gladstone, S. A. Effect of posture and prolonged rest on cardiac output and related functions. *Amer. J. Physiol.* 112:705, 1935a.

Gladstone, S. A. Factor of recirculation in acetylene method for determination of output. *Proc. Soc. Exp. Biol. Med.* 32:1319, 1935b.

Gladstone, S. A. Output and related functions under basal and post-prandial conditions; clinical study. *Arch. Intern. Med.* 55:533, 1935c.

Glaviano, V. V., and M. A. Klouda. Myocardial catecholamines and stimulation of the stellate ganglion in hemorrhagic shock. *Amer. J. Physiol.* 209:751, 1965.

Glenert, J., and S. M. Pedersen. Albumin transfer from blood to small intestine during exsanguination hypotension. *Acta Chir. Scand.* 133:96, 1967.

Glenn, T. M., and A. M. Lefer. Role of lysosomes in the pathogenesis of splanchnic ischemia shock in cars. *Circ. Res.* 26:783, 1970.

Glenn, T. M., A. M. Lefer, J. B. Martin, W. I. Lovett, J. N. Morris, and S. L. Wangensteen. Production of a myocardial depressant factor in cardiogenic shock. *Amer. Heart J.* 82:78, 1971.

Glick, G., W. H. Plauth, Jr., and E. Braunwald. Role of the autonomic nervous system in the circulatory response to acutely induced anemia in unanesthetized dogs. *J. Clin. Invest.* 43:2112, 1964.

Glover, W. E., I. C. Roddie, and R. G. Shanks. The effect of intraarterial potassium chloride infusions on vascular reactivity in the human forearm. *J. Physiol.* (London) 163:22P, 1963.

Gold, H., McK. Catell, T. Greiner, L. W. Hanlon, N. Kwit, W. Modell, E. Cotlove, J. Benton, and H. L. Otto. Clinical pharmacology of digoxin. *J. Pharmacol. Exp. Ther.* 109:45, 1953.

Goldsmith, G. Output in polycythemia vera. *Arch. Intern. Med.* 58:1041, 1936.

Golenhofen, K., and G. Hilderbrandt. Die Reaktion der menschlichen Muskelgafafe auf Durchblutungsdrosselelung. *Pflüger's Arch. ges. Physiol.* 264:492, 1957.

Gomez, O. A., and W. F. Hamilton. Functional cardiac deterioration during development of hemorrhagic circulatory deficiency. *Circ. Res.* 14:336, 1964.

Goodwin, R. S., and L. A. Sapirstein. Measurement of cardiac output in dogs by a conductivity method after single intravenous injections of autogenous plasma. *Circ. Res.* 5:531, 1957.

Gordon, J. W. On certain molar movements of the human body produced by the circulation of the blood. *J. Anat. Physiol.* 11:533, 1877.

Gorlin, R., and S. G. Gorlin. Hydraulic formula for calculation of the area of the stenotic mitral valve, other cardiac valves, and central circulatory shunts. *Amer. Heart J.* 41:1, 1951.

Gorlin, R., and B. M. Lewis. Circulatory adjustments to hypoxia in dogs. *J. Appl. Physiol.* 7:180, 1954.

Gorten, R. J., and J. C. Stauffer. A study of the techniques and sources of error in the clinical application of the external counting method of estimating cardiac output. *Amer. J. Med. Sci.* 238:274, 1959.

Gorten, R., J. C. Gunnells, A. M. Weissler, and E. A. Stead, Jr. Effects of atropine and isoproterenol on cardiac output, central venous pressure, and mean transit time of indicators placed at three different sites in the nervous system. *Circ. Res.* 9:979, 1961.

Gorten, R. J. A small lightweight precordial counter for determination of cardiac output. *J. Appl. Physiol.* 20:1365, 1965.

Gott, V. L., J. D. Wiffen, D. E. Koepke, R. L. Daggett, W. C. Boake, and W. P. Young. Techniques of applying a graphite-benzalkonium-heparin coating to various plastics and metals. *Trans. Amer. Soc. Artif. Intern. Organs* 10:213, 1964.

Goult, J. H., J. Ross, Jr., and E. Braunwald. The contractile state of the left ventricle in man: Instantaneous tension-velocity-length relations in patients with and without disease of the left ventricular myocardia. *Circ. Res.* 22:451, 1968.

Gowdey, C. W. Anemia-induced changes in cardiac output in dogs treated with dechlorisoproterenol. *Circ. Res.* 10:354, 1962.

Graettinger, J. S., J. J. Muenster, C. S. Checchia, and J. A. Campbell. Correlation of clinical and hemodynamic studies in patients with thyroid disease. *Clin. Res. Proc.* 4:120, 1956.

Grahn, A. R., M. H. Paul, and H. U. Wessel. Design and evaluation of a new linear thermistor velocity probe. *J. Appl. Physiol.* 24:236, 1968.

Grahn, A. R., M. H. Paul, and H. U. Wessel. A new direction-sensitive probe for catheter-tip thermal velocity measurement. *J. Appl. Physiol.* 27:407, 1969.

Granger, H. J., and A. C. Guyton. Autoregulation of the total systemic circulation following destruction of the central nervous system in the dog. *Circ. Res.* 25:379, 1969.

Gray, F. D., Jr., R. J. Bind, and L. Vandam. An evaluation of a method involving carbon dioxide equilibration for determining cardiac output. *Amer. J. Physiol.* 151:245, 1947.

Gray, S. D., J. Lundvall, and S. Mellander. Regional hyperosmolality in relation to exercise hyperemia. *Acta Physiol. Scand.* 73:11A, 1968.

Green, H. D., R. N. Lewis, N. D. Nickerson, and A. L. Heller. Blood flow, peripheral resistance and vascular tonus, with observations on the relationship between blood flow and cutaneous temperature. *Amer. J. Physiol.* 141:518, 1944.

Green, H. D. Circulation—blood flow measurement. In *Methods in Medical Research.* Chicago: Year Book Publishers, 1948, Vol. 1, p. 66.

Green, H. D. Circulatory system: physical principles. In Otto Glasser. *Medical Physics.* Chicago: Year Book Publishers, 1950, Vol. 2, p. 231.

Green, H. D., and J. H. Kepchar. Control of peripheral resistance in major systemic vascular beds. *Physiol. Rev.* 39:617, 1959.

Green, H. D., and C. E. Rapela. Blood flow in passive vascular beds. *Circ. Res.* 15: Suppl. II, p. 11, 1964.

Greene, D. G., R. Carlisle, G. Grant, and I. L. Bunnell. Estimation of left ventricular volume by one-plane cineangiography. *Circulation* 35:61, 1967.

Greenfield, J. C., Jr., and D. J. Patel. Relation between pressure and diameter in the ascending aorta of man. *Circ. Res.* 10:778, 1962.

Greer, A. P. Comparison of electrokymography with dimensional recording devices in situ. *Fed. Proc.* 17:60, 1958.

Greganti, F. P., and A. C. Guyton. Right

ventricle as physiological level for reference of pressure in circulatory system. *Amer. J. Physiol.* 183:622, 1955.

Gregerson, M. I., and R. A. Rawson. Blood volume. *Physiol. Rev.* 39:307, 1959.

Gregg, D. E., and H. D. Green. Effects of viscosity, ischemia, cardiac output and aortic pressure on coronary blood flow measured under a constant perfusion pressure. *Amer. J. Physiol.* 130:108, 1940.

Gregg, D. E., and R. E. Shipley. Augmentation of left coronary inflow with elevation of left ventricular pressure and observations of the mechanism for increased coronary inflow with increased cardiac load. *Amer. J. Physiol.* 142:44, 1944.

Gregg, D. E. Thermostromuhr. In *Methods in Medical Research*. Chicago: Year Book Publishers, 1948, Vol. 1, p. 89.

Gregg, D. E., and L. C. Fisher. Blood supply to the heart. In W. F. Hamilton, and P. Dow (Eds.). *Handbook of Physiology. Circulation*. Washington, D.C., 1963, American Physiological Society, Sect. 2, Vol. II, Chap. 44, p. 1517.

Grehant, H., and C. E. Quinquaud. Recherches experimentales sur la mesure du volume de sang qui traverse les poumons en un temps donne. *Compt. Rend. Soc. Biol.* 30:159, 1886.

Greisheimer, E. M., D. W. Ellis, H. N. Baier, G. C. Ring, L. Makarenko, and J. Graziano. Cardiac output by cuvette oximeter under thiopental. *Amer. J. Physiol.* 175:171, 1953.

Greisheimer, E. M., D. W. Ellis, D. L. Webber, H. N. Baier, and P. R. Lynch. Cardiac output by cuvette oximeter under cyclopropane-oxygen anesthesia. *Amer. J. Physiol.* 177:489, 1954a.

Greisheimer, E. M., D. W. Ellis, D. L. Webber, F. Nawara, J. G. Baker, and M. R. Wester. Cardiac output by cuvette oximeter under ether anesthesia. *Amer. J. Physiol.* 177:493, 1954b.

Greisheimer, E. M., D. W. Ellis, G. Stewart, L. Makarenko, K. T. Thompson, and N. Oleksyshyn. Cardiac output by cuvette oximeter under thiopental sodium and cyclopropane-oxygen anesthesia. *Amer. J. Physiol.* 182:145, 1955a.

Greisheimer, E. M., D. W. Ellis, G. Stewart, D. L. Webber, L. Makarenko, K. T. Thompson, M. G. Resinski, and W. K. Frankenburg. Cardiac output by cuvette oximeter under cyclopropane-oxygen and ether anesthesia. *Amer. J. Physiol.* 180: 357, 1955b.

Greisheimer, E. M., D. W. Ellis, G. Stewart, L. Makarenko, M. Oleksyshyn, and K. T. Thompson. Cardiac output by the dye dilution technique under thiopental sodium oxygen and ether anesthesia. *Amer. J. Physiol.* 186:101, 1956.

Gribbe, P., L. Hirvonen, J. Lind, and C. Wegelius. Cineangiocardiographic recordings of the cyclic changes in volume of the left ventricle. *Cardiologia* 34:348, 1959.

Gribbe, P. Comparison of the angiocardiographic and the direct Fick methods in determining cardiac output. *Cardiologia* 36:20, 1960.

Griffin, G. D. J., E. H. Wood, and H. E. Essex. Variability of direct Fick values and validity of right atrial blood samples in determining cardiac output of anesthetized dogs. *Amer. J. Physiol.*, 164:583, 1951.

Griggs, D. M., Jr., F. R. Holt, and R. B. Case. Serial pressure-volume studies in the excised canine heart. *Amer. J. Physiol.* 198: 336, 1960.

Grimby, G., N. J. Nilsson, and H. Sanne. Repeated serial determination of cardiac output during 30 min exercise. *J. Appl. Physiol.* 21:1750, 1966.

Grimm, A. F., R. Kubota, and W. V. Whitehorn. Properties of myocardium in cardiomegaly. *Circ. Res.* 12:118, 1963.

Grishman, A., and A. M. Master. Cardiac output in occlusion studied by Wezler-Boeger physical method. *Proc. Soc. Exp. Biol. Med.* 48:207, 1941.

Grodins, F. S. Integrative cardiovascular physiology: a mathematical synthesis of cardiac and blood vessel hemodynamics. *Quart. Rev. Biol.* 34:93, 1959.

Grodins, F. S., W. H. Stuart, and R. L. Veenstra. Performance characteristics of the right heart bypass preparation. *Amer. J. Physiol.* 198:552, 1960.

Grollman, A. The effect of the ingestion of food on the cardiac output, pulse rate, blood pressure, and oxygen consumption of man. *Amer. J. Physiol.* 89:366, 1929a.

Grollman, A. The determination of the cardiac output of man by the use of acetylene. *Amer. J. Physiol.* 88:432, 1929b.

Grollman, A. A comparison of the triple extrapolation (Fick principle) and the acetylene (foreign gas principle) methods for the determination of the cardiac output of man. *Amer. J. Physiol.* 93:116, 1930a.

Grollman, A. Effect of high altitude on cardiac output of man and its related functions; account of experiments conducted on summit of Pike's Peak, Colorado. *Amer. J. Physiol.* 93:19, 1930b.

Grollman, A. Variations in cardiac output in man; effect of variations in environmental temperature on pulse rate, blood pressure, oxygen consumption, arterio-venous oxygen difference, and cardiac output of normal individuals. *Amer. J. Physiol.* 95:263, 1930c.

Grollman, A. Variations in cardiac output of man; pulse rate, blood pressure, oxygen consumption, arterio-venous oxygen difference, and cardiac output of man during normal nocturnal sleep. *Amer. J. Physiol.* 95:274, 1930d.

Grollman, A. *The Cardiac Output in Health and Disease*. Springfield, Illinois: Charles C Thomas, Publisher, 1932, Chap. 19, p. 32.

Groom, A. C., B. M. A. Löfving, S. Rowlands, and H. W. Thomas. The effect of lowering the pulse pressure in the carotid arteries on the cardiac output in the cat. *Acta Physiol. Scand.* 54:116, 1962.

Gross, R. E., and R. Mittermaier. Untersuchungen über das minute Volumen des Herzens. *Pflüger's Arch. ges. Physiol.* 212:136, 1926.

Grossman, J., R. E. Weston, and L. Leiter. A method for determining cardiac output by the direct Fick principle without gas analysis. *J. Clin. Invest.* 32:161, 1953.

Gunnells, J. C., and R. Gorten. Effect of varying indicator injection sites on values for cardiac output. *J. Appl. Physiol.* 16:261, 1961.

Guntheroth, W. G., and S. Chakmakjian. Active changes in tone in the canine vena cava. *Circ. Res.* 28:554, 1971.

Gupta, P. D., J. P. Henry, R. Sinclair, and R. Von Baumgarten. Responses of atrial and aortic baroreceptors to nonhypotensive hemorrhage and to transfusion. *Amer. J. Physiol.* 211:1429, 1966.

Guyton, A. C. Measurement of the respiratory volumes of laboratory animals. *Amer. J. Physiol.* 150:70, 1947a.

Guyton, A. C. Analysis of respiratory patterns in laboratory animals. *Amer. J. Physiol.* 150:78, 1947b.

Guyton, A. C., J. E. Lindley, R. N. Touchstone, C. M. Smith, Jr., and H. M. Batson, Jr. Effects of massive transfusion and hemorrhage on blood pressure and fluid shifts. *Amer. J. Physiol.* 163:525, 1950.

Guyton, A. C., H. M. Batson, Jr., and C. M. Smith, Jr. Adjustments of the circulatory system following very rapid transfusion or hemorrhage. *Amer. J. Physiol.* 164:351, 1951a.

Guyton, A. C., W. M. Gillespie, Jr., and G. G. Armstrong, Jr. Continuous recording of circulatory hemoglobin. *Rev. Sci. Instr.* 22:205, 1951b.

Guyton, A. C. and J. Satterfield. Factors concerned in electrical defibrillation of the heart through the unopened chest. *Amer. J. Physiol.* 167:81, 1951c.

Guyton, A. C., and L. H. Adkins. Relationship of abdominal pressure to venous pressure in the lower body. *Amer. J. Physiol.* 171:731, 1952a.

Guyton, A. C., L. J. Scanlon, and G. G. Armstrong, Jr. Effect of pressoreceptor reflex and Cushing reflex on urinary output. *Fed. Proc.* 11:61, 1952b.

Guyton, A. C., J. H. Satterfield, and J. W. Harris. Dynamics of central venous resistance with observations on static blood pressure. *Amer. J. Physiol.* 169:691, 1952c.

Guyton, A. C., and L. H. Adkins. Quantitative aspects of the collapse factor in relation to venous return. *Amer. J. Physiol.* 177:523, 1954a.

Guyton, A. C., A. W. Lindsey, and J. J. Gilluly. The limits of right ventricular compensation following acute increase in pulmonary circulatory resistance. *Circ. Res.* 2:326, 1954b.

Guyton, A. C., D. Polizo, and G. G. Armstrong, Jr. Mean circulatory filling pressure measured immediately after cessation of heart pumping. *Amer. J. Physiol.* 179:261, 1954c.

Guyton, A. C. Determination of cardiac output by equating venous return curves with cardiac response curves. *Physiol. Rev.* 35:123, 1955a.

Guyton, A. C., A. W. Lindsey, and B. Kaufmann. Effect of mean circulatory filling pressure and other peripheral circulatory factors on cardiac output. *Amer. J. Physiol.* 180:463, 1955b.

Guyton, A. C. Factors which determine the rate of venous return to the heart. In *World Trends in Cardiology.* New York: Paul B. Hoeber, 1956a, p. 32.

Guyton, A. C., G. G. Armstrong, Jr., and P. L. Chipley. Pressure-volume curves of the entire arterial and venous systems in the living animal. *Amer. J. Physiol.* 184:253, 1956b.

Guyton, A. C., and F. P. Greganti. A physiologic reference point for measuring circulatory pressures in the dog—particularly venous pressure. *Amer. J. Physiol.* 185:137, 1956c.

Guyton, A. C., A. W. Lindsey, and G. G. Armstrong, Jr. Relationship of total peripheral resistance to the pressure gradient from the arteries to the veins. *Amer. J. Physiol.* 186:294, 1956d.

Guyton, A. C., C. A. Farish, and R. J. Nichols. Continuous recording of cardiac output by the Fick method. *Clin. Res. Proc.* 5:94, 1957a.

Guyton, A. C., A. W. Lindsey, J. B. Abernathy, and T. Richardson. Venous return at various right atrial pressures and the normal venous return curve. *Amer. J. Physiol.* 189:609, 1957b.

Guyton, A. C., R. J. Nichols, and C. A. Farish. An arteriovenous oxygen difference recorder. *J. Appl. Physiol.* 10:158, 1957c.

Guyton, A. C. La circulation veineuse. *Symposia from the IIIrd World Congress of Cardiology,* 1958a, p. 109.

Guyton, A. C. The venous system and its role in the circulation. *Mod. Conc. Cardiovasc. Dis.* 27:483, 1958b.

Guyton, A. C., A. W. Lindsey, J. B. Abernathy, and J. B. Langston. Mechanism of the increased venous return and cardiac output caused by epinephrine. *Amer. J. Physiol.* 192:126, 1958c.

Guyton, A. C., A. W. Lindsey, B. N. Kaufmann, and J. B. Abernathy. Effect of blood transfusion and hemorrhage on cardiac output and on the venous return curve. *Amer. J. Physiol.* 194:263, 1958d.

Guyton, A. C. Cardiac output and venous return in heart failure. In *Cardiology.* New

York: McGraw-Hill Book Company, 1959a, Vol. 4, p. 18.

Guyton, A. C., J. B. Abernathy, J. B. Langston, B. N. Kaufmann, and H. M. Fairchild. Relative importance of venous and arterial resistances in controlling venous return and cardiac output. *Amer. J. Physiol.* 196:1008, 1959b.

Guyton, A. C., and A. W. Lindsey. Effect of elevated left atrial pressure and decreased plasma protein concentration on the development of pulmonary edema. *Circ. Res.* 7:649, 1959c.

Guyton, A. C., C. A. Farish, and J. W. Williams. An improved arteriovenous oxygen difference recorder. *J. Appl. Physiol.* 14:145, 1959d.

Guyton, A. C., and C. A. Farish. A rapidly responding continuous oxygen consumption recorder. *J. Appl. Physiol.* 14:143, 1959e.

Guyton, A. C., C. A. Farish, and J. B. Abernathy. A continuous cardiac output recorder employing the Fick principle. *Circ. Res.* 7:661, 1959f.

Guyton, A. C., and T. Q. Richardson. Effect of hematocrit on venous return. *Circ. Res.* 9:157, 1961a.

Guyton, A. C., and K. Sagawa. Compensations of cardiac output and other circulatory functions in areflex dogs with large A-V fistulae. *Amer. J. Physiol.* 200:1157, 1961b.

Guyton, A. C., and J. W. Crowell. Dynamics of the heart in shock. *Fed. Proc.* 20:51 (Part III), 1961c.

Guyton, A. C., J. B. Langston, and O. Carrier. Decrease of venous return caused by right atrial pulsation. *Circ. Res.* 10:188, 1962a.

Guyton, A. C., B. H. Douglas, J. B. Langston, and T. Q. Richardson. Instantaneous increase in mean circulatory pressure and cardiac output at onset of muscular activity. *Circ. Res.* 11:431, 1962b.

Guyton, A. C. Venous return. In W. F. Hamilton and P. Dow (Eds.). *Handbook of Physiology. Circulation.* Washington, D.C., 1963a, American Physiological Society, Sect. 2, Vol. II, Chap. 32, p. 1099.

Guyton, A. C. A concept of negative interstitial fluid pressure based on pressures in implanted perforated capsules. *Circ. Res.* 12:399, 1963b.

Guyton, A. C., J. M. Ross, O. Carrier, Jr., and J. R. Walker. Evidence for tissue oxygen demand as the major factor causing autoregulation. *Circ. Res.* 14:Suppl. I, p. 60, 1964.

Guyton, A. C., and T. G. Coleman. Long-term regulation of the circulation: interrelationships with body fluid volumes. In E. B. Reeve and A. C. Guyton (Eds.). *Physical Bases of Circulatory Transport: Regulation and Exchange.* Philadelphai: W. B. Saunders Company, 1967, pp. 179–201.

Guyton, A. C., T. G. Coleman, J. C. Fourcade, and L. G. Navar. Physiologic control of arterial pressure. *Bull. N.Y. Acad. Med.* 45:811, 1969a.

Guyton, A. C., and T. G. Coleman, Quantitative analysis of the pathophysiology of hypertension. *Circ. Res.* 24:Suppl. I, p. 1, 1969b.

Guyton, A. C., H. J. Granger, and T. G. Coleman. Autoregulation of the total systemic circulation and its relation to control of cardiac output and arterial pressure. *Circ. Res.* 28:Suppl. I, p. 93, 1971.

Guyton, A. C., T. G. Coleman, and H. J. Granger. Circulation: overall regulation. *Ann. Rev. Physiol.* 34:13, 1972.

Guyton, A. C., T. G. Coleman, A. W. Cowley, Jr., R. A. Norman, Jr., R. D. Manning, Jr., and J. F. Liard. Relationship of fluid and electrolytes to arterial pressure control and hypertension: quantitative analysis of an infinite gain feedback system. To be published.

Hackel, D. B., and W. T. Goodale. Effects of hemorrhagic shock on the heart and circulation of intact dogs. *Circulation* 11:628, 1955.

Haddy, F. J., J. B. Scott, and J. I. Molnar. Mechanism of volume replacement and vascular constriction following hemorrhage. *Amer. J. Physiol.* 208:169, 1965.

Haddy, F. J., and J. B. Scott. Metabolically linked vasoactive chemicals in local regulation of blood flow. *Physiol. Rev.* 48:688, 1968.

Haldane, J. S., and J. G. Priestley. The regulation of the lung-ventilation. *J. Physiol.* 32:225, 1905.

Hallerman, F. J., F. C. Rastelli, and H. J. C. Swan. Comparison of left ventricular volumes by dye dilution and angiographic methods in the dog. *Amer. J. Physiol.* 204:446, 1963.

Hamer, J., R. Emanuel, J. Norman, and M. Burgess. Use of a computer in the calibration of dye dilution curves by a dynamics method. *Brit. Heart J.* 28:147, 1966.

Hamilton, W. F., J. W. Moore, J. M. Kinsman, and R. G. Spurling. Simultaneous determination of the greater and lesser circulation times, of the mean velocity of blood flow through the heart and lungs, of the cardiac output and an approximation of the amount of blood actively circulating in the heart and lungs. *Amer. J. Physiol.* 85:377, 1928a.

Hamilton, W. F., J. W. Moore, J. M. Kinsman, and R. G. Spurling. Simultaneous determination of the pulmonary and systemic circulation times in man and of a figure related to the cardiac output. *Amer. J. Physiol.* 84:338, 1928b.

Hamilton, W. F., J. W. Moore, J. M. Kinsman, and R. G. Spurling. Studies on the circulation. IV. Further analysis of the injection method, and of changes in hemodynamics under physiological and pathological conditions. *Amer. J. Physiol.* 99:534, 1932.

Hamilton, W. F. Heart output. In Otto Glasser. *Medical Physics.* Chicago: Year Book Publishers, 1944, Vol. I, p. 575.

Hamilton, W. F. Development of physiology of cardiac output. *Fed. Proc.* 4:183, 1945a.

Hamilton, W. F., P. Dow, and J. W. Remington. The relationship between the cardiac ejection curve and the ballistocardiographic forces. *Amer. J. Physiol.* 144:557, 1945b.

Hamilton, W. F., and J. W. Remington. Comparison of the time concentration curves in arterial blood of diffusible and non-diffusible substances when injected at a constant rate and when injected instantaneously. *Amer. J. Physiol.* 148:35, 1947a.

Hamilton, W. F., and J. W. Remington. The measurement of the stroke volume from the pressure pulse. *Amer. J. Physiol.* 148:14, 1947b.

Hamilton, W. F., R. L. Riley, A. M. Attyah, A. Cournand, D. M. Fowell, A. Himmelstein, R. P. Noble, J. W. Remington, D. W. Richards, Jr., N. C. Wheeler, and A. C. Witham. Comparison of Fick and dye injection methods of measuring cardiac output in man. *Amer. J. Physiol.* 153:309, 1948.

Hamilton, W. F. Cardiac output in normal pregnancy as determined by Cournand right heart catherization technic. *J. Obst. Gynaecol. Brit. Empire* 56:548, 1949.

Hamilton, W. F. The Lewis A. Connor memorial lecture: the physiology of the cardiac output. *Circulation* 8:527, 1953.

Hamilton, W. F., R. G. Ellison, R. G. Pickering, E. E. Hague, and J. T. Rucker. Hemodynamic and endocrine responses to experimental mitral stenosis. *Amer. J. Physiol.* 176:445, 1954.

Hamilton, W. F. Measurement of the cardiac output. *Handbook of Physiology.* Washington: American Physiological Society, 1962, Section 2, Vol. I, p. 551.

Hamrick, L. W., Jr., and J. D. Myers. The effect of subfebrile doses of bacterial pyrogens on splanchnic metabolism and cardiac output. *J. Lab. Clin. Med.* 45:568, 1955.

Handbook of Circulation. Edited by P. L. Altman. Philadelphia: W. B. Saunders Company, 1959.

Handley, C., H. Huggins, and E. Hay. Changes in extracellular fluid and cardiac output in hemorrhagic shock. *Amer. Surgeon* 16:673, 1950.

Hansen, J. T., and N. Pace. Apparatus for automatic dye dilution measurement of cardiac output. *J. Appl. Physiol.* 17:163, 1962.

Hara, H. H., and J. W. Bellville. On-line computation of cardiac output from dye dilution curves. *Circ. Res.* 12:379, 1963.

Hardy, J. D., and L. Godfrey, Jr. Effect of intravenous fluids on dehydrated patients and on normal subjects; cardiac output, stroke volume, pulse rate, and blood pressure. *J.A.M.A.* 126:23, 1944.

Hardy, J. D., W. A. Neely, F. C. Wilson, Jr., J. R. Lovelace, and E. Jabbour. Thermal burns in man. V. Cardiac output during early therapy. *Surg. Gynec. Obstet.* 101:94, 1955.

Harlan, J. C., E. E. Smith, and T. Q. Richardson. Pressure-volume curves of systemic and pulmonary circuit. *Amer. J. Physiol.* 213:1499, 1967.

Harmison, L. T. Totally implantable nuclear heart assist and artificial heart. A report of the National Heart and Lung Institute, 1972.

Harris, C. W. *Neural Control of the Pituitary Gland.* Baltimore: The Williams and Wilkins Co., 1955.

Harris, S. The spread of excitation in turtle, dog, cat, and monkey ventricles. *Amer. J. Physiol.* 134:319, 1941.

Harrison, T. R., W. Dock, and E. Holman. Experimental studies in arteriovenous fistulae: cardiac output. *Heart* 11:337, 1924.

Harrison, T. R., W. G. Harrison, J. A. Calhoun, and J. P. Marsh. Congestive heart failure. *Arch. Intern. Med.* 50:690, 1932.

Harrison, T. R. Arterial and venous pressure factors in circulatory failure. *Physiol. Rev.* 18:86, 1938.

Harvey, R. M., M. I. Ferrer, R. T. Cathcart, and J. K. Alexander. Some effects of digoxin on the heart and circulation in man. Digoxin in enlarged hearts not in clinical congestive failure. *Circulation* 4:366, 1951.

Hastings, F. W., W. H. Potter, and J. W. Holter. Artificial intracorporeal heart. *Trans. Amer. Soc. Artif. Intern. Organs.* 7:323, 1961.

Hatakeyama, I. On the analysis of blood pressure regulation by means of a pressure amplifier. *Yokohama Med. Bull.* 12:171, 1961.

Hatcher, J. D., F. A. Sunahara, O. G. Edholm, and J. M. Woolner. The circulatory adjustments to posthemorrhagic anemia in dogs. *Circ. Res.* 2:499, 1954.

Hawthorne, E. W., S. L. C. Perry, M. Gaspar, G. Thomson, W. Pitts, and W. G. Pogue. Relationship between left ventricular stroke work and end-diastolic diameter at different filling pressures in anesthetized normal dogs and dogs with atrial septal defects (ASD). *Fed. Proc.* 17:67, 1958.

Hayasaka, E. On the minute volume of the heart in hypertension. *Tohoku J. Ep. Med.* 9:401, 1927.

Haynes, B. W., Jr. The alterations of cardiac output and plasma volume in normal subjects with the administration of concentrated human serum albumin. *Proc. Amer. Fed. Clin. Res.* 2:74, 1945.

Haynes, B. W., Jr., G. C. Morris, Jr., J. H. Moyer, and H. B. Snyder. Effects of controlled hypotension on glomerular filtration and renal plasma flow in man. *Surg. Forum* 4:443, 1953.

Heald, C. B., and W. S. Tucker. Recoil curves as shown by the hot-wire microphone. *Proc. Roy. Soc. (London), Series B* 93:281, 1922.

Heller, S., W. Lochner, and W. Schoedel. Die Bestimmung des Herzzeitvolumens mittel Injektions-methode bei fortlaufender photometrischer Registrierung der Zeit-Konzentrationskurven. *Pflüger's Arch. ges. Physiol.* 253:181, 1951.

Hellerbrandt, F. A., and E. B. Franseen. Physiological study of the vertical stance of man. *Physiol. Rev.* 23:220, 1943.

Henderson, Y. The mass-movements of the circulation as shown by a recoil curve. *Amer. J. Physiol.* 14:287, 1905.

Henderson, Y., and T. B. Barringer, Jr. The influence of respiration upon the velocity of the blood stream. *Amer. J. Physiol.* 31:399, 1913.

Henderson, Y., and A. L. Prince. Applications of gas analysis. II. the CO_2 tension of the venous blood and the circulation rate. *J. Biol. Chem.* 32:325, 1917.

Henderson, Y. Volume changes of the heart. *Physiol. Rev.* 3:165, 1923.

Henderson, Y., and H. W. Haggard. The circulation and its measurement. *Amer. J. Physiol.* 73:193, 1925.

Henderson, Y., and H. W. Haggard. The validity of the ethyl iodide method for measuring the circulation. *Amer. J. Physiol.* 82:497, 1927a.

Henderson, Y., H. W. Haggard, and F. S. Dolley. The efficiency of the heart, and the significance of rapid and slow pulse rates. *Amer. J. Physiol.* 82:523, 1927b.

Henriques, V. Über die Verteilung des Blutes vom linken Herzen zwichen dem Herzen und dem übrigen Organismus. *Biochem. Z.* 56:230, 1913.

Henry, W. L., C. Ploeg, S. L. Kountz, and D. C. Harrison. An improved hydraulic vascular occluder for chronic electromagnetic blood flow measurements. *J. Appl. Physiol.* 25:790, 1968.

Heringman, E. C., H. A. Davis, and J. D. Ribes. Effect of acute A-V fistula on circulation time and auricular pressure in dogs. *Proc. Soc. Exp. Biol. Med.* 60:371, 1945.

Hermansen, L., B. Ekblom, and B. Saltin. Cardiac output during submaximal and maximal treadmill and bicycle exercise. *J. Appl. Physiol.* 29:82, 1970.

Hernandez, A., Jr., D. Goldring, M. Ter-Pogossian, and J. Eichling. New technique for determing cardiac output with the use of a miniature esophageal scintillation detector. *Circulation* 35:55, 1967.

Herndon, C. W., and K. Sagawa. Combined effects of aortic and right atrial pressures on aortic flow. *Amer. J. Physiol.* 217:65, 1969.

Herrick, J. F., J. H. Grindlay, E. J. Baldes, and F. C. Mann. Effect of exercise on the blood flow in the superior mesenteric, renal and common iliac arteries. *Amer. J. Physiol.* 128:338, 1940.

Herrick, J. F., and J. A. Anderson. Ultrasonic flowmeter. In Otto Glasser. *Medical Physics.* Chicago: Year Book Publishers, 1960, Vol. III, p. 181.

Hershey, S. G. Dynamics of peripheral vascular collapse in shock. In S. G. Hershey (Ed.). *Shock.* Boston: Little, Brown and Company, 1964, p. 185.

Hertzman, A. B. Vasomotor regulation of cutaneous circulation. *Physiol. Rev.* 39:280, 1959.

Hetzel, P. S., H. J. Swan, and E. H. Wood. Influence of injection site on arterial dilution curves of T-1824. *J. Appl. Physiol.* 7:66, 1954.

Hetzel, P., H. J. Swan, A. A. Ramirez de Arellano, and E. H. Wood. Estimation of cardiac output from first part of arterial dye-dilution curves. *J. Appl. Physiol.* 13:92, 1958.

Heymans, C., and E. Neil. *Reflexogenic Areas of the Cardiovascular System.* Boston: Little, Brown and Company, 1958, p. 37.

Hickam, J. B., and W. H. Cargill. Effects of exercise on cardiac output and pulmonary arterial pressure in normal persons and in patients with cardiovascular disease and pulmonary emphysema. *J. Clin. Invest.* 27:10, 1948a.

Hickam, J. B., W. H. Cargill, and A. Golden. Cardiovascular reactions to emotional stimuli; effect on cardiac output, arteriovenous oxygen difference, arterial pressure, and peripheral resistance. *J. Clin. Invest.* 27:290, 1948b.

Hickam, J. B., R. P. McCullough, and R. J. Reeves. Normal and impaired function of the leg veins. *Amer. Heart J.* 37:1017, 1949.

Hickam, J. B., and W. W. Pryor. Cardiac output in postural hypotension. *J. Clin. Invest.* 30:401, 1951.

Hift, H., and J. G. Strawitz. Structure and function of mitochondria in irreversible hemorrhagic shock. *Proc. Soc. Exp. Biol. Med.* 98:235, 1958.

Hilger, H.-H., and H. Brechtelsbauer. Erfahrungen über Stromungsmessung mit verschiedenen Typen elektrisch registrierender Rotameter. *Pflüger's Arch. ges. Physiol.* 263:615, 1956.

Hill, A. V. The beat of shortening and the dynamic constants of muscle. *Proc. Roy. Soc. (London)* Sec. B 126:136, 1938.

Hilton, J. G., D. M. Kanter, D. R. Hays, E. H. Bowen, J. R. Golub, J. H. Keatings, and R. Wegria. The effect of acute arteriovenous fistulae on renal functions. *J. Clin. Invest.* 34:732, 1955.

Hilton, S. M. Hypothalamic regulation of the cardiovascular system. *Brit. Med. Bull.* 22:243, 1966.

Hinshaw, L. Arterial and venous pressure-resistance relationships in perfused leg and intestine. *Amer. J. Physiol.* 203:271, 1962.

Hinshaw, L., T. E. Emerson, Jr., and D. A. Reins. Cardiovascular responses of the primate in endotoxin shock. *Amer. J. Physiol.* 210:335, 1966.

Hitzig, W. M., F. H. Kind, and A. M. Fishberg. Circulation time in failure of left side of heart. *Arch. Intern. Med.* 55:112, 1935.

Hlastala, M. P., B. Wranne, and C. J. Lenfant. "Breath by breath" determination of cardiac output. *Proc. Int. Union. Physiol. Sci.* 9:251, 1971.

Hochrein, M., and K. Matthes. Verschiedenheiten der Schlagvolumina und Ungleichmässigkeiten der Leistung beider Ventrikel in ihrer Auswirking auf Lungendepot und Herzdurchblutung. *Pflüger's Arch. ges. Physiol.* 231:207, 1932.

Hockman, C. H., J. Talesnik, and K. E. Livingston. Central nervous system modulation of baroreceptor reflexes. *Amer. J. Physiol.* 217:1681, 1969.

Hodges, F. J. The roentgenographic measurement of cardiac output in man; a preliminary report. *Radiology* 10:122, 1928.

Hoff, E. C., and H. D. Green. Cardiovascular reactions induced by electrical stimulation of the cerebral cortex. *Amer. J. Physiol.* 117:411, 1936.

Hoff, E. C., J. F. Keli, and M. N. Carroll, Jr. Effects of cortical stimulation and lesions on cardiovascular function. *Physiol. Rev.* 43:68, 1963.

Hohnen, H. W., and H. Klensch. Ballistische Bestimmung des Schlagvolumens bei Verminderung des intrapulmonalen Druckes. *Pflüger's Arch. ges Physiol.* 265:199, 1957.

Hojensgard, I. C., and H. Sturup. Static and dynamic pressures in superficial and deep veins of the lower extremity in man. *Acta Physiol. Scand.* 27:49, 1952.

Hollenberg, N. K., J. R. Waters, M. R. Toews, R. O. Davies, and M. Nickerson. Nature of cardiovascular decompensation during hemorrhagic hypotension. *Amer. J. Physiol.* 219:1476, 1970a.

Hollenberg, N. K., and M. Nickerson. Changes in pre- and postcapillary resistance in pathogenesis of hemorrhagic shock. *Amer. J. Physiol.* 219:1483, 1970b.

Holman, D. V., and I. H. Page. Cardiac output in arterial hypertension produced by constricting renal arteries in unanesthetized and anesthetized (pentobarbital) dogs. *Amer. Heart J.* 16:321, 1938.

Holmgren, A., B. Jonsson, M. Levander, H. Linderholm, and T. Sjöstrand. Low physical working capacity in suspected heart cases due to inadequate adjustments of peripheral blood flow (vasoregulatory asthenia). *Acta Med. Scand.* 158:413, 1957.

Holmgren, A., P. Karlberg, and B. Pernnow. Circulatory adaptation at rest and during muscular work in patients with complete heart block. *Acta Med. Scand.* 164:119, 1959.

Holt, J. P. The collapse factor in the measurement of venous pressure. *Amer. J. Physiol.* 134:292, 1941.

Holt, J. P. The effect of positive and negative intra-thoracic pressure on peripheral venous pressure in man. *Amer. J. Physiol.* 139:208, 1943.

Holt, J. P. The effect of positive and negative intra-thoracic pressure on cardiac and venous pressure in the dog. *Amer. J. Physiol.* 142:594, 1944a.

Holt, J. P., and P. K. Knoefel. Changes in plasma volume and cardiac output following intravenous injection of gelatin, serum, and physiologic saline solution. *J. Clin. Invest.* 23:657, 1944b.

Holt, J. P. Estimation of the residual volume of the ventricle of the dog's heart by two indicator dilution technics. *Circ. Res.* 4:187, 1956.

Holt, J. P. Regulation of the degree of emptying of the left ventricle by the force of ventricular contraction. *Circ. Res.* 5:281, 1957.

Holt, J. P. Flow of liquids through "collapsible" tubes. *Circ. Res.* 7:342, 1959.

Hood, W. P., W. J. Thomson, C. E. Rackley, and E. L. Rolett. Comparison of calculations of left ventricular wall stress in man from thin-walled and thick-walled ellipsoidal models. *Circ. Res.* 24:574, 1969.

Horvath, S. M., and E. A. Farrand. Aortic obstruction and cardiac output. *Amer. Heart J.* 55:631, 1958.

Hosie, K. F. Thermal-dilution technics. *Circ. Res.* 10:491, 1962.

Houston, C. S., T. Akutsu, and W. J. Kolff. Pendulum type of artificial heart within the chest. *Amer. Heart J.* 59:723, 1960.

Hovarth, S. M., and C. D. Howell. Organ systems in adaptation: the circulatory system. In D. B. Dill (Ed.). *Handbook of Physiology.* Baltimore, The Williams and Wilkins Co., 1964, Section 4.

Howard, A. R., W. F. Hamilton, and I. Dow. Limitations of the continuous infusion method for measuring cardiac output by dye dilution. *Amer. J. Physiol.* 175:173, 1953.

Howarth, S. J. McMichael, and E. P. Sharpey-Schafer. Effects of venesection in low output heart failure. *Clin. Sci.* 6:41, 1948.

Howell, C. D., and S. M. Horvath. Reproducibility of cardiac output measurements in the dog. *J. Appl. Physiol.* 14:421, 1959.

Hubay, C. A., R. C. Waltz, G. A. Brecher, J. Praglin, and R. A. Hingson. Circulatory dynamics of venous return during positive-negative pressure respiration. *Anesthesiology* 15:445, 1954.

Huckabee, W. E., and W. E. Judson. The role of anaerobic metabolism in the performance of mild muscular work. I. Relationship of oxygen consumption and cardiac output, and the effect of congestive heart failure. *J. Clin. Invest.* 37:1577, 1958.

Huckabee, W. E. Circulatory response to cytochrome oxidase inhibition *in vivo*. *Fed. Proc.* 19:119, 1960.

Huerkamp, B., and E. Opitz. Die Blutgefässe des Augenhintergrundes bei höhenangepassten Kaninchen. *Pflüger's Arch. ges. Physiol.* 252:129, 1950.

Huff, R. L., D. D. Feller, O. J. Judd, and G. M. Bogardus. Cardiac output of men and dogs measured by *in vivo* analysis of iodinated (I-131) human serum albumin. *Circ. Res.* 3:564, 1955.

Hugenholtz, P. G., W. J. Gamble, G. Monroe, and M. Polanyi. The use of fiberoptics in clinical catheterization. II. In vivo dye-dilution curves. *Circulation* 31:344, 1965.

Hugenholtz, P. G., H. R. Wagner, W. J. Gamble, and M. L. Polanyi. Direct readout of cardiac output by means of the fiberoptic indicator dilution method. *Amer. Heart J.* 77:178, 1969.

Huggins, R. A., C. A. Handley, and M. LaForge. Comparison of cardiac outputs determined by direct Fick and pressure pulse methods. *Proc. Soc. Exp. Biol. Med.* 68:543, 1948.

Huggins, R. A., E. L. Smith, and M. A. Sinclair. Comparison of cardiac output by direct Fick and pressure pulse contour methods in open-chest dogs. *Amer. J. Physiol.* 159:385, 1949.

Huggins, R. A., E. L. Smith, and M. A. Sinclair. Comparison between the cardiac output measured with a rotameter and output determined by the direct Fick method in open-chest dogs. *Amer. J. Physiol.* 160:183, 1950.

Humphreys, G. H., R. L. Moore, H. C. Maier, and V. Apgar. Cardiac output of anesthetized dogs during continuous and intermittent inflation of lungs. *J. Thorac. Surg.* 7:438, 1938.

Hurlimann, A., and C. J. Wiggers. The effects of progressive general anoxia on the pulmonary circulation. *Circ. Res.* 1:231, 1953.

Hurthle, K. Ueber eine Methode zur Registrierung des arteriellen Blutdrucks beim Menschen. *Deut. Med. Wochschr.* 22:574, 1896.

Huxley, H. E. Contractile structure of cardiac and skeletal muscle. *Circulation* 24:328, 1961.

Hyman, C., R. L. Paldino, and E. Zimmerman. Local regulation of effective blood flow in muscle. *Circ. Res.* 12:176, 1963.

Imai, S., A. L. Riley, and R. M. Berne. Effect of ischemia on adenine nucleotides

in cardiac and skeletal muscle. *Circ. Res.* 15:443, 1964.

Ingraham, R. C., and H. C. Wiggers. Alkalinizing agents and fluid priming in hemorrhagic shock. *Amer. J. Physiol.* 144:505, 1945.

Iriuchijima, J., M. E. Soulsby, and M. F. Wilson. Participation of cardiac sympathetics in carotid occlusion pressor reflex. *Amer. J. Physiol.* 215:1111, 1968.

Isaacs, J. P., E. Berglund, and S. J. Sarnoff. Ventricular function. III. The pathologic physiology of acute cardiac tamponade studied by means of ventricular function curves. *Amer. Heart J.* 48:66, 1954.

Isschutz, B., Jr. Effect of sympathomimetic drugs on cardiac output. *Arch. Intern. Pharmacodynamie* 77:145, 1948.

Jacobowitz, D., T. Cooper, and H. B. Barner. Histochemical and chemical studies of the localization of adrenergic and cholinergic nerves in normal and denervated cat hearts. *Circ. Res.* 20:289, 1967.

Jalavisto, E., O. Martens, and W. Schoedel. Zur Steuerung der Muskeldurchblutung nach rhythmischer Tatigkeit. *Pflüger's Arch. ges. Physiol.* 249:167, 1948.

Jernerus, R., G. Lundin, and D. Thomson. Cardiac output in health subjects determined with a CO_2 rebreathing method. *Acta Physiol. Scand.* 59:390, 1963.

Jepson, R. P. The effects of vascular occlusion and local cooling on fringe skin blood flow. *Clin. Sci.* 13:259, 1954.

Jochim, K. E. Electromagnetic flowmeter. In *Methods in Medical Research*. Chicago: Year Book Publishers, 1948, Vol. 1.

Johnson, G. S., and A. Blalock. Experimental shock. XII. A study of the effects of hemorrhage, or trauma to muscles, of trauma to the intestines, of burns and of histamine on the cardiac output and on blood pressure of dogs. *Arch. Surg.* 23:855, 1931.

Johnson, P. C. Autoregulation of intestinal blood flow. *Amer. J. Physiol.* 199:311, 1960.

Johnson, P. C. Origin, localization, and homeostatic significance of autoregulation in the intestine. *Circ. Res.* 15:Suppl. I, p. 225, 1964.

Johnson, S. E. Roentgen kymography considered in relation to heart output and a new heart index. *Amer. J. Roentgen.* 37:167, 1937.

Johnston, C. I., J. O. Davis, C. A. Robb, and J. W. Mackenzie. Plasma renin in chronic experimental heart failure and during renal sodium "escape" from mineralocorticoids. *Circ. Res.* 22:113, 1968.

Jones, J. W. L. Left ventricular volumes in valvular heart disease. *Circulation* 29:887, 1964a.

Jones, R. D., and R. M. Berne. Intrinsic regulation of skeletal muscle blood flow. *Circ. Res.* 14:126, 1964b.

Jones, R. D., and R. M. Berne. Evidence for

a metabolic mechanism in autoregulation of blood flow in skeletal muscle. *Circ. Res.* 17:540, 1965.

Jones, N. L., E. J. M. Campbell, G. J. R. McHardy, B. E. Higgs, and M. Clode. The estimation of carbon dioxide pressure of mixed venous blood during exercise. *Clin. Sci.* 32:311, 1967.

Jones, C. E., J. W. Crowell, and E. E. Smith. A cause-effect relationship between oxygen deficit and irreversible hemorrhagic shock. *Surgery* 127:93, 1968a.

Jones, W. B., and Reeves, T. J. Total cardiac output response during four minutes of exercise. *Amer. Heart J.* 76:209, 1968b.

Jones, C. E., H. L. Bethea, E. E. Smith, and J. W. Crowell. Effect of a coronary vasodilator on the development of irreversible hemorrhagic shock. *Surgery* 68:356, 1970.

Jose, A. D., and F. Stitt. Effects of hypoxia and metabolic inhibitors on the intrinsic heart rate and myocardial contractility in dogs. *Circ. Res.* 25:53, 1969.

Judson, W. E., W. Hollander, J. D. Hatcher, H. H. Halperin, and I. H. Friedman. Cardiohemodynamic effects of venous congestion of legs or of phlebotomy in patients with and without congestive heart failure. *J. Clin. Invest.* 34:614, 1955.

Kaada, B. R. Somato-motor, autonomic and electrocorticographic responses to electrical stimulation of rhinencephalic and other structures in primates, cat, and dog. *Acta Physiol. Scand.* 24:Suppl. 83, p. 1, 1951.

Kabat, H., H. W. Magoun, and S. W. Ranson. Electrical stimulation of points in the forebrain and midbrain. *Arch. Neurol. Psychiat.* 34:931, 1935.

Kagan, A. Dynamic responses of the right ventricle following extensive damage by cauterization. *Circulation* 5:816, 1952.

Kahler, R. L., T. E. Gaffney, and E. Braunwald. The effects of autonomic nervous system inhibition on the circulatory response to muscular exercise. *J. Clin. Invest.* 41:1981, 1962a.

Kahler, R. L., A. Goldblatt, and E. Braunwald. The effects of acute hypoxia on the systemic venous and arterial systems and on myocardial contractile force. *J. Clin. Invest.* 41:1553, 1962b.

Kalmus, H. P. Electronic flowmeter system. *Rev. Sci. Instr.* 25:201, 1954.

Kao, F. F., and L. H. Ray. Respiratory and circulatory responses of anesthetized dogs to induced muscular work. *Amer. J. Physiol.* 179:249, 1954.

Katori, M., and R. M. Berne. Release of adenosine from anoxic hearts: Relationship to coronary flow. *Circ. Res.* 19:420, 1966.

Kattus, A. A., A. U. Rivin, A. Cohen, and C. S. Sofio. Cardiac output and central volume as determined by dye dilution curves: resting values in normal subjects and patients with cardiovascular disease. *Circulation* 11:447, 1955.

Katz, A. M. The descending limb of the Starling curve and the failing heart. *Circulation* 32:871, 1965.

Katz, L. N. Relation of initial volume and initial pressure to dynamics of the ventricular contraction. *Amer. J. Physiol.* 87:348, 1928.

Katz, L. N. The role played by the ventricular relaxation process in filling the ventricle. *Amer. J. Physiol.* 95:542, 1930.

Katz, L. N., and A. Kolin. The flow of blood in the carotid artery of the dog under various circumstances as determined with the electromagnetic flowmeter. *Amer. J. Physiol.* 122:788, 1938.

Katz, L. N., A. M. Katz, and F. L. Williams. Metabolic adjustments to alterations of cardiac work in hypoxemia. *Amer. J. Physiol.* 181:539, 1955.

Katz, L. N., and H. Feinburg. The relation of cardiac output to myocardial oxygen consumption and coronary flow. *Circ. Res.* 6:656, 1958.

Katz, L. N., Feinberg, H., and A. B. Shaffer. Hemodynamic aspects of congestive heart failure. *Circulation* 21:95, 1960.

Kawai, C., and W. H. Abelmann. Transient myocardial damage secondary to extravasation of contrast material during left ventricular angiocardiography. *Circulation.* 30:897, 1964.

Keefer, C. S. The beriberi heart. *Arch. Intern. Med.* 45:1, 1930.

Kelley, D. T., H. M. Spotnitz, G. D. Beiser, J. E. Pierce, and S. E. Epstein. Effects of chronic right ventricular volume and pressure loading on left ventricular performance. *Circulation* 44:403, 1971.

Kelly, W. D., and M. B. Visscher. Effect of sympathetic nerve stimulation on cutaneous small vein and small artery pressures, blood flow and hindpaw volume in the dog. *Amer. J. Physiol.* 185:453, 1956.

Kennedy, J. W., W. A. Baxley, M. M. Figley, H. T. Dodge, and J. R. Blackman. Quantitative angiocardiography: I. The normal left ventricle in man. *Circulation* 34:272, 1966.

Kenner, H. M., and E. H. Wood. Intrapericardial, intrapleural, and intracardiac pressures during acute heart failure in dogs studied without thoracotomy. *Circ. Res.* 19:1071, 1966.

Kenney, R. A., E. Neil, and A. Schweitzer. Carotid sinus reflexes and cardiac output in dogs. *J. Physiol.* 114:27, 1951.

Keroes, J., R. R. Ecker, and E. Rapaport. Ventricular function curves in the exercising dog. *Circ. Res.* 25:557, 1969.

Kerwin, A. J. Observations on the heart size of natives living at high altitudes. *Amer. Heart J.* 28:69, 1944.

Kester, N. C., A. W. Richardson, and H. D. Green. Effect of controlled hydrogen ion concentration on peripheral vascular tone and blood flow in innervated hind leg of the dog. *Amer. J. Physiol.* 169:678, 1952.

Keys, A., and H. L. Friedell. Measurement of the stroke volume of the human heart from roentgenograms; simultaneous roentgenkymographic and acetylene rebreathing experiments. *Amer. J. Physiol.* 126:741, 1939.

Keys, A. Estimation by foreign-gas method of net (systemic) cardiac output in conditions where there is recirculation through lungs (in patent ductus arteriosus). *Amer. J. Physiol.* 134:268, 1941.

Keys, A., J. P. Stapp, and A. Violante. Responses in size, output, and efficiency of human heart to acute alteration in composition of inspired air. *Amer. J. Physiol.* 138:763, 1943.

Kezdi, P., and W. Spickler. The evidence for resetting of the baroreceptors in hypertension. In P. Kezdi (Ed.) *Baroreceptors and Hypertension.* Pergamon Press, 1967.

Khalil, H. H. Determination of cardiac output in man by a new method based on thermodilution. Lancet 1:1352, 1963a.

Khalil, H. H. Determination of cardiac output in man by a new method based on thermodilution. Fed. Proc. 22:400, 1963b.

Khalil, H. H., T. O. Richardson, and A. C. Guyton. Measurement of cardiac output by thermal-dilution and direct Fick methods in dogs. *J. Appl. Physiol.* 21:1131, 1966.

Khouri, E. M., D. E. Gregg, and C. R. Rayford. Effect of exercise on cardiac output, left coronary flow and myocardial metabolism in the unanesthetized dog. *Circ. Res.* 17:427, 1965.

Khouri, E. M., and D. E. Gregg. An inflatable cuff for zero determination in blood flow studies. *J. Appl. Physiol.* 23:395, 1967.

Kidd, B. S., and S. M. Lyons. The distensibility of the blood vessels of the human calf determined by graded venous congestion. *J. Physiol.* 140:122, 1958.

Kilburn, K. H. Hemodynamic effects of continuous positive and negative pressure breathing in normal man. *Circ. Res.* 8:660, 1960.

Kilburn, K. H. Muscular origin of elevated plasma potassium during exercise. *J. Appl. Physiol.* 21:675, 1966.

Kim, T. S., H. Rahn, and L. E. Farhi. Estimation of true venous and arterial P_{CO_2} by gas analysis of a single breath. *J. Appl. Physiol.* 21:1338, 1966.

Kinnen, E. Thermistor tipped catheter instrumentation for measuring pulsatile blood flow. *Proc. Ann. Conf. Eng. Med. Biol.* 19:110, 1966.

Kinsman, J. M., J. W. Moore, and W. F. Hamilton. Studies on the circulation: I. Injection method. Physical and mathematical considerations. *Amer. J. Physiol.* 89:322, 1929.

Kjellberg, S. R., U. Rudhe, and T. Sjöstrand. The effect of adrenaline on the contraction of the human heart under normal circulatory conditions. *Acta Physiol. Scand.* 24:333, 1952.

Kjellmer, I. Some aspects of work hyperemia in skeletal muscles. *Acta Physiol. Scand.* 50:Suppl. 175, p. 85, 1960.

Kjellmer, I. The role of potassium ions in exercise hyperemia. *Med. Exp.* (Basel) 5:56, 1961.

Kjellmer, I. The potassium ion as a vasodilator during muscular exercise. *Acta Physiol. Scand.* 63:460, 1964.

Kjellmer, I., and H. Odelram. The effect of some physiological vasodilators on the vascular bed of skeletal muscle. *Acta Physiol. Scand.* 63:94, 1965.

Klausen, K. Comparison of CO_2 rebreathing and acetylene methods for cardiac output. *J. Appl. Physiol.* 20:763, 1965.

Kleiber, M. Body size and metabolic rate. *Physiol. Rev.* 27:511, 1947.

Klein, O. Zur Bestimmung des zirkulatorischen Minutenvolums beim Menschen nach den Fickschen Prinzip mittels Herzsondierung. *Münch. Med. Wochschr.* 77:1311, 1930.

Klensch, H., and W. Eger. Ein neues Verfahren der physikulischen Schlagvolumenbestimmung (quantitative Ballistographie). *Pflüger's Arch. ges. Physiol.* 263:459, 1956.

Klensch, H., and H. W. Hohnen. Bestimmung von Schlag- und Minutevolumen nach Arbeitsleistung mit der ballistischen Methode. *Pflüger's Arch. ges. Physiol.* 265: 207, 1957.

Klepzig, H. Untersuchungen über die Arbeitsweise des menschlichen Herzens bei vermehrter Belastung. *Arch. Kreislaufforsch.* 23:96, 1955.

Klocke, F. J., D. G. Greene, and R. C. Koberstein. Indicator-dilution measurement of cardiac output with dissolved hydrogen. *Circ. Res.* 22:841, 1968.

Kloster, F. E., J. D. Bristow, and H. E. Griswold. Cardiac output determination from precordial isotope-dilution curves during exercise. *J. Appl. Physiol.* 26:465, 1969.

Klussman, F. W., W. Koenig, and A. Lutcke. Uber die "thermodilution Methode zur Bestimmung des Herzzeitvolumens aus narkotisierten und unnarkotisierten Hund. *Arch. Ges. Physiol.* 269:392, 1959.

Knebel, R., and D. Wick. Über den Einfluss der Atmung auf den zentralen Venendruck. *Z. Kreislaufforsch.* 47:623, 1958.

Knowlton, F. P., and E. H. Starling. The influence of variations in temperature and blood pressure on the performance of the isolated mammalian heart. *J. Physiol.* 44: 206, 1912.

Kolff, W. J., T. Akutsu, B. Dreyer, and H. Norton. Artificial heart in the chest and use of polyurethane for making hearts, valves, and aortas. *Trans. Amer. Soc. Artif. Intern. Organs* 5:298, 1959.

Kolin, A. An electromagnetic flowmeter. Principle of the method and its application to blood flow measurement. *Proc. Soc. Exp. Biol. Med.* 35:53, 1936.

Kolin, A. An A. C. induction flowmeter for measurement of blood flow in intact blood vessels. *Proc. Soc. Exp. Biol. Med.* 46:235, 1941a.

Kolin, A., J. L. Weissberg, and L. Gerber. Electromagnetic measurement of blood flow and sphygmomanometry in intact animal. *Proc. Soc. Exp. Biol. Med.* 47:324, 1941b.

Kolin, A. An alternating field induction flowmeter of high sensitivity. *Rev. Sci. Instr.* 16:109, 1945.

Kolin, A. Improved apparatus and technique for electromagnetic determination of blood flow. *Rev. Sci. Instr.* 23:235, 1952.

Kolin, A. Blood flow determination by electromagnetic method. In Otto Glasser. *Medical Physics.* Chicago: Year Book Publishers, 1960, Vol. III, p. 141.

Kontos, H. A., D. W. Richardson, and J. L. Patterson, Jr. Effects of hypercapnia on human forearm blood vessels. *Amer. J. Physiol.* 212:1070, 1967.

Kontos, H. A., D. W. Richardson, and J. L. Patterson, Jr. Vasodilator effect of hypercapnic acidosis on human forearm blood vessels. *Amer. J. Physiol.* 215:1403, 1968.

Kontos, H. A. Role of hypercapnic acidosis in the local regulation of blood flow in skeletal muscle. *Circ. Res.* 28:Suppl. I, p. 98, 1971.

Korner, P. I., and I. D. Smith. Cardiac output in normal unanesthetized and anesthetized rabbits. *Aust. J. Exp. Biol.* 32:499, 1954.

Korner, P. I. Circulatory adaptations in hypoxia. *Physiol. Rev.* 39:687, 1959.

Korner, P. I. Some factors influencing the dispersion of indicator substances in the mammalian circulation. *Progr. in Biophys.* 11:111, 1961.

Korner, P. I. The effect of section of the carotid sinus and aortic nerves on the cardiac output of the rabbit. *J. Physiol.* (London) 180:266, 1965.

Korner, P. I., and J. B. Uther. Dynamic characteristics of the cardiovascular autonomic effects during severe arterial hypoxia in the unanesthetized rabbit. *Circ. Res.* 24:671, 1969.

Korner, P. I., and J. B. Uther. Stimulus cardiorespiratory effects response profile during arterial hypoxia in the unanesthetized rabbit. *Aust. J. Exp. Biol. Med. Sci.* 48:663, 1970.

Kot, P. A., C. S. Nunez, E. D. Freis, and J. C. Rose. Cardiac versus peripheral effects of left stellate ganglion stimulation. *Amer. J. Physiol.* 205:576, 1963.

Kovalcik, V. The response of the isolated ductus arteriosus to oxygen and anoxia. *J. Physiol.* 169:185, 1963.

Kowalski, H. J., W. H. Abelmann, W. F. McNeely, N. R. Frank, and L. B. Ellis. The cardiac output of normal subjects determined by the dye-injection method at rest and during exercise. *Amer. J. Med. Sci.* 228:622, 1954.

Kozawa, S. The mechanical regulation of the heart beat in the tortoise. *J. Physiol.* 49:233, 1915.

Knowles, J. H., W. Newman, and W. O. Fenn. Determination of oxygenated mixed venous blood CO_2 tension by a breath method. *J. Appl. Physiol.* 15:225, 1960.

Krames, B., and D. W. Northup. Isometric tension development in the hypertrophied heart. *Fed. Proc.* 23:358, 1964.

Krasney, J. A. Cardiovascular responses to cyanide in awake sinoaortic denervated dogs. *Amer. J. Physiol.* 220:1361, 1971.

Krayer, O. Über die Beziehung zwischen Pulsfrequenz, Minutenvolumen und Venendruck am isolierten Saugetierherzen. *Arch. Exp. Pathol. Pharmakol.* 157:90, 1930.

Krayer, O. Versuche am insuffizienten Herzen. *Arch. Exp. Pathol. Pharmakol.* 162:1, 1931.

Krieger, E. M. Time course of baroreceptor resetting in acute hypertension. *Amer. J. Physiol.* 218:486, 1970.

Kroetz, C. Messung der Kreislaufminutenvolumens mit einem neuen Kohlensäurevefahren. *Zentr. inn. Med.,* p. 275, 1930.

Krogh, A., and J. Lindhard. Measurements of the blood flow through the lungs of man. *Skand. Arch. Physiol.* 27:100, 1912.

Krogh, A., and J. Lindhard. The regulation of respiration and circulation during the initial stages of muscular work. *J. Physiol.* 47:131, 1913.

Krug, H., and L. Schlicher. *Die Dynamik des Venösen Rückstromes.* Leipzig: Veb Georg Thieme, 1960.

Kubicek, W. G., F. J. Kottke, D. J. Laker, and M. B. Vischer. Adaptation in the pressoreceptor reflex mechanisms in experimental neurogenic hypertension. *Amer. J. Physiol.* 175:380, 1953.

Kuhn, H. W., and J. H. Weaver. *Elementary College Algebra.* New York: The Macmillan Company, 1935.

Kuhn, L. A., H. J. Kline, A. J. Marano, Jr., R. I. Hamby, J. Cestero, L. J. Cohn, H. Weinrauch, and M. Berger. Mechanical increase of vascular resistance in experimental myocardial infarction with shock. *Circ. Res.* 19:1086, 1966.

Kumada, M., and K. Sagawa. Aortic nerve activity during blood volume changes. *Amer. J. Physiol.* 218:961, 1970.

Kunkel, P., E. A. Stead, Jr., and S. Weiss. Blood flow and vasomotor reactions in hand, forearm, foot, and calf in response to physical and chemical stimuli. *J. Clin. Invest.* 18:225, 1939.

Kunz, A. L., and C. W. Smith. Theory and design of an on-line cardiac output computer. *J. Appl. Physiol.* 23:784, 1967.

Lacy, W. W., C. Ugaz, and E. V. Newman. The use of indigo carmine for dye dilution curves. *Circ. Res.* 3:570, 1955.

Lagerlöf, H., H. Bucht, L. Werkö, and A. Holmgren. Determination of the cardiac output and the blood volume in the lungs and in the right and left heart by means of dye dilution curves. *Acta Med. Scand.* 239:Suppl., p. 149, 1950.

Lahey, W. J. Physiologic observations on a case of beriberi heart disease, with a note on the acute effects of thiamine. *Amer. J. Med.* 14:248, 1953.

Landis, E. M. Capillary pressure and capillary permeability. *Physiol. Rev.* 14:404, 1934.

Landis, E. M., E. Brown, M. Fauteux, and C. Wise. Central venous pressure in relation to cardiac "competence," blood volume and exercise. *J. Clin. Invest.* 25:237, 1946.

Landis, E. M., and J. C. Hortenstine. Functional significance of venous blood pressure. *Physiol. Rev.* 30:1, 1950.

Landowne, M., and L. N. Katz. Circulatory system: Heart; work and failure, vol. II. In Otto Glasser. *Medical Physics.* Chicago: Year Book Publishers, 1950.

Lange, R. L., C. Smith, and H. H. Hecht. Arterial blood flow patterns in human subjects and their effect on indicator dilution curves from various arterial sites. *J. Clin. Invest.* 39:1413, 1960.

Langston, J. B., A. C. Guyton, and W. J. Gillespie. Acute effect of changes in renal arterial pressure and sympathetic blockade on kidney function. *Amer. J. Physiol.* 197:595, 1959.

Langston, J. B., A. C. Guyton, C. G. Hull, and G. G. Armstrong. Further evidence for the unimportance of renal autoregulation. *Amer. J. Physiol.* 201:495, 1961.

Langston, J. B., A. C. Guyton, B. H. Douglas, and P. E. Dorsett. Effect of changes in salt intake on arterial pressure and renal function in partially nephrectomized dogs. *Circ. Res.* 12:508, 1963.

Lassen, N. A. Cerebral blood flow and oxygen consumption in man. *Physiol. Rev.* 39:183, 1959.

Laurell, H., and B. Pernow. Effect of exercise on plasma potassium in man. *Acta Physiol. Scand.* 66:241, 1966.

Lawrence, J. H., R. L. Huff, L. R. Wasserman, and T. G. Hennessy. A physiological study in the Peruvian Andes. *Acta Med. Scand.* 142:117, 1952.

Lawrence, J. S., L. M. Hurxthal, and A. V. Bock. Variation in blood flow with changes in position in normal and pathologic subjects. *J. Clin. Invest.* 3:613, 1927.

Lawson, H. C., W. F. Cantrell, J. E. Shaw, D. L. Blackburn, and S. Adams. Measurement of cardiac output in the dog by the simultaneous injection of dye and radioactive red cells. *Amer. J. Physiol.* 170:277, 1952.

Lawson, H. C., H. D. Mellette, and E. S. Coleman. The transport of radioactive inorganic phosphate by the pulmonary circulation. *Circ. Res.* 2:248, 1954a.

Lawson, H. C., O. W. Shadle, E. S. Coleman, and D. E. Holtgrave. A comparison of intracardiac and intravenous injections for the measurement of cardiac output by the dilution technic. *Circ. Res.* 2:251, 1954b.

Leeds, S. E. Effects of occlusion of experimental chronic patent ductus arteriosus on cardiac output, pulse, and blood pressure of dogs. *Amer. J. Physiol.* 139:451, 1943.

Lefer, A. M., G. B. Craddock, R. Cowgill, and E. D. Brand. Performance of papillary muscles isolated from cats in postoligemic shock. *Amer. J. Physiol.* 211:687, 1966.

Lefer, A. M., R. Cowgill, F. F. Marshall, L. M. Hail, and E. D. Brand. Characterization of a myocardial depressant factor present in hemorrhagic shock. *Amer. J. Physiol.* 213:492, 1967.

Lefer, A. M., and J. Martin. Origin of myocardial depressant factor in shock. *Amer. J. Physiol.* 218:1423, 1970.

Lefer, A. M., T. M. Glenn, T. J. O'Neill, W. L. Lovett, W. J. Geissinger, and S. L. Wangensteen. Inotropic influence on hemorrhagic pancreatitis. *Surgery* 69:220, 1971.

LePage, G. A. The effects of hemorrhage on tissue metabolites. *Amer. J. Physiol.* 147:446, 1946.

Lequime, J. Le débit cardiaque; études expérimentales et cliniques. *Acta Med. Scand.* 107:Suppl., p. 1, 1940.

Lequime, J., and H. Denolin. Modifications du débit cardiaque lors de l'effort chez les sujets normaux et chez les patients atteints de cardiopathies diverses. *Cardiologia* 32:65, 1958.

Leusen, I., G. Demeester, and J. J. Bouckaert. Influence des réflexes sinocarotidiens sur le débit cardiaque et la résistance périphérique après hémorragie. *Arch. Intern. Physiol.* 62:535, 1954.

Leusen, I., G. Demeester, and J. J. Bouckaert. Presso-récepteurs arteriels et débit cardiaque au cours de l'exercise musculaire. *Arch. Intern. Physiol.* 64:564, 1956a.

Leusen, I., G. Demeester, and J. J. Bouckaert. Influence des pressorécepteurs des sinus carotidiens sur le débit cardiaque. *Arch. Intern. Physiol.* 64:489, 1956b.

Levy, M. N., and R. M. Berne. Effects of acute reduction of cardiac output upon the mechanisms of sodium excretion in the dog. *Amer. J. Physiol.* 166:262, 1951.

Levy, M. N., and L. Share. The influence of

erythrocyte concentration upon the pressure-flow relationships in the dog's hind limb. *Circ. Res.* 1:247, 1953.

Levy, M. N., and S. H. Brind. Influence of l-norepinephrine upon cardiac output in anesthetized dogs. *Circ. Res.* 5:85, 1957.

Levy, M. N., M. Ng, P. Martin, and H. Zieske. Sympathetic and para-sympathetic interactions upon the left ventricle of the dog. *Circ. Res.* 19:5, 1966a.

Levy, M. N., M. Ng, R. I. Lipman, and H. Zieske. Vagus nerves and baroreceptor control of ventricular performance. *Circ. Res.* 18:101, 1966b.

Levy, M. N., M. L. Ng, and H. Zieske. Cardiac response to cephalic ischemia. *Amer. J. Physiol.* 215:169, 1968.

Levy, M. N., and H. Zieske. Autonomic control of cardiac pacemaker activity and atrioventricular transmission. *J. Appl. Physiol.* 27:465, 1969a.

Levy, M. N., and H. Zieske. Effect of enhanced contractility of the left ventricular response to vagus nerve stimulation in dogs. *Circ. Res.* 24:303, 1969b.

Lewis, A. E. Measurement of thoracic visceral plasma volume. *Amer. J. Physiol.* 172: 195, 1953a.

Lewis, A. E. Computation of cardiac output from dye dilution curves. *J. Appl. Physiol.* 6:93, 1953b.

Lewis, D. H., M. Cardenas, and H. Sandberg. Effect of ganglionic blockade on venous pressure and blood volume: Further evidence in favor of increased venomotor tone in congestive heart failure. *Amer. Heart J.* 57:897, 1959.

Lewis, J. M., A. C. Montero, S. A. Kinard, E. W. Dennis, and J. K. Alexander. Hemodynamic response to exercise in isolated pulmonary stenosis. *Circulation* 29:85, 1964.

Lewis, T., and A. N. Drury. Observations relating to arteriovenous aneurysm. *Heart* 10:301, 1923.

Lewis, T. *The Blood Vessels of the Human Skin and Their Responses.* New Haven: Yale University Press, 1924, p. 133.

Liljestrand, G., and N. Stenström. Clinical studies on the work of the heart during rest. I. Blood flow and blood pressure in exophthalmic goiter. *Acta Med. Scand.* 63:99, 1925.

Linden, R. J., and J. H. Mitchell. Relation between left ventricular diastolic pressure and myocardial segment length and observations on the contribution of atrial systole. *Circ. Res.* 8:1092, 1960.

Lindhard, J. Funktionsuntersuchungen an den Lungen des Menschen mittels gasanalytischer Methoden. *Abderhaldens Handb. der biol. Arbeitsmethoden*, Abt. V, Teil 4II, p. 1581, 1925.

Lindsey, A. W., B. F. Banahan, R. N. Cannon, and A. C. Guyton. Pulmonary blood volume of the dog and its changes in acute

heart failure. *Amer. J. Physiol.* 190:45, 1957.

Lindsey, A. W., and A. C. Guyton. Continuous recording of pulmonary blood volume, and pulmonary pressure and volume changes during acute right or left ventricular failure. *Amer. J. Physiol.* 197: 959, 1959.

Liotta, D., T. Taliani, A. H. Giffoniella, A. H. Deheza, S. Liotta, R. Lizarraga, L. Tolocka, J. Panano, and E. Bianciotti. Artificial heart in the chest: Preliminary report. *Trans. Amer. Soc. Artif. Intern. Organs* 7:318, 1961.

Linzbach, A. J. Heart failure from the point of view of quantitative anatomy. *Amer. J. Cardiol.* 5:370, 1960.

Little, R. C. The cardiodynamics of tricuspid insufficiency. *Proc. Soc. Exp. Biol. Med.* 68:602, 1948.

Lochner, W., and H. dal Ri. Die Abhangigkeit der Wirkung einer explosiven Dekompression vom absoluten Druck. *Pflüger's Arch. ges. Physiol.* 264:543, 1957.

Loeb, H. S., R. J. Pietras, J. R. Tobin, Jr., and R. M. Gunnar. Hypovolemia in shock due to acute myocardial infarction. *Circulation* 40:653, 1969.

Loewy, A., and H. von Schrotter. Ein Verfahren zur Bestimmung der Blutgasspannungen, der Kreislaufeschwindigkeit und des Herzschlagvolumens am Menschen. *Arch. Anat. u. Physiol.* Physiol. Abt. 394:1903.

Loewy, A., and H. von Schrotter. Untersuchungen über die Blutcirculation beim Menschen. *Z. Exp. Pathol. Therapy.* 1:197, 1905.

Longino, F. H., and D. E. Gregg. Comparison of cardiac stroke volume as determined by pressure pulse contour method and by a direct method using a rotameter. *Amer. J. Physiol.* 167:721, 1951.

Longnecker, D., and F. L. Abel. Peripheral vascular response to simulated hemorrhagic shock during cardiopulmonary bypass in dogs. *Circ. Res.* 25:107, 1969.

Loo, A. V., and E. C. Heringham. Circulatory changes in the dog produced by acute arteriovenous fistula. *Amer. J. Physiol.* 158: 103, 1949.

Love, W. D., and G. E. Burch. A simple new method for estimating cardiac output. *J. Lab. Clin. Med.* 52:515, 1958.

Lovegrove, T. D., C. W. Gowdy, and J. A. F. Stevenson. Sympathoadrenal system and response of heart to acute exchange anemia. *Circ. Res.* 5:659, 1957.

Lovett, W. L., S. Wangensteen, T. M. Glenn, and A. M. Lefer. Presence of a myocardial depressant factor in patients in circulatory shock. *Surgery* 70:223, 1971.

Lowe, R. D., and J. W. Thompson. The effect of intra-arterial potassium chloride infusion upon forearm blood flow in man. *J. Physiol.* (London) 162:62P, 1962.

Lundgren, O., J. Lundwall, and S. Mellander. Range of sympathetic discharge and reflex vascular adjustments in skeletal muscle during hemorrhagic hypotension. *Acta Physiol. Scand.* 62:380, 1964.

Lundholm, L., and E. Mahme-Lundholm. Energetics of isometric and isotonic contraction in isolated vascular smooth muscle under anaerobic conditions. *Acta Physiol. Scand.* 64:275, 1965.

Lundvall, J., S. Mellander, and T. White. Hyperosmolality and vasodilatation in human skeletal muscle. *Acta Physiol. Scand.* 77:224, 1969.

MacCanon, D. M., and S. M. Horvath. Determinations of cardiac outputs and pulmonary blood volumes by modified tracer dilution procedure. *J. Appl. Physiol.* 7:413, 1955.

MacIntyre, W. J., J. P. Storaasli, H. Krieger, W. Pritchard, and H. L. Friedell. I^{131}-labeled serum albumin: its use in the study of cardiac output and peripheral vascular flow. *Radiology* 59:849, 1952.

MacIntyre, W. J., W. H. Pritchard, and T. W. Moir. The determination of cardiac output by the dilution method without arterial sampling. I. Analytical concepts. *Circulation* 18:1139, 1958.

Mack, R. E., H. J. Wells, and R. Pollack. An in vivo method for the determination of cardiac output. *Radiology* 68:245, 1957.

MacMaster, P. D. The pressure and interstitial resistance prevailing in the normal and edematous skin of animals and man. *J. Exp. Med.* 84:473, 1946.

Maloney, J. V., Jr., and S. W. Handford. Circulatory responses to intermittent positive and alternating positive-negative pressure respirators. *J. Appl. Physiol.* 6:453, 1954.

Maltby, A. B. Cardiac output in Pick syndrome. *Proc. Soc. Exp. Biol. Med.* 31:853, 1934.

Maltby, A. B., and J. E. Williams. Attempts to apply acetylene method of determining output to dog. *J. Lab. Clin. Med.* 21:354, 1936.

Manning, J. W., Jr., and C. N. Peiss. Cardiovascular responses elicited by electrical stimulation of the hypothalamus. *Fed. Proc.* 17:104, 1958.

Manning, J. W. Cardiovascular reflexes following lesions in medullary reticular formation. *Amer. J. Physiol.* 208:283, 1965.

Markoff, I., F. Muller, and N. Zuntz. Neue Methode zur Bestimmung der im menschlichen Korper umlaufenden Blutmenge. *Z. für Balneologie* 4:373, 1911.

Markwalder, J., and E. H. Starling. On the constancy of systolic output under varying conditions. *J. Physiol.* 48:348, 1914.

Marshall, E. K., and A. Grollman. A method for the determination of the circulatory minute volume in man. *Amer. J. Physiol.* 86:117, 1928.

Marshall, R. J., and J. T. Shepherd. Effect of injections of hypertonic solutions on blood flow through the femoral artery of the dog. *Amer. J. Physiol.* 197:951, 1959.

Marshall, R. J., M. J. Allwood, E. W. O. Keck, and J. T. Shepherd. Measurement of cardiac output and "central" blood volume by various systems. *J. Appl. Physiol.* 16:541, 1961.

Mason, D. T. Usefulness and limitation of the rate of rise of intraventricular pressure (dp/dt) in the evaluation of myocardial contractility. *Amer. J. Cardiol.* 23:516, 1969.

Mateeff, D., and C. Petroff. Gravitationsshock beim Menschen nach Muskelarbeit. *Z. ges. Exp. Med.* 85:115, 1932.

Mateeff, D. Der orthostatische Kreislaufkollaps — Gravitationsshock (gravity shock) — beim Menschen nach körperlicher Arbeit. *Arbeitsphysiologie* 8:595, 1935.

Mauck, H. P., Jr., W. Shapiro, and J. L. Patterson. Pulmonary venous (wedge) pressure. Correlation with onset and disappearance of dyspnea in acute left ventricular heart failure. Amer. J. Cardiol. 13:301, 1963.

Mayerson, H. S., and G. E. Burch. Relationships of tissue (subcutaneous and intramuscular) and venous pressures to syncope induced in man by gravity. *Amer. J. Physiol.* 128:258, 1939.

Mayerson, H. S. Roentgenkymographic determination of cardiac output in syncope induced by gravity. *Amer. J. Physiol.* 138:630, 1943.

McCrea, F. D., J. A. E. Eyster, and W. J. Meek. The effect of exercise upon diastolic heart size. *Amer. J. Physiol.* 83:678, 1928.

McCredie, M. Measurement of pulmonary edema in valvular heart disease. *Circulation* 36:381, 1967.

McCubbin, J. W., J. H. Green, and I. H. Page. Baroreceptor function in chronic renal hypertension. *Circ. Res.* 4:205, 1956.

McGregor, M., P. Sekelj, and W. Adam. Measurement of cardiac output in man by dye dilution curves using simultaneous ear oximeter and whole blood cuvette techniques. *Circ. Res.* 9:1083, 1961.

McGuire, J., R. Shore, V. Hauenstein, and F. Goldman. Cardiac output in compensation and decompensation in same individual. *Amer. Heart J.* 16:449, 1938.

McGuire, J. R. Shore, V. Hauenstein, and F. Goldman. Influence of exercise on cardiac output in congestive heart failure. *Arch. Intern. Med.* 63:469, 1939a.

McGuire, J., R. Shore, V. Hauenstein, and F. Goldman. Relation of cardiac output to congestive heart failure. *Arch. Intern. Med.* 63:290, 1939b.

McKee, F. W., J. A. Schilling, G. H. Tishkoff, and R. E. Hyatt. Experimental ascites; effects of sodium chloride and protein intake on protein metabolism of dogs with constricted inferior vena cava. *Surg. Gynec. Obstet.* 89:529, 1949.

McMichael, J., and E. P. Sharpey-Schafer. Cardiac output in man by direct Fick method; effects of posture, venous pressure change, atropine and adrenaline. *Brit. Heart J.* 6:33, 1944.

McMichael, J. Cardiac output methods. *Fed. Proc.* 4:212, 1945.

McMichael, J., and J. P. Shellingford. Role of valvular incompetence in heart failure. *Brit. Med. J.* 1:537, 1957.

Meakins, J., and H. W. Davies. The influence of circulatory disturbances on the gaseous exchange in the blood. II. A method of estimating the circulation rate in man. *Heart* 9:191, 1922.

Meek, W. J., and J. A. E. Eyster. Cardiac size and output in man during rest and moderate exercise. *Amer. J. Physiol.* 63:400, 1923.

Meerson, F. Z., and M. G. Pshennikova. Effect of myocardial hypertrophy on cardiac contractility. *Fed. Proc.* (Translation Suppl.) 24:957, 1965.

Meier, P., and K. L. Zierler. On the theory of the indicator-dilution method for measurement of blood flow and volume. *J. Appl. Physiol.* 6:731, 1954.

Mellander, S. Venous blood flow recorded with an isothermal flowmeter. *Fed. Proc.* 17:394, 1958.

Mellander, S. Comparative studies on the adrenergic neuro-hormonal control of resistance and capacitance blood vessels in the cat. *Acta Physiol. Scand.* 50:Suppl. 176, 1960a.

Mellander, S., and R. F. Rushmer. Venous blood flow recorded with an isothermal flowmeter. *Acta Physiol. Scand.* 48:13, 1960b.

Mellander, S., and D. H. Lewis. Effect of hemorrhagic shock on the reactivity of resistance and capacitance vessels and on capillary filtration transfer in cat skeletal muscle. *Circ. Res.* 13:105, 1963.

Mellander, S., B. Johansson, S. Gray, O. Jonsson, J. Lundvall, and B. Ljung. Effects of hyperosmolarity on intact and isolated vascular smooth muscle: possible role in exercise hyperemia. *Angiologica* 4:310, 1967.

Mellette, H. C., R. W. Booth, J. M. Ryan, and G. F. Rieser. The use of bromsulphalein (B.S.P.) as an indicator for the determination of cardiac output by the dye dilution technique. *J. Lab. Clin. Med.* 51:441, 1958.

Meneely, G. R., M. Stahlman, F. R. McCrea, L. E. Smith, and H. J. Smith, Jr. Ischemic and anoxemic damage to myocardial capillaries and its relation to shock, angina pectoris, and myocardial infarction. *Fed. Proc.* 5:226, 1946.

Mercker, H., and M. Schneider. Über Capillarveränderungen des Gehirns bei Hohenanpassung. *Pflüger's Arch. ges Physiol.* 251:49, 1949.

Merrill, E. W. Rheology of blood. *Physiol. Rev.* 49:863, 1969.

Merriman, J. E., G. M. Wyant, G. Bray, and W. McGeachy. Serial cardiac output determinations in man. *Canad. Anaesth. Soc. J.* 5:375, 1958.

Merritt, F. L., and A. M. Weissler. Reflex venomotor alterations during exercise and hyperventilation. *Amer. Heart J.* 58:382, 1959.

Metcalfe, J., J. W. Woodbury, V. Richards, and C. S. Burwell. Studies in experimental pericardial tamponade; effects on intravascular pressures and cardiac output. *Circulation* 5:518, 1952.

Miller, A. T., and D. M. Hale. Increased vascularity of brain, heart, and skeletal muscle of polycythemic rats. *Amer. J. Physiol.* 219:702, 1970.

Miller, D. E., W. L. Gleason, R. E. Whalen, J. J. Morris, and H. D. McIntosh. Effect of ventricular rate on the cardiac output in the dog with chronic heart block. *Circ. Res.* 10:658, 1962.

Miller, G. A. H., and H. J. C. Swan. Effect of chronic pressure and volume overload on left heart volumes in subjects with congenital heart disease. *Circulation* 30:205, 1964.

Miller, G. A. H., J. W. Kirklin, and H. J. C. Swan. Myocardial function and left ventricular volumes in acquired valvular insufficiency. *Circulation* 31:374, 1965.

Mills, C. J. A catheter tip electromagnetic velocity probe. *Phys. Med. Biol.* 11:323, 1966.

Mills, C. J., and J. P. Shillingford. A catheter tip electromagnetic velocity probe and its evaluation. *Cardiovasc. Res.* 1:263, 1967.

Milnor, W. R., S. A. Talbot, W. P. McKeever, R. B. Marye, and E. V. Newman. A photoelectric ear densitometer for continuously recording the arterial concentration of T-1824 in the dye-dilution method. *Circ. Res.* 1:117, 1953.

Milnor, W. R., A. D. Jose, and C. J. McGaff. Pulmonary vascular volume, resistance, and compliance in man. *Circulation* 22:130, 1960.

Mirkovitch, V., T. Akutsu, W. Seidel, and W. J. Kolff. Study of thrombosis on plastics placed inside the heart resulting in a mitral valve with chordae tendinae. *Trans. Amer. Soc. Artif. Intern. Organs* 7:345, 1961.

Mirsky, I. Left ventricular stresses in the intact human heart. *Biophys. J.* 9:189, 1969.

Mixter, G., Jr. Respiratory augmentation of inferior vena caval flow demonstrated by a low-resistance phasic flowmeter. *Amer. J. Physiol.* 172:446, 1953.

Mohammed, S., C. J. Imig, E. J. Greenfield, and J. W. Eckstein. Thermal indicator sampling and injection sites for cardiac output. *J. Appl. Physiol.* 18:742, 1963.

Monroe, R. G., W. J. Gamble, C. G. LaFarge, A. E. Kumar, and F. J. Manasek. Left ventricular performance at high end-diastolic pressures in isolated, perfused dog hearts. *Circ. Res.* 26:85, 1970.

Moody, N. E., H. D. Barber, B. A. Holmlund, and J. E. Merriman. A cardiac output computer for the rapid analysis of indicator dilution curves. *Digest of the 1961 Conference on Medical Electronics.* New York, July, 1971, p. 179.

Moore, J. W., J. M. Kinsman, W. F. Hamilton, and R. G. Spurling. Studies on the circulation. II. Cardiac output determinations: Comparison of the injection method with the direct Fick procedure. *Amer. J. Physiol.* 89:331, 1929.

Moreno, A. H., A. R. Burchell, R. Van Der Woude, and J. H. Burke. Respiratory regulation of splanchnic and systemic venous return. *Amer. J. Physiol.* 213:455, 1967.

Morgan, B. C., F. L. Abel, G. L. Mullins, and W. G. Guntheroth. Flow patterns in cavae, pulmonary artery, pulmonary vein, and aorta in intact dog. *Amer. J. Physiol.* 210: 903, 1966.

Morhardt, P. E. Collapsus et syncopes par arrêt de la circulation en retour. *Vie Méd.* 16:109, 1935.

Motley, H. L., A. Cournand, L. Werkö, D. T. Dresdale, A. Himmelstein, and D. W. Richards, Jr. Intermittent positive pressure breathing. *J.A.M.A.* 137:370, 1948.

Mueller, H., S. M. Ayres, J. J. Gregory, S. Giannelli, Jr., and W. J. Grace. Hemodynamics, coronary blood flow, and myocardial metabolism in coronary shock; response to l-norepinephrine and isoproterenol. *J. Clin. Invest.* 49:1885, 1970.

Muiesan, G., C. A. Sorbini, C. Valori, V. Grassi, E. Solinas, and V. Renzini. La metodica del rebreathing applicata alla determinazione incruenta della portata circolatoria. *Cuore Circolaz.* 49:136, 1965.

Muiesan, G., C. A. Sorbini, E. Solinas, V. Grassi, G. Casucci, and E. Petz. Comparison of CO_2 − rebreathing and direct Fick methods for determining cardiac output. *J. Appl. Physiol.* 24:424, 1968.

Müller, A., L. Laszt, and L. Pircher. Über ein Menbrannanometer mit elektrischer Transmission zur Druck- und Geschwindigkeitsmessung. *Helv. Physiol. Pharmacol. Acta* 6:783, 1948.

Müller, A. Über die Verwendung des Castelliprinzips zur Geschwindigkeitsmessung. *Helv. Physiol. Pharmacol. Acta* 12:300, 1954a.

Müller, A. Über die Verwendung des Pitotrohres zur Geschwindigkeitsmessung. *Helv. Physiol. Pharmacol. Acta* 12:98, 1954b.

Murphy, G. W., G. Glick, B. F. Schreiner, and P. N. Yu. Cardiac output in acute myocardial infarction. Serial determination by precordial radioisotope dilution curves. *Amer. J. Cardiol.* 11:587, 1963.

Murphy, Q. R., Jr., B. S. Guillixson, C. H. Kratochvil, and J. S. Silva, Jr. Circulatory and renal adjustments to acute femoral arteriovenous fistulas. *Circ. Res.* 6:710, 1958.

Murray, J. F., and I. M. Young. Regional bloodflow and cardiac output during acute hypoxia in the anesthetized dog. *Amer. J. Physiol.* 204:963, 1963a.

Murray, J. F., P. Gold, and B. L. Johnson, Jr. The circulatory effects of hematocrit variations in normovolemic and hypervolemic dogs. *J. Clin. Invest.* 42:1150, 1963b.

Murray, J. F., E. Escobar, and E. Rapaport. Viscosity and the circulatory changes in acute anemia. *Clin. Res.* 14:163, 1966.

Murray, J. F., and E. Escobar. Circulatory effects of blood viscosity: comparison of methemoglobinemia and anemia. *J. Appl. Physiol.* 25:594, 1968.

Murray, J. F., R. B. Carp, and J. A. Nadel. Viscosity effects on pressure-flow relations and vascular resistance in dogs' lungs. *J. Appl. Physiol.* 27:336, 1969a.

Murray, J. F., E. Escobar, and E. Rapaport. Effects of blood viscosity on hemodynamic responses in acute normovolemic anemia. *Amer. J. Physiol.* 216:638, 1969b.

Musshoff, K., H. Reindell, H. Klepzig, and H. W. Kirchkoff. Herzvolumen, Schlagvolumen und körperliche Leistungsfähigkeit. *Cardiologia* 31:359, 1957.

Musshoff, K., H. Reindell, and H. Klepzig. Stroke volume, arterio-venous difference, cardiac output and physical working capacity, and their relationship to heart volume. *Acta Cardiol.* 14:427, 1959.

Mylrea, K. C., and P. H. Albrecht. Hematologic responses of mice subjected to continuous hypoxia. *Amer. J. Physiol.* 218: 1145, 1970.

Nadas, A. S., and A. J. Hauck. Pediatric aspects of congestive heart failure. *Circulation* 21:424, 1960.

Nahas, G. G., F. J. Haddy, and M. B. Visscher. Discrepancies of cardiac output measured by two applications of the direct Fick principle. *Amer. J. Physiol.* 171:752, 1952.

Nahas, G. G., M. B. Visscher, and F. J. Haddy. Discrepancies in cardiac output measurement by two applications of the direct Fick principle. *J. Appl. Physiol.* 6:292, 1953.

Navar, L. G., and P. G. Baer. Renal autoregulatory and glomerular filtration responses to gradated ureteral obstruction. *Nephron* 7:301, 1970a.

Navar, L. G. Minimal preglomerular resistance and calculation of normal glomerular pressure. *Amer. J. Physiol.* 219: 1658, 1970b.

Navar, L. G., J. B. Uther, and P. G. Baer. Pressure diuresis in dogs with diabetes insipidus. *Nephron* 8:97, 1971.

Nealon, T. F., Jr., R. T. Cathcart, W. W. Framow, E. D. McLaughlin, and J. H. Gibbon, Jr. The effect of mean endotracheal pressure on the cardiac output of patients undergoing intrathoracic operations. *J. Thor. Cardiovasc. Surg.* 38:449, 1959.

Neely, W. A., F. C. Wilson, Jr., J. P. Milnor, J. D. Hardy, and H. Wilson. Cardiac output: a clinical comparison of the direct Fick, dye, and ballistocardiographic methods. *Surgery* 35:22, 1954.

Neill, W. A., J. M. Oxendine, and S. C. Moore. Acute and chronic cardiovascular adjustments to induced anemia in dogs. *Amer. J. Physiol.* 217:710, 1969.

Nelson, P. J. Vascular pneumatic constrictor for in vivo calibration of electromagnetic flowmeters. *J. Appl. Physiol.* 22:818, 1967.

Nerlich, W. E. Determinants of impairment of cardiac filling during progressive pericardial effusion. *Circulation* 3:377, 1951.

Newberry, P. D., and A. C. Bryan. Effect on venous compliance and peripheral vascular resistance of headward (+ G_z) acceleration. *J. Appl. Physiol.* 23:150, 1967.

Newman, E. V., M. Merrell, A. Genecin, C. Monge, W. R. Milnor, and W. P. McKeever. The dye-dilution method for describing the central circulation. An analysis of factors shaping the time-concentration curves. *Circulation* 4:735, 1951.

Newman, M. M., E. B. Bay, and W. E. Adams. Ballistocardiography in experimental mitral insufficiency. *Amer. J. Physiol.* 165:497, 1951.

Nicholson, J. W., III, and E. H. Wood. Estimation of cardiac output and Evans blue space in man, using an oximeter. *J. Lab. Clin. Med.* 38:588, 1951.

Nickerson, J. L., Symposium on cardiac output; low frequency, critically damped ballistocardiography. *Fed. Proc.* 4:201, 1945.

Nickerson, J. L., J. V. Warren, and E. S. Brannon. Cardiac output in man; studies with low frequency, critically damped ballistocardiograph and method of right atrial catheterization. *J. Clin. Invest.* 26:1, 1947.

Nickerson, J. L., F. W. Cooper, Jr., R. Robertson, and J. V. Warren. Arterial, atrial and venous pressure changes in the presence of an arteriovenous fistula. *Amer. J. Physiol.* 167:426, 1951a.

Nickerson, J. L., D. C. Elkin, and J. V. Warren. The effect of temporary occlusion of arteriovenous fistulas on heart rate, stroke volume, and cardiac output. *J. Clin. Invest.* 30:215, 1951b.

Nickerson, J. L. Estimation of stroke volume by means of the ballistocardiograph. *Amer. J. Cardiol.* 2:642, 1958.

Nicoll, P. A., and R. L. Webb. Vascular patterns and active vasomotor as determiners of flow through minute vessels. *Angiology* 6:291, 1955.

Nielsen, H. E. Clinical investigations into cardiac output of patients with compensated heart disease during rest and during muscular work. *Acta Med. Scand.* 91:223, 1937.

Noble, M. I. M., T. E. Bowen, and L. L. Hefner. Force-velocity relationship of cat cardiac muscle, studied by the isotonic and quick-release techniques. *Circ. Res.* 25:821, 1969.

Noble, M. I. M. Problems concerning the application of concepts of muscle mechanics to the determination of the contractile state of the heart. *Circulation* 45:252, 1972.

Norton, S. H., T. Akutsu, and W. J. Kolff. Artificial heart with anti-vacuum bellows. *Trans. Amer. Soc. Artif. Intern. Organs* 8:131, 1962.

Nylin, G. On the amount of, and changes in, the residual blood of the heart. *Amer. Heart J.* 25:598, 1943.

Öberg, B., T. Q. Richardson, and A. C. Guyton. Effect of sodium cyanide on cardiac output. *Physiologist* 4:84, 1961.

Öberg, B. Effects of cardiovascular reflexes on net capillary fluid transfer. *Acta Physiol. Scand.* 62:Suppl. 229, p. 1, 1964.

O'Brien, L. J. Negative diastolic pressure in the isolated hypothermic dog heart. *Circ. Res.* 8:956, 1960.

Ohara, I., and T. Sakai. Cardiovascular responses during interruption of the thoracic inferior vena cava; an experimental study. *Tohoku J. Exp. Med.* 66:79, 1957.

Okura, T., S. Tjonneland, P. S. Free, and A. Kantrowitz. A U-shaped mechanical auxiliary ventricle. *Arch. Surg.* 95:821, 1967.

Olmsted, F. Improved electromagnetic flowmeter; phase detection, a new principle. *J. Appl. Physiol.* 16:197, 1961.

Olson, R. M. In vivo blood viscosity and hindrance. *Amer. J. Physiol.* 206:955, 1964.

Olsson, R. A. Changes in content of purine nucleoside in canine myocardium during coronary occlusion. *Circ. Res.* 26:301, 1970.

Opdyke, D. F., and C. J. Wiggers. Studies of right and left ventricular activity during hemorrhagic hypotension and shock. *Amer. J. Physiol.* 147:270, 1946.

Opdyke, D. F., H. F. VanNoate, and G. A. Brecher. Further evidence that inspiration increases right atrial inflow. *Amer. J. Physiol.* 162:259, 1950.

Opdyke, D. F. Genesis of the pressure pulse contour method for calculating cardiac stroke index. *Fed. Proc.* 11:732, 1952.

Opitz, E., and M. Schneider. Über die Sauerstoffvesorgung ges gehirns und den mechanismus von mangelwirkungen. *Ergeb. Physiol.* 46:126, 1950.

Oriol, A. Determination of cardiac output,

using Dow's Formula. *J. Appl. Physiol.* 22:588, 1967.

O'Rourke, M. F., and M. G. Taylor. Vascular impedence of the femoral bed. *Circ. Res.* 18:126, 1966.

O'Rourke, R. A., D. P. Fischer, E. E. Escobar, V. S. Bishop, and E. Rapaport. Effect of acute pericardial tamponade on coronary blood flow. *Amer. J. Physiol.* 212:549, 1967.

Osher, W. J. Pressure-flow relationships of the coronary system. *Amer. J. Physiol.* 172: 403, 1951.

Otis, A. B., H. Rann, and W. O. Fenn. Venous pressure changes associated with positive intrapulmonary pressures; their relationship to the distensibility of the lung. *Amer. J. Physiol.* 146:307, 1946a.

Otis, A. B., H. Rahn, M. Brontman, L. J. Mullins, and W. O. Fenn. Ballistocardiographic study of changes in cardiac output due to respiration. *J. Clin. Invest.* 25:413, 1946b.

Ouellet, Y., S. C. Poh, and M. R. Becklake. Circulatory factors limiting maximal aerobic exercise capacity. *J. Appl. Physiol.* 27:874, 1969.

Overbeck, H. W., J. I. Molnar, and F. J. Haddy. Resistance to blood flow through the vascular bed of the dog forelimb: Local effects of sodium, potassium, calcium, magnesium, acetate, hypertonicity, and hypotonicity. *Amer. J. Cardiol.* 8:533, 1961.

Overbeck, H. W., and G. J. Grega. Response of the limb vascular bed in man to intrabrachial arterial infusions of hypertonic dextrose or hypertonic sodium chloride solutions. *Circ. Res.* 26:717, 1970.

Pace, J. B. Influence of carotid chemoreceptor stimulation on ventricular dynamics. *Amer. J. Physiol.* 218:1687, 1970a.

Pace, J. B., and W. F. Keefe. Influence of efferent vagosympathetic nerve stimulation on right ventricular dynamics. *Amer. J. Physiol.* 218:811, 1970b.

Page, E. B., J. B. Hickam, H. O. Sieker, H. D. McIntosh, and W. W. Pryor. Reflex venomotor activity in normal persons and in patients with postural hypotension. *Circulation* 11:262, 1955.

Pappenheimer, J. R. Passage of molecules through capillary walls. *Physiol. Rev.* 33:387, 1953.

Parker, J. O., R. O. West, J. R. Ledwich, and S. D. Georgi. The effect of acute digitalization on the hemodynamic response to exercise in coronary artery disease. *Circulation* 40:453, 1969.

Parmley, W. W., D. L. Brutsaert, and E. H. Sonnenblick. Effects of altered loading on contractile events in isolated cat papillary muscle. *Circ. Res.* 24:521, 1969.

Patel, D. J., and A. C. Burton. Reactive hyperemia in the human finger. *Circ. Res.* 4:710, 1956.

Patel, D. J., F. M. de Freitas, and D. M. Fry. Hydraulic input impedence to aorta and pulmonary artery in dogs. *J. Appl. Physiol.* 18:134, 1963.

Patterson, G. C., and R. F. Whelan. Reactive hyperemia in the human forearm. *Clin. Sci.* 14:197, 1955.

Patterson, G. C. The role of intravascular pressure in the causation of reactive hyperemia in the human forearm. *Clin. Sci.* 15:17, 1956.

Patterson, S. W., E. H. Piper, and E. H. Starling. The regulation of the heart beat. *J. Physiol.* 48:465, 1914a.

Patterson, S. W., and E. H. Starling. On the mechanical factors which determine the output of the ventricles. *J. Physiol.* 48: 357, 1914b.

Patz, A. Effect of oxygen on immature retinal vessels. *Invest. Ophthal.* 4:988, 1965.

Pavek, K., D. E. Boska, and F. V. Selecky. Measurement of cardiac output by thermodilution with constant rate injection of indicator. *Circ. Res.* 15:311, 1964.

Payne, J. P., D. Gardiner, and I. R. Verner. Cardiac output during halothane anaesthesia. *Brit. J. Anaesthesia* 31(2):87, 1959.

Pearce, M. L., W. P. McKeever, P. Dow, and E. V. Newman. The influence of injection site upon the form of dye dilution curves. *Circ. Res.* 1:112, 1953.

Penna, M., F. Linares, and L. Caceres. Mechanism for cardiac stimulation during hypoxia. *Amer. J. Physiol.* 208:1237, 1965.

Pentecost, B. L., D. W. Irving, and J. P. Shillingford. The effects of posture on the blood flow in the inferior vena cava. *Clin. Sci.* 24:149, 1963.

Pentecost, B. L., and W. G. Austen. Beta-adrenergic blockade in experimental myocardial infarction. *Amer. Heart J.* 72: 790, 1966.

Peters, J. P., and D. D. Van Slyke. *Quantitative Clinical Chemistry.* Methods. Baltimore: The Williams & Wilkins Company, 1932, Vol. II.

Peterson, L. H. Some characteristics of certain reflexes which modify the circulation in man. *Circulation* 2:351, 1950.

Peterson, L. H. Participation of the veins in active regulation of circulation. *Fed. Proc.* 10:104, 1951.

Peterson, L. H. Certain aspects of reflex and mechanical influences upon venous circulation. *Fed. Proc.* 11:122, 1952.

Peterson, L. H., M. Helrich, L. Greene, C. Taylor, and G. Choquette. Measurement of left ventricular output. *J. Appl. Physiol.* 7:258, 1954.

Phinney, A. O., Jr., W. P. C. Clason, P. V. Stoughton, and C. E. McLean. Measurement of cardiac output using the photoelectric earpiece: a comparison with simultaneous Fick measurements. *Circ. Res.* 13:80, 1963.

Pickering, Sir G. Starling and the concept of heart failure. *Circulation* 21:323, 1960.

Pitts, R. F., M. G. Larrabee, and D. W. Bronk. An analysis of hypothalmic cardiovascular control. *Amer. J. Physiol.* 134:359, 1941.

Plesch, J. Hemodynamische studien. *Z. Exp. Pathol. Therap.* 6:380, 1909.

Pollack, A. A., B. E. Taylor, T. T. Myers, and E. H. Wood. The effect of exercise and body position in patients having venous valvular defects. *J. Clin. Invest.* 28:559, 1949a.

Pollack, A. A., and E. H. Wood. Venous pressure in the saphenous vein at the ankle in man during exercise and changes in posture. *J. Appl. Physiol.* 1:649, 1949b.

Pollock, P., M. H. Harmel, and R. E. Clark. Estimation of cardiac output by the ballistocardiograph during thiopental-nitrous oxide-oxygen anesthesia. *Anesthesiology* 16:970, 1955.

Polosa, C., and G. Rossi. Cardiac output and peripheral blood flow during occlusion of carotid arteries. *Amer. J. Physiol.* 200:1185, 1961.

Pool, R. E., and E. Braunwald. Fundamental mechanisms in congestive heart failure. *Amer. J. Cardiol.* 22:7, 1968.

Porciuncula, C. I., G. G. Armstrong, Jr., A. C. Guyton, and H. L. Stone. Delayed compliance in external jugular vein of the dog. *Amer. J. Physiol.* 207:728, 1964.

Porciuncula, C., and J. W. Crowell. Quantitative study of intestinal fluid loss in irreversible hemorrhagic shock. *Amer. J. Physiol.* 205:261, 1963.

Post, R. J. Decrease of cardiac output by acute pericardial effusion and its effect on renal hemodynamics and electrolyte excretion. *Amer. J. Physiol.* 165:278, 1951.

Praglin, J., and G. A. Brecher. Amplifier for 5734-tube bristle flowmeter. *Rev. Sci. Inst.* 26:385, 1955.

Prather, J. W., A. E. Taylor, and A. C. Guyton. Effect of blood volume, mean circulatory pressure, and stress relaxation on cardiac output. *Amer. J. Physiol.* 216:467, 1969.

Prec, K. J., and D. E. Cassels. Dye-dilution curves and cardiac output determinations in newborn infants. *A.M.A. J. Diseases Children* 86:346, 1953.

Prec, K. J., and D. E. Cassels. Dye dilution curves and cardiac output in newborn infants. *Circulation* 11:789, 1955.

Prime, F. J., and T. C. Gray. Difficulties in the application of the Fick principle to the determination of cardiac output in anesthesia. *Anesth. Analg.* 31:347, 1952.

Prinzmetal, M., E. Corday, H. C. Bergman, L. Schwartz, and R. J. Spritzler. Radiocardiography; new method for studying blood flow through chambers of heart in human beings. *Science* 108:340, 1948.

Priola, B. V., and R. L. Fulton. Positive and negative inotropic responses of the atria and ventricles to vagosympathetic stimulation in the isovolumic canine heart. *Circ. Res.* 25:265, 1969.

Pritchard, W. H., W. J. MacIntyre, W. C. Schmidt, B. L. Brofman, and D. J. Moore. The determination of cardiac output by a continuous recording system utilizing iodinated (I^{131}) human serum albumin. II. Clinical studies. *Circulation* 6:572, 1952.

Pritchard, W. H., W. J. MacIntyre, and T. W. Moir. The determination of cardiac output by the dilution method without arterial sampling. II. Validation of precordial recording. *Circulation* 18:1147, 1958.

Quilligan, E. J., C. H. Hendricks, and R. Hingson. Cardiac output: the acute effects of various anesthetic agents and techniques as measured by the pulse-pressure method. *Anesth. Analg.* 36:33, 1957.

Rackley, C. E., H. T. Dodge, T. D. Coble, and R. E. Hay. A method for determining left ventricular mass in man. *Circulation* 29:666, 1964.

Rackley, C. E., V. S. Behar, R. E. Whalen, and H. D. McIntosh. Biplane cineangiographic determinations of left ventricular function: pressure–volume relationships. *Amer. Heart J.* 74:766, 1967.

Rahimtoola, S. H., J. P. Duffy, and H. J. C. Swan. Ventricular performance after angiocardiography. *Circulation* 35:70, 1967.

Rainer, W. G., C. S. Houston, J. P. Newby, and W. R. Coppinger. Experimental artificial heart implantation. *Amer. J. Surg.* 106:645, 1963.

Ralston, H. J., W. D. Collings, A. N. Taylor, and E. Ogden. Venous return in absence of cardiac drive. *Amer. J. Physiol.* 145:441, 1946.

Ramirez de Arellano, A. A., P. S. Hetzel, and E. H. Wood. Measurement of pulmonary blood flow using the indicator-dilution technic in patients with a central arteriovenous shunt. *Circ. Res.* 4:400, 1956.

Randall, W. C., and H. McNally. Augmentor action of the sympathetic cardiac nerves in man. *J. Appl. Physiol.* 15:629, 1960.

Randall, W. C., D. V. Priola, and J. B. Pace. Responses of individual cardiac chambers to stimulation of the cervical vagosympathetic trunk in atropinized dogs. *Circ. Res.* 20:534, 1967.

Randall, W. C., J. S. Wechsler, J. B. Pace, and M. Szentivanyi. Alterations in myocardial contractility during stimulation of the cardiac nerves. *Amer. J. Physiol.* 214:1205, 1968.

Randall, D. C., J. A. Armour, and W. C. Randall. Dynamic responses to cardiac nerve stimulation in the baboon. *Amer. J. Physiol.* 220:526, 1971.

Rapela, C. E., and H. D. Green. Autoregulation of canine cerebral blood flow. *Circ. Res.* 15:Suppl. I, p. 205, 1964.

Raper, A. J., H. A. Kontos, and J. L. Patterson, Jr. Response of pial precapillary vessels to changes in arterial carbon dioxide tension. *Circ. Res.* 28:518, 1971.

Rashkind, W. T., and J. H. Morton. Comparison of constant and instantaneous injection technics for determining cardiac output. *Amer. J. Physiol.* 159:389, 1949.

Rashkind, W. T., D. H. Lewis, J. B. Henderson, D. F. Heiman, and R. B. Dietrick. Venous return as affected by cardiac output and total peripheral resistance. *Amer. J. Physiol.* 175:415, 1953.

Read, R. C., H. Kuida, and J. A. Johnson. Effect of alterations in vasomotor tone on pressure-flow relationships in the totally perfused dog. *Circ. Res.* 5:676, 1957.

Reed, J. H., Jr., and E. H. Wood. Use of dichromatic earpiece densitometry for determination of cardiac output. *J. Appl. Physiol.* 23:373, 1967.

Reeve, E. B. Regulation of blood volume (symposium on regulation of the cardiovascular system in health and disease). *Circulation* 21:1176, 1960.

Reeves, J. T., R. F. Grover, G. F. Filley, and S. G. Blount, Jr. Cardiac output in normal resting man. *J. Appl. Physiol.* 16:276, 1961a.

Reeves, J. T., R. F. Grover, S. G. Blount, Jr., and G. F. Filley. Cardiac output response to standing and treadmill walking. *J. Appl. Physiol.* 16:283, 1961b.

Regan, T. J., F. M. LaForce, D. Teres, J. Block, and H. K. Hellems. Contribution of left ventricle and small bowel in irreversible hemorrhagic shock. *Amer. J. Physiol.* 176:439, 1954.

Reichsman, F., and H. Grant. Some observations on the pathogenesis of edema in cardiac failure. *Amer. Heart J.* 32:438, 1946.

Reid, M. R., and J. McGuire. Arteriovenous aneurysms. *Ann. Surg.* 108:643, 1938.

Rein, H. Die Thermo-Stromuhr. *Z. Biol.* 87:394, 1928.

Rein, H. Vasomotorische regulationen. *Ergebn. Physiol.* 32:28, 1931.

Reiner, L., A. Mazzoleni, F. L. Rodriguez, and R. R. Freudenthal. The weight of the human heart. *Arch. Path.* 68:58, 1959.

Reiss, R. A., and J. R. DiPalma. Right and left heart failure: unilateral rises in right and left auricular pressure in hypervolemic cats following near lethal doses of quinidine, auricular fibrillation and epinephrine. *Amer. J. Physiol.* 155:336, 1948.

Remington, J. W., W. F. Hamilton, and P. Dow. Some difficulties involved in the prediction of the stroke volume from the pulse wave velocity. *Amer. J. Physiol.* 144:536, 1945a.

Remington, J. W., and W. F. Hamilton. The construction of a theoretical cardiac ejection curve from the contour of the aortic pressure pulse. *Amer. J. Physiol.* 144:546, 1945b.

Remington, J. W., and W. F. Hamilton. Quantitative calculation of the time course of cardiac ejection from the pressure pulse. *Amer. J. Physiol.* 148:25, 1947.

Remington, J. W., C. R. Noback, W. F. Hamilton, and J. J. Gold. Volume elasticity characteristics of the human aorta and prediction of the stroke volume from the pressure pulse. *Amer. J. Physiol.* 153:298, 1948.

Remington, J. W., W. F. Hamilton, N. C. Wheeler, and W. F. Hamilton, Jr. Validity of pulse contour method for calculating cardiac output of dog, with notes on effect of various anesthetics. *Amer. J. Physiol.* 159:379, 1949.

Remington, J. W., W. F. Hamilton, G. H. Boyd, Jr., W. F. Hamilton, Jr., and H. M. Caddell. Role of vasoconstriction in the response of the dog to hemorrhage. *Amer. J. Physiol.* 161:116, 1950a.

Remington, J. W., W. F. Hamilton, H. M. Caddell, G. H. Boyd, Jr., and W. F. Hamilton, Jr. Some circulatory responses to hemorrhage in the dog. *Amer. J. Physiol.* 161:106, 1950b.

Remington, J. W., W. F. Hamilton, H. M. Caddell, G. H. Boyd, Jr., and R. W. Pickering. Vasoconstriction as a precipitating factor in traumatic shock in the dog. *Amer. J. Physiol.* 161:125, 1950c.

Remington, J. W. Volume quantitation of the aortic pressure pulse. *Fed. Proc.* 11:750, 1952.

Resnik, H., Jr., B. Friedman, and T. R. Harrison. Effect of certain therapeutic measures on cardiac output of patients with congestive heart failure. *Arch. Intern. Med.* 56:891, 1935.

Reubi, F., and A. Schmid. Le débit cardiaque peut-il être déterminé par la methode de Starr (1954). *Cardiologia* 28:197, 1956.

Richards, D. W., Jr., A. Cournand, R. C. Darling, W. H. Gillespie, and E. DeF. Baldwin. Pressure of blood in the right auricle, in animals and in man: under normal conditions and in right heart failure. *Amer. J. Physiol.* 136:115, 1942.

Richards, D. W., Jr. Cardiac output by catheterization technique in various clinical conditions. *Fed. Proc.* 4:215, 1945.

Richardson, A. W., A. B. Denison, and H. D. Green. A newly modified electromagnetic blood flowmeter capable of high fidelity flow registration. *Circulation* 5:430, 1952.

Richardson, D. W., E. M. Wyso, A. M. Hecht, and D. P. Fitzpatrick. Value of continuous photoelectric recording of dye curves in the estimation of cardiac output. *Circulation* 20:1111, 1959.

Richardson, D. W., H. A. Kontos, A. J. Raper, and J. L. Patterson, Jr. Modification by beta-adrenergic blockade of the circulatory responses to acute hypoxia in man. *J. Clin. Invest.* 46:77, 1967.

Richardson, T. Q., and A. C. Guyton. Effects of polycythemia and anemia on cardiac output and other circulatory factors. *Amer. J. Physiol.* 197:1167, 1959.

Richardson, T. Q., J. O. Stallings, and A. C. Guyton. Pressure-volume curves in live, intact dogs. *Amer. J. Physiol.* 201:471, 1961.

Richardson, T. Q., and J. D. Fermoso. Elevation of mean circulatory pressure in dogs with cerebral ischemia-induced hypertension *J. Appl. Physiol.* 19:1133, 1964.

Richardson, T. Q., J. D. Fermoso, and G. O. Pugh. Effect of acutely elevated intracranial pressure on cardiac output and other circulatory factors. *J. Surg. Res.* 5:318, 1965.

Richman, H. G., and L. Wyborny. Adenine nucleotide degradation in the rabbit heart. *Amer. J. Physiol.* 207:1139, 1964.

Ring, G. C., M. Balaban, and M. J. Oppenheimer. Measurements of heart output by electrokymography. *Amer. J. Physiol.* 157:343, 1949.

Ring, G. C., E. M. Greisheimer, H. N. Baier, M. J. Oppenheimer, A. Sokalchuk, D. Ellis, and S. J. Friday. Electrokymograph for estimation of heart output: comparison with direct Fick in dogs. *Amer. J. Physiol.* 161:231, 1950a.

Ring, G. C., A. Sokalchuk, H. N. Baier, H. Rudel, M. J. Oppenheimer, S. J. Friday, and G. Navis. Electrokymograph for estimation of heart output: comparison with Stewart in dogs. *Amer. J. Physiol.* 161:236, 1950b.

Ring, G. C., M. J. Oppenheimer, H. N. Baier, J. H. Long, A. Sokalchuk, L. L. Bell, D. W. Ellis, P. R. Lynch, L. J. Shapiro, and L. D. Ichtiarowa. Estimation of heart output from electrokymographic measurements in human subjects. *J. Appl. Physiol.* 5:99, 1952.

Ringer, M., and M. Altschule. Cardiac output in diseases of heart, and under influence of digitalis therapy. *Amer. Heart J.* 5:305, 1930.

Robb, J. S., and R. D. Robb. The normal heart, anatomy and physiology of the structural units. *Amer. Heart J.* 23:455, 1942.

Robbins, B. H., and J. H. Baxter, Jr. Cardiac output in dogs under cyclopropane anesthesia. *J. Pharmacol. Exp. Therap.* 62:179, 1938.

Robinson, B. F., S. E. Epstein, G. D. Beiser, and E. Braunwald. Control of heart rate by the autonomic nervous system. Studies in man on the interrelationship between baroreceptor mechanisms and exercise. *Circ. Res.* 19:400, 1966.

Robinson, B. F., S. E. Epstein, R. L. Kahler, and E. Braunwald. Circulatory effects of acute expansion of blood volume: studies during maximal exercise and at rest. *Circ. Res.* 19:26, 1966.

Rochester, D. F., J. Durand, J. O. Parker, H. W. Fritts, Jr., and R. M. Harvey. Estimation of right ventricular output in man using radioactive krypton (Kr^{85}). *J. Clin. Invest.* 40:643, 1961.

Rodbard, S., and W. Stone. Distribution of blood flow through the vena cavae in intracranial compression. *Amer. J. Physiol.* 177:504, 1954.

Rodes, N. D., J. M. Lemley, A. B. Dale, S. E. Stephenson, Jr., and G. R. Meneely. Extracellular water content of the heart in dogs subjected to hemorrhagic shock measured with the radioactive isotope of sodium. *Amer. J. Physiol.* 157:254, 1949.

Rodrigo, F. A. Estimation of valve area and "valvular resistance." *Amer. Heart J.* 45:1, 1953.

Roos, A., and J. R. Smith. Production of experimental heart failure in dogs with intact circulation. *Amer. J. Physiol.* 153:558, 1948.

Root, R. W. *Handbook of Respiration.* Philadelphia: W. B. Saunders Company, 1958, Table 67.

Root, W. S., Walcott, W. W., and M. I. Gregersen. Effects of muscle trauma and of hemorrhage upon cardiac output of dog. *Amer. J. Physiol.* 151:34, 1947.

Rose, J. C., S. J. Cosimano, Jr., C. A. Hufnagel, and E. A. Massullo. The effects of exclusion of the right ventricle from the circulation in dogs. *J. Clin. Invest.* 34:1625, 1955.

Rose, J. C. The Fick principle and the cardiac output. *G. P.* 14:115, 1956.

Rosen, I. T., and H. L. White. The relation of pulse pressure to stroke volume. *Amer. J. Physiol.* 78:168, 1926.

Rosenblueth, A., J. Alania, R. Rubio, and G. Pilar. Relations between coronary flow and work of the heart. *Amer. J. Physiol.* 200:243, 1961.

Rosenthal, A., D. G. Nathan, A. T. Marty, L. N. Button, O. S. Miettinen, and A. S. Nadas. Acute hemodynamic effects of red cell volume reduction in polycythemia of cyanotic congenital heart disease. *Circulation* 42:297, 1970.

Ross, C. A. Cardiovascular responses of unanesthetized rats during traumatic and endotoxin shock. *Proc. Soc. Exp. Biol. Med.* 96:582, 1957.

Ross, J. M., H. M. Fairchild, J. F. Weldy, and A. C. Guyton. Autoregulation of blood flow by oxygen lack. *Amer. J. Physiol.* 202:21, 1962.

Ross, J. Jr., J. W. Linhart, and E. Braunwald. Effects of changing heart rate in man by electrical stimulation of the right atrium: Studies at rest, during exercise, and with isoproterenol. *Circulation* 32:549, 1965.

Ross, J., Jr., J. W. Covell, E. H. Sonnenblick, and E. Braunwald. Contractile state of the heart characterized by force-velocity relations in variably afterloaded and isovolumic beats. *Circ. Res.* 18:149, 1966.

Ross, J., E. H. Sonnenblick, J. W. Covell, G. A. Kaiser, and D. Spiro. The architecture of the heart in systole and diastole. *Circ. Res.* 21:409, 1967a.

Ross, J., Jr., J. W. Covell, and E. H. Sonnenblick. The mechanics of left ventricular contraction in acute experimental cardiac failure. *J. Clin. Invest.* 46:299, 1967b.

Rost, E., Jr. Beitrag zur Kenntuis der Kreislaufverhaltnisse bei Wiederbelebung durch Veranderung des intrapulmonalen Druckes. *Z. Ges. Exp. Med.* 82:255, 1932.

Rothe, C. F., and L. A. Sapirstein. A Rapid blood sample collector for use in the determination of cardiac output. *Amer. Heart J.* 48:141, 1954.

Rothe, C. F., J. R. Love, and E. E. Selkurt. Control of total vascular resistance in hemorrhagic shock in the dog. *Circ. Res.* 12:667, 1963.

Rothe, C. F., and E. E. Selkurt. Cardiac and peripheral failure in hemorrhagic shock in the dog. *Amer. J. Physiol.* 207:203, 1964.

Rothe, C. F. Cardiac and peripheral failure in hemorrhagic shock treated with massive transfusions. *Amer. J. Physiol.* 210:1347, 1966.

Rotta, A. Physiologic condition of the heart in the natives of high altitudes. *Amer. Heart J.* 33:669, 1949.

Roughton, F. J. W., and P. F. Scholander. Microgasometric estimation of blood gases: I. Oxygen. *J. Biol. Chem.* 148:541, 1943.

Rowlands, D. J., and D. E. Donald. Sympathetic vasoconstrictive responses during exercise- or drug-induced vasodilatation. *Circ. Res.* 23:45, 1968.

Roy, C. S. The elastic properties of the arterial wall. *J. Physiol.* 3:125, 1881.

Roy, S. B., M. L. Bhatia, V. S. Mathur, and S. Virman. Hemodynamic effects of chronic severe anemia. *Circulation* 28:346, 1963.

Rubin, A. L., N. Spritz, A. W. Mead, R. A. Herrmann, W. S. Braveman, and E. H. Luckey, The use of L-lysine monohydrochloride in combination with mercurial diuretics in the treatment of refractory fluid retention. *Circulation* 21:332, 1960.

Rubio, R., R. M. Berne, and M. Katori. Release of adenosine in reactive hyperemia of the dog heart. *Amer. J. Physiol.* 216:56, 1969a.

Rubio, R., and R. M. Berne. Release of adenosine by the normal myocardium in dogs and its relationship to the regulation of coronary resistance. *Circ. Res.* 25:407, 1969b.

Rushmer, R. F., and N. Thal. Mechanics of ventricular contraction. A cinefluorographic study. *Circulation* 4:219, 1951.

Rushmer, R. F., D. K. Crystal, C. Wagner, R. M. Ellis, and A. A. Nash. Continuous measurements of left ventricular dimensions in intact, unanesthetized dogs. *Circ. Res.* 2:14, 1954.

Rushmer, R. F. Length-circumference relations of the left ventricle. *Circ. Res.* 3:639, 1955.

Rushmer, R. F. Pressure-circumference relations of left ventricle. *Amer. J. Physiol.* 186:115, 1956a.

Rushmer, R. F., D. Franklin, and R. Ellis. Left ventricular dimensions recorded by sonocardiometry. *Circ. Res.* 4:684, 1956b.

Rushmer, R. F., and T. C. West. Role of autonomic hormones on left ventricular performance continuously analyzed by electronic computers. *Circ. Res.* 5:240, 1957.

Rushmer, R. F. Autonomic balance in cardiac control. *Amer. J. Physiol.* 192:631, 1958.

Rushmer, R. F., and D. A. Smith, Jr. Cardiac control. *Physiol. Rev.* 39:41, 1959.

Rushmer, R. F. *Cardiovascular Dynamics.* Philadelphia: W. B. Saunders Company, 1961, Chapter 3.

Ryder, H. W., W. E. Molle, and E. B. Ferris, Jr. The influence of the collapsibility of veins on venous pressure, including a new procedure for measuring tissue pressure. *J. Clin. Invest.* 23:333, 1944.

Sagawa, K., J. M. Ross, and A. C. Guyton. Quantitation of the cerebral ischemic pressor response in dogs. *Amer. J. Physiol.* 200:1164, 1961a.

Sagawa, K., A. E. Taylor, and A. C. Guyton. Dynamic performance and stability of cerebral ischemic-pressor response. *Amer. J. Physiol.* 201:1164, 1961b.

Sagawa, K., O. Carrier, and A. C. Guyton. Elicitation of theoretically predicted feedback oscillation in arterial pressure. *Amer. J. Physiol.* 203:141, 1962.

Sagawa, K., and K. Watenabe. Summation of bilateral corotid sinus signals in the barostatic reflex. *Amer. J. Physiol.* 209:1278, 1965.

Sagawa, K. Cardiac output as a function of arterial pressure. *Fed. Proc.* 25:268, 1966.

Sagawa, K. Analysis of the ventricular pumping capacity as a function of input and output pressure loads. In E. B. Reeve and A. C. Guyton (Eds.). *Physical Bases of Circulatory Transport: Regulation and Exchange.* Philadelphia: W. B. Saunders Company, 1967, p. 141.

Sagawa, K. Analysis of the CNS ischemic feedback regulation of the circulation. In E. B. Reeve and A. C. Guyton (Eds.). *Physical Bases of Circulatory Transport: Regulation and Exchange.* Philadelphia: W. B. Saunders Company, 1967, p. 129.

Salisbury, P. F., C. E. Cross, K. Katsuhara, and P. A. Rieben. Factors which initiate or influence edema in the isolated dog's heart. *Circ. Res.* 9:601, 1961.

Salisbury, P. F., C. E. Cross, P. A. Rieben and D. Sodi-Pallares. Physiologic and electrocardiographic correlations in experimental left heart failure. *Amer. J. Physiol.* 209: 928, 1965.

Samet, P., W. H. Bernstein, and A. Medow. Effect of site of injection upon left ventricular indicator-dilution output. *Amer. Heart J.* 69:241, 1965.

Sanchez, C., C. Marino, and M. Figallo. Simultaneous measurement of plasma volume and cell mass in polycythemia of high altitude. *J. Appl. Physiol.* 28:775, 1970.

Sandler, H., and H. T. Dodge. Left ventricular tension and stress in man. *Circ. Res.* 13:91, 1963.

Sandler, H. H., R. R. Dodge, and W. A. Baxley. Calculation of left ventricular volume from single plan (A-P) angiocardiograms. *J. Clin. Invest.* 44:1094, 1965.

Sanmarco, M. E., K. Fronek, C. M. Phillips, and J. C. Davila. Continuous measurement of left ventricular volume in dogs. II. Comparison of washout and radiographic techniques with the external dimension method. *Amer. J. Cardiol.* 18:584, 1966a.

Sanmarco, M. E., and H. B. Stuart. Measurement of left ventricular volume in the canine heart by biplane angiocardiography; accuracy of the method using different model analogies. *Circ. Res.* 19:11, 1966b.

Sapirstein, L. A., R. W. Greene, M. J. Mandel, and H. B. Hull. A constant infusion technique for the determination of cardiac output. *Amer. J. Physiol.* 177:134, 1954a.

Sapirstein, L. A., M. J. Mandel, A. Pultz, R. W. Greene, and C. H. Hendricks. Determination of cardiac output by a constant infusion technique in man; its employment to validate infusion-slope measurement of para-amino hippuric acid and space clearance. *J. Appl. Physiol.* 6: 753, 1954b.

Sapirstein, L. A., and F. A. Hartman. Cardiac output and its distribution in the chicken. *Amer. J. Physiol.* 196:751, 1959.

Sapirstein, L. A., E. H. Sapirstein, and A. Bredemeyer. Effect of hemorrhage on the cardiac output and its distribution in the rat. *Circ. Res.* 8:135, 1960.

Sarnoff, S. J., E. Berglund, and P. E. Waithe. Measurement of systemic blood flow. *Proc. Soc. Exp. Biol. Med.* 79:414, 1952.

Sarnoff, S. J., and E. Berglund. Potter electroturbinometer. An instrument for recording total systemic blood flow in the dog. *Circ. Res.* 1:331, 1953.

Sarnoff, S. J., and E. Berglund. Ventricular function. I. Starling's law of the heart studied by means of simultaneous left and right ventricular function curves in the dog. *Circulation* 9:706, 1954a.

Sarnoff, S. J., R. B. Case, E. Berglund, and L. C. Sarnoff. Ventricular function. V.

The circulatory effects of aramine; mechanism of action of "vasopressor" drugs in cardiogenic shock. *Circulation* 10:84, 1954b.

Sarnoff, S. J. Myocardial contractility as described by ventricular function curves. *Physiol. Rev.* 35:107, 1955.

Scarbrough, W. R., E. F. Folk, III, P. M. Smith, and J. H. Condon. The nature of records from ultra-low frequency ballistocardiographic systems and their relation to circulatory events. *Amer. J. Cardiol.* 2: 613, 1958.

Scheel, K. W., D. G. Watson, and P. H. Lehan. An improved on-line calibrator for dye-dilution curves. *J. Appl. Physiol.* 26: 667, 1969.

Scheel, K. W., M. Banet, C. Ott, and P. H. Lehan. A quantitative approach to collateral and antegrade flows after coronary occlusion. *Amer. J. Physiol.* 222:687, 1972.

Schenk, W. G., Jr., B. A. Portin, and M. B. Leslie. The electronic measurement of cardiac output. *Surgery* 44:333, 1958.

Scher, A. M., T. H. Weigert, and A. C. Young. Compact flowmeters for use in the unanesthetized animal, an electronic version of Chauveau's hemodrometer. *Science* 118:82, 1953.

Scher, A. M., and A. C. Young. Servoanalysis of peripheral vascular responses to carotid sinus pressure. *Proc. International Union Physiol. Sci.,* Vol. 2, Abstract 158. Amsterdam: Excerpta Medica Foundation, 1962.

Schmid, A., and F. Reubi. Vergleichende Herzminutenvolumen bestimmung mit der Wezler-Böger Pulswellenmethode undrach dem direkten Fickschen Prinzip. *Cardiologia* 19:42, 1951.

Schmid, A., F. Reubi, and V. Settler. Simultane Herzminutenvolumenbestimmung nach Fick und mit der Pulswellenmethode nach Wezler-Böger unter Hydrazinophthalazin (Apresolin). *Cardiologia* 23:90, 1953.

Schmidt, C. F. *The Cerebral Circulation in Health and Disease.* Springfield, Illinois: Charles C Thomas, Publisher, 1950.

Schnabel, T. G., Jr., H. Eliasch, B. Thomasson, and L. Werkö. Effect of experimentally induced hypervolemia on cardiac function in normal subjects and patients with mitral stenosis. *J. Clin. Invest.* 38:117, 1959.

Schneider, E. C., and C. B. Crampton. A comparison of some respiratory and circulatory reactions of athletes and nonathletes. *Amer. J. Physiol.* 129:165, 1940.

Schneider, E. G., J. O. Davis, C. A. Robb, and J. S. Baumber. Hepatic clearance of renin in canine experimental models for low- and high-output heart failure. *Circ. Res.* 24:213, 1969.

Schreiner, B. F., Jr., G. W. Murphy, G. Glick, and P. N. Yu. Effect of exercise on the pulmonary blood volume in patients with acquired heart disease. *Circulation* 27:559, 1963.

Schröder, G., and L. Werkö. Hemodynamic studies and clinical experience with nethalide, a beta-adrenergic blocking agent. *Amer. J. Cardiol.* 15:58, 1965.

Scott, J. C. Cardiac output in standing position. *Amer. J. Physiol.* 115:268, 1936.

Scott, J. C., H. C. Bazett, and G. C. Machie. Climatic effects on cardiac output and circulation in man. *Amer. J. Physiol.* 129: 102, 1940.

Scott, J. B., R. M. Daugherty, Jr., J. M. Dabney, and F. J. Haddy. Role of chemical factors in regulation of flow through kidney, hindlimb, and heart. *Amer. J. Physiol.* 208:813, 1965.

Scott, J. B., M. Rudko, D. Radawski, and F. J. Haddy. Role of osmolarity, K^+, H^+, Mg^{++} and O_2 in local blood flow regulation. *Amer. J. Physiol.* 218:338, 1970.

Seely, R. D. Dynamic effect of inspiration on the simultaneous stroke volume of the right and left ventricles. *Amer. J. Physiol.* 154:273, 1948.

Seely, R. D., and D. E. Gregg. A technique for measuring cardiac output directly by cannulation of the pulmonary artery. *Proc. Soc. Exp. Biol. Med.* 73:269, 1950a.

Seely, R. D., W. E. Nerlich, and D. E. Gregg. Comparison of cardiac output determined by the Fick procedure and a direct method using the rotameter. *Circulation* 1:1261, 1950b.

Seidel, W., T. Akutsu, V. Mirkovitch, F. Brown, and W. J. Kolff. Air-driven artificial hearts inside the chest. *Trans. Amer. Soc. Artif. Intern. Organs* 7:378, 1961.

Sekelj, P., W. Jegier, and A. L. Johnson. Automatic electronic computer for the estimation of arterial concentration of Evans blue dye. *Amer. Heart J.* 55:485, 1958a.

Sekelj, P., D. V. Bates, A. L. Johnson, and W. Jegier. Estimation of cardiac output in man by dye dilution method using an automatic computing oximeter. *Amer. Heart J.* 58:810, 1958b.

Sekelj, P., K. R. Shankar, J. Doman, I. P. Sukumar, and W. H. Palmer. Trichromatic ear densitometer for estimation of cardiac output using inodcyanine green. *J. Appl. Physiol.* 29:249, 1970.

Seldon, W. A., J. B. Hickie, and E. P. George. Measurement of cardiac output using a radioisotope and a scintillation counter. *Brit. Heart J.* 21:401, 1959.

Seligman, A. M., H. A. Frank, and J. Fine. Traumatic shock: XII. Hemodynamic effects of alterations of blood viscosity in normal dogs and in dogs in shock. *J. Clin. Invest.* 25:1, 1946.

Selkurt, E. E. Relationship of renal blood flow to effective arterial pressure in the intact kidney of the dog. *Amer. J. Physiol.* 147:537, 1946.

Selzer, A., and R. B. Sudrann. Reliability of the determination of cardiac output in man by means of the Fick principle. *Circ. Res.* 6:485, 1958.

Sevelius, G., and P. C. Johnson. Blood flow determined by the use of radioiodinated serum albumin and an externally placed scintillator detector. *Southern Med. J.* 52: 1058, 1959.

Severinghaus, J. W., and N. Lassen. Step hypocapnia to separate arterial from tissue Pco_2 in the regulation of cerebral blood flow. *Circ. Res.* 20:272, 1967.

Seymour, W. B., W. H. Pritchard, L. P. Langley, and J. M. Hayman, Jr. Cardiac output, blood, and interstitial fluid volumes, total circulating serum protein, and kidney function during cardiac failure and after improvement. *J. Clin. Invest.* 21:229, 1942.

Shadle, O. W., T. B. Ferguson, D. E. Gregg, and S. R. Gilford. Evaluation of a new cuvette densitometer for determination of cardiac output. *Circ. Res.* 1:200, 1953.

Shadle, O. W., M. Zukof, and J. Diana. Translocation of blood from the isolated dog's hindlimb during levarterenol infusion and sciatic nerve stimulation. *Circ. Res.* 6:326, 1958.

Shapiro, W., A. J. Wasserman, and J. L. Patterson, Jr. Mechanism and pattern of human cerebrovascular regulation after rapid changes in blood CO_2 tension. *J. Clin. Invest.* 45:913, 1966a.

Shapiro, W., A. J. Wasserman, and J. L. Patterson. Human cerebrovascular response to combined hypoxia and hypercapnia. *Circ. Res.* 19:903, 1966b.

Sharp, J. T., I. L. Bunnell, J. F. Holland, G. T. Griffith, and D. C. Green. Hemodynamics during induced cardiac tamponade in man. *Amer. J. Med.* 29:640, 1960.

Sharpey-Schafer, E. P. Cardiac output in severe anemia. *Clin. Sci.* 5:125, 1944.

Shepherd, A. P., Jr., H. J. Granger, E. E. Smith, and A. C. Guyton. Local control of tissue oxygen delivery and its contribution to the regulation of cardiac output. In press.

Shepherd, J. T., D. Bowers, and E. H. Wood. Measurement of cardiac output in man by injection of dye at a constant rate into the right ventricle or pulmonary artery. *J. Appl. Physiol.* 7:629, 1955.

Shepherd, J. T. Behavior of resistance and capacity vessels in human limbs during exercise. *Circ. Res.* 20:Suppl. I, p. 70, 1967.

Sheppard, C. W. Synthesis of dye dilution curves. *Amer. J. Physiol.* 171:767, 1952.

Sheppard, C. W. *Basic Principles of the Tracer Method.* New York: John Wiley and Sons, 1962.

Shipley, R. E., and E. C. Crittenden, Jr.

Optical recording rotameter for measuring blood flow. *Proc. Soc. Exp. Biol. Med.* 56:103, 1944.

Shipley, R. E., and D. E. Gregg. The cardiac response to stimulation of the stellate ganglia and cardiac nerves. *Amer. J. Physiol.* 143:396, 1945.

Shipley, R. E. Rotameter. In: Potter, V. R. *Methods in Medical Research.* Chicago: Year Book Publishers, 1948, Vol. 1, p. 96.

Shipley, R. E., and C. Wilson. An improved recording rotameter. *Proc. Soc. Exp. Biol. Med.* 78:725, 1951.

Shore, R., J. P. Holt, and P. K. Knoefel. Determination of cardiac output in the dog by the Fick procedure. *Amer. J. Physiol.* 143:709, 1945.

Shubin, H. Shock mechanisms and therapy. In H. G. Lasch (Ed.). *Microcirculation, Hemostasis and Shock.* New York: F. K. Schattauer Verlag, 1969, p. 129.

Shuler, R. H., C. Ensor, R. E. Gunning, W. G. Moss, and V. Johnson. The differential effects of respiration on the left and right ventricles. *Amer. J. Physiol.* 137:620, 1942.

Siegel, H. W., and S. E. Downing. Contributions of coronary perfusion pressure, metabolic acidosis and adrenergic factors to the reduction of myocardial contractility during hemorrhagic shock in the cat. *Circ. Res.* 27:875, 1970.

Sikand, R., P. Cerretelli, and L. E. Farhi. Effects of $\dot{V}$ and $\dot{V}_a/\dot{Q}$ distribution and of time on the alveolar plateau. *J. Appl. Physiol.* 21:1331, 1966.

Simeone, F. A. Experimental hemorrhagic shock and irreversibility. In L. C. Mills and J. H. Moyer (Eds.). *Shock and Hypotension.* New York: Grune & Stratton, Inc., 1965, p. 588.

Simonson, E., and N. Enzer. Physiology of muscular exercise and fatigue in disease. *Medicine* 21:345, 1942.

Sinclair, J. E., W. F. Sutterer, I. J. Fox, and E. H. Wood. Apparent dye-dilution curves produced by injection of transparent solutions. *J. Appl. Physiol.* 16:669, 1961.

Sinclair, S., J. H. Duff, and L. D. MacLean. Use of a computer for calculating cardiac output. *Surgery* 57:414, 1965.

Singh, N., A. J. Ranieri, Jr., N. R. Vest, Jr., D. L. Bowers, and J. F. Dammann, Jr. Simultaneous determinations of cardiac output by thermal dilution, fiberoptic and dye-dilution methods. *Amer. J. Cardiol.* 25:579, 1970.

Skinner, R. L., and D. K. Gehmlich. Analog computer aids heart ailment diganosis. *Electronics* 32:56, 1959.

Skinner, N. S., Jr., and W. J. Powell, Jr. Action of oxygen and potassium on vascular resistance of dog's skeletal muscle. *Amer. J. Physiol.* 212:533, 1967a.

Skinner, N. S., Jr., and W. J. Powell, Jr.

Regulation of skeletal muscle blood flow during exercise. *Circ. Res.* 21:59, 1967b.

Skinner, N. S., Jr., and J. C. Costin. Role of O_2 and K^+ in abolition of sympathetic vasoconstriction in dog skeletal muscle. *Amer. J. Physiol.* 217:438, 1969.

Skinner, N. S., Jr., and J. C. Costin. Interactions of vasoactive substances in exercise hyperemia: O_2, K^+, and osmolality. *Amer. J. Physiol.* 219:1386, 1970.

Skinner, N. S., and J. C. Costin. Interactions between oxygen, potassium, and osmolality in regulation of skeletal muscle blood flow. *Circ. Res.* 29:Suppl. I, p. 73, 1971.

Skovborg, R., A. V. Nielsen, and J. Schlichtkrull. Blood viscosity and vascular flow rate. *Scand. J. Clin. Lab. Invest.* 21:83, 1968.

Sleator, W., Jr., J. O. Elam, W. N. Elam, and H. L. White. Oximetric determinations of cardiac output responses to light exercise. *J. Appl. Physiol.* 3:649, 1951.

Smirk, F. H. Observations on the causes of edema in congestive heart failure. *Clin. Sci.* 2:317, 1936.

Smith, D. J., and J. R. Vane. Effects of oxygen tension on vascular and other smooth muscle. *J. Physiol.* 186:284, 1966.

Smith, E. E., and J. W. Crowell. Influence of hematocrit ratio on survival of unacclimatized dogs at simulated high altitude. *Amer. J. Physiol.* 205:1172, 1963.

Smith, E. E., and J. W. Crowell. Role of an increased hematocrit in altitude acclimatization. *Aerospace Med.* 38:39, 1967a.

Smith, E. E., and J. W. Crowell. Influence of hypoxia on mean circulatory pressure and cardiac output. *Amer. J. Physiol.* 212:1967b.

Smith, E. E., J. W. Crowell, C. J. Moran, and R. A. Smith. Intestinal fluid loss in dogs during irreversible hemorrhagic shock. *Surg. Gynec. Obstet.* 125:45, 1967c.

Smith, E. L., and R. A. Huggins. Effect of dibenamine on blood flow and cardiac output in dog. *Proc. Soc. Exp. Biol. Med.* 71:106, 1949.

Smith, E. L., R. A. Huggins, R. W. Randall, and G. A. Jeffrey. Hemodynamic changes resulting from insertion of a rotameter in the venous circulation of a dog. *Texas Repts. Biol. Med.* 10:674, 1952.

Smith, H. W. *Principles of Renal Physiology.* New York: Oxford University Press, 1956.

Smith, O. A., Jr., and M. A. Nathan. Inhibition of the carotid sinus reflex by stimulation of the inferior olive. *Science* 154:674, 1966.

Smith, W. M., A. N. Damato, and J. G. Galante. Response of the heart to exercise. *Clin. Res.* 12:81, 1964.

Smulyan, H., R. P. Cuddy, W. A. Vincent, U. Kashemsant, and R. H. Eich. Initial hemodynamic responses to mild exercise in trained dogs. *Amer. J. Physiol.* 20:437, 1965.

Snyder, G. K. Influence of temperature and hematocrit on blood viscosity. *Amer. J. Physiol.* 220:1667, 1971.

Snyder, J., and E. H. Wood. Effect of heart rate on atrial contribution to cardiac performance in dogs with complete heart block. *Fed. Proc.* 21:137, 1962.

Sodeman, W. A. *Pathologic Physiology.* Philadelphia: W. B. Saunders Company, 1961.

Sokoloff, L., and S. S. Kety. Regulation of cerebral circulation. *Physiol. Rev.* 40:38, 1960.

Solis, R. T., and S. E. Downing. Effects of *E. coli* endotoxemia on ventricular performance. *Amer. J. Physiol.* 211:307, 1966.

Soloff, L. A., J. Zatuchni, and G. E. Mark, Jr. Relationship of left atrial volume to pulmonary artery and wedge pressures in mitral stenosis. *Circulation* 13:334, 1956.

Soloff, L. A. On measuring left ventricular volume. *Amer. J. Cardiol.* 18:2, 1966.

Sonnenblick, E. H. Force-velocity relation in mammalian heart muscle. *Amer. J. Physiol.* 202:931, 1962a.

Sonnenblick, E. H. Implications of muscle mechanics in the heart. *Fed. Proc.* 21:975, 1962b.

Sonnenblick, E. H., D. Spiro, and T. S. Cottrell. Five structural changes in heart muscle in relation to the length-tension curve. *Proc. Nat. Acad. Sci.* 49:193, 1963.

Sonnenblick, E. H. Series elastic and contractile elements in heart muscle: Changes in muscle length. *Amer. J. Physiol.* 207:1330, 1964.

Sonnenblick, E. H. Instantaneous force-velocity-length determinants in the contraction of heart muscle. *Circ. Res.* 16:441, 1965a.

Sonnenblick, E. H., E. Braunwald, J. F. Williams, Jr., and G. Glick. Effects of exercise on myocardial force-velocity relations in intact unanesthetized man: relative roles of changes in heart rate, sympathetic activity, and ventricular dimensions. *J. Clin. Invest.* 44:2051, 1965b.

Sonnenblick, E. H., Ross, J., Jr., J. W. Covell, H. M. Spotnitz, and D. Spiro. The ultrastructure of the heart in systole and diastole: Changes in sarcomere length. *Circ. Res.* 21:423, 1967a.

Sonnenblick, E. H. Active state in heart muscle: Its delayed onset and modification by inotropic agents. *J. Gen. Physiol.* 50:661, 1967b.

Spann, J., Jr., C. A. Chidsey, P. E. Pool, and E. Braunwald. Mechanism of norepinephrine depletion in experimental heart failure produced by aortic constriction in the guinea pig. *Circ. Res.* 17:312, 1965.

Spann, J. F., Jr., R. A. Buccino, E. H. Sonnenblick, and E. Braunwald. Contractile state of the myocardium in ventricular hypertrophy and heart failure. *Circulation* 34:Suppl. III, p. 222, 1966.

Spann, J. F., Jr., R. A. Buccino, E. H. Son-nenblick, and E. Braunwald. Contractile state of cardiac muscle obtained from cats with experimentally produced ventricular hypertrophy and heart failure. *Circ. Res.* 21:341, 1967.

Spencer, M. P., and A. B. Denison. The aortic flow pulse as related to differential pressure. *Circ. Res.* 4:476, 1956.

Spencer, M. P., A. B. Denison, Jr., and C. A. Barefoot. Continuous measurement of cardiac output in conscious dogs by means of an indwelling magnet and the square-wave magnetic flowmeter. *Fed. Proc.* 17:154, 1958.

Spencer, M. P. Differential pressure measurement; paired transducer system. In: *Methods in Medical Research.* Chicago: Year Book Publishers, 1960a, Vol. 8, p. 341.

Spencer, M. P., and A. B. Denison, Jr. Square-wave electromagnetic flowmeter for surgical and experimental application. In: *Methods in Medical Research.* Chicago: Year Book Publishers, 1960b, Vol. 8, p. 321.

Spencer, M. P., and F. C. Greiss. Dynamics of ventricular ejection. *Circ. Res.* 10:274, 1962.

Spink, W. W., J. Reddin, S. J. Zak, M. Peterson, B. Starzecki, and E. Seljeskog. Correlation of plastic catecholamine levels with hemodynamic changes in canine endotoxin shock. *J. Clin. Invest.* 45:78, 1966.

Spiro, D., and E. H. Sonnenblick. Comparison of ultrastructural basis of contractile process in heart and skeletal muscle. *Circ. Res.* 15:Suppl. 2, pp. 14–37, 1964.

Spotnitz, H. M., E. H. Sonnenblick, and D. Spiro. Relation of ultrastructure to function in the intact heart: Sarcomere structure relative to pressure–volume curves of intact left ventricles of dog and cat. *Circ. Res.* 18:49, 1966.

Stainsby, W. N. Autoregulation of blood flow in skeletal muscle during increased metabolic activity. *Amer. J. Physiol.* 202:273, 1962.

Stainsby, W. N., and A. B. Otis. Blood flow, blood oxygen tension, oxygen uptake and oxygen transport in skeletal muscle. *Amer. J. Physiol.* 206:858, 1964a.

Stainsby, W. N. Autoregulation in skeletal muscle. *Circ. Res.* 15:Suppl. I, p. 39, 1964b.

Stainsby, W. N., and M. J. Fregly. Effect of plasma osmolality on resistance to blood flow through skeletal muscle. In: *Proceedings of the International Symposium on Circulation in Skeletal Muscle.* Smolenice, Czech, 1968, p. 315.

Starling, E. H. On the mode of action of lymphagogues. *J. Physiol.* 17:30, 1894.

Starling, E. H. Some points in the pathology of heart disease. *Lancet* 1:652, 1897.

Starling, E. H. *The Linacre Lecture on the Law of the Heart.* London and New York: Longman, Green, and Co., 1918.

Starling, E. H., and M. B. Visscher. The

regulation of the energy output of the heart. *J. Physiol.* 62:243, 1927.

Starmer, C. F., and D. O. Clark. Computer computations of cardiac output using the gamma function. *J. Appl. Physiol.* 28:219, 1970.

Starr, I., Jr., and C. J. Gamble. A method for the determination of minute amounts of ethyl iodide in air, water, and blood by means of its reaction with silver nitrate; and experiments bearing on the determination of blood flow by means of ethyl iodide. *J. Biol. Chem.* 71:509, 1927.

Starr, I., Jr., and C. J. Gamble. An improved method for the determination of cardiac output in man by means of ethyl iodide. *Amer. J. Physiol.* 87:450, 1928.

Starr, I., Jr., and L. H. Collins. Estimations of the velocity and amount of blood flowing through the shorter paths of the systemic circulation. *Amer. J. Physiol.* 93:690, 1930.

Starr, I., Jr., L. H. Collins, Jr., and F. C. Wood, Basal work and output of heart in clinical conditions. *J. Clin. Invest.* 12:13, 1933.

Starr, I., Jr., J. S. Donal, A. Margolies, R. Shaw, L. H. Collins, and C. J. Gamble. Heart and circulation in disease; estimations of basal cardiac output, metabolism, heart size, and blood pressure in 235 subjects. *J. Clin. Invest.* 13:561, 1934.

Starr, I., Jr., and C. J. Gamble. Cardiac output in common clinical conditions; diagnosis of myocardial insufficiency by cardiac output methods. *Ann. Intern. Med.* 9:569, 1935.

Starr, I., A. J. Rawson, H. A. Schroder, and N. R. Joseph. Studies on the estimation of cardiac output in man, and of abnormalities in cardiac function, from the heart's recoil and the blood's impacts; the ballistocardiogram. *Amer. J. Physiol.* 127:1, 1939.

Starr, I. Role of the "static blood pressure" in abnormal increments of venous pressure, especially in heart failure. II. Clinical and experimental studies. *Amer. J. Med. Sci.* 199:40, 1940a.

Starr, I., and A. J. Rawson. Role of the "static blood pressure" in abnormal increments of venous pressure, especially in heart failure. I. Theoretical studies on an improved circulation schema whose pumps obey Starling's law of the heart. *Amer. J. Med. Sci.* 199:27, 1940b.

Starr, I., W. A. Jeffers, and R. H. Meade. The absence of conspicuous increments of venous pressure after severe damage to the right ventricle of the dog, with a discussion of the relation between clinical congestive failure and heart disease. *Amer. Heart J.* 26:291, 1943.

Starr, I. Present status of ballistocardiograph as means of measuring cardiac output. *Fed. Proc.* 4:195, 1945.

Starr, I. Clinical tests of the simple method of estimating cardiac stroke volume from blood pressure and age. *Circulation* 9:664, 1954a.

Starr, I., and A Schild. A rough cardiac output method so simple that it could be performed by any doctor with the apparatus he now has. *Trans. Ass. Amer. Physicians* 67:192, 1954b.

Starr, I., T. G. Schnabel, Jr., S. I. Askovitz, and A. Schild. Studies made by simulating systole at necropsy. IV. On the relation between pulse pressure and cardiac stroke volume, leading to a clinical method of estimating cardiac output from blood pressure and age. *Circulation* 9:648, 1954c.

Stead, E. A., Jr., J. V. Warren, A. J. Merrill, and E. S. Brannon. Cardiac output in male subjects as measured by technic of right atrial catheterization; normal values with observations on effect of anxiety and tilting. *J. Clin. Invest.* 24:326, 1945.

Stead, E. A., Jr., J. B. Hickam, and J. V. Warren. Mechanism for changing cardiac output in man. *Trans. Assoc. Amer. Physicians* 60:74, 1947a.

Stead, E. A., Jr., and J. V. Warren. Cardiac output in man; analysis of mechanisms varying cardiac output based on recent clinical studies. *Arch. Intern. Med.* 80:237, 1947b.

Stead, E. A., Jr., J. V. Warren, and E. S. Brannon. Cardiac output in congestive heart failure; analysis of reasons for lack of close correlation between symptoms of heart failure and resting cardiac output. *Amer. Heart J.* 35:529, 1948.

Stead, E. A., Jr. Role of cardiac output in mechanisms of congestive heart failure. *Amer. J. Med.* 6:232, 1949.

Stead, E. A., Jr., J. D. Myers, P. Scheinberg, W. H. Cargill, J. B. Hickam, and B. A. Levitan. Studies of cardiac output and of blood flow and metabolism of splanchnic area, brain, and kidney. *Trans. Assoc. Amer. Physicians* 63:241, 1950.

Stegall, H. F. Muscle pumping in the dependent leg. *Circ. Res.* 19:180, 1966.

Stewart, G. N. Researches on the circulation time and on the influences which affect it. IV. The output of the heart. *J. Physiol.* 22:159, 1897.

Stewart, G. N. The output of the heart in dogs. *Amer. J. Physiol.* 57:27, 1921a.

Stewart, G. N. The pulmonary circulation time, the quantity of blood in the lungs and the output of the heart. *Amer. J. Physiol.* 58:20, 1921b.

Stewart, H. J., and A. E. Cohn. Action of digitalis on output of blood from normal hearts and from hearts in heart failure with congestion in human beings. *J. Clin. Invest.* 11:917, 1932a.

Stewart, H. J., and A. E. Cohn. Action of

digitalis on output of hearts of dogs subject to artificial auricular fibrillation. *J. Clin. Invest.* 11:897, 1932b.

Stewart, H. J., N. F. Crane, R. F. Watson, C. H. Wheeler, and J. E. Deitrick. Cardiac output in organic heart disease. *Ann. Intern. Med.* 13:2323, 1940.

Stone, H. L., V. S. Bishop, and A. C. Guyton. Cardiac function after embolization of coronaries with microspheres. *Amer. J. Physiol.* 204:16, 1963.

Stone, H. L., V. S. Bishop, and A. C. Guyton. Progressive changes in cardiovascular function after unilateral heart irradiation. *Amer. J. Physiol.* 206:289, 1964.

Stone, H. L., V. S. Bishop, and A. C. Guyton. Ventricular function following radiation damage of the right ventricle. *Amer. J. Physiol.* 211:1209, 1966.

Stone, H. L., V. S. Bishop, and E. Dong. Ventricular function in cardiac-denervated and cardiac-sympathectomized conscious dogs. *Circ. Res.* 20:587, 1967.

Stone, H. L., and V. S. Bishop. Ventricular output in conscious dogs following acute vagal blockade. *J. Appl. Physiol.* 24:782, 1968.

Stow, R. W., and P. S. Hetzel. An empirical formula for indicator-dilution curves as obtained in human beings. *J. Appl. Physiol.* 7:161, 1954.

Straub, H. Dynamik des Säugetierherzens. *Deut. Arch. Klin. Med.* 115:531, 1914.

Streeter, D. D., Jr., and P. L. Bassett. Engineering analysis of myocardial fiber orientation in pig's left ventricle in systole. *Anat. Rec.* 155:503, 1966.

Streeter, D. D., H. M. Spotnitz, D. D. Patel, J. Ross, Jr., and E. H. Sonnenblick. Fiber orientation in the canine left ventricle during diastole and systole. *Circ. Res.* 24:339, 1969.

Sturkie, P. D., and J. A. Vogel. Cardiac output, central blood volume, and peripheral resistance in chickens. *Amer. J. Physiol.* 197:1165, 1959.

Stydom, N. B. Changes in cardiac output with progressive work. *S. African J. Med. Sci.* 17:37, 1952.

Suárez, J. R. E., J. C. Fasciolo, and O. C. Taquine. Cardiac output in heart failure. *Amer. Heart J.* 32:339, 1946.

Suckling, E. E., and A. Vogel. Thermistor bridge for blood flow measurements. *J. Appl. Physiol.* 15:966, 1960.

Sugimoto, T., K. Sagawa, and A. C. Guyton. Effect of tachycardia on cardiac output during normal and increased venous return. *Amer. J. Physiol.* 211:288, 1966.

Sugimoto, T., K. Sagawa, and A. C. Guyton. Quantitative effect of low coronary pressure on left ventricular performance. *Jap. Heart J.* 9:46, 1968.

Sunahara, F. A., and L. Beck. Cardiovascular effects of acutely produced anemia in the normal dog. *Amer. J. Physiol.* 176:139, 1954.

Sunahara, F. A., J. D. Hatcher, L. Beck, and C. W. Gowdey. Cardiovascular responses in dogs to intravenous infusions of whole blood plasma, and plasma followed by packed erythrocytes. *Can. J. Biochem. Physiol.* 33:349, 1955.

Sundt, T. M., and A. G. Waltz. Cerebral ischemia and reactive hyperemia: Studies of cortical blood flow and microcirculation before, during, and after temporary occlusion of middle cerebral artery of squirrel monkeys. *Circ. Res.* 28:426, 1971.

Sutherland, N. G., G. Bounous, and F. N. Gurd. Role of intestinal mucosal lysosomal enzymes in the pathogenesis of shock. *J. Trauma* 8:350, 1968.

Sutterer, W. F., and E. H. Wood. A compensated dichromatic densitometer for indocyanine green. *IRE Trans. Bio. Med. Electron.* 9:133, 1962.

Sweeney, H. M., and H. S. Mayerson. Effect of posture on cardiac output. *Amer. J. Physiol.* 120:329, 1937.

Swigart, R. H. Polycythemia and right ventricular hypertrophy. *Circ. Res.* 17:30, 1965.

Tabakin, B. S., J. S. Hanson, T. W. Merriam, Jr., and E. J. Caldwell. Hemodynamic response of normal men to graded treadmill exercise. *J. Appl. Physiol.* 19:457, 1964.

Takano, H., H. Takagi, M. D. Turner, E. C. Henson, J. W. Crowell, and T. Akutsu. Problems in artificial heart. *Trans. Amer. Soc. Artif. Intern. Organs.* 17:449, 1971.

Takaro, T., H. E. Essex, and H. B. Burchell. Experimental pulmonary arteriovenous fistula. *Amer. J. Physiol.* 165:513, 1951.

Talbot, S. A. Biophysical aspects of ballistocardiography. *Amer. J. Cardiol.* 2:395, 1958.

Tanner, J. M. Construction of normal standards for cardiac output in man. *J. Clin. Invest.* 28:567, 1949a.

Tanner, J. M. Fallacy of per-weight and per-surface area standards and their relation to spurious correlation. *J. Appl. Physiol.* 2:1, 1949b.

Taquini, A. C., J. D. Fermoso, and P. Aramendia. Behavior of the right ventricle following acute constriction of the pulmonary artery. *Circ. Res.* 8:315, 1960.

Taquini, A. C., J. D. Fermoso, and P. Aramendia. The effects of bleeding and tilting in congestive heart failure. *Malattie Cardiovascolari* 2(4):461, 1961.

Tarazi, R. C., H. J. Melsher, H. P. Dustan, and E. D. Frohlich. Plasma volume changes with upright tilt: studies in hypertension and syncope. *J. Appl. Physiol.* 28:121, 1970.

Taylor, H. L., and K. Tiede. Comparison of estimation of basal cardiac output from linear formula. *J. Clin. Invest.* 31:209, 1952.

Taylor, R. R., J. W. Covell, and J. Ross, Jr. Left ventricular function in experimental aorta-caval fistula with circulatory congestion and fluid retention. *J. Clin. Invest.* 47:1333, 1968.

Taylor, S. H., K. W. Donald, and J. M. Bishop. Circulatory studies in hypertensive patients at rest and during exercise, with a note on the Starling relationship in the left ventricle in essential hypertension. *Clin. Sci.* 16:351, 1957.

Theilen, E. O., D. E. Gregg, M. H. Paul, and S. R. Gilford. Determination of cardiac output with the cuvette densitometer in the presence of reduced arterial oxygen saturation. *J. Appl. Physiol.* 8:330, 1955a.

Theilen, E. O., D. E. Gregg, and A. Rotta. Exercise and cardiac work response at high altitude. *Circulation* 12:383, 1955b.

Thomasson, B. Cardiac output in normal subjects under standard basal conditions; the repeatability of measurements by the Fick method. *Scand. J. Clin. Lab. Invest.* 9:365, 1957.

Thorburn, G. D. Estimates of cardiac output from forward part of indicator dilution curves. *J. Appl. Physiol.* 16:891, 1961.

Thorsen, A. H. Ballistocardiographic methods of calculating cardiac output in man; reliability and limitations of methods. *Scand. J. Clin. Lab. Invest.* 7:Suppl. 20, p. 87, 1955.

Threefoot, S., T. Gibbons, and G. Burch. Relationship of weight, venous pressure and radiosodium (Na^{22}) excretion in chronic congestive heart failure. *Proc. Soc. Exp. Biol. Med.* 66:369, 1947.

Tichy, V. L., and B. W. Shaw. Augmentation of femoral venous flow in dog by electrical stimulation of muscles. *Proc. Soc. Exp. Biol. Med.* 69:368, 1948.

Torrance, H. B. Control of the hepatic arterial circulation. *J. Roy. Coll. Surg. Edinb.* 4:147, 1958.

Trapold, J. H. Role of venous return in the cardiovascular response following injection of ganglion-blocking agents. *Circ. Res.* 5:444, 1957.

Tsagaris, T. J., M. Gani, and R. L. Lange. Central blood volume during endotoxin shock in dogs. *Amer. J. Physiol.* 212:498, 1967.

Tsakiris, A. G., R. A. Vandenberg, N. Banchero, R. E. Sturm, and E. H. Wood. Variations of left ventricular and diastolic pressure, volume, and ejection fraction with changes in outflow resistance in anesthetized intact dogs. *Circ. Res.* 23:213, 1968.

Ueda, H., Y. Uchida, H. Yasuda, and T. Takeda. Reflex control of blood pressure by the right subclavian baroreceptor in experimental renal hypertension of rabbit. *Jap. Heart J.* 7:543, 1966.

Uther, J. B., S. N. Hunyor, J. Shaw, and P. I. Korner. Bulbar and suprabulbar control of the cardiovascular effects during arterial hypoxia in the rabbit. *Circ. Res.* 26:491, 1970.

Uvnäs, B. Sympathetic vasodilator outflow. *Physiol. Rev.* 34:608, 1954.

Uvnäs, B. Cholinergic vasodilator innervation to skeletal muscles. *Circ. Res.* 20:Suppl. I, p. 83, 1967.

Valdivia, E. *Mechanisms of Natural Acclimatization: Capillary Studies at High Altitudes.* Randolph Air Force Base, Texas: School of Aviation Medicine, Rept. No. 55–101, June, 1956.

Valdivia, E. Right ventricular hypertrophy in guinea pigs exposed to simulated high altitude. *Circ. Res.* 5:612, 1957.

Valdivia, E. Total capillary bed in striated muscle of guinea pig native to the Peruvian mountains. *Amer. J. Physiol.* 194:585, 1958.

Valdivia, E., M. Watson, and C. M. Dass. Histologic alterations in muscles of guinea pigs during chronic hypoxia. *Arch. Pathol.* 69:199, 1960.

Van Citters, R. L., and D. L. Franklin. Cardiovascular performance of Alaska sled dogs during exercise. *Circ. Res.* 24:33, 1969.

Vandenberg, M. B., G. L. Donnelly, K. W. MacLeod, and I. Monk. Aneurysm of the right ventricle caused by selective angiocardiography. *Circulation* 30:902, 1964.

Van Der Feer, Y., J. H. Douma, and W. Klip. Cardiac output measurement by the injection method without arterial sampling. *Amer. Heart J.* 56:642, 1958.

Van Der Werf, T. Directe en indirecte Stroommeting in het Hart en de grote Bloedvaten (doctoral dissertation). Groningen, Netherlands: University of Groningen, 1965.

Van Liere, E. J., and J. C. Stickney. *Hypoxia.* Chicago: University of Chicago Press, 1963.

Van Thiel, E., C. Libert, F. Desmet, and H. Denolin. Continued registration of T-1824 concentrations in blood by photometric method. *Acta Cardiol. (Brux.)* 13:433, 1958.

Vatner, S. E., D. Granklin, and R. L. Van Citters. Simultaneous comparison and calibration of the Doppler and electromagnetic flowmeters. *J. Appl. Physiol.* 29:907, 1970.

Verel, D. Blood volume changes in cyanotic congenital heart disease and polycythemia rubra vera. *Circulation* 23:749, 1961.

Vidt, D. G., G. Hanusek, J. F. Schieve, H. B. Hull, and L. A. Sapirstein. Spontaneous variability of cardiac output in the dog. *Amer. J. Physiol.* 181:337, 1955.

Vidt, D. G., A. Bredemeyer, E. Sapirstein, and L. A. Sapirstein. Effect of ether anesthesia on the cardiac output, blood pressure, and distribution of blood flow in the albino rat. *Circ. Res.* 7:759, 1959.

Visscher, M. B., and J. A. Johnson. The Fick principle: Analysis of potential errors in its conventional application. *J. Appl. Physiol.* 5:635, 1953.

Vleeschhouwer, G. R. de, R. Pannier, and

A. L. Delaunois. Sinus carotidiens et débit cardiaque. *Arch. Internat. Pharmacodynamie* 83:149, 1950.

Vogel, J. A., and C. W. Harris. Cardiopulmonary responses of resting man during early exposure to high altitude. *J. Appl. Physiol.* 22:1124, 1967.

Wagner, H. R., W. J. Gamble, W. H. Albers, and P. G. Hugenholtz. Fiberoptic dye dilution method for measurement of cardiac output. *Circulation* 37:694, 1968.

Wagoner, G. W., and A. E. Livingston. Application of venturimeter to measurement of blood flow in vessels. *J. Pharmacol. Exp. Therap.* 32:171, 1928.

Walcott, W. W. Blood volume in experimental hemorrhagic shock. *Amer. J. Physiol.* 143:247, 1945.

Walker, A. J., and C. J. Longland. Venous pressure measurement in the foot in exercise as an aid to investigation of venous disease in the leg. *Clin. Sci.* 9:101, 1950.

Walker, J. R., and A. C. Guyton. Influence of blood oxygen saturation on pressure flow curve of dog hindleg. *Amer. J. Physiol.* 212:506, 1967.

Wall, P. D., and G. D. Davis. Three cerebral cortical systems affecting autonomic function. *J. Neurophysiol.* 14:507, 1951.

Wang, Y., R. J. Marshall, and J. T. Shepherd. Effect of changes in posture and of graded exercise on stroke volume in man. *J. Clin. Invest.* 39:1051, 1960.

Wang, Y., G. Blomquist, L. B. Rowell, and H. L. Taylor. Central blood volume during upright exercise in normal subjects. *Fed. Proc.* 21:124, 1962.

Wangensteen, S. L., W. T. Geissinger, W. L. Lovett, T. M. Glenn, and A. M. Lefer. Relationship between splanchnic blood flow and a myocardial depressant factor in endotoxin shock. *Surgery* 69:410, 1971.

Ward, R. J., F. Danziger, J. J. Bonica, G. D. Allen, and A. G. Tolas. Cardiovascular effects of changes of posture. *Aerospace Med.* 37:257, 1966.

Warner, H. R., J. H. C. Swan, and E. H. Wood. Quantitation of rapid stroke volume changes in man from aortic pulse pressure changes. *Amer. J. Physiol.* 171:777, 1952a.

Warner, H. R., and E. H. Wood. Simplified calculation of cardiac output from dye dilution curves recorded by oximeter. *J. Appl. Physiol.* 5:111, 1952b.

Warner, H. R., J. H. C. Swan, D. C. Connolly, R. G. Tompkins, and E. H. Wood. Quantitation of beat-to-beat changes in stroke volume from the aortic pulse contour in man. *J. Appl. Physiol.* 5:495, 1953.

Warner, H. R. The use of an analog computer for analysis of control mechanisms in the circulation. *Proc. I.R.E.* 47:1913, 1959.

Warner, H. R. The control of heart rate by sympathetic efferent information. *The Physiologist* 3:173, 1960a.

Warner, H. R., and A. F. Toronto. Regulation of cardiac output through stroke volume. *Circ. Res.* 8:549, 1960b.

Warner, H. R., and R. O. Russell. Effect of combined sympathetic and vagal stimulation on heart rate in the dog. *Circ. Res.* 24:567, 1969.

Warren, J. V., A. J. Merrill, and E. A. Stead, Jr. The role of the extracellular fluid in the maintenance of a normal plasma volume. *J. Clin. Invest.* 22:635, 1943.

Warren, J. V., and E. A. Stead, Jr. Fluid dynamics in chronic congestive heart failure. *Arch. Intern. Med.* 73:138, 1944.

Warren, J. V., E. S. Brannon, E. A. Stead, Jr., and A. J. Merrill. The effect of venesection and the pooling of blood in the extremities on the atrial pressure and cardiac output in normal subjects with observations on acute circulatory collapse in three instances. *J. Clin. Invest.* 24:337, 1945.

Warren, J. V., E. A. Stead, Jr., and E. S. Brannon. The cardiac output in man: A study of some of the errors in the method of right heart catheterization. *Amer. J. Physiol.* 145:458, 1946.

Warren, J. V. Determination of cardiac output in man by right heart catheterization. In: *Methods in Medical Research.* Chicago: Year Book Publishers, 1948a, p. 224.

Warren, J. V., E. S. Brannon, H. S. Weens, and E. A. Stead, Jr. Effect of increasing blood volume and right atrial pressure on circulation of normal subjects by intravenous infusions. *Amer. J. Med.* 4:193, 1948b.

Warren, J. V., D. C. Elkin, and J. L. Nickerson. The blood volume in patients with arteriovenous fistulas. *J. Clin. Invest.* 30:220, 1951a.

Warren, J. V., J. L. Nickerson, and D. C. Elkin. The cardiac output in patients with arteriovenous fistulas. *J. Clin. Invest.* 30:210, 1951b.

Warren, J. V., A. M. Weissler, and J. J. Leonard. Observations on the determinants of cardiac output. *Trans. Ass. Amer. Physicians* 70:268, 1957.

Warren, J. V. Dye method for determining cardiac output. In: *Methods in Medical Research.* Chicago: Year Book Publishers, 1958, Vol. 7, p. 62.

Wassen, A. The use of bromsulphalein for determination of the cardiac output. *Scand. J. Clin. Lab. Invest.* 8:189, 1956.

Wasserman, K., J. D. Joseph, and H. S. Mayerson. Kinetics of vascular and extravascular protein exchange in unbled and bled dogs. *Amer. J. Physiol.* 184:175, 1956.

Wasserman, K., and J. H. Comroe, Jr. A method for estimating instantaneous pulmonary capillary blood flow in man. *J. Clin. Invest.* 41:401, 1961.

Weale, F. E. Standard experimental shock and post-mortem cardiac arrest. *J. Appl. Physiol.* 13:283, 1958.

Weber, E. H. *Ber Verhandl. sächs. Akad. Wiss.* 196. (Quoted from Grodins, 1959.)

Webster, M. E., N. S. Skinner, Jr., and W. J. Powell, Jr. Role of the kinins in vasodilatation of skeletal muscle of the dog. *Amer. J. Physiol.* 212:553, 1967.

Wegria, R., R. A. Guevara, and C. J. Wiggers. A study of spontaneous fulminant shock in a heart-lung dog preparation. *Amer. J. Physiol.* 138:212, 1943.

Wegria, R., C. W. Frank, G. A. Misrahy, R. S. Sioussat, L. S. Sommer, and G. H. McCormack, Jr. Effect of auricular fibrillation on cardiac output, coronary blood flow and mean arterial blood pressure. *Amer. J. Physiol.* 163:135, 1950.

Wegria, R., G. Muelheims, R. Jreissaty, and J. Nakano. Effect of acute mitral insufficiency of various degrees on mean arterial blood pressure, coronary blood flow, cardiac output and oxygen consumption. *Circ. Res.* 6:301, 1958.

Weinberg, S. L., G. R. Grove, R. E. Zipp, D. C. Daniels, and J. P. Murphy. Normal response curve to exercise of relative cardiac output measured with radioiodinated serum albumin. *Circulation* 19:590, 1959.

Weiss, S., R. W. Wilkins, and F. W. Haynes. The nature of circulatory collapse induced by sodium nitrite. *J. Clin. Invest.* 16:73, 1937.

Weisse, A. B., F. M. Carlton, H. Kuida, and H. H. Hecht. Hemodynamic effects of normovolemic polycythemia in dogs at rest and during exercise. *Amer. J. Physiol.* 207:1361, 1964.

Weisse, A. B., T. J. Regan, M. Nadimi, and H. K. Hellems. Late circulatory adjustments to acute normovolemic polycythemia. *Amer. J. Physiol.* 211:1413, 1966.

Weissler, A. M., J. J. Leonard, and J. V. Warren. Effects of posture and atropine on the cardiac output. *J. Clin. Invest.* 36:1656, 1957a.

Weissler, A. M., J. V. Warren, E. H. Estes, Jr., H. D. McIntosh, and J. J. Leonard. Vasodepressor syncope; factors influencing cardiac output. *Circulation* 15:875, 1957b.

Wells, H. S., J. B. Youmans, and D. G. Miller, Jr. Tissue pressure (intracutaneous, subcutaneous, and intramuscular) as related to venous pressure, capillary filtration and other factors. *J. Clin. Invest.* 17:489, 1938.

Werkö, L., H. Lagerlöf, H. Buch, B. Wehle, and A. Holmgren. Comparison of the Fick and Hamilton methods for the determination of the cardiac output in man. *Scand. J. Clin. Lab. Invest.* 1:109, 1949a.

Werkö, L., G. Berseus, and H. Lagerlöf. Comparison of direct Fick and Grollman methods for determination of cardiac output in man. *J. Clin. Invest.* 28:516, 1949b.

Werkö, L., R. Sannerstedt, E. Varnauskas, and G. Bojs. Experimentally induced hypervolemia during ganglionic blockage. *Scand. J. Clin. Lab. Invest.* 14:289, 1962.

Werle, J. M., R. S. Cosby, and C. J. Wiggers. Observations on hemorrhagic hypotension and hemorrhagic shock. *Amer. J. Physiol.* 136:401, 1942.

Wessel, H. U., C. F. Hepner, G. W. James, and P. Kezdi. Performance of a new on-line computer for indicator-dilution curves. *J. Appl. Physiol.* 19:1024, 1964.

Wessel, H. U., M. H. Paul, G. W. James, and A. R. Grahn. Limitations of thermal dilution curves for cardiac output determinations. *J. Appl. Physiol.* 30:643, 1971.

Westersten, A., E. Rice, C. R. Brinkman, and N. S. Assali. A balanced field-type electromagnetic flowmeter. *J. Appl. Physiol.* 26:497, 1969.

Wetterer, E. Eine neue methode zur registrierung der blutstromungsgeschwindigkeit am uneroffneten. *Z. Biol.* 98:26, 1937.

Wetterer, E., and D. Deppe. Vergleichende tierexperimentelle untersuchungen zur physikalischen schlagvolumenbestimmung (2. Mitteilung): Kaminchen und Katzen. *Z. Biol.* 99:320, 1939.

Wetterer, E. Quantitative beziehungen zwischen stromstarke und druck im naturlichen kreislauf bei zeitlich variabler elastizitat des arteriellen windkessels. *Z. Biol.* 100:260, 1940.

Wever, R. Die verteilung des diathermiestromes im blutgefass bei der thermostromuhr messung. *Pflüger's Arch. ges. Physiol.* 262:1, 1956a.

Wever, R., and J. Aschoff. Durchflussemessung mit der diathermie-thermostromuhr bei pulsierender stromung. *Pflüger's Arch. ges Physiol.* 262:152, 1956b.

Wexler, L., D. H. Bergel, I. T. Gabe, G. S. Makin, and C. J. Mills. Velocity of blood flow in normal human venae cavae. *Circ. Res.* 23:349, 1968.

Wezler, K., and A. Böger. Die dynamik des arteriellen systems. *Ergeb. Physiol.* 41:292, 1939.

Whalen, W. J., and P. Nair. Intracellular PO_2 and its regulation in resting skeletal muscle of the Guinea pig. *Circ. Res.* 21:251, 1967.

Whelan, R. F. Control of the peripheral circulation in man. Springfield, Illinois: Charles C Thomas, Publisher, 1967, p. 234.

White, H. L. Measurement of cardiac output by a continuously recording conductivity method. *Amer. J. Physiol.* 151:45, 1947.

Whitehorn, W. V., A. Edelmann, and F. A.

Hitchcock. The cardiovascular responses to the breathing of 100 per cent oxygen at normal barometric pressure. *Amer. J. Physiol.* 146:61, 1946.

Whittaker, S. R. F., and F. R. Winton. The apparent viscosity of blood flowing in the isolated hindlimb of the dog, and its variation with corpuscular concentration. *J. Physiol.* 78:339, 1933.

Widimsky, J., E. Berglund, and R. Malmberg. Effect of repeated exercise on the lesser circulation. *J. Appl. Physiol.* 18:983, 1963.

Wiederhielm, C. Amplifier for linear recording of oxygen saturation and dye dilution curves. *Circ. Res.* 4:450, 1956.

Wieting, D. W., C. W. Hall, D. Liotta, and M. E. DeBakey. Dynamic flow behavior of artificial heart valves. In L. A. Brewer (Ed.). *Prosthetic Heart Valves.* Springfield, Illinois, Charles C Thomas, Publisher, 1969, p. 34.

Wiggers, C. J. The electrocardiogram: its relation to cardiodynamic events. *Arch. Intern. Med.* 20:93, 1917.

Wiggers, C. J., and H. Feil. Cardiodynamics of mitral insufficiency. *Heart* 9:149, 1922a.

Wiggers, C. J., and L. Katz. The contour of the ventricular volume curves under different conditions. *Amer. J. Physiol.* 58:439, 1922b.

Wiggers, C. J., and J. M. Werle. Cardiac and peripheral resistance factors as determinants of circulatory failure in hemorrhagic shock. *Amer. J. Physiol.* 136:421, 1942.

Wiggers, C. J. The failure of transfusions in irreversible hemorrhagic shock. *Amer. J. Physiol.* 144:91, 1945.

Wiggers, C. J. Myocardial depression in shock. *Amer. Heart J.* 33:633, 1947a.

Wiggers, C. J., M. N. Levy, and G. Graham. Regional intrathoracic pressures and their bearing on calculation of effective venous pressures. *Amer. J. Physiol.* 151:1, 1947b.

Wiggers, C. J. *Physiology of Shock.* New York: The Commonwealth Fund, 1950, p. 253.

Wiggers, H. C. Cardiac output and total peripheral resistance measurements in experimental dogs. *Amer. J. Physiol.* 140:519, 1944a.

Wiggers, H. C., and S. Middleton. Cardiac output and total peripheral resistance in post-hemorrhagic hypotension and shock. *Amer. J. Physiol.* 140:677, 1944b.

Wildenthal, K. D., S. Mierzwiak, N. S. Skinner, Jr., and J. H. Mitchell. Potassium-induced cardiovascular and ventilatory reflexes from the dog hindlimb. *Amer. J. Physiol.* 215:542, 1968.

Wildenthal, K., D. S. Mierzwiak, and J. H. Mitchell. Influence of vagal stimulation on left ventricular end-diastolic distensibility. *Amer. J. Physiol.* 217:1446, 1969a.

Wildenthal, K., D. S. Mierzwiak, H. L. Wyatt, and J. H. Mitchell. Influence of efferent vagal stimulation on left ventricular function in dogs. *Amer. J. Physiol.* 216:577, 1969b.

Wilkins, R. W., F. W. Haynes, and S. Weiss. The role of the venous system in circulatory collapse induced by sodium nitrite. *J. Clin. Invest.* 16:85, 1937.

Wilkins, R. W., S. Weiss, and F. W. Haynes. The effect of epinephrine in circulatory collapse induced by sodium nitrite. *J. Clin. Invest.* 17:41, 1938.

Williams, J. C. P., T. P. B. O'Donovan, and E. H. Wood. A method for the calculation of areas under indicator-dilution curves. *J. Appl. Physiol.* 21:695, 1966.

Williams, J. C. P., R. E. Sturm, A. G. Tsakiris, and E. H. Wood. Biplane videoangiography. *J. Appl. Physiol.* 24:724, 1968.

Wilson, F. C., Jr. W. A. Neely, and J. D. Hardy. The blue dyemethod for the measurement of cardiac output. *Surg. Forum* 4:88, 1953.

Wise, H. M., Jr., A. T. Knecht, Jr., G. S. Beals, and M. Yessis. Observations of the cardiovascular system in experimental traumatic shock. I. General hemodynamics. *Surgery* 46:543, 1959.

Wolf, A. V. *Thirst.* Springfield, Illinois: Charles C Thomas, Publisher, 1958.

Wolff, H. P., D. R. Koczorek, and E. Buchborn. Hyperaldosteronism in heart disease. *Lancet* 1:63, 1957.

Wong, A. Y. K., and R. M. Rautaharju. Stress distribution within the left ventricular wall approximated as a thick ellipsoidal shell. *Amer. Heart J.* 15:649, 1968.

Wood, E. H., D. Bowers, J. T. Shepherd, and I. J. Fox. O_2 content of mixed venous blood in man during various phases of the respiratory and cardiac output cycles in relation to possible errors in measurement of cardiac output by conventional application of the Fick method. *J. Appl. Physiol.* 7:621, 1955.

Wood, J. E., J. Litter, and R. W. Wilkins. The mechanism of limb segment reactive hyperemia in man. *Circ. Res.* 3:581, 1955.

Wright, D. L., and R. R. Sonnenschein. Relations among activity, blood flow, and vascular state in skeletal muscle. *Amer. J. Physiol.* 208:782, 1965.

Yagi, S., D. M. Kramsch, I. M. Madoff, and W. Hollander. Plasma renin activity in hypertension associated with coarctation of the aorta. *Amer. J. Physiol.* 215:605, 1968.

Yonce, L. R., and W. F. Hamilton. Oxygen consumption in skeletal muscle during reactive hyperemia. *Amer. J. Physiol.* 197:190, 1959.

Yoshida, K., J. S. Meyer, K. Sakamoto, and J. Handa. Autoregulation of cerebral blood flow: electromagnetic flow measurements during acute hypertension in the monkey. *Circ. Res.* 19:726, 1966.

Zelis, R., D. J. Mason, J. F. Spann, and E. A.

Amsterdam. The effects of angiocardiographic dye on cardiac contractility and the peripheral circulation in man. *Amer. J. Cardiol.* 25:131, 1970.

Zierler, K. L. Circulation times and the theory of indicator-dilution methods for determining blood flow and volume. *Handbook of Physiology.* Washington: Am. Physiological Society, 1962, Section 2, Vol. 1, p. 585.

Zimmerman, B. G., M. J. Brody, and L. Beck. Mechanism of the cardiac output reduction by hexamethonium. *Amer. J. Physiol.* 199:319, 1960.

Zimmerman, B. G. Separation of responses of arteries and veins to sympathetic stimulation. *Circ. Res.* 18:429, 1966.

Zingher, D., and F. S. Grodins. Effect of carotid baroreceptor stimulation upon the forelimb vascular bed of the dog. *Circ. Res.* 14:392, 1964.

Zipf, R. E., T. F. McGuire, J. M. Webber, and G. R. Grove. Determination of cardiac output by means of external monitoring of radioisotope injected intravenously. *Amer. J. Clin. Pathol.* 28:134, 1957.

Zitnik, R. S., F. S. Rodich, H. W. Marshall, and E. H. Wood. Continuously recorded changes of thoracic aortic blood flow in man in response to leg exercise in supine position. *Circ. Res.* 17:97, 1965.

Zoll, P. M., S. Wessler, and M. J. Schlesinger. Interarterial coronary anastomoses in the human heart with particular reference to anemia and relative cardiac anoxia. *Circulation* 4:797, 1951.

Zuehlke, V., W. du Mesnil de Rochemont, S. Gudbjarnason, and R. J. Bing. Inhibition of protein synthesis in cardiac hypertrophy and its relation to myocardial failure. *Circ. Res.* 18:558, 1966.

Zuntz, N., and O. Hagemann. Untersuchungen über den stoffwechsel des pferdes bei ruhe und arbeit. Landwirtschaftliche jahrbucher. *Z. wissenschaftliche landwirtsch.* erganzunbsband II. 27:1, 1898.

INDEX